Disorders of Hemostasis and Thrombosis

A CLINICAL GUIDE

SECOND EDITION

Disorders of Hemostasis and Thrombosis

A CLINICAL GUIDE

Scott H. Goodnight, MD

Professor of Medicine and Pathology
Director of the Hemostasis and Thrombosis Laboratory
Oregon Health Sciences University
Portland, Oregon

William E. Hathaway, MD

Professor Emeritus of Pediatrics
Mountain States Regional Hemophilia and Thrombosis Center
University of Colorado
Denver, Colorado

The McGraw-Hill Companies
Medical Publishing Division
New York   St. Louis   San Francisco   Auckland   Bogotá   Caracas   Lisbon
London   Madrid   Milan   Montreal   New Delhi   Paris   San Juan
Singapore   Sydney   Tokoyo   Toronto

McGraw-Hill

A Division of The **McGraw·Hill** *Companies*

3 4 5 6 7 8 9 0 DOC DOC 0 9 8 7 6 5 4 3 2

ISBN 0-07-134834-4

This book was set in Palatino by North Market Street Graphics, Lancaster, PA.
The editors were Andrea Seils, Katherine McCullough, and Karen G. Edmonson.
The production supervisor was Richard Ruzycka.
The cover and text were designed by José Fonfrias.
The index was prepared by Kathy Unger.
R.R. Donnelley & Sons Company was printer and binder.

This book is printed on acid-free paper.
Library of Congress Cataloging-in-Publication Data
CIP information is on file at the Library of Congress.

To the students, technologists,

residents, fellows and colleagues

who keep asking the critical questions—

and who have helped provide new answers.

Contributors

Lynn K. Boshkov, MDCM
Associate Professor of Pathology
Director of Transfusion Medicine
Oregon Health Sciences University

Edwin G. Bovill, MD, FCAP, FRCS (EDIN)
Professor and Chair
Department of Pathology and Laboratory Medicine
Director of Clinical Laboratories
University of Vermont College of Medicine

James B. Bussel, MD
Associate Professor of Pediatrics
Weill Medical College of Cornell University

Mary Cushman, MD, MSc
Assistant Professor of Medicine and Pathology
University of Vermont College of Medicine

Thomas G. DeLoughery, MD
Associate Professor of Medicine
Oregon Health Sciences University

Donna M. DiMichele, MD
Assistant Professor of Pediatrics
Director, Regional Comprehensive Hemophilia Diagnostic
and Treatment Center
Weill Medical College of Cornell University

Jeffrey S. Dlott, MD
Associate Medical Director
Midwest Hemostasis and Thrombosis Laboratories

Scott H. Goodnight, MD
Professor of Medicine and Pathology
Director, Hemostasis and Thrombosis Laboratory
Oregon Health Sciences University

Barbara W. Grant, MD
Associate Professor of Medicine
University of Vermont College of Medicine

William E. Hathaway, MD
Professor Emeritus of Pediatrics
Mountain States Regional Hemophilia and Thrombosis Center
University of Colorado School of Medicine

Marilyn J. Manco-Johnson, MD
Professor of Pediatrics
Director, Mountain States Regional Hemophilia and Thrombosis Center
University of Colorado School of Medicine

Robert R. Montgomery, MD
Professor and Vice Chair for Research
Department of Pediatrics
Medical College of Wisconsin
Senior Investigator
Blood Research Institute
The Blood Center of Southeastern Wisconsin

Amy D. Shapiro, MD
Medical Director
Indiana Hemophilia & Thrombosis Center, Inc.

Russell P. Tracy, PhD
Professor of Biochemistry and Pathology
Director of the Laboratory for Clinical Biochemistry Research
Interim Dean of Research
University of Vermont College of Medicine

Douglas A. Triplett, MD
Assistant Dean and Professor of Pathology
Indiana University School of Medicine
Vice President and Director of Medical Education
Ball Memorial Hospital
Director, Midwest Hemostasis and Thrombosis Laboratories

Contents

ix

Preface

For many years as teachers, researchers, clinicians, consultants, and directors of coagulation laboratories, we have been asked many difficult but stimulating questions about hemostasis and thrombosis. These questions and the resulting dialogues have involved medical students, medical technologists, residents, and fellows oriented to hematology and oncology, academic and clinical colleagues and, very frequently, members of the practicing medical community. As a result of these conversations we realized that a need existed for concise information which could be easily understood and readily assimilated by the questioners, who were not always experts in thrombotic and bleeding disorders. Indeed, during the academic careers of the authors and particularly in the last several years, the field has exploded with new information, both basic and clinical, which has made it necessary for even the so-called "experts" to constantly review and struggle to place all of these new findings in perspective. Our efforts have been to try to capture this burst of knowledge and to provide the student and clinician a readily usable resource in the care of patients and their problems of thrombosis and hemostasis.

In the second edition we have tried to retain the readability and concise nature of the first edition, despite the need to extensively revise most of the chapters and to add some new ones. We had the very good fortune to recruit some outstanding individuals to help in the review and revision of several of the chapters; we will be forever grateful to them for their precise and patient help and advice.

This book, therefore, is the result of the collaborative efforts of the authors and their colleagues, who have attempted to combine their collective experiences to address important bleeding and clotting problems that affect all ages—from the newborn to the elderly. The attempts to be comprehensive but still remain current and concise have resulted in a selection of examples of particular defects and modes of therapy rather than an exhaustive review. For the same reason, a limited number of key references have been included for each topic. We hope these references will stimulate the reader to delve deeper into the subject if desired.

Acknowledgments

For Scott H. Goodnight: The Hemostasis and Thrombosis Laboratory at the Oregon Health Sciences University (including Melinda Heuschkel, Shelley Keenan, Maryann Renwick, and Diana Nelson); my colleagues Dr. Tom DeLoughery and Dr. Jody Kujovich; Judy Jensen and Sherri Brenner for their help with the manuscript; and most of all to my family—Cecelia, Kate and Tracy for their patience and unflagging support.

For William E. Hathaway: The personnel of the Coagulation Laboratory of University Hospital, in particular Susan Clarke and Jerry Lefkowitz, M.D.; the staff of the Mountain States Regional Hemophilia and Thrombosis Center, in particular Linda Jacobson, Marilyn Manco-Johnson, M.D. and Rachelle Nuss, M.D.; and Helen Sue Hathaway, M.D.

Disorders of Hemostasis and Thrombosis

A CLINICAL GUIDE

SECOND EDITION

Hemostasis and Thrombosis— General Considerations

CHAPTER 1

Mechanisms of Hemostasis and Thrombosis

GENERAL CONSIDERATIONS

Hemostasis may be defined as the arrest of blood flow from or within a blood vessel. Clinical hemostasis or the control of bleeding from an injury site involves (1) the interaction of the blood vessel and supporting structures, (2) the circulating platelet and its interaction with the disrupted vessel, (3) the formation of fibrin by the coagulation system, (4) the regulation of the extension of the blood clot by coagulation factor inhibitors and the fibrinolytic system, and (5) the remodeling and repair of the injury site after arrest of bleeding. Thrombosis may be defined as the formation and propagation of a blood clot within the vasculature. Clinical thrombosis involves: (1) blood flow and the blood vessels, (2) platelet-vessel interactions related to disruption of the endothelium, and (3) the coagulation system, and in particular the natural anticoagulants and the fibrinolytic system. This chapter presents an overview of the physiologic basis for hemostasis and thrombosis to set the stage for more detailed discussions of pathophysiology related to specific disorders.

OVERVIEW

The same basic mechanisms are involved in the generation of a hemostatic plug that arrests bleeding and the formation of an occlusive thrombus leading to obstruction to blood flow and possible tissue infarction. When a blood vessel is damaged and the normal endothelial cell (EC) barrier is disrupted, exposing tissue factor and collagen, platelets are recruited (by adhesion and aggregation mediated by von Willebrand factor and fibrinogen) from the circulating blood to form an occlusive plug and provide surfaces for blood coagulation reactions. In addition, the coagulation system is triggered because factor VII combines with tissue factor leading to a stepwise activation of a series of proenzymes to produce thrombin.

Thrombin and other agonists activate platelets leading to exposure of negatively charged phospholipids (phosphatidylserine, PS) on their surfaces for clotting factor assembly (from plasma coagulation factors trapped in the plug and released by the platelets) further fostering thrombin formation. Importantly, thrombin converts soluble fibrinogen to insoluble fibrin which is then cross-linked (factor XIII) and anchored into place by the process of clot retraction. Thus, the formation of the platelet-fibrin plug or clot is mediated by adhesive proteins and their receptors (the platelet-vessel interaction) as well as proenzymes and their activators (the coagulation system).

This complex but precise process is regulated by antithrombins, antithrombin (AT) and thrombomodulin, tissue factor pathway inhibitor (TFPI), and the protein C-protein S system which inactivate the accelerators of thrombin formation (factor Va and VIIIa). Subsequently, the clot is lysed by plasmin formed through the fibrinolytic system and the repair process continues. Each component of this hemostatic process is discussed separately even though all are dynamically intertwined.

PLATELET-VESSEL INTERACTION

The Vessel

The blood vasculature forms a circuit, free of leaks, which maintains blood in a fluid state. If a vessel is disrupted and blood loss occurs, the platelets and the coagulation system temporarily close the rent until the cells in the vessel wall permanently repair the leak. Blood vessels are composed of ECs and subendothelial basement membrane (intima), layers of smooth muscle cells and their extracellular matrix (media) surrounded by fibroblasts and their extracellular matrix (adventitia). The blood vessel exhibits many properties that contribute to hemostasis or arrest of hemorrhage as well as prevention of thrombosis. The media and adventitia provide mechanical strength and enable blood vessels to constrict or dilate. The subendothelial basement membranes contain several EC-derived adhesive proteins (collagen microfibrils, laminin, thrombospondin, fibronectin, elastin, vitronectin, and von Willebrand factor) which provide binding sites for platelets and leukocytes. As part of the remodeling process after injury, these extracellular matrix proteins are degraded by over 20 specific matrix metalloproteinases (MMP) such as collagenases, gelatinases, etc. The zymogen MMPs are activated by organomercurial compounds and several proteinases such as kallikrein, trypsin and plasmin (see Figure 1-1).

Endothelial Cells

Endothelial cells have multiple mechanisms to help ensure blood flow. They exhibit vasoconstrictive properties by secreting renin, which produces angiotensin, by inactivating bradykinins, and by secreting endothelin, a potent vasoconstrictor peptide. ECs synthesize PAF (platelet activating factor) which when exposed on the cell surface act as vasoconstrictors and promote leukocyte adhesion. ECs can induce vasodilatation by synthesizing and releasing endothelium-derived relaxing factor (EDRF) which is nitric oxide (NO), and PGI_2 (prostacyclin), a potent vasodilator and inhibitor of platelet function.

Some anticoagulant properties of ECs include the presence of mucopolysaccharides (heparin sulfate, dermatan sulfate), which accelerate the inhibitory effects of AT and heparin cofactor II on the coagulation mechanism as well as an EC surface protein, thrombomodulin, which binds thrombin and enhances the activation of protein C and thrombin activatable fibrinolysis inhibitor (TAFI). ECs also prevent thrombin formation by synthesis and release of the TFPI which inhibits tissue factor (TF).

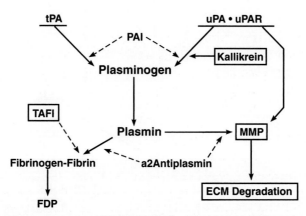

FIGURE 1-1 The fibrinolytic system. Solid arrows indicate activation; dotted line arrows indicate inhibition. tPA, tissue plasminogen activator; uPA, urokinase; uPAR, cellular urokinase receptor; PAI, plasminogen activator inhibitor; FDP, fibrinogen-fibrin degradation products; MMP, matrix metalloproteinases; ECM, extracellular matrix; TAFI, thrombin activatable fibrinolysis inhibitor. See text for description of connections of the fibrinolytic system to the ECM and contact factor system.

In addition to their antithrombotic properties, ECs exhibit many pro-coagulant mechanisms for the arrest of hemorrhage from the injured vessel. The initial step in the formation of thrombin is the expression of tissue factor (TF) on the cell surface only when the cell is perturbed (see Figure 1-2). Newly formed thrombin binds to a thrombin receptor (termed protease-activated receptor-1, PAR-1) on the EC and leads to expression of other important prothrombotic and and antithrombotic molecules (TF, PGI_2, NO, PAF and platelet adhesion receptors). Receptors for the fibrinolytic system (t-PA, u-PA, PAI-1) can be expressed by the EC and its matrix, see Figure 1-1. The ECs secrete several substances that modulate vascular repair by altering smooth muscle and fibroblast proliferation and function: platelet-derived growth factor (PDGF), vascular

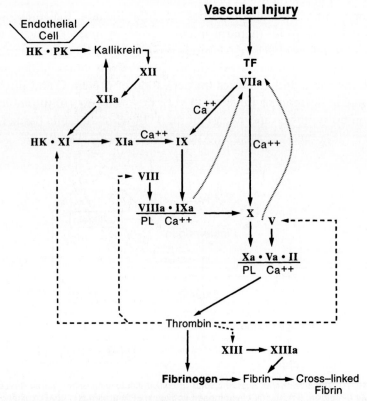

FIGURE 1-2 The procoagulant system and formation of a fibrin clot. Vascular injury initiates the coagulation process by exposure of tissue factor (TF); the dashed lines indicate thrombin actions in addition to clotting of fibrinogen. The finely dotted lines indicate the feedback activation of the VII-TF complex by Xa and IXa.

permeability factor, and fibroblast growth factor. For details of the physiology of the endotheial cell, see the Cines reference.

The Platelet

The circulating platelet is a small anuclear discoid cell (1.5 to 3μ) that arises from megakaryocytes with a maturation time of 4 to 5 days and a circulating life span of 9 to 10 days. The bone marrow reserve of platelets is limited and can be rapidly depleted after sudden platelet loss or destruction. Newly formed platelets are larger in size and termed megathrombocytes. The morphology of a nonactivated platelet is shown diagrammatically in Fig. 1-3.

When the EC surface of a blood vessel is injured or disrupted, a platelet and fibrin hemostatic plug is formed, which halts the bleeding

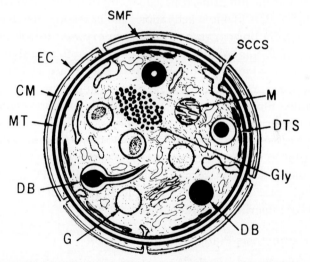

FIGURE 1-3 Platelet (equatorial plane) structure as seen by electron microscopy. The surface membrane shows extensive invagination by an open canalicular system (SCCS), which forms an interconnecting network throughout the cell. The canaliculi provide ready access to the interior of the platelet for plasma proteins and facilitate secretion from the cytoplasmic granules during the release reaction. The cytoskeleton of the platelet which is responsible for the disc shape and the alterations in shape induced by activation (spherical with pseudopodia), is comprised of a circumferential band of microtubules (MT), submembrane filaments (SMF), and cytosolic actin and myosin microfilaments. Typical mitochondria (M), Golgi bodies, ribosomes, peroxisomes, and glycogen masses (GLY) are seen within the platelets as well as three types of granules: lysosomes, dense bodies (DB) and α-granules (G). Both dense bodies and α-granules can fuse with the surface connecting system and release their contents to the platelet exterior during contraction. EC, exterior coat, glycocalyx; CM, triaminar unit membrane; SMF, submembrane area; DTS, dense tubular system. (Used with permission from White JG, Gerrard JM: Ultrastructural features of abnormal blood platelets. A review. Am J Pathol 83:590, 1976.)

and allows repair processes to begin. The events mediated by platelets that are part of the hemostatic plug formation include platelet adhesion, activation and shape change, secretion or release reaction, and support of local coagulation (fibrin formation and clot retraction), (see Figure 1-4).

In the past several years much information has accumulated about the mediators of these events. The platelet surface membrane contains multiple agonist/antagonist G-protein receptors as well as adhesion receptors or integrins. Integrins are composed of α and β tramsmembrane heterodimeric subunits which are responsible for adhesive interactions and signal transduction pathways. The most abundant platelet adhesion receptor is integrin $\alpha_{IIb}\beta_3$ or glycoprotein (GP) IIb/IIIa. Integrin $\alpha_{IIb}\beta_3$, a calcium-dependent heterodimer, is a receptor for the ligands fibrinogen, fibronectin, vitronectin, von Willebrand factor (vWf) and thrombospondin, and mediates platelet adhesion, spreading and aggregation. Other adhesive receptors and their ligands include the GPIb-V-IX complex (vWf) and the integrins, $\alpha_2\beta_1$ (collagen), $\alpha_5\beta_1$ and GPVI (collagen).

Integrin $\alpha_{IIb3}\beta_3$ is in a low activation state in resting platelets and does not bind soluble fibrinogen or vWf. When exposed to soluble agonists (thrombin, ADP, epinephrine, thromboxane A_2) or to adhesive proteins in the subendothelial matrix (collagen, vWf), the affinity and avidity for its ligands increase rapidly. The soluble agonists and their membrane receptors include: thrombin (PAR1, PAR2), ADP (purinoreceptors, P2Y1, P2X1), epinephrine (α_2-adrenergic receptors), and thromboxane A_2 (TP receptor). Each of these agonists acts on its heterotrimeric G-protein coupled receptor to induce its own intracellular signaling pathways. Counteracting these stimuli are certain protaglandins (PGI_2, PGG_2), nitric oxide and possibly platelet-derived growth factor, PDGF. See Shattil reference for details of integrin signaling pathways.

Primary Hemostasis-Platelet Plug Formation

Figure 1-4 illustrates platelet hemostatic plug formation on injured or exposed subendothelium. A similar process is thought to initiate thrombosis. Although each part of the hemostatic plug will be discussed under separate headings, the process is a continuous and dynamic interaction of vessel, platelet and plasma components which is completed in a few minutes.

Adhesion. Under conditions of high shear at the vessel wall, circulating platelets contact exposed subendothelial components (collagen) in a rolling fashion and adhere by interaction between GPIb-V-IX and vWf (A1 domain) deposited on the subendothelium. Platelets tethered to the

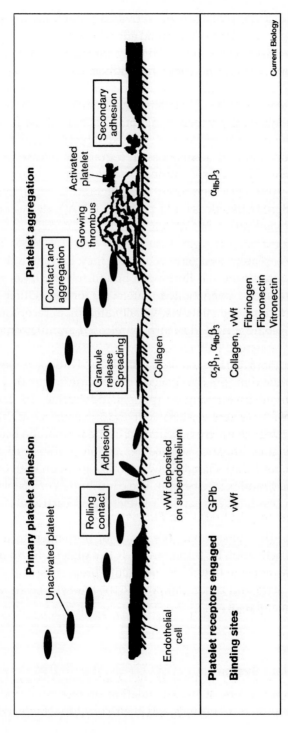

FIGURE 1-4 Platelet adhesion, activation and aggregation on exposed subendothelium at a wound site. See text for details. Used with permission from Clemetson KJ: Primary haemostasis: sticky fingers cement the relationship. Current Biology 9:R110, 1999.

vessel wall move less rapidly, become activated (soluble agonists and collagen) and bind to the vWf (C1 domain) deposited on collagen through the activated $\alpha_{IIb}\beta_3$ and to collagen directly through the $\alpha_2\beta_1$ receptors; thus a temporary "tether" becomes a firm adherence.

Shape Change and Secretion. Platelets next undergo a shape change (cytoskeletal activation) by becoming more spherical with extended pseudopods thus spreading over the exposed subendothelium. The contents of the platelet granules are released: α-granules release fibrinogen, vWf, thrombospondin, factor V, vitronectin and other proteins; the dense bodies release ADP, ATP, serotonin and calcium. Cytoplasmic events include activation of the eicosanoid pathway (TXA$_2$), decreased cAMP and increased mobilization of Ca^{++}.

Aggregation. As platelets become activated, they become adhesive for other platelets interacting via fibrinogen bound to their $\alpha_{IIb}\beta_3$ receptors and a microthrombus of aggregated platelets is formed. Other platelets bind to the surface-bound platelets via activated $\alpha_{IIb}\beta_3$ receptors and fibrinogen and become activated in turn by released granule contents.

Platelet-associated coagulation. During platelet activation, under control of a transport mediating protein called "scramblase", activated by Ca^{++}, negatively charged phospholipids (phosphatidylserine, PS and phosphatidylethanolamine) are translocated to the outer surface of the plasma membrane. In addition, microvesiculation of the membrane occurs. The microvesicles further enhance surface expression of PS which acts as a binding surface for factor Va and Xa which in conjunction with Ca^{++} is the prothrombinase complex (see below). The contribution of platelets to the coagulation process has been called "platelet factor 3 activity".

Clot retraction. The subsequent conversion of fibrinogen to fibrin and further platelet activation by thrombin leads to a platelet-fibrin mass that undergoes retraction mediated by contractile properties of the platelet (interaction of actin and other components of the cytoskeleton with fibrin, fibrinogen and $\alpha_{IIb}\beta_3$).

COAGULATION

The Procoagulant System

The procoagulant system of the coagulation process is composed of a series of serine protease enzymes and their cofactors (Table 1-1) which interact on a phospholipid surface (platelet membrane or damaged EC) to form a stable fibrin clot (see Figure 1-2). Historically, the system has been divided into an extrinsic pathway (tissue factor-factor VII) and an intrinsic pathway (surface-contact factors). Present evidence suggests that the process be considered in stages rather than pathways. The vascular injury-tissue factor stage is critical to the initiation of fibrin formation, whereas the XIa-IXa-VIIIa activation stage plays a role in the continued formation of fibrin.

The blood procoagulant cascade is activated when tissue factor, expressed on damaged or stimulated cells (vascular cells or monocytes), comes in contact with circulating factor VIIa (1-2% of circulating plasma factor VII has been cleaved at Arg 152 to yield VIIa) and forms a complex in the presence of calcium ions. Factor VII is converted to a serine protease by minor proteolysis (possible from trace factor Xa or other protease). The now active factor VIIa-tissue factor complex then converts factor IX to IXa and factor X to Xa. The newly generated IXa forms a complex with VIIIa (activated by traces of thrombin generated slowly by Xa) in the presence of calcium and membrane phospholipid and subsequently also activates factor X to Xa. The complex is called "tenase". Factor Xa binds to Va (again activated by thrombin) which with calcium and the phospholipid is called "prothrombinase", the complex that rapidly converts prothrombin to thrombin.

The initial TF-VIIa complex is enhanced by feedback activation of VII by factors Xa and IXa; however, the complex is quickly inhibited by TFPI (tissue factor pathway inhibitor), a high affinity, low abundance protein found in plasma and on vascular cells. By this time the thrombin that has been produced activates factor XI as well as factors V and VIII and therefore augments the formation of tenase and ultimately the production of more thrombin. Thus, both the initial stage (TF-VIIa) and subsequent enhancement by intrinsic tenase are necessary to achieve optimal activation of the procoagulant system. As shown in Figure 1-2, factor XI can also be activated by factor XIIa formed from the HK-prekallikrein complex on endothelial cells; however, this contribution to physiologic hemostasis is minimal as indicated by the absence of clinical bleeding in individuals severely deficient in factor XII, prekallikrein or HK. The ultimate function of thrombin (IIa) is to cleave fibrinogen to fibrin and activate factor XIII that results in the cross-linked stable clot.

In addition to its role as the structural framework of a thrombus and a site for cell attachment during the repair process, fibrin has several other cofactor and regulatory activities (see Chap. 18). Examples include modulating thrombin activity, regulating cross-linking activity by factor XIII,

TABLE 1-1

Hemostatic Factors

Name	Description	Concentration in Plasma
Procoagulants		
Contact Factors		
XII (Hageman)	Mr 80,000; single-chain serine protease	30 µg/mL (0.375 µM)
HK	Mr 110,000; single-chain cofactor; complexed with prekallikrein and XI	70 µg/mL (0.7 µM)
Prekallikrein (Fletcher)	Mr 85,000; single-chain serine protease complexed with HK	40 µg/mL (0.45 µM)
XI (plasma thromboplastin antecedent, PTA)	Mr 160,000; two identical sulfide-linked chains; serine protease complexed with HK	6 µg/mL (0.03 µM)
Vitamin K-dependent		
II (prothrombin)	Mr 72,500; single-chain-glycoprotein; 10 Gla residues	100 µg/mL (1400 nM)
VII (proconvertin)	Mr 48,000; single-chain glycoprotein: VIIa activates X and IX	0.5 µg/mL (10 nM)
IX (plasma thromboplastin component, PTC)	Mr 57,100; single-chain glycoprotein; 12 Gla residues	5 µg/mL (90 nM)
X (Stuart-Prower)	Mr 54,800; two-chain glycoprotein serine protease: 11 Gla residues	10 µg/mL (170 nM)
Others		
I (fibrinogen)	Mr 340,000; glycoprotein: $A\alpha_2B\beta_{2\gamma2}$	300 mg/dL
V (proaccelerin)	Mr 350,000; single-chain nonenzymatic cofactor; activated by thrombin	200 ng/mL (20 nM)
Tissue factor (TF)	Mr 35,000; single-chain glycoprotein complexed to phospholipids	—

Component	Description	Concentration
VIII (AHF)	Mr 285,000; complexed with von Willebrand factor in plasma	0.15 µg/mL (1.0 nM)
Von Willebrand factor	Mr: multimers of 800,000 to 12×10^6 (subunit 250,000); glycoprotein	8 µg/mL
XIII (fibrin-stabilizing factor)	Mr 320,000; zymogen for a transamidating enzyme (A, B subunits)	20 µg/mL
Fibrinolytic System		
Plasminogen	Mr 92,000; glycoprotein (Glu, Lys)	1.5–2 µMol/L; 21 mg/dL
Tissue plasminogen activator (t-PA)	Mr 68,000 serine protease	4–7 µg/dL
α_2-antiplasmin	Mr 70,000 glycoprotein; specific inhibitor of plasmin (1:1)	1 µM; 7 mg/dL
Plasminogen activator inhibitor-1 (PAI-1)	Mr 52,000; glycoprotein serpin; complexes with t-PA, u-PA	5 µg/dL
Plasminogen activator inhibitor-2 (PAI-2)	Mr 70,000; glycoprotein serpin; complexes with t-PA, u-PA	Trace
Anticoagulants, inhibitors		
Tissue factor pathway inhibitor (TFPI)	Mr 33,000; inhibits VIIa/TF catalytic activity	60–80 ng/mL (2–5 nM)
Protein C	Mr 62,000; two-chain serine protease, vitamin K dependent; 11 Gla residues	2–6 µg/mL (60 nM)
Protein S	Mr 75,000; single-chain cofactor for activated protein C; vitamin K dependent	25 µg/mL (300 nM)
Thrombomodulin	Mr 450 kD; endothelial cell surface receptor for thrombin	—
Antithrombin (heparin cofactor I)	Mr 58,000; single-chain glycoprotein; forms complexes (1:1) with thrombin, Xa, IXa, XIa, XIIa	3–5 µM; 18–30 mg/dL
Heparin cofactor II	Mr 65,000; forms covalent 1:1 molar complex with thrombin	0.47–1.02 µM; 31–67 µg/mL
C1-esterase inhibitor	Mr 105,000; single-chain 1:1 inhibitor of kallikrein, plasmin, C1, and XIIa	1.7 µM; 18 mg/dL

TABLE 1-1 CONTINUED

Hemostatic Factors

Name	Description	Concentration in Plasma
Protein C inhibitor	Mr 57,000; 1:1 complex with APC; accelerated by heparin	5.3 µg/mL
Thrombin-activated fibrinolysis inhibitor (TAFI)	Mr 60,000; inhibits Glu-plasminogen activation	73 nM
Protein Z	Mr 62,000, vitamin K dependent cofactor for protein Z dependent protease inhibitor (ZPI) of Xa	
α_1-Antitrypsin	Mr 60,000; inhibits plasma trypsin, chymotrypsin, XIa and tissue proteases	45 µM; 250 mg/dL
α_2-Macroglobulin	Mr 725,000; dimeric protein; inhibits plasmin, kallikrein, thrombin	3.5 µM; 250 mg/dL
Fibronectin	Mr 440,000; adhesive matrix glycoprotein; mediator of tissue repair	150–700 µg/mL
Vitronectin	Mr 65,000; adhesive glycoprotein; unfolded vitronectin binds heparin; binds PAI-1 and increases $T^{1/2}$	0.25–0.45 ng/mL
Thrombospondin	Mr 420,000; adhesive glycoprotein in many cells including a-granules of platelets; $T1/2 = 9$ h; acute phase reactant	0–3 ng/mL

and enhancing fibrinolysis by binding α_2-antiplasmin (α_2-AP), tissue plasminogen activator (t-PA), and plasminogen.

REGULATION OF BLOOD COAGULATION

The natural anticoagulant mechanism regulates and localizes the formation of the hemostatic plug or thrombus to the site of injury to blood vessels. The majority of the coagulation factor inhibitors or natural anticoagulants are directed against the formation or action of thrombin and include antithrombins and the protein C system (Fig. 1-5). Antithrombin inactivates thrombin and other serine proteases (VIIa, XIIa, XIa, Xa, IXa) by binding irreversibly through an arginine residue to the active serine site of the protease (serine protease inhibitor or serpin). In the absence of heparin, the rate of inactivation is relatively slow, but when heparin or vessel wall heparan sulfate binds to a lysine residue on the AT

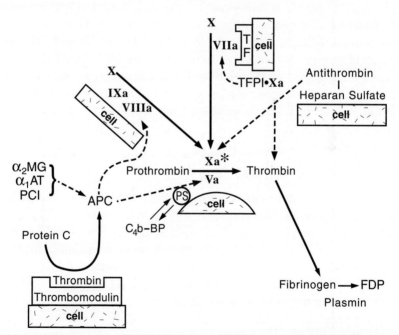

FIGURE 1-5 The physiologic blood coagulation regulatory system. Solid lines indicate activation; dashed lines indicate inhibition. TFPI, tissue factor pathway inhibitor; APC, activated protein C; PS, protein S; TF, tissue factor; C4b-BP, C4b-binding protein; α_2MG, α_2-macroglobin; α_1AT, α_1-antitrypsin; PCI, protein C inhibitor. Additional inhibitor actions include: (1) antithrombin inhibits VIIa-TF, IXa and XIa; (2) Xa is also inhibited by a protein Z dependent protease inhibitor complex (PZ-ZPI) as shown by *; (3) α_2MG provides backup inactivation of Xa and thrombin as well as additional inhibition of APC in conjunction with α_1AT and PCI. (4) XIa is also inhibited by α_1AT. (Adapted from Bauer KA, Rosenberg RD: Role of antithrombin III as a regulator of in vitro coagulation. Semin Hematol 28:10, 1991.

molecule, a conformational change occurs in the AT, resulting in almost instantaneous inactivation of thrombin. AT is therefore called heparin cofactor I. Heparin cofactor II, a second inhibitor, can also be activated by heparin (although larger amounts are needed) on another vessel wall glycosaminoglycan, dermatan sulfate, to inactive thrombin. Thrombin may also be bound to the endothelial or platelet surface by the thrombomodulin receptor and removed from the circulation. Other serpins such as α_1-antitrypsin and α_2-macroglobulin serve a backup role in thrombin inactivation. Protein Z (PZ), a vitamin K dependent protein, serves as a cofactor for the inhibition of factor Xa by a protein called PZ-dependent protease inhibitor (ZPI).

The protein C (PC) pathway is a major mechanism for limiting the coagulation response to injury. The pathway is initiated when thrombin binds to thrombomodulin (TM). The thrombin-TM complex is a potent activator of PC and has little ability to activate platelets or clot fibrinogen. Activated PC (APC) is enhanced by the endothelial cell PC receptor (EPCR) which increases the affinity of the thrombin-TM complex for PC. Once formed, APC proteolytically inactivates factors Va and VIIIa with the critical help of the cofactor protein S (PS). The thrombin-TM complex is rapidly inactivated by PC inhibitor (PCI) and AT. However, APC is relatively resistant to plasma protease inhibitors; its approximate 15 minute half-life is determined by a combined inhibition by α_1-AT, α_2-MG and PCI.

THE FIBRINOLYTIC SYSTEM

The fibrinolytic system and its relation to remodeling of the ECM is depicted in figure 1-1. Plasminogen, which circulates partly (50 percent) in a reversible complex with histidine-rich glycoprotein (HRG), a competitive inhibitor, is converted to the two-chain active plasmin molecule by cleavage of a single peptide bond. Native plasminogen has Glu 1 as the NH2 terminal amino acid (Glu-plasminogen) but due to catalytic degradation the terminal 76 residues are cleaved resulting in the more active (in vitro) Lys 77 form (Lys-plasminogen). In physiologic circumstances, the activation of plasminogen is mainly by t-PA synthesized and released from vascular endothelial cells. The activity of t-PA is enhanced when it is bound to the surface of fibrin, facilitating the conversion of clot bound plasminogen to plasmin. After stimulation of t-PA release by exercise, stasis, or desmopressin (DDAVP), its half-life in the circulation is very short (about 5 min) due to inhibition by PAI-1 and clearance in the liver.

Another activator, urokinase (u-PA), is produced in the kidney and is found mostly in the urine. However, trace amounts of plasma prourokinase or single-chain u-PA (scuPA) can be converted to active form through the contact system by kallikrein. Plasma uPA complexed with its cell receptor, uPAR, activates the matrix metalloproteases (MMP), a family of zinc endopeptidases, which along with plasmin degrade tissue fibronectin, laminin, collagen and gelatins.

The fibrinolytic process is regulated at each enzymatic step by specific protease inhibitors. The plasminogen activators are rapidly inhibited by PAI-1 (sources are platelets, ECs, plasma) and PAI-2 produced in the placenta and neutrophils. PAI-1 is an acute phase reactant that may result in high levels following stress. PAI-1 is quickly inactivated by physiologic conditions (neutral pH and 37°C) resulting in a half-life of about 2 h; the molecule is stable at pH 5.5 and 0°C. PAI-2 is found in the plasma usually only during pregnancy.

Plasmin is rapidly inhibited by α_2-antiplasmin (α_2-AP), backed up by α_2-macroglobulin. These inhibitors protect the normal constituents in plasma (fibrinogen, factor VIII, factor V) from proteolysis by unopposed plasmin. However α_2-AP is not an efficient inhibitor of plasmin at or near the fibrin surface of a clot (fibrin-bound plasmin covers the lysine sites and slows the reaction with α_2-AP), thus allowing fibrinolytic activity where it is most useful. The newly described thrombin activatable fibrinolysis inhibitor (TAFI) is a carboxypeptidase B-like enzyme that down regulates fibrinolysis by removing C-terminal lysines from partially degraded fibrin thus preventing the binding of plasminogen and t-PA. TAFI activation is related to the thrombin-TM complex.

Plasmin has fibrinogen and fibrin as its major substrates leading to the production of specific fragments collectively called fibrinogen-fibrin degradation products (FDP). Cleavage of fibrinogen first produces X fragments (237 to 246 Kd) which are clottable and are often measured as fibrinogen in standard assays. The transiently produced X fragment continues to degrade into smaller D and E fragments or a transient Y fragment composed of a D-E core. Plasmin cleavage of intact fibrinogen also produces Bβ peptide 1-42 that has been used as a clinical marker for primary fibrinolysis.

Fibrin lysis by plasmin leads to a different pattern of fragments because of the cross-linking of the molecule by factor XIII after clotting by thrombin (even though the plasmin cleavage sites are generally the same). These unique fragments such as DD (D-dimer), DY, and YY are characteristic of fibrin breakdown. In addition, non-cross-linked fibrin (fibrin I or early polymers) may complex with fibrinogen and early proteolytic products (X, Y) to produce large macromolecular complexes. Under physiologic conditions fibrinogen is spared plasmin action more than fibrin because of the circulating plasmin inhibitors; however, during pathologic proteolysis (disseminated intravascular coagulation, liver disease, and thrombolytic therapy) significant fibrinogenolysis may occur. Accumulation of FDP in the circulation is associated with inhibition of fibrin formation as reflected in prolongation of screening tests (activated partial thromboplastin time [APTT], prothrombin time [PT], thrombin time) and with decreased platelet function.

Details of FDP production and their application to detection of disease states are discussed in Chapter 24.

BIBLIOGRAPHY

Bajaj SP, Joist JH: New insights into how blood clots: implications for the use of APTT and PT as coagulation screening tests and in monitoring of anticoagulation therapy. *Semin Thromb Hemost* 25:407, 1999.

Blann AD, Taberner DA: Annotation. A reliable marker of endothelial cell dysfunction: does it exist? *Brit J Haematol* 90:244, 1995.

Bouma BN, Meijers JCM: Fibrinolysis and the contact system: a role for factor XI in the down-regulation of fibrinolysis. *Thromb Haemost* 82:243, 1999.

Butenas S et al: "Normal" thrombin generation. *Blood* 94:2169, 1999.

Calvete JJ: Platelet integrin GPIIb/IIIa: structure-function correlations. An update and lessons from other integrins. *Proc Soc Exper Med Biol* 222:29, 1999.

Cattaneo M, Gachet C: ADP receptors and clinical bleeding disorders. *Arterioscler Thromb Vasc Biol* 19:2281, 1999.

Cines DB et al: Endothelial cells in physiology and in the pathophysiology of vascular disorders. *Blood* 91:3527, 1998.

Clemetson KJ: Primary haemostasis: sticky fingers cement the relationship. *Current Biology* 9:R110, 1999.

Collen D: The plasminogen (fibrinolytic) system. *Thromb Haemost* 82:259, 1999.

Esmon CT et al: Endothelial protein C receptor. *Thromb Haemost* 82:251, 1999.

Fox JEB: Platelet activation: new aspects. *Haemostasis* 26 (Suppl 4):102, 1996.

Han X et al: The protein Z-dependent protease inhibitor is a serpin. *Biochemistry* 38:11073, 1999.

Kaufman RJ: Post-translational modifications required for coagulation factor secretion and function. *Thromb Haemost* 79:1068, 1998.

Rapaport SI: The extrinsic pathway inhibitor: A regulator of tissue factor dependent blood coagulation. *Thromb Haemost* 66:6, 1991.

Ruggeri ZM: Mechanisms initiating platelet thrombus formation. *Thromb Haemost* 78:611, 1997.

Schmaier AH et al: Activation of the plasma kallikrein/kinin system on cells: a revised hypothesis. *Thromb Haemost* 82:226, 1999.

Shattil SJ: Signaling through platelet integrin IIb3: inside-out, out-side in, and side-ways. *Thromb Haemost* 82:318, 1999.

Solum NO: Procoagulant expression in platelets and defects leading to clinical disorders. *Arterioscler Thromb Vasc Biol* 19:2841, 1999.

Tuffin DP: The platelet surface membrane: Ultrastructure, receptor binding and function. In: Page CP (ed): The Platelet in Health and Disease, London, Blackwell Scientific Publications, 1991, pp 10–60.

CHAPTER 2

Laboratory Measurements of Hemostasis and Thrombosis

The accurate and efficient diagnosis and monitoring of disorders of hemostasis and thrombosis depend on a high-quality hematology laboratory. This laboratory, often designated for "special coagulation," is essential for optimal diagnosis and management of hemorrhagic and thrombotic disorders, and the measurement of hemostatic variables in solving basic and applied research problems. These tests are discussed below and in subsequent chapters.

PLATELET–VESSEL INTERACTION (PRIMARY HEMOSTASIS)

Several measurements can be made of platelets and their interaction with key components of the vessel wall (endothelial cell and plasma components), as it occurs in physiologic platelet plug formation. Platelets may be enumerated and their morphology observed on peripheral blood smear or electron microscopy. Platelet aggregation to standard agonists can be measured using photo-optical instruments and recorded over time (platelet-aggregation tests). More specific measures can be made of platelet adhesive receptors and their ligands including glycoprotein Ib-IX-V and von Willebrand factor, and GPIIb-IIIa and fibrinogen; each component of which may be quantitated by specific assays. The bleeding-time test, an in vivo measurement of platelet plug formation reflecting platelet number and function, is commonly used in clinical practice. However, new instruments to evaluate platelet function have recently been introduced, including the PFA-100® that measures platelet function at high shear stress. In this test, citrated whole blood is aspirated through a capillary to the central aperture of a membrane coated with collagen and either ADP or epinephrine. The formation of a platelet plug is reflected by the closure time. The test is sensitive to platelet defects such as mild von Willebrand disease and aspirin effect.

SCREENING TESTS, CONTROLS, STANDARDS, AND PREDICTIVE VALUE

Screening or global tests of hemostasis are usually performed on citrated plasma samples and are designed to measure a portion of the coagulation scheme (both procoagulant and acquired inhibitory activities). These simple, one-stage clotting tests (APTT, PT, thrombin clotting time [TCT], etc.) are discussed in detail in Chapter 4. The results of these tests are usually expressed as clotting time in seconds and are compared to the range as calculated from the mean ± 2 or 3 standard deviations (SD) of test values in a group of normal adults (at least 25 subjects). The test result and the "normal range" (usually ± 2 SD) are supplied to the clinician. In addition, a "normal control," which ensures the reproducibility of the test system, is performed on standard normal or reference plasma, frozen or prepared from lyophilized normal pooled plasma. Other abnormal "controls" besides the normal reference plasma are often used to indicate the ability of the test system to detect mild abnormalities.

The *predictive value* (ability of a test to detect an abnormality) is the interaction of test sensitivity and test specificity. *Sensitivity* refers to the percentage of positive results in patients with a known defect. A sensitivity of 95 percent means that 95 percent of patients with the defect will be detected by the test (true positives, TP) and 5 percent of patients with the defect will have false negative (FN) results.

$$\text{Sensitivity} = \frac{\text{TP}}{\text{TP} + \text{FN}} \times 100$$

Specificity refers to the percentage of negative test results in persons without the defect. A specificity of 95 percent means that 95 percent of persons without the defect will test negative (true negatives, TN) and 5 percent of patients without the defect will have false positive results (FP):

$$\text{Specificity} = \frac{TN}{TN + FP} \times 100$$

The predictive value of a laboratory measurement depends on sensitivity, specificity, and *prevalence* (the frequency of patients with a certain disease in the group being tested). For example, these parameters can be used to compute receiver operating characteristic curves (ROC) for measurements like the bleeding time (Rodgers ref). The ROC method assumes that values above a predetermined precision level (cutoff point) are considered abnormal (e.g., a prolonged bleeding time) and those below it are normal. The sensitivity of the bleeding time is the fraction of abnormal (diseased) subjects that have an abnormal test result and the specificity is the fraction of nondiseased subjects classified by the test as normal. Combined with prevalence information these measurements allow estimation of the positive and negative predictive power of the test. Sensitivity and specificity summarize the performance of the test when prior knowledge of the state of the test subjects is available, whereas positive and negative predictive values provide information about a "patient" given prior experience with the test.

WHOLE-BLOOD CLOT FORMATION

Whole blood (native or without anticoagulation) or anticoagulated whole blood may be studied for time of clot formation with (activated clotting time) or without (whole-blood clotting time) particulate activators, as well as for the dynamics of fibrin formation and lysis by instruments such as the thromboelastograph (TEG) or Sonoclot®. Platelet-rich plasma or platelet-poor plasma prepared by appropriate centrifugation of anticoagulated whole blood is used in procedures such as the thrombin generation test or the platelet-rich plasma clotting time to detect the influence of platelets on fibrin formation. When native blood is allowed to clot, the centrifuged supernatant or serum can be used in tests such as the prothrombin consumption test (tests platelet factor 3, factor VIII, and factor IX contribution to prothrombinase) and the thromboplastin generation test, which is sometimes used as the basis of a method for factor VIII assays. Tests using whole blood have an advantage over plasma clotting tests because they measure platelet, leukocyte, and erythrocyte contributions to coagulability. However, they frequently lack sensitivity in the detection of mild to moderate abnormalities of the coagulation system; e.g., the whole-blood clotting time is not abnormal when levels of factor VIII are above 2 percent. At present, the most frequent use of whole-blood clotting tests are in assessing the degree of heparinization during renal dialysis and cardiovascular surgery, and the detection of severe hypocoagulability and fibrinolysis during liver transplantation (TEG).

QUALITATIVE OR FUNCTIONAL ASSAYS OF SPECIFIC COAGULATION FACTORS

Qualitative coagulation factor activity assays are of two major types: clotting assays and chromogenic substrate assays. Clotting-time assays use a reagent system depleted of the factor activity to be measured by using a specific congenitally deficient or artificially factor-depleted plasma. The length of the time for final clot formation is therefore indirectly proportional to the concentration of the coagulation factor in question (see Fig. 2-1). Chromogenic (amidolytic) assays take advantage of the principle that clotting proteases or enzymes generally act specifically toward their natural substrates. Chromogenic substrates are synthetic short peptide chains that mimic the natural substrate and are attached to color markers such as p-nitroaniline. Fluorogenic, luminogenic, and radioactive markers are also feasible. The rate and magnitude of color generated on release of the chromophore is proportional to the enzyme activity. Commonly used chromogenic substrates are S-2222 (thrombin), S-2302 (kallikrein), S-2251 (plasmin), and S-2336 (activated protein C).

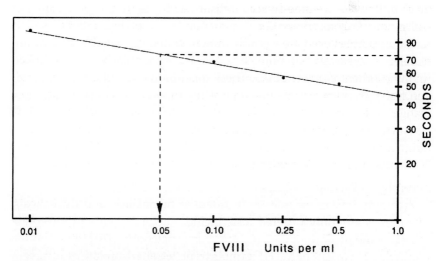

FIGURE 2-1 The standard normal curve used to determine factor VIII activity from clotting times of mixtures of diluted "pooled normal plasma" or "unknown plasma" in the assay system. When the unknown or patient plasma was assayed at a dilution equal to 1.0 U/mL of standard, the clotting time was 75 s or (as the dashed line indicates) 0.05 U/mL.

Both the clotting activity and the chromogenic assays must be standardized and related to a calibration curve of normal enzymes (see Fig. 2-1). The reference plasma used to develop the standard curve is a critical determinant of the overall accuracy of the assay. Pooled (at least 25 donors) normal adult plasma preferably measured against a known standard (World Health Organization or College of American Pathologists) is assigned a 100 percent value. Clotting-time assays may be automated using various instruments that utilize electromechanical detection of fibrin strands formed during clotting, interruption of a light path to detect a clot, photometric detection of increased turbidity, or centrifugal analysis with nephelometric detection of increased turbidity as endpoints. Kinetic spectrophotometry is used for chromogenic assays. These qualitative assays measure enzyme function available under test conditions, regardless of the amount of protein present. That is, nonfunctional proteins may have normal amounts of protein (antigen) as measured by a quantitative assay, but reduced or nondetectable amounts of enzyme (activity) as measured by the qualitative tests.

QUANTITATIVE ASSAYS OF SPECIFIC COAGULATION FACTORS (ANTIGENIC TESTS)

The measurement of the total amount of a clotting protein (procoagulant, anticoagulant, fibrinolytic components, or activation peptides, fragments or complexes) is frequently accomplished with immunologic techniques using heterologous, monoclonal, or naturally occurring antibodies. The major techniques used are agglutination of antibody-coated beads, immunoelectrophoresis, radioimmunoassay, and most popularly, enzyme-linked immunosorbent assay (ELISA). These quantitative tests (also called antigen tests) do not measure function of the protein. New assays are now being developed to measure coagulation proteins using quantitative flow cytometry (e.g., anticardiolipin antibodies, platelet glycoproteins).

Molecular Diagnostic Testing

Recently, molecular diagnosis using DNA technology has played an increasingly important role in disorders of hemostasis and thrombosis. The most commonly ordered tests include factor V Leiden (nucleotide G1691A), the prothrombin gene mutation (nucleotide G20210A), and the thermolabile variant of MTHFR (methylene tetrahydrofolate reductase—nucleotide C677T). Genetic defects in other coagulation genes (e.g., factor VIII, factor IX, vWF, protein C, protein S) can also be identified using this technology, but is more difficult because of the many different mutations affecting these genes. However, if the mutation is known, family studies and prenatal diagnoses can be accomplished with the help of highly specialized laboratories.

ACTIVATION PEPTIDES, FRAGMENTS, AND COMPLEXES

In addition to the assay of specific clotting-factor levels, measurements of fragments or peptides released during the clotting process (activation peptides, enzyme–inhibitor complexes, clot lysis products) or abnormally formed during synthesis (noncarboxylated proteins) can be obtained. Examples of these products include prothrombin fragment 1.2, thrombin–antithrombin complexes, fibrinopeptide A, D-dimer and other fibrin degradation products, and noncarboxylated prothrombin (see Chap. 22). Most of these circulating protein fragments are detected by sensitive immunoassays (often ELISA).

COAGULATION TESTS ARE NO BETTER THAN THE TEST SPECIMEN

An important axiom of clinical hemostasis is that the results of a coagulation test or assay is only as good as the sample collection. Adherence to the details of sample collection and processing is essential if the results are to be meaningful. Unusual or spurious results are often related to problems with blood procurement. Artifacts that must be avoided are discussed below.

Correction for Hematocrit

Several investigators have stressed the necessity of proportionately decreasing the anticoagulant used when the subject's hematocrit is elevated above the normal adult values, as it frequently is in the term infant (preterm infants have hematocrit levels comparable to those of normal adults) and in polycythemic children (congenital heart disease) and adults (Hellum ref). The volume of anticoagulant in the collection tube is decreased to avoid excess citrate, which binds more calcium and prolongs the clotting time. A nomogram based on hematocrit and amount of anticoagulant to use is available and representative values to maintain a constant ratio of anticoagulant to plasma volume are given in Table 2-1. Anemia (unless extremely severe) does not significantly influence the clotting tests.

TABLE 2-1

Values to Maintain a Constant Ratio of Anticoagulant in Blood of 1:10

Hematocrit	Anticoagulant (mL)	Final volume (mL)
70	0.30	5
60	0.37	5
50	0.45	5
40	0.50	5
70	0.12	2
60	0.15	2
50	0.18	2
40	0.20	2

Anticoagulation and Plasma Preparation

To maintain the pH of the blood near physiologic values and to bind calcium, a buffered citrate (three parts, 0.1 mol/L of sodium citrate to two parts, 0.1 mol/L of citric acid) anticoagulant or its equivalent is used. Currently, the use of 3.2% citrate (instead of 3.8%) as the anticoagulant for routine testing is strongly recommended. The collection tube is plastic or silicone coated and is kept covered at 4°C during processing by centrifugation at 1400g (minimum) to remove platelets. The time and temperature of sample storage is less critical for screening tests such as the PT, TCT, or fibrinogen. APTT values may be higher after prolonged storage at room temperature or above. Various inhibitors may be added to the basic citrate anticoagulant to prevent proteolytic changes during transport and storage of sample (EDTA, adenosine, heparin, aprotinin).

Tissue "Juice" Contamination

Whenever possible, a two-syringe venipuncture technique or free-flowing (without squeezing) puncture technique should be used to avoid contamination of the specimen by procoagulant materials (tissue factor or thrombin). Traumatic and repeated punctures as well as slow flow of blood may produce this artifact, which characteristically shortens the APTT and elevates fibrin monomer, or even produces fibrin clots in the specimen.

Heparin Contamination of Specimens

Heparin contamination of specimens obtained from indwelling arterial and venous catheters is a common problem. Others have studied this problem and have concluded that at least 4 to 6 mL blood (or five to six times the volume of the catheter dead space) must be withdrawn through a catheter to prevent heparin contamination of the specimen. The blood should be drawn slowly from the catheter. After the sample arrives in the laboratory, neutralization of heparin by protamine, polybrene, or anion-exchange resins is difficult and may give unreliable results. However, the use of heparinase (e.g., Dade-Behring Hepzyme) reliably removes heparin from plasma samples prior to screening tests and coagulation assays. Recognition of heparin contamination can also be difficult in the infant; characteristically, heparin prolongs the partial thromboplastin time (APTT) and TCT with more minor effects on the PT. In vitro mixtures of cord blood plasma with heparin gave the results listed in Table 2-2. The reptilase time (not affected by heparin) can be helpful in determining whether a prolonged TCT is due to heparin.

In Vitro Fibrinolysis

Specimens of plasma or serum to be tested for presence of degradation products of fibrinogen or fibrin should be collected in tubes containing a fibrinolytic inhibitor such as ε-aminocaproic acid, soybean trypsin inhibitor, tranexamic acid, or aprotinin to prevent in vitro fibrinolysis, which is particularly apt to occur in cord or newborn blood samples.

Cord Blood Collection

Two techniques have proven adequate for collection of cord blood to be used for coagulation assays. As soon as the infant is delivered, the cord is

TABLE 2-2

Effect of Heparin on Screening Tests (in Vitro Mixtures). Cord Studies Performed with Kaolin PTT (Normal range = 37–50 sec)

Heparin Concentration (U/mL)		APTT (s)	PT (s)	TCT(s)
Adult plasma				
	2.0	>150	15	>55
	1.0	>150	12	>55
	0.5	105	11	>55
	0.3	67	11	>55
	0.1	33	10	20
	0.05	29	10	13.5
	0	28	10	12
Cord Plasma				
	0.5	>300	22	>120
	0.25	165	18.5	>120
	0.10	96	17	90
	0.05	78	16.5	19
	0	70	15	13

clamped with two clamps and is cut between them; the infant is removed from the field, and immediately before separation of the placenta, the umbilical vein is punctured and the sample is withdrawn. Alternatively, as soon as the infant is delivered, a segment of cord is double-clamped with four clamps (Fig. 2-2) and is cut between each pair, freeing a long cord segment, which is given to another member of the team to procure the specimen. Both techniques are done with a two-syringe technique with the anticoagulant in the second syringe. Five to ten mL of blood can be obtained in this manner. The amount of anticoagulant necessary for a hematocrit of 55 percent is used in term deliveries. The first procedure is faster but requires that aseptic technique be observed by the blood procurer; the second procedure is a few seconds slower but allows the cord segment to be handed to the blood procurer, who may work in an adjacent area.

Micromethods

The need to evaluate hemostatic problems in small infants has led to many attempts to establish "micromethodology." The components of these efforts are efficient and safe sample procurement, and the ability to perform multiple tests on a small sample. Our own experience has caused us to use methods that require very small amounts of plasma from blood obtained by venipuncture, indwelling catheters, or occasionally arterial punctures (rather than "capillary" samples). Four to six clot-

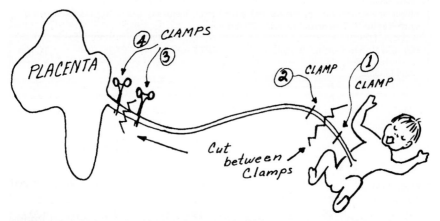

FIGURE 2-2 Cord blood collection. Clamps are placed immediately after delivery of infant in order shown (1 through 4) and cord is cut as illustrated to free segment for blood procurement.

ting factor assays can be done on 100 µL of plasma when appropriately diluted. When screening tests like the PT, TCT, APTT, or fibrinogen are needed, undiluted plasma samples must be used, and the minimal amount of plasma is 500 µL, which requires a whole blood sample up to 2 mL depending on the infant's hematocrit. In special situations blood can be obtained by heel stick (warmed heel, B-D microlance) directly into plastic collection tubes (B-D microcontainer containing the anticoagulant). As discussed in the Hathaway reference, the successful use of micromethods is directly proportional to the energy and effort input of the personnel responsible for the procedures.

BIBLIOGRAPHY

Adcock D et al: The effect of time and temperature variables on routine coagulation tests. *Blood Coag Fibrinol* 9:463, 1998.

Castillo JB et al: Prothrombin times and clottable fibrinogen determination on an automated coagulation laboratory (ACL-810). *Thromb Res* 55:213, 1989.

Cattaneo M et al: Evaluation of PFA-100 system in the diagnosis of therapeutic monitoring of patients with von Willebrand disease. *Thromb Haemost* 82:35, 1999.

Cumming AM et al: In vitro neutralization of heparin in plasma prior to the activated partial thromboplastin time test: An assessment of four heparin antagonists and two anion exchange resins. *Thromb Res* 41:43, 1986.

Friberger P: Synthetic peptide substrate assays in coagulation and fibrinolysis and their application on automates. *Semin Thromb Hemost* 9:281, 1983.

Harrison P et al: Performance of the platelet function analyzer PFA-100 in testing abnormalities of primary hemostasis. *Blood Coag Fibrinolysis* 10:25, 1999.

Hathaway WE, Bonnar J: *Hemostatic Disorders of the Pregnant Woman and Newborn Infant.* Elsevier, New York, Chap. 1, 1987.

Johnston J, Zipursky A: Microtechnology for the study of the blood coagulation system in newborn infants. In: Lusher JM, Barnhart MI (eds): *Acquired Bleeding Disorders in Children,* Masson, New York, pp 133–148, 1981.

Kundu S et al: Description of an in vitro platelet function analyzer—PFA-100®. *Semin Thromb Hemost* 21:Suppl 2 106, 1995.

Molyneaux RD Jr et al: Coagulation studies and the indwelling heparinized catheter. *Heart Lung* 16:20, 1987.

Collection, Transport, and Processing of Blood Specimens for Coagulation Testing and Performance of Coagulation Assays-Second Edition. NCCLS Document H21-A2, Vol. 11, No. 23:1–12, 1991.

Peterson P, Gottfried EL: The effects of inaccurate blood sample volume on prothrombin time (PT) and activated partial thromboplastin time (APTT). *Thromb Hemost* 47:101, 1982.

Rodgers RP, Levin J: A critical reappraisal of the bleeding time. *Semin Thromb Hemost* 16:1, 1990.

Triplett DA: Laboratory evaluation of coagulation. Chicago, *American Society of Clinical Pathology Press*, 1982.

CHAPTER 3

Normal Values for the Hemostatic System

Normal values for measurements of the hemostatic system can be tabulated according to age and other physiologic alterations, such as development, pregnancy, stress, or exercise. Values (taken from the recent literature) for each of the biologic subsets are shown in Table 3-1. Comparisons were made with adult pooled plasma obtained from young males and females aged 20 to 40 years (normal adult). In Table 3-1, the lower limit of normal is minus 2 SD and therefore will exclude 2.5 percent of the values. However, this lower limit provides practical help in deciding what is abnormal and deserving of further evaluation. Whenever possible the values used are based on functional or activity tests that in most instances are equal to quantitative or immunologic values. Examples of discrepancies between activity and antigen for the clotting protein are occasionally seen in the fetus and newborn (fetal proteins as noted below), and during exercise (activation of factors VIII and VII). Certain generalizations may be made from study of Table 3-1 and are discussed below.

FETUS AND NEWBORN

Guidelines (see Hathaway and Corrigan reference) for obtaining normal data in the newborn infant have stressed the need for selection of gestational-age matched subgroups of well infants in whom careful attention is paid to specimen procurement. Of interest, only a few clotting factors display unique characteristics that suggest structural and functional differences from the mature "adult" protein. Examples of such "fetal" pro-

TABLE 3-1

Physiologic Alterations in Measurements of the Hemostatic System

Measurement	Normal Adults	Fetus (20 wk)	Preterm (25–32 wk)	Term Infant	Infant (6 mo)	Pregnancy (term)	Exercise (acute)	Aging (70–80 y)
Platelets								
Count µL/10^3	250	107–297	293	332	—	260	↑18–40%	225
Size (fl)	9.0	8.9	8.5	9.1	—	9.6	↑	—
Aggregation ADP	N	+→	→	→	—	↑	↓15%	N
Collagen	N	→	→	→	—	N	↓60%	—
Ristocetin	N	—	→	←	—	N	↓10%	—
BT (min)	2–9	—	3.6±2	3.4±1.8	—	9.0±1.4	—	5.6
Procoagulant System								
PTT*	1	4.0	3	1.3	1.1	1.1	↓15%	→
PT*	1.00	2.3	1.3	1.1	1	0.95	N	—
TCT*	1	2.4	1.3	1.1	1	0.92	N	—
Fibrinogen mg/dL	278 (0.61)	96 (50)	250 (100)	240 (150)	251 (160)	450 (100)	↓25%	↑15%
II, U/mL	1 (0.7)	0.16 (0.10)	0.32 (0.18)	0.52 (0.25)	0.88 (0.6)	1.15 (0.68–1.9)	—	N
V, U/mL	1.0 (0.6)	0.32 (0.21)	0.80 (0.43)	1.00 (0.54)	0.91 (0.55)	0.85 (0.40–1.9)	—	N
VII, U/mL	1.0 (0.6)	0.27 (0.17)	0.37 (0.24)	0.57 (0.35)	0.87 (0.50)	1.17 (0.87–3.3)	↑200%	↑25%
VIIIc, U/mL	1.0 (0.6)	0.50 (0.23)	0.75 (0.40)	1.50 (0.55)	0.90 (0.50)	2.12 (0.8–6.0)	↑250%	1.50
vWF, U/mL	1.0 (0.6)	0.65 (0.40)	1.50 (0.90)	1.60 (0.84)	1.07 (0.60)	1.7	↑75–200%	↑
IX, U/mL	1.0 (0.5)	0.10 (0.05)	0.22 (0.17)	0.35 (0.15)	0.86 (0.36)	0.81–2.15	↑25%	1.0–1.40
X, U/mL	1.0 (0.6)	0.19 (0.15)	0.38 (0.20)	0.45 (0.3)	0.78 (0.38)	1.30	—	N
XI, U/mL	1 (0.6)	0.13 (0.08)	0.2 (0.12)	0.42 (0.20)	0.86 (0.38)	0.7	—	N

XII, U/mL	1.0 (0.6) (0.55)	0.15 (0.08)	0.22 (0.09)	0.44 (0.16)	0.77 (0.39)	1.3 (0.82)	—	↑16%
XIII, U/mL	1.04	0.30	0.4	0.61 (0.36)	1.04 (0.50)	0.96	—	—
PreK, U/mL	1.12 (0.06)	0.13 (0.08)	0.26 (0.14)	0.35 (0.16)	0.86 (0.56)	1.18	—	↑27%
HK, U/mL	0.92 (0.48)	0.15 (0.10)	0.28 (0.20)	0.64 (0.50)	0.82 (0.36)	1.6	—	↑32%
Anticoagulant System								
AT-U/mL	1.0	0.23	0.35	0.56	1.04	1.02	↑14%	N
α_2MG, U/mL	1.05 (0.79)	0.18 (0.10)	—	1.39 (0.95)	1.91 (1.49)	1.53 (0.85)	—	—
C1IN, U/mL	1.01	—	—	0.72	1.41	—	—	—
PC, U/mL	1.0	0.10	0.29	0.50	0.59	0.99	N	N
Total PS, U/mL	1.0 (0.6)	0.15 (0.11)	0.17 (0.14)	0.24 (0.1)	0.87 (0.55)	0.89	—	N
Free PS, U/mL	1.0 (0.5)	0.22 (0.13)	0.28 (0.19)	0.49 (0.33)	—	0.25	—	—
Heparin cofactor II, U/mL	1.01 (0.73)	0.10 (0.06)	0.25 (0.10)	0.49 (0.33)	0.97 (0.59)	—	—	↓15%
TFPI, ng/mL	73	21	20.6	38	—	—	—	—
Fibrinolytic System								
Plasminogen U/mL	1.0	0.20	0.35 (0.20)	0.37 (0.18)	0.90	1.39	↓10%	N
t-PA, ng/mL	4.9	—	8.48	9.6	2.8	4.9	↑300%	N
α_2-AP, U/mL	1.0	1.0	0.74 (0.5)	0.83 (0.65)	1.11 (0.83)	0.95	N	N
PAI-1, U/mL	1.0	—	1.5	1.0	1.07	4.0	↓5%	N
Overall Fibrinolysis	N	↑	↑	↑	—	→	—	N →

Except as otherwise indicated values are mean ±2 SD or values in () are lower limits (−2SD or lower range); +, positive or present; ↓, decreased; ↑, increased; N, normal or no change; *, values as ratio or subject/mean of reference range; BT, bleeding time; TCT, thrombin clotting time; PreK, prekallikrein; HK, high molecular weight kinnogen; PC, protein C; PS, protein S; t-PA, tissue plasminogen activator; PAI, plasminogen activator inhibitor; vWF, von Willebrand factor; AT, antithrombin; ADP, adenosine diphosphate; α_2AP, α_2-antiplasmin; α_2MG, α_2-macroglobulin; C1IN, C1 esterase inhibitor; TFPI, tissue factor pathway inhibitor. Overall fibrinolysis is measured by euglobulin lysis time.

teins and the differences include: (1) fibrinogen (represents a postsynthetic modification of the fibrinogen molecule resulting in increased phosphorous and sialic acid content, associated with a prolonged reptilase and thrombin time); (2) plasminogen (adult amino acid sequence but increased mannose and sialic acid content producing decreased activation kinetics); (3) von Willebrand factor (altered multimeric structure with increased high molecular weight forms producing increased reactivity with ristocetin); and (4) protein C (altered migration in agarose gel).

In the fetus and newborn infant, the procoagulant system shows decreased levels of the contact and vitamin K-dependent factors inversely related to gestational age; that is, the younger the fetus, the lower the factor. However, cofactors such as factor VIII and V, as well as fibrinogen, are within the normal adult range even in the small preterm infant. Most of the naturally occurring anticoagulants (antithrombin [AT], proteins C and S) are decreased in activity; an exception is an elevation of α_2-macroglobulin. Neonatal whole blood clots faster than the blood of adults even though the plasma screening tests (especially the APTT) are prolonged. Regarding the fibrinolytic system, plasminogen is decreased, tissue plasminogen activator (t-PA) activity and antigen are increased; plasminogen activator inhibitor (PAI-1) and α_2-antiplasmin are normal to increased; and overall plasmin generation is increased in cord blood but decreases during the first few days of life. The platelet count is normal, and despite reduced platelet aggregation the bleeding time of the infant is shorter than that of adults, probably due to the increased hematocrit and altered von Willebrand factor of the newborn. Despite these paradoxical changes, the normal infant is not a "bleeder" and shows no undue thrombotic tendency. However, the balance of the coagulation system appears to be weighted toward hypercoagulability and potential thrombosis in the sick infant.

The decreased hemostatic factors (note that von Willebrand factor is elevated and associated with a slight increase in factor VIII in the term infant) of the newborn infant gradually reach normal adult levels during the first 3 to 6 months of life. A notable exception is protein C, which does not reach the adult range until puberty. The mean activity is slightly lower for several factors (V, II, VII, IX, X, XI, XII) throughout childhood. The upper limit of the bleeding time is slightly longer in children (see Chap. 4).

PREGNANCY

During pregnancy, major changes occur in the coagulation system and to a lesser extent in platelets and their interaction with blood vessels. Levels of most procoagulants (factors VII, VIII, IX, XII, and fibrinogen) rise during pregnancy and are associated with laboratory evidence of enhanced thrombin generation (increased $F_{1.2}$, TAT, and FPA). The anticoagulants AT and protein C remain at normal levels while the protein S level falls. Apparently, to secure hemostasis at the uteroplacental level, systemic fibrinolysis is deficient during pregnancy (prolonged euglobulin lysis time [ELT], normal t-PA, and plasminogen with increased levels of PAI of both endothelial cell type [PAI-1] and placental-derived type [PAI-2]). At delivery, the coagulation system is activated and overall fibrinolytic activity is increased. Coagulation changes similar to those seen during pregnancy (except that fibrinolysis is normal and AT III is decreased) are observed after the use of oral contraceptive agents. These changes are dose-dependent with ethinyl estradiol and mestranol.

STRESS OR INFLAMMATION

Stimuli such as cell injury, inflammation, and pregnancy promote the production of increased levels of a heterogeneous group of proteins called acute-phase reactants. In addition to C-reactive protein and complement components including C4b-binding protein and ceruloplasmin, several coagulation proteins also behave as acute-phase reactants: fibrinogen, von Willebrand factor, factor VIII, factor V, α_1-antitrypsin, PAI-1, t-PA, α_2-macroglobulin, plasminogen, and factor VII. Stress, whether in the form of strenuous exercise, high altitude, or mental stress, is associated with an increase in some acute-phase reactants (fibrinogen, factor VIII, von Willebrand factor, and factor VII) and enhanced thrombin generation with an activation of the fibrinolytic system (increased t-PA, decreased plasminogen and α_2-AP, increased fibrinogen degradation products). Platelet number may increase and the bleeding time is shortened.

EFFECT OF POLYMORPHISMS OF COAGULATION FACTOR GENES ON LEVELS OF CLOTTING FACTORS

In recent years, several common variants for many coagulation genes have been demonstrated. Although these polymorphisms are silent in many instances, sometimes they are associated with increased and decreased plasma levels of clotting factors, and thereby could alter the "normal ranges" listed in Table 3-1, and can be observed as deficiencies of certain factors. Since these genetic variants are rather common in some population groups, the clinician should be aware of the possibility that abnormal values may be due to a polymorphism. For example, an isolated low factor VII could produce a mildly prolonged PT, while low factor XII activity could prolong the APTT. Table 3-2 lists several examples.

THE ELDERLY

Studies of hemostasis in the elderly have shown shortening of the bleeding time and APTT, and an increase in factors VIII, X, high molecular weight kininogen, and prekallikrein (see Table 3-1). Fibrinogen is increased and fibrinolysis may be decreased. In addition, markers of increased coagulation such as VIIa and activation peptides of prothrombin, FIX, FX, and thrombin–antithrombin gradually increase with age until they reach strikingly high levels in centenarians. Enhanced formation of fibrin and secondary fibrinolysis (elevated D-dimer and plasmin–antiplasmin com-

TABLE 3-2			
Polymorphisms in Coagulation Factor Genes Which Effect Plasma Factor Levels			
Coagulation Factor	**Location of Polymorphism**	**Effect on Plasma Level**	**Clinical Relevance**
Fibrinogen	G455A-Bβ gene	Carrier A allele increase levels over baseline in stress and exercise	Risk factor for vascular disease
Factor VII	Arg353Gln	Decreased levels PT in 20–40% heterozygotes	Mildly prolonged PT
	Promoter region: 10bp insertion	Decreased level	
	G/T substitution-401	Decreased level	
	G/A substitution-402	Increased level	Risk factor for vascular disease
Prothrombin	G/A substitution at 20210 position 3′ untranslated region	Increased FII levels 2% of population	Risk factor for venous thrombosis
PAI-1	Single bp insertion-deletion 4G/5G in promoter region	Common frequency; increase levels	Relation to venous thrombosis, osteonecrosis
Factor XII	46C/T substitution in 5′ untranslated region	Decr FXII levels, more in Orientals than in Caucasians	Unknown
von Willebrand factor	Promotor region: C/T-1234; A/G-1185; G/A-1051	TT/GG/AA genotype has low (mean vWF 0.77 μ/mL) Levels in group O	Diagnostic implications for mild vWD

plexes) are also seen. However, these changes in the very elderly do not necessarily indicate a high risk of thrombosis.

Evaluation of patients with hemorrhagic or thrombotic tendencies should be accomplished in the resting state whenever possible, and the results should be interpreted in light of age-related normal values. The resting state for both patients and normal controls refers to a consistent time of day (preferably morning), prior to eating, following a night's rest without early morning exercise. The effects of oral contraceptive agents and pregnancy must also be considered.

BIBLIOGRAPHY

Anwar R et al: Genotype/phenotype correlations for coagulation factor XIII: specific normal polymorphisms are associated with high or low factor XIII specific activity. *Blood* 93:897, 1999.

Andrew M, Brooker LA: Hemostatic disorders in newborns. Polin RA, Fox WW. *Fetal and Neonatal Physiology*, Vol. 2. Philadelphia, WB Saunders, 1998, p 1803.

Andrew M et al: Maturation of the hemostatic system during childhood. *Blood* 80:1998, 1992.

Bremme K et al: Enhanced thrombin generation and fibrinolytic activity in normal pregnancy and the puerperium. *Obstet Gynecol* 80:132, 1992.

Edelberg JM et al: Neonatal plasminogen displays altered cell surface binding and activation kinetics, correlation with increased glycosylation of the protein. *J Clin Invest* 86:107, 1990.

Ferrer-Atunes C: Polymorphisms of coagulation factor genes—a review. *Clin Chem Lab Med* 36:897, 1998.

Glueck CJ et al: The plasminogen inhibitor-1 gene, hypofibrinolysis, and osteonecrosis. *Clin Orthopaedics and Related Research* 366:133, 1999.

Greffe BS et al: Neonatal protein C: Molecular composition and distribution in normal term infants. *Thromb Res* 56:91, 1989.

Hathaway W, Corrigan J: Report of Scientific and Standardization Subcommittee on Neonatal Hemostasis. Normal coagulation data for fetuses and newborn infants. *Thromb Haemost* 65:323, 1991.

Hathaway WE, Bonnar J: *Hemostatic Disorders of the Pregnant Woman and Newborn Infant.* New York, Elsevier Science, 1987.

van't Hooft FM et al: Two common functional polymorphisms in the promoter region of the coagulation factor VII gene determining plasma factor VII activity and mass concentration. *Blood* 93:3432, 1999.

Jern C et al: Changes of plasma coagulation and fibrinolysis in response to mental stress. *Thromb Haemost* 62:767, 1989.

Kamphuisen PW et al: Increased levels of factor VIII and fibrinogen in patients with venous thrombosis are not caused by acute phase reactions. *Thromb Haemost* 81:680, 1999.

Kanaji T et al: A common genetic polymorphism (46 C to T substitution) in the 5'-untranslated region of the coagulation factor XII gene is associated with low translation efficiency and decrease in plasma factor XII level. *Blood* 91:2010, 1998.

Keightley AM et al: Variation at the von Willebrand factor (vWF) gene locus is associated with plasma vWF: Ag levels: identification of three novel single nucleotide polymorphisms in the vWF gene promoter. *Blood* 93:4277, 1999.

Kurachi S et al: Genetic mechanisms of age regulation of human coagulation factor IX. *Science* 285:739, 1999.

Lane DA, Grant PJ: Role of hemostatic gene polymorphisms in venous and arterial thrombotic disease. *Blood* 95:1517, 2000.

Lin X et al: Activation and disturbance of blood haemostasis following strenuous physical exercise. *Int J Sports Med* 20:149, 1999.

Lopez Y et al: Measurement of prethrombotic markers in the assessment of acquired hypercoagulable states. *Thromb Res* 93:71, 1999.

Lowe GD et al: Epidemiology of coagulation factors, inhibitors and activation markers: the Third Glasgow MONICA Survey. I. Illustrative reference ranges by age, sex and hormone use. *Br J Haematol* 97:775, 1997.

Macpherson CR, Jacobs P: Bleeding time decreases with age. *Arch Pathol Lab Med* 111:328, 1987.

Mannucci PM et al: Gene polymorphisms predicting high plasma levels of coagulation and fibrinolysis proteins. A study in centenarians. *Arterioscler Thromb Vasc Biol* 17:755, 1997.

Mari D et al: Hypercoagulability in centenarians: the paradox of successful aging. *Blood* 85:3144, 1995.

Prisco D et al: Evaluation of clotting and fibrinolytic activation after protracted physical exercise. *Thromb Res* 89:73, 1998.

Reverdiau-Moalic P et al: Evolution of blood coagulation activators and inhibitors in the healthy human fetus. *Blood* 88:900, 1996.

Rock G et al: Coagulation factor changes following endurance exercise. *Clin J Sport Med* 7:94, 1997.

Stout RW et al: Seasonal changes in haemostatic factors in young and elderly subjects. *Age Aging* 25:256, 1996.

Trusen B et al: Whole blood clot lysis in newborns and adults after adding different concentrations of recombinant tissue plasminogen activator (Rt-PA). *Sem Thromb Hemost* 24:599, 1998.

Tygart SG et al: Longitudinal study of platelet indices during normal pregnancy. *Am J Obstet Gynecol* 154:883, 1986.

Hemorrhagic Disorders

CHAPTER 4

Screening Tests of Hemostasis

When historical or physical examination assessment indicates that a bleeding tendency should be evaluated, appropriate laboratory tests are performed. These tests, called hemostatic screening tests, are designed to detect both severe and mild defects and should lead to a definitive diagnosis (which may require further procedures and assays). The initial screening tests are selected and performed as a group depending on the age and clinical condition of the patient. The use of the screening tests will be discussed further for the bleeding infant (see Chap. 7), ambulatory patients with history of bleeding (see Chap. 5), and ill in-patients who are bleeding (see Chap. 6).

PLATELET COUNT AND SIZE

At all ages the normal platelet count ranges from 150,000 to 450,000/μL. Any instances of thrombocytopenia (platelet count <150,000/μL) should be confirmed by an estimation of platelets from a stained peripheral blood smear. Examination of the blood smear is particularly important because most laboratories use an electronic counter that counts particles by size and that may over- or underestimate the true platelet count. For example, a measured platelet count higher than actual may be caused by microspherocytes, fragmented red blood cells, leukocyte fragments, Pappenheimer bodies, and bacteria. Conversely, pseudothrombocytopenia may be caused by poor collection techniques (blood clotting in the specimen), EDTA-dependent platelet agglutination (EDTA anticoagulant plus a plasma factor such as an IgG or IgM platelet antibody), platelet cold agglutinins, or platelet satellitism (platelet adherence to neutrophils or monocytes). Platelet aggregates may mimic leukocytes, resulting in concomitant pseudoleukocytosis. In these instances, an accurate platelet count can usually be obtained by performing a phase-contrast count on a freshly obtained finger-stick blood sample.

Several methods based on platelet size have been used to help the clinician decide whether a low platelet count is caused by decreased production (small- or normal-sized platelets) or increased destruction (large platelets). Estimation of megathrombocytes on the peripheral blood smear has been correlated with bone marrow megakaryocyte number. The mean platelet volume (by electronic counter, MPV) is a better index of platelet production, i.e., an MPV greater than 10 fL is often seen in immune thrombocytopenias. However, since the MPV is influenced by cell debris and fragments, a better discriminant of platelet production may be the "maximum" of platelet volume distribution on the histogram provided by the Coulter System (usually greater than 7 fL in hyperproduction states). Extremes of platelet size are also indicative of hereditary defects of platelet number and function (see Chap. 8). Recently, a method has been developed to assess platelet maturity that uses flow cytometry and thiazole orange to detect RNA content of platelets (reticulated platelets). Clinical use has shown good discrimination between acute ITP and non-ITP patients.

BLEEDING TIME

In 1910 Duke described a bleeding time method in which a small cut was made in the lobe of the ear (normal bleeding time, 1 to 3 min), and related bleeding time prolongation to thrombocytopenia. The sensitivity was improved by Ivy, who used a puncture wound of the forearm while a blood pressure cuff was applied. The Ivy bleeding time was further "standardized" by use of a 9 mm by 1 mm template (Mielke)-guided cut (normal, up to 10 min). Currently, modifications of the template bleeding time are widely used (Simplate, Surgicut); the upper limit of normal is approximately 9 min. The bleeding time has been widely used as a screening test for primary hemostasis or platelet–vessel interaction and hemostatic "plug" formation and, as such, is a measurement of platelet number and intrinsic function in relation to vessel and endothelial cell components, von Willebrand factor, and other coagulation factors (fibrinogen, factor V), as well as leukocytes and erythrocytes.

Variables Influencing the Bleeding Time

Many factors affect the skin bleeding time, not the least of which are the technical variables in performance of the test (skin temperature and patient age, direction and depth of the incision, excessive wiping of the wound, marked anxiety, variations in cuff pressure). The bleeding time (Simplate) may be slightly longer in children ages 1 through 12, with the upper limits of normal being 10 to 12 minutes. Although there is an approximate relationship between the BT and the platelet count, many conditions prolong the BT out of proportion to the number of platelets: uremia, liver disease, chronic myeloproliferative disorders, paraproteinemia, and anemia. Drugs and medications such as ASA, nonsteroidal anti-inflammatory drugs (NSAIDs), β-blockers, alcohol, and antibiotics may prolong the BT. When carefully standardized, the prolonged BT is associated with a bleeding tendency in conditions like uremia, liver disease, and myeloproliferative disorders, as well as NSAID-induced gastrointestinal hemorrhage. Disorders like vWD, Glanzmann's thrombasthenia, Bernard-Soulier syndrome, and other hereditary platelet function disorders usually display a prolonged BT (except the mildest forms).

Clinical Use of the Bleeding Time

The BT has been frequently used in three clinical situations: (1) as part of the diagnostic screening tests for evaluation of primary hemostasis in suspected bleeding disorders; (2) to determine a bleeding tendency prior to an invasive procedure; and (3) the evaluation of a bleeding risk in patients taking ASA or NSAIDs. Recently a position paper from the College of American Pathologists and American Society of Clinical Pathologists has addressed the excessive use of the BT for indications (2) and (3) as follows.

1. In the absence of a history of a bleeding disorder, the BT is not a useful predictor of the risk of hemorrhage associated with invasive procedures.
2. A normal BT does not exclude the possibility of excessive hemorrhage associated with invasive procedures.
3. The BT cannot be used to reliably identify patients who may have recently ingested aspirin or non-steroidal anti-inflammatory agents or those who have a platelet defect attributable to these drugs.

However, the BT continues to be a useful test in the evaluation of primary hemostasis in ambulatory children and adults with an undiagnosed bleeding condition. When the BT is prolonged, additional diagnostic tests are indicated; when normal, these additional tests may or may not be indicated depending on the history (personal, family; see Chap. 5).

Other Tests of Primary Hemostasis

As many diagnostic laboratories do fewer bleeding times and rely less on the BT as a screening test, the search for substitute tests for evaluation of primary hemostasis has been intensified. One approach, even though quite expensive, is to use more specific tests of components of platelet plug formation, such as a functional test of vWF and/or platelet aggregation procedures using a battery of agonists. More promising is a global test of primary hemostasis, the Platelet Function Analyzer (PFA-100). The PFA-100™ is an in vitro system of detection of platelet dysfunction and vWD using anticoagulated whole blood. The system comprises a microprocessor-controlled instrument and a disposable test cartridge containing a membrane coated with collagen and epinephrine or ADP through which a small amount (0.4 mL) of whole blood is aspirated until an aperture is occluded, i.e., the closure time (CT). The system has been evaluated in multiclinical laboratory trials of both adults and children with various platelet-related defects and vWD. The instrument was better than the BT and as good as more detailed tests (platelet aggregometry, vWF screening tests) in diagnosis of platelet function disorders and moderate to severe vWD.

ACTIVATED PARTIAL THROMBOPLASTIN TIME

The partial thromboplastin time (PTT) has been used as a screening test for coagulation factor deficiencies since the early 1950s. The modern test, a recalcification clotting time of citrated plasma with added surface contact activation (kaolin, celite, ellagic acid) and a source of phospholipid (the "partial" thromboplastin), is especially sensitive to coagulation abnormalities of the "intrinsic" pathway (factors XII, XI, IX, and VIII) and less sensitive to deficiencies of prothrombin and fibrinogen. The test is usually designated as APTT (activated PTT). The range of APTT values for normal subjects and the sensitivity of the test in detecting factor deficiencies, inhibitors, or bleeding tendency in postsurgical dilutional coagulopathy vary considerably depending on the reagents (activator, phospholipid) used and should be determined for each clinical laboratory, especially when reagents or equipment are changed.

Prolongation of the APTT indicates a deficiency of one or more coagulation factors (prekallikrein; high molecular weight kininogen; factors XII, XI, IX, VIII, X, V, II; or fibrinogen) or inhibition of the coagulation process by heparin, the lupus anticoagulant (LA), fibrin-fibrinogen degradation products, or specific factor inhibitors. When a prolonged APTT plasma is mixed with normal plasma in the proportion of equal parts (1:1) and the resultant APTT is within the normal range, a factor deficiency is suggested; if "correction" is not complete, then an inhibitor is suspected. This 1:1 mixing is often the first step in the investigation of a prolonged APTT of unknown cause.

Recent studies have shown that an abnormally short APPT is associated with thrombotic events, bleeding, and subsequent death in hospitalized patients.

Factor Deficiencies

The APTT is commonly used to screen for disorders of the "intrinsic pathway," that is, contact factor deficiencies and hemophilia A (factor VIII deficiency), hemophilia B (factor IX deficiency), and hemophilia C (factor XI deficiency). Several studies (Fig. 4-1) have demonstrated that the APTT is abnormal with factor deficiencies of <0.3 to 0.4 U/mL. Since the minimal hemostatic level of factors VIII, IX, and XI is approximately 30 percent, the APTT is particularly useful as a hemostatic screening test. However, some APTT procedures, in particular with actin FS and actin FSL reagents have failed to detect mild hemophilia at levels of 25 to 30 percent of normal. Therefore, specific factor assays should be performed when there is strong suspicion of mild hemophilia even when the APTT is normal. The degree of prolongation of the APTT reflects the level of factor VIII in most patients with hemophilia A (the rare exception may be certain hereditary variants, see Chap. 13). The correlation of factor level and APTT prolongation is less precise in patients with factor IX and factor XI deficient hemophilia and von Willebrand disease (Table 4-1).

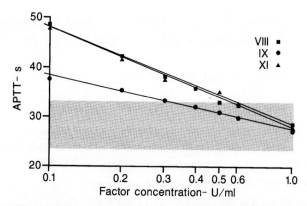

FIGURE 4-1 APTT sensitivity curves. Each curve represents the APTT (s) for the various in vitro mixtures of normal plasma in factor XI-, IX-, or VIII-deficient plasma. The shaded area indicates the normal range for the APTT.

TABLE 4-1	
Representative APTTs in Various Conditions	
Condition	**APTT (s)**
Normal adult (range)	23.5–33.0
Term infant	30.0–54.0
Factor VIII deficient hemophilia	
Severe (VIII = <0.01 U/mL)	82.5
Moderate (VIII = 0.03 U/mL)	57.5
Mild (VIII = 0.18 U/mL)	35.0
Acquired factor VIII inhibitor (VIII = <0.01 U/mL)	64.0
von Willebrand disease (VIII = 0.02 U/mL)	55.0
von Willebrand disease (VIII = 0.25 U/mL)	36.0
Factor IX deficient hemophilia	
Severe (IX = <0.01 U/mL)	55.6
Mild (IX = 0.20 U/mL)	34.0
Factor XI deficient hemophilia	
Severe (XI = <0.01 U/mL)	86.0
Mild (XI = 0.50 U/mL)	40.0
Factor XII deficiency	
Severe (XII = <0.01 U/ml)	200.0
Mild (XII = 0.32 U/mL)	37.0
Lupus anticoagulant	72.0
Heparin therapy	
0.1 U/mL	34.0
0.3 U/mL	66.0

* APTT performed with micronized silica in a photo-optical detecting instrument.

"Normal" children may have a slightly prolonged APTT depending on the method for screening. The role of a mild LA and the physiologic decreased levels of some coagulation factors (IX, XI, XII) still needs further evaluation before establishing a separate normal range for children.

Inhibitors

The APTT is a screening test for inhibitors such as the LA when a sensitive reagent is used. The inhibitory effects of fibrin degradation products (FDP) in disseminated intravascular coagulation (DIC) may prolong the APTT. In addition, depending on the reagent system used, heparin effect (therapeutic or sample contamination) can be detected in amounts as low as 0.05 U/mL (see Chap. 59). Specific factor inhibitors such as factor VIII antibodies may prolong the APTT by reducing the level of the clotting factor. In these instances, the 1:1 mixture may "correct" immediately but is prolonged after incubation for 1 to 2 h at 37°C.

Artifacts

A spuriously prolonged APTT may be observed in several clinical situations: (1) a polycythemic adult or infant when the citrate/plasma ratio has not been corrected during blood procurement; severe anemia does not have an effect on the APTT and PT when drawn into 3.8% citrate (2) partially filled blood collection tubes (excess citrate), (3) other pretesting variables such as prolonged storage or warming of samples before processing, (4) a clotted sample, and (5) heparin contamination. An incompletely characterized deficiency state with a prolonged APTT has been reported in some bleeding and non-bleeding patients (Passovoy deficiency); however, the commercially available deficient plasma used in evaluation may have been procured from a LA-positive patient.

PROTHROMBIN TIME

The prothrombin time (PT), first introduced by Quick in 1935, is performed by adding brain tissue thromboplastin and calcium to citrated plasma and recording the clotting time. The PT is a measure of the "extrinsic" system and reflects the procoagulant activity of factors VII, X, V, and II. The test is usually not prolonged by low fibrinogen unless the level is <100 mg/dL.

The PT is particularly useful in monitoring the effect of coumarin-type agents (dicumarol, warfarin) during anticoagulant therapy (see INR, Chap. 60) or in screening for vitamin K deficiency from other causes. The PT is less sensitive to nonspecific inhibition by FDP and heparin than the PTT or thrombin time. The PT is abnormally prolonged when the level of one or more factors (VII, X, V, or II) is below 0.4 to 0.5 U/mL. A major cause of an isolated prolongation (2 to 3 sec) of the PT is heterozygous factor VII deficiency or factor VII gene polymorphisms (see Chap. 17). In addition, a LA may prolong the PT by a few seconds but usually in association with prolongation of the APTT.

THROMBIN CLOTTING TIME

The thrombin clotting time (TCT), performed by adding thrombin (usually of bovine or human origin) to citrated plasma (with or without added calcium), measures the amount and quality of fibrinogen and the rate of conversion of fibrinogen to fibrin. Depending on the dilutions of added thrombin, the clotting time of normal plasma may vary from 10–12 sec to 20–30 sec ("dilute TCT"). A prolonged TCT may indicate a deficiency of normal fibrinogen (usually <100 mg/dL) as seen in congenital hypofibrinogenemia or afibrinogenemia. The TCT may rarely be prolonged in conditions with abnormally high levels of fibrinogen (inflammation) or, more commonly, qualitatively abnormal fibrinogen (hereditary dysfibrinogenemia, cirrhosis, hepatocellular carcinoma, newborn infants). Substances interfering with the thrombin-induced fibrinogen conversion to fibrin are associated with a prolonged TCT (heparin, antithrombin antibodies after exposure to bovine thrombin), proteolytic products of fibrin and fibrinogen (FDP), procainamide-induced anticoagulant, systemic amyloidosis, abnormal serum proteins). Combinations of these mechanisms producing an increased TCT are seen in renal diseases and DIC. A TCT reported as an infinite clotting time usually means heparin effect or afibrinogenemia. The snake venom Bathrop's atrox (Reptilase) clots fibrinogen in the presence of heparin and therefore can be used to identify heparin as the cause of a prolonged TCT.

FIBRINOGEN

Fibrinogen, the clotting factor present in highest concentration in plasma, is significantly reduced in both acquired (DIC, liver dysfunction, fibrinolytic states) and hereditary (afibrinogenemia, dysfibrinogenemia, and hypofibrinogenemia) coagulopathies. Although the normal adult level ranges from 175 to 400 mg/dL, the commonly used screening tests (APTT, PT, thrombin time) usually are not prolonged until the fibrinogen level falls to <100 mg/dL. Therefore a specific assay for fibrinogen, best done by a functional assay, must be included in the basic screening tests. A fibrinogen level that is low by a functional method (thrombin clotting) but near normal by an immunologic or heat precipitation method is suggestive of a dysfibrinogenemia. The minimal level for normal hemostasis is approximately 75 to 100 mg/dL.

EUGLOBULIN LYSIS TIME

The euglobulin lysis time (ELT) is a screening test for accelerated fibrinolytic activity of blood. The euglobulin fraction of citrated plasma (prepared by acidification of dilute plasma) is clotted and the time for spontaneous lysis of the clot at 37°C is recorded (normal range is 60 to 300 min). The test should be performed on freshly drawn platelet-poor plasma or on samples stored at –80°C for 24 hours. A shortened lysis time may be detected after severe stress or DDAVP infusion in normal individuals and during hyperfibrinolytic states (liver disease, α_2-antiplasmin deficiency, plasminogen activator inhibitor-1 [PAI-1] deficiency, postplasminogen activator infusions) or systemic fibrinolysis. Only rarely is the test abnormally decreased in DIC or secondary fibrinolysis. Prolonged lysis times have been observed in venous thrombosis (in association with increased PAI-1 levels) and renal disease.

FIBRINOGEN-FIBRIN DEGRADATION PRODUCTS

The major screening tests for detection of fibrinogen-fibrin degradation products (FDP) are variations of the D-dimer assay (performed on citrated plasma, detects D-dimer). These and similar tests are frequently used to screen for or confirm the diagnosis of DIC in a sick patient. Their use is further discussed in Chapter 24.

USE OF THE SCREENING TESTS IN COMBINATION

When determining the etiology of a bleeding diathesis, the use of the screening tests as a group or "battery" is recommended, even though the tests included in each battery will vary according to the clinical situation. In outpatients with a history of bleeding or potential bleeding, the following tests are routinely performed: platelet count, bleeding time or PFA-100™, APTT, PT, TCT, and fibrinogen. In-patients who are ill and bleeding usually have the same tests plus a determination for FDP and consideration of the ELT; the bleeding time is less commonly done. Bleeding newborn infants have the platelet count, PT, fibrinogen, and FDP performed; the bleeding time and APTT are seldom indicated. The rationale and strategy of using these groups of tests will be discussed in the following three chapters.

Another advantage of using the tests together is the diagnostic help provided when only one or two tests are abnormal with the other tests in the group being normal. For example, if only the APTT is abnormal, consider factor XII, XI, IX, or VIII deficiency; if only the PT is abnormal, consider factor VII deficiency; if both PT and APTT are abnormal, consider early liver disease or vitamin K deficiency; if only the bleeding time is abnormal, platelet-function defects should be considered.

BIBLIOGRAPHY

Abshire TC et al: The prolonged thrombin time of nephrotic syndrome. *J Pediatr Hematol Oncol* 17:156, 1995.

Boberg KM et al: Is a prolonged bleeding time associated with an increased risk of hemorrhage after liver biopsy? *Thromb Haemost* 81:378, 1999.

Brancaccio V et al: A rapid screen for lupus anticoagulant with good discrimination from oral anticoagulants, congenital factor deficiency and heparin, is provided by comparing a sensitive and an insensitive APTT reagent. *Blood Coag Fibrinol* 8:155, 1997.

Chouhan VD et al: Simultaneous occurrence of human antibodies directed against fibrinogen, thrombin, and factor V following exposure to bovine thrombin: effects on blood coagulation, protein C activation and platelet function. *Thromb Haemost* 77:343, 1997.

Day JP et al: Reversible prolonged skin bleeding in acute gastrointestinal bleeding presumed due to NSAIDs. *J Clin Gastroenterol* 22:96, 1996.

Finazzi G et al: Bleeding time and platelet function in essential thrombocythemia and other myeloproliferative syndromes. *Leuk Lymphoma* 22:Suppl 1, 71, 1996.

Galanakis DK et al: Circulating thrombin time anticoagulant in a procainamide-induced syndrome. *JAMA* 239:1873, 1978.

Gallistl S et al: Longer aPTT values in healthy children than adults: no single cause. *Thromb Res* 88:355, 1997.

Gastineau DA et al: Inhibitor of the thrombin time in systemic amyloidosis: A common coagulation abnormality. *Blood* 77:2637, 1991.

Hathaway WE et al: Activated partial thromboplastin time and minor coagulopathies. *Am J Clin Pathol* 71:22, 1979.

Kovacs MJ et al: Assessment of the validity of the INR system for patients with liver impairment. *Thromb Haemost* 71:727, 1994.

Lawrie AS et al: Assessment of Actin FS and Actin FSL sensitivity to specific clotting factor deficiencies. *Clin Lab Haematol* 20:179, 1998.

Mammen EF et al: PFA-100™ system: a new method for assessment of platelet dysfunction. *Sem Thromb Hemost* 24:195, 1998.

Murray D et al: Variability of prothrombin time and activated partial thromboplastin time in the diagnosis of increased surgical bleeding. *Transfusion* 39:56, 1999.

Niethammar AG, Forman EN: Use of the platelet histogram maximum in evaluating thrombocytopenia. *Am J Hematol* 60:19, 1999.

Peterson P, Gottfried EL: The effects of inaccurate blood sample volume on prothrombin time (PT) and activated partial thromboplastin time (aPTT). *Thromb Haemost* 47:101, 1982.

Prisco D et al: Euglobulin lysis time in fresh and stored samples. *Am J Clin Pathol* 102:794, 1994.

Rand ML et al: Use of the PFA-100® in the assessment of primary platelet-related hemostasis in a pediatric setting. *Sem Thromb Hemost* 24:523, 1998.

Reddy NM et al: Partial thromboplastin time-prediction of adverse events and poor prognosis by low abnormal values. *Arch Intern Med* 159:2706, 1999.

Rodgers RP, Levin J: A critical reappraisal of the bleeding time. *Sem Thromb Hemost* 16:1, 1990.

Saxon BR et al: Reticulated platelet counts in the diagnosis of acute immune thrombocytopenic purpura. *J Pediatr Hematol/Oncol* 20:44, 1998.

Schrezenmeier H et al: Anticoagulant-induced pseudothrombocytopenia and pseudoleucocytosis. *Thromb Haemost* 73:506, 1995.

Siegel JE et al: Effect (or lack of it) of severe anemia on PT and APTT results. *Am J Clin Pathol* 110:106, 1998.

Sutor AH: The bleeding time in pediatrics. *Sem Thromb Hemost* 24:531, 1998.

Triplett DA: Evaluation of the minimally prolonged APTT: Passovoy factor or lupus anticoagulant? *J Pediatr Hematol Oncol* 18:247, 1996.

CHAPTER 5

Evaluation of Bleeding Tendency in the Outpatient Child and Adult

The clinician is frequently asked to evaluate the cause of acute or chronic bleeding or to determine the potential for excess bleeding prior to invasive diagnostic or surgical procedures. The patient evaluation includes assessment of historical information (Table 5-1), physical examination, and performance of basic hemostatic screening tests; depending on the initial assessment, additional tests and procedures are done to confirm the diagnosis. With the advent of many new therapies, a precise diagnosis is essential to the successful management of the bleeding patient.

HISTORY

Obtaining a meaningful history of excessive hemorrhage can be more difficult than it sounds. Many individuals are convinced that they or their children are "bleeders" or have a bleeding tendency even though no real defect can be determined. Others consider significant episodes of bleeding as "normal." A carefully taken history covering the areas listed in Table 5-1 should be interpreted to answer the following questions: Does the patient display excessive, prolonged, recurrent, or delayed bleeding? Has the patient ever had the opportunity to bleed excessively (physical trauma, skin lacerations, surgery)? Is there a family history of significant bleeding?

TABLE 5-1
The Hemostatic History Questionnaire: Historical Information to be Obtained from Patient or Parent

1. Abnormal bruising (ecchymoses or petechiae): Are bruises extensive (larger than quarter, indurated), located where trauma is unlikely or unexplained by minor injury? Are petechiae ever seen? Gum bleeding?
2. Prolonged bleeding after laceration or surgery: Has there been prolonged (hours) or recurrent bleeding after lacerations (cuts, oral injury), surgery (circumcision, skin biopsy, tonsillectomy), tooth extractions, or childbirth? Poor wound healing? List all operations and significant trauma.
3. Epistaxis or menorrhagia: Has there been prolonged and heavy menstrual bleeding or severe or recurrent epistaxis? If so, was anemia present or need for iron therapy or transfusion?
4. Soft tissue or joint hemorrhage: Is there a history of unusual hematomas or unexplained "arthritis" or joint swelling?
5. Has there been hematemesis, melena, hematuria, hemoptysis without obvious cause?
6. Family history: Has any blood relative had a problem with excessive bleeding as noted in questions 1–4?
7. General health: Is there evidence for a disorder known to be associated with a bleeding tendency (chronic liver or renal disease, connective tissue disorder, malabsorption syndrome, systemic lupus erythematosus, myeloproliferative disorder, leukemia, amyloidosis)? Is there evidence for abuse or self-inflicted injury?
8. Drugs or medications: Has aspirin, an antibiotic, or warfarin been taken in last 10–14 days? Has vitamin K been used? History of transfusion?

PHYSICAL EXAMINATION

Bleeding manifestations can be the presenting symptoms and signs of an underlying disorder that may be suggested by certain physical findings. Consider, for example, petechiae in thrombocytopenia, palpable purpura in anaphylactoid purpura, enlarged spleen and lymph nodes in chronic infections or malignancies, signs of liver decompensation, telangiectasias in Osler-Weber-Rendu disease, albinism in Hermansky-Pudlak syndrome, mitral valve prolapse and von Willebrand disease, hyperextensible joints and paper-thin scars in Ehlers-Danlos syndrome, Noonan syndrome and factor XI-platelet function defects, skin plaques and scalloped tongue in amyloidosis, and musculoskeletal abnormalities in the hemophilias.

HEMOSTATIC SCREENING TESTS

The basic screening tests are performed as a group and include:

- Platelet count and blood smear
- Bleeding time or other test of primary hemostasis

- Activated partial thromboplastin time
- Prothrombin time
- Thrombin clotting time
- Fibrinogen

Each of these tests may be the single abnormal test in bleeding disorders present in an outpatient (Table 5-2). In particular, disorders of primary hemostasis should be screened for by an appropriate test if the bleeding time is omitted (see Table 5-4).

STRATEGY FOR EVALUATION OF BLEEDING TENDENCY

Figure 5-1 outlines the strategy used for the diagnosis of the potential bleeder. With the information obtained through the history and physical examination, the patient is classified as positive or negative for a potential bleeding disorder. In addition, some patients may be subject to certain high-bleeding–risk procedures (these procedures are associated with considerable bleeding in "normal" persons: tonsillectomy, complicated cardiovascular surgery, scoliosis corrective surgery, CNS surgery, prostatectomy, closed needle biopsies of liver and kidney). Depending on the age (young children may not have had enough challenges to initiate bleeding) and general health, including drug history, the screening tests are recommended for those with a potential for hemorrhage. For instance, children prior to tonsillectomy and adenoidectomy should have these tests. Adults prior to cardiovascular surgery should at least have a APTT, PT, and platelet count for baseline values.

TABLE 5-2						
Abnormal Screening Tests in Various Hemorrhagic Disorders						
	Screening Tests					
Disorder	**Platelet Count**	**Bleeding Time**	**APTT**	**PT**	**TCT**	**Fibrinogen**
Thrombocytopenia	X					
Platelet dysfunction		X				
Hemophilia			X			
Factor VII deficiency				X		
Dysfibrinogenemia (mild)					X	
Hypofibrinogenemia						X

* X, abnormal tests. Note that only one test is abnormal in each disorder. This observation emphasizes the need to perform the tests as a group since omission of one test may miss a disorder.

Patients with a definite history of bleeding and a negative hemostatic screening battery should have further diagnostic evaluation to consider mild hemophilia, von Willebrand disease, factor XIII deficiency, α_2-antiplasmin, plasminogen activator inhibitor-1 deficiencies, and primary hemostatic defects. Frequently, von Willebrand factor testing is initially performed and often repeated to establish the diagnosis in mild cases. Rarely a mild hemophilic patient has a normal APTT (especially if factor IX deficient) and specific factor assays are indicated if the history is suspicious.

Preoperative Hemostatic Evaluation

The routine preoperative performance of bleeding screening tests such as the APTT and bleeding time has not been demonstrated to be significantly predictive of hemorrhagic complications or cost effective. With the more sensitive APTT reagents, the test has been shown to be misleading in determining a bleeding tendency in children prior to open heart surgery (see Wojtkowski reference).

As indicated in Fig. 5-1, basic screening laboratory tests are reserved for those patients with a positive assessment or who are at higher risk of bleeding because of special circumstances. For example, the basic screening tests are indicated in all young children prior to tonsillectomy and adenoidectomy because the procedure has a significant incidence of postoperative bleeding, and a personal history of bleeding may not be available in the young child (no previous hemostatic stress).

Easy Bruising

Complaints or signs of easy bruising are common in children and many elderly people. Small bruises (smaller than the size of a quarter) are frequently seen on the lower extremities of active youngsters; up to 30 percent of children report bruises as often as weekly. However, it is rare for children less than the age of one year to show bruising. Trauma (accidental, nonaccidental, or self-inflicted) should be considered as a cause of multiple or unusual bruises at any age. A positive family history for hemorrhagic tendencies or the suspicion of nonaccidental trauma is an indication for basic screening tests in patients with easy bruising. Large (> 2 inches in diameter) or indurated purpuric lesions of the skin evoke the differential diagnosis of skin purpura (see Chap. 21).

Chronic Epistaxis

Chronic or habitual epistaxis may be the only indication of a mild bleeding disorder. Recurrent brief nosebleeds are frequently seen in

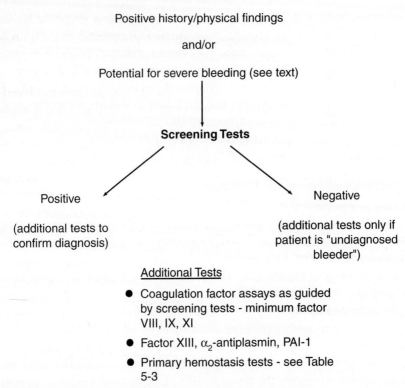

Positive history/physical findings

and/or

Potential for severe bleeding (see text)

Screening Tests

Positive

(additional tests to confirm diagnosis)

Negative

(additional tests only if patient is "undiagnosed bleeder")

Additional Tests

- Coagulation factor assays as guided by screening tests - minimum factor VIII, IX, XI
- Factor XIII, α_2-antiplasmin, PAI-1
- Primary hemostasis tests - see Table 5-3

FIGURE 5-1 Diagnostic evaluation of potential bleeding disorders.

children; nosebleeds that occur every 1 to 2 months, last longer than 10 min, involve both nares, and require medical attention or transfusion are suspicious of a bleeding defect. As many as 25 percent of these patients may have an underlying hemostatic defect, particularly of the platelet-vessel interaction type (platelet dysfunction, von Willebrand disease).

MENORRHAGIA

In a recent study of 150 women with estimated menstrual blood loss of more than 80 mL and a normal pelvic examination, an inherited bleeding disorder was diagnosed in 26 (17%). Both this report and others suggest using blood samples at days 5–10 of the menstrual cycle to confirm the diagnosis of the most common disorder, von Willebrand disease.

MILD BLEEDING DISORDERS

The evaluation of a bleeding tendency in an ambulatory setting is often the differential diagnosis of the mild bleeding disorder. Older children and young adults who are otherwise healthy will present with a history of easy bruising, epistaxis, excessive postoperative or postpartum bleeding, menorrhagia, gingival bleeding, excessive bleeding after a tooth extraction, or the concern of a positive family history for excess bleeding. The diagnoses most frequently confirmed in the patient with a mild bleeding disorder (incidence ranging from 3 to 50/100,000) are von Willebrand disease, mild hemophilia A or B, platelet function disorder, or factor XI deficiency. Frequently these patients delay seeking medical attention and may only be diagnosed after persistent postoperative or postdental extraction bleeding. A precise diagnosis of the mild defect is difficult and sometimes requires repeated testing using the most sensitive tests and assays available. Often the most cost-effective method is referral to a reference or consulting laboratory if the initial screening battery is inconclusive.

ISOLATED PROLONGATION OF THE ACTIVATED PARTIAL THROMBOPLASTIN TIME

A challenging clinical problem is the investigation of a prolonged APTT in a person who does not have an obvious bleeding diathesis but in whom a surgical procedure is contemplated. Complete hemostatic screening tests (PT, TCT, platelet count, bleeding time, fibrinogen level) are normal except for a slight or moderately prolonged APTT. The approach to this problem is outlined in Fig. 5-2. The most common causes of the prolongation of the APTT are mild factor XII deficiency or the presence of lupus anticoagulant, both of which are not usually associated with a bleeding tendency (see Table 5-3). Normal levels of factors XI, IX, and VIII are indications that the patient should not bleed in excess at time of surgery.

ISOLATED PROLONGATION OF THE BLEEDING TIME

Occasionally only the bleeding time will be prolonged or borderline abnormal in patients with otherwise normal hemostatic screening tests. The platelet count is usually normal and examination of the blood smear reveals no abnormal platelet size or staining. The diagnostic possibilities

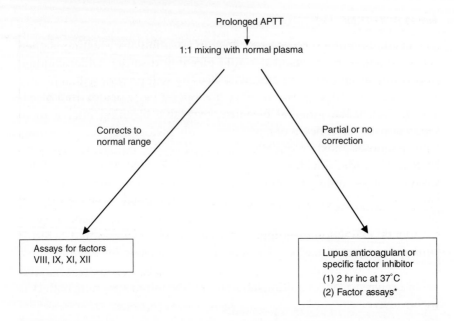

FIGURE 5-2 Evaluation of APTT when other screening tests are normal and heparin effect has been eliminated. *Do complete standard curves and look for inhibitor effect.

include von Willebrand disease, platelet function disorders, congenital heart disease, connective tissue disorders, and acquired disorders such as uremia, paraproteinemias, myelodysplasia, and drug effects. An approach to the evaluation of these defects in primary hemostasis is outlined in Table 5-4.

TABLE 5-3

Causes of an Isolated Prolonged APTT in an Ambulatory Patient

No Bleeding

Factor XII deficiency
(probable heterozygote)

Lupus anticoagulant

Potential Bleeding

Mild hemophilia (factors VIII, IX, XI deficiency)

Mild von Willebrand disease

TABLE 5-4
Evaluation of Possible Defect in Primary Hemostasis

Clinical Manifestations:

Mucocutaneous bleeding such as bruising, petechiae, epistaxis, menorrhagia, prolonged oozing after tooth extraction or minor oral mucosal injury; increased bleeding after aspirin intake.

Laboratory Screening Tests:

Normal or mildly decreased platelet count, prolonged or normal BT, abnormal PFA-100 test.

Additional Tests to Perform

1) vWF activity (ristocetin cofactor assay), vWF antigen, FVIII assay, vWF multimeric analysis
2) Platelet aggregations to ADP, collagen, ristocetin, arachidonic acid
3) PFA-100 tests
4) Platelet sizing and morphology

BIBLIOGRAPHY

Burk CD et al: Preoperative history and coagulation screening in children undergoing tonsillectomy. *Pediatrics* 89:691, 1992.

Gamba G et al: Bleeding tendency of unknown origin and protein Z levels. *Thromb Res* 90:291, 1998.

Harley JR: Disorders of coagulation misdiagnosed as nonaccidental bruising. *Pediatr Emerg Care* 13:347, 1997.

Harrison P et al: Performance of the platelet function analyser PFA-100 in testing abnormalities of primary hemostasis. *Blood Coag Fibrinol* 10:25, 1999.

Houry S et al: A prospective multicenter evaluation of preoperative hemostatic screening tests. The French Associations for Surgical Research. *Am J Surg* 170:19, 1995.

Kadir RA et al: Frequency of inherited bleeding disorders in women with menorrhagia. *Lancet* 351:485, 1998.

Katsanis E et al: Prevalence and significance of mild bleeding disorders in children with recurrent epistaxis. *J Pediatr* 113:73, 1988.

Lusher JM: Screening and diagnosis of coagulation disorders. *Am J Obstet Gynecol* 175:778, 1996.

Kitchens CS: Prolonged activated partial thromboplastin time of unknown etiology: A prospective study of 100 consecutive cases referred for consultation. *Am J Hematol* 27:38, 1988.

de Moerloose P: Laboratory evaluation of hemostasis before cardiac operations. *Ann Thorac Surg* 62:1921, 1996.

Nosek-Cenkowska B et al: Bleeding/bruising symptomatology in children with and without bleeding disorders. *Thromb Haemost* 65:237, 1991.

Preston FE: Laboratory diagnosis of hereditary bleeding disorders: external quality assessment. *Haemophilia* 4 Suppl 2:12, 1998.

Singer ST et al: Bleeding disorders in the Noonan syndrome: three case reports and a review of the literature. *J Pediatr Hematol Oncol* 19:130, 1997.

Werner EJ et al: Relative value of diagnostic studies for von Willebrand disease. *J Pediatr* 121:34, 1992.

Wojkowski TA et al: The clinical impact of increased sensitivity PT and APTT coagulation assays. *Am J Clin Pathol* 112:225, 1999.

CHAPTER 6

Evaluation
of Bleeding in the
Hospitalized Patient

GENERAL APPROACH

Excessive bleeding in hospitalized patients is a common and challenging clinical problem. Most of the time, the bleeding is surgical and quickly controlled with a few well-placed sutures. All too frequently, however, the bleeding is accentuated by generalized hemostatic defects that require prompt identification and therapy. A correct diagnosis can usually be rapidly made using data gathered from the patient's history, the physical examination, and the laboratory. A general approach to these patients is outlined in Tables 6-1 and 6-2. Note that the laboratory studies should be obtained early, so that results are available by the time the rest of the evaluation is complete.

HISTORY AND MEDICAL RECORD

Data must be collected from several sources, including the patient, family, nurses, the medical record, and the laboratory information system. If there is extensive data from a long or complex hospital course, a simple flow sheet should be constructed to include key test results, major clinical events (e.g., surgery, episodes of bleeding), changes in medications, and blood product administration. While the new laboratory studies are pending, the information gathered from these sources should be reviewed to determine:

Has the bleeding been prolonged, delayed, or recurrent; or is it simply more rapid than normal?

TABLE 6-1
An Approach to the Actively Bleeding Hospitalized Patient
See the patient; make an initial assessment ↓ Draw screening tests of hemostasis ↓ Collect historical data: history medical record laboratory information system construct a flow sheet (if needed) ↓ Do the physical exam ↓ Analyze the data Make a presumptive diagnosis Construct a plan of action ↓ Write orders for therapy and/or further diagnostic tests

In general, brisk bleeding from a site of obvious trauma suggests a local vascular defect. In contrast, bleeding that is prolonged, delayed, or recurrent is characteristic of a generalized hemostatic disorder. Sudden resumption of bleeding from a previously injured site raises the possibility of systemic fibrinolysis.

Is the bleeding from a single site or from several different locations?

Bleeding from multiple sites strongly suggests a generalized hemostatic disorder, whereas hemorrhage from a single location is more likely due to a local defect.

Is the bleeding appropriate for the injury?

Although rather subjective, extensive bleeding from small injuries (e.g., venipuncture sites, nasogastric tubes) suggests a hemostatic disorder.

TABLE 6-2
Key Questions
■ Is the bleeding serious or trivial? ■ Is the bleeding due to a generalized disorder of hemostasis or to a local vascular defect? ■ Is the disorder hereditary or acquired? ■ What is the relationship of the bleeding to medical or surgical management? ■ What is the urgency of the situation?

Is there a past history of bleeding?

Bleeding symptoms could be lifelong (suggesting a hereditary defect) or associated with an illness (more likely an acquired disorder).

What medications have been given?

Particular attention should be directed toward antiplatelet agents (aspirin, nonsteroidal anti-inflammatory drugs), anticoagulants, and antibiotics.

Are diseases present that are associated with known hemorrhagic syndromes?

Examples include the combinations of acute promyelocytic leukemia and disseminated intravascular coagulation (DIC), liver disease and systemic fibrinolysis, antibiotic therapy and vitamin K deficiency, or trauma and a dilutional coagulopathy.

Is there a family history of bleeding?

Although most hemostatic defects in hospitalized patients are acquired, underlying hereditary disorders may become manifest in the hospital setting. For example, von Willebrand disease might be discovered because of hemorrhage after a surgical procedure.

PHYSICAL EXAMINATION

The objective of the physical examination is to determine whether bleeding seems appropriate for the injury and whether single or multiple sites are involved. A careful examination may also uncover diseases associated with hemostatic defects (e.g., splenomegaly in myeloproliferative disease, lymphadenopathy in malignancy, hepatomegaly in liver disease). Areas to examine with particular care are wounds, intravenous or other catheter sites, fluid collection bags (urine, gastric, wound drainage, pleural fluid), and the patient's clothing and bedding. The skin should be examined in detail seeking oozing or bleeding from previous finger or heel sticks, and injection or bleeding time sites. Petechiae, particularly in dependent locations, and ecchymoses should be sought. The patient should be turned to one side to seek evidence of bruising over the flank (suggesting retroperitoneal hemorrhage). Ultrasound or MRI scans can be useful for the identification of deep-seated hematomas.

LABORATORY STUDIES

After an initial assessment of the clinical situation, laboratory tests of hemostasis should be obtained as soon as possible in patients who are actively bleeding, without waiting for the completion of the history, medical record review, and physical examination. Platelet function, coagulation, DIC, and systemic fibrinolysis must be assessed (Table 6-3). The tests should be ordered as a battery to save time and to obtain an overview of all facets of hemostasis. Often, the bleeding time is not routinely obtained and is reserved for patients suspected of a platelet function defect in which bleeding persists even with a near-normal platelet count. Alternatively, other screening tests of platelet function can be used (e.g., PFA-100; see Chap. 2). The euglobulin lysis time (ELT) is usually limited to patients with known liver disease or those suspected of complex coagulopathies. Based on the results of the screening tests, more definitive assays should be ordered as needed.

Care must be taken in obtaining, labeling, and processing the blood samples. Generally, in adults one or two citrate (blue top) tubes are needed for coagulation tests, with an EDTA (lavender top) tube for the complete blood and platelet counts. Smaller volumes are collected from pediatric patients. Ideally, the blood samples should be obtained from a separate clean venipuncture with efforts made to avoid contamination with heparin or dilution by intravenous fluids, and then transported promptly to the laboratory for analysis.

Some comments about the use and interpretation of the laboratory screening tests are listed below.

Isolated prolongation of the PT by 2 to 3 sec (INR up to 1.2) is seen frequently in adults who have undergone major surgery or trauma or who are seriously ill. Although possibly related to a fall in factor VII, the mechanisms are unknown. Considerations include early liver insufficiency or vitamin K deficiency. In adults, excessive bleeding is unusual when the sole laboratory abnormality is a mild prolongation of the PT. In children, a prolonged PT more often reflects a propensity for hemorrhage, especially when associated with a long APTT.

- If both the PT and APTT are prolonged, and the disorder is acquired, then the cause is more likely to involve multiple clotting factor defi-

TABLE 6-3	
Screening Tests of Hemostasis for Hospitalized Patients	
Coagulation disorders	PT, APTT, TCT, fibrinogen
Platelet function defects	Platelet count, bleeding time or PFA-100
Disseminated intravascular coagulation	Fibrin degradation products (e.g., D-dimer)
Systemic fibrinolysis	Euglobulin lysis time

ciencies (as in liver disease, vitamin K deficiency, or DIC) than a single abnormality of factor X, V, or prothrombin.

- The TCT is mildly prolonged in both renal and liver disease, but when it is greatly prolonged (e.g., >>100 sec), severe hypofibrinogenemia or heparin effect is likely.

- A separate measurement of fibrinogen is always warranted because the PT and APTT are not sensitive to moderate hypofibrinogenemia. The fibrinogen concentration is an excellent reflection of the severity of DIC, systemic fibrinolysis, or liver disease.

- In acutely ill hospitalized patients, the bleeding time is of less diagnostic value if the platelet count is <50,000/μL. In general, if the bleeding time is normal (and the patient does not have von Willebrand's disease), bleeding is unlikely to be due to a platelet function defect. However, a prolonged bleeding time does not always predict future hemorrhage. Recently, platelet function analyzers such as the PFA-100 are being studied to determine the relationship between abnormal results and bleeding at surgery or other invasive procedures.

- Bleeding times are infrequently performed in sick children. The PFA-100 has been studied in children and neonates and has been shown to be useful for identifying hereditary defects of platelet plug formation (e.g., von Willebrand disease).

- Modern tests for fibrin degradation products (FDP); e.g., D-dimer, make the older paracoagulation tests for fibrin monomer (protamine or ethanol gel tests) less useful in patients suspected of DIC.

- A shortened ELT is a sensitive measure of systemic fibrinolysis but is not always predictive of fibrinolytic bleeding. Additional tests to evaluate fibrinolysis include plasmin–antiplasmin complexes and α_2-antiplasmin assays.

Once results of the initial battery of laboratory tests have been obtained, then consideration should be given to follow-up testing to guide therapy in an actively bleeding patient. Serial hematocrits will be needed, as well as the PT, APTT, fibrinogen, and platelet count. The bleeding time, D-dimer test, and ELT are usually not repeated unless they are abnormal. Intervals between tests may be as short as hourly in a severely injured trauma patient with massive hemorrhage or as infrequently as daily in patients with less severe but persistent bleeding.

ANALYSIS OF THE DATA

A limited number of hemorrhagic defects account for most of the bleeding in hospitalized patients. These disorders are usually acquired rather than hereditary and involve multiple rather than single hemostatic defects (Table 6-4). In children, with a less informative past history, bleeding after surgery or other trauma suggests a hereditary disorder (see Chap. 5).

Vitamin K Deficiency

Seriously ill patients can easily become deficient in vitamin K due to poor nutrition or long-term antibiotic therapy. Because vitamin K deficiency reduces the activity of clotting factors II, VII, IX, and X, the PT and APTT are both prolonged, but the fibrinogen concentration and TCT are normal. The PT lengthens before the APTT because of the short half-life of factor VII (5 hr).

Liver Disease

Because the liver is the site of synthesis of most of the clotting factors, the PT and APTT are often prolonged in advanced liver disease. As in vita-

---

TABLE 6-4

Representative Test Results for Common Bleeding Disorders in Hospitalized Patients

	PT	APTT	TCT	Fibrinogen	Platelet Count	D-Dimer	ELT
Normal Range	11–13.5 s	25–35 s	<30 s	150–450 mg/dL	150–350 K/μL	<0.5 μg/mL	<60 min
Vitamin K deficiency							
Early	18	32	21	225	250	<0.5	>60
Late	26	58	21	225	250	<0.5	>60
Liver disease							
Early	16	32	23	225	185	<0.5	>60
Late	22	63	45	75	60	1.0	30
Disseminated intravascular coagulation							
Mild	12.5	22	36	190	250	1.5	>60
Severe	24	86	45	65	40	4–8	>60
Systemic fibrinolysis							
Mild	12.5	32	35	225	250	<0.5	15
Severe	22	72	60	55	250	<0.5	<15
Dilutional coagulopathy							
Mild	16	38	21	150	125	<0.5	>60
Severe	28	90	21	55	25	1.0	>60
Heparin							
Small	12.5	36	>100	225	250	<0.5	>60
Large	18	>100	>100	225	250	<0.5	>60

min K deficiency, the PT is first to increase. The TCT is often mildly prolonged, which is most likely a result of hepatic synthesis of a dysfunctional fibrinogen or inhibition of fibrin polymerization by circulating FDP. As liver failure becomes more profound, the concentration of fibrinogen begins to fall. The platelet count can be low due to hypersplenism. The bleeding time is often mildly or moderately prolonged although the mechanism is unclear. The ELT is shortened in up to 40 percent of patients with end-stage liver disease due to circulating fibrinolytic enzymes that are not cleared by the liver or are ineffectively neutralized by α_2-antiplasmin.

Disseminated Intravascular Coagulation

The classic pattern of laboratory abnormalities in acute severe DIC includes low concentrations of fibrinogen (<100 mg/dL), high levels of FDP (>2 µg/mL), prolonged PT and APTT, thrombocytopenia, and a prolonged bleeding time. The ELT will be normal in most patients with DIC. In mild DIC, fibrinogen concentrations are often normal since synthesis is increased due to acute phase reactions, but this is balanced by accelerated consumption of fibrinogen. The APTT can be short, presumably due to circulating activated clotting factors. Concentrations of FDP are almost always elevated (see Chap. 24).

Systemic Fibrinolysis

Bleeding due to circulating fibrinolytic enzymes occurs with some regularity in two clinical situations: (1) as a complication of therapeutic thrombolysis and (2) in patients with advanced liver disease, particularly in conjunction with trauma or surgery. In both of these settings, the ELT is short. If fibrinolysis is severe, fibrinogen concentrations are low, and the PT, APTT, and TCT are mildly to moderately prolonged. Concentrations of D-dimer are usually normal, but have been reported to be elevated in some patients with severe systemic fibrinolysis due to plasmin digestion of circulating soluble fibrin.

Dilutional Coagulopathy

In patients with extensive trauma or surgery, blood loss is often temporarily replaced with large volumes of intravenous fluids, which produces substantial dilution of clotting factors and platelets (see Chap. 26). This "washout" syndrome may be enhanced by consumption of clotting factors and platelets at sites of massive tissue injury. Almost all screening tests of hemostasis are abnormal due to depletion of clotting factors and platelets. D-dimer is usually normal or only slightly elevated, except in cases of DIC in patients with brain injury or prolonged hypotension. The ELT is normal except in some patients with advanced liver disease.

Heparin Excess

The presence of heparin in plasma commonly causes confusion in the interpretation of coagulation tests. The blood sample may be contaminated by residual heparin in central venous or arterial lines, which produces abnormal laboratory tests, but not bleeding. Rarely, heparin may be inadvertently administered to patients, producing both bleeding and abnormal laboratory studies. Heparin in the plasma may be strongly suspected if the TCT and APTT are greatly prolonged, particularly if the fibrinogen concentration is >100 mg/dL. Other tests used to identify heparin include the reptilase time (normal in the presence of heparin when the TCT is prolonged). In case of doubt, the most practical approach is to redraw the sample using a peripheral venipuncture site. Alternatively, the plasma can be passed through a heparin-retaining filter, or the heparin neutralized prior to repeating the coagulation screening tests (see Chap. 2).

The conditions described above represent a large proportion of the serious hemostatic defects in hospitalized patients. Other disorders necessitate more specific laboratory assays. For example, a patient with a spontaneous inhibitor to factor VIII will require mixing studies and quantification of the circulating anticoagulant. In children, specific assays for hereditary disorders of hemostasis may be necessary. However, in the great majority of patients, simple screening tests are usually sufficient for a presumptive diagnosis and can serve as guides for clotting factor and platelet replacement therapy to treat the bleeding.

BIBLIOGRAPHY

Bowie EJW, Owen CA: Hemostatic failure in clinical medicine. *Semin Hematol* 14:341, 1977.

Bowie EJW, Owen CA: The significance of abnormal preoperative hemostatic tests. *Prog Hemost Thromb* 5:179, 1980.

Carcao MD et al: The platelet function analyzer (PFA-100): A novel in-vitro system for evaluation of primary haemostasis in children. *Br J Haematol* 101:70, 1998.

Coller BS, Schneiderman PI: Clinical evaluation of hemorrhagic disorders: The bleeding history and differential diagnosis of purpura. In: Hoffman R, et al. (eds): *Hematology. Basic Principles and Practice*, New York, Churchill Livingstone, 3rd ed, pp 1783–1803, 2000.

DeCaterina R et al: Bleeding time and bleeding: An analysis of the relationship of the bleeding time test with parameters of surgical bleeding. *Blood* 84:3363, 1994.

Feinstein DI: Diagnosis and management of disseminated intravascular coagulation: The role of heparin therapy. *Blood* 60:284, 1982.

Francis CW, Kaplan KL: Hematologic problems in the surgical patient: Bleeding and thrombosis. In: Hoffman R, et al. (eds): *Hematology. Basic Principles and Practice,* New York, Churchill Livingstone, 3rd ed, pp 2381–2391, 2000.

Harker LA, Slichter SJ: The bleeding time as a screening test for evaluation of platelet function. *N Engl J Med* 287:155, 1972.

Lind SE: The bleeding time does not predict surgical bleeding. *Blood* 77:2547, 1991.

Mammen EF et al: PFA-100 system: A new method for assessment of platelet dysfunction. *Sem Thromb Haemost* 24:195, 1998.

Manco-Johnson MJ et al: Heparin neutralization is essential for accurate measurement of factor VIII activity and inhibitor assays in blood samples drawn from implanted venous devices. *J Lab Clin Med* 136:74, 2000.

Rapaport SI: Preoperative hemostatic evaluation: Which test if any? *Blood* 61:229, 1983.

Suchman AL, Griner PF: Diagnostic uses of the activated partial thromboplastin time and prothrombin time. *Ann Intern Med* 104:810, 1986.

CHAPTER 7

Evaluation of Bleeding in the Newborn

The evaluation of a bleeding tendency in the newborn infant demands a different approach from that taken for older children or adults. The neonate manifests physiologic alterations of the developing hemostatic system that are reflected in unique normal values (see Chap. 3) for blood samples and result in a number of hemorrhagic disorders that are specific to the perinatal period.

A meticulous family and obstetrical history is mandatory. Familial bleeding disorders that may affect the neonate include the hemophilias, rare autosomal recessive coagulation disorders, and familial thrombocytopenia, which may be best diagnosed using a cord blood sample obtained at the time of delivery (see Chap. 2). Such planning prevents the need for subsequent vessel puncture, which may lead to excessive bleeding if the infant is affected with a hemorrhagic disorder. If the mother has immune thrombocytopenic purpura (ITP), a fetal scalp sample for a platelet count may be indicated. If a previous infant was thrombocytopenic, platelet alloimmunization should be considered. Prenatal and obstetric complications that should alert the physician to potential bleeding in the infant include maternal medications (anticonvulsants and warfarin), intrauterine hypoxia, abruptio placenta, and dead twin fetus (disseminated intravascular coagulation, DIC).

Routine screening tests used in the newborn include the platelet count, PT, APTT, and TCT or fibrinogen. Because physiologic alterations in the contact factors result in a significant prolongation of the APTT (especially in preterm infants), this test is often not helpful. If heparin contamination of the sample is suggested, heparinase in a concentration of 25 mg/mL added *in vitro* enzymatically degrades heparin in the sample (up to

2 U/mL) and confirms heparin as the cause of the prolongation. If hemophilia is suspected, factor assays should be performed because the APTT may not be reliable as a screening test. The precise role of the bleeding time or other tests of platelet-vessel interaction remains to be established. Recent advances in whole blood platelet function analyzers (e.g., PFA-100) may yield useful information for the rare infant in whom a platelet function defect requires immediate diagnosis. Unless there are urgent reasons (i.e., the need for specific therapy), it is more practical to defer the bleeding time and associated studies until 6 months of age or later in suspected cases of von Willebrand disease or platelet function disorders. Determinations of fibrin degradation products (FDP) such as D-dimer are usually done routinely in sick infants since it is a most useful test for DIC. Table 7-1 summarizes the results of screening tests in the newborn infant. The values shown demonstrate the relative differences for these tests in the neonate as compared to the adult.

DIFFERENTIAL DIAGNOSIS OF THE BLEEDING INFANT

Figure 7-1 presents an algorithm for the differential diagnosis of a bleeding infant. The assessment is based on the history and physical findings, which allows classification into "well" and "sick." The well-appearing infant is usually of term gestation, with normal vital signs and physical assessment apart from bleeding from one or more orifices (oral or rectal bleeding, hematuria), skin purpura or petechiae, cephalohematoma, or persistent oozing after the trauma of skin punctures or minor surgery (circumcision). One or more of these manifestations may occur in an otherwise well-appearing infant.

TABLE 7-1

Mean Values for Newborn Screening Tests

	Adult	Term Infant (≥37 Weeks Gestation)	Preterm Infant (<33 Week Gestation)
Platelet count (no./μL)	250,000	330,000	290,000
Bleeding time (Simplate, min)	5.5	3.5	3.5
APTT, (sec)	28	36	45
PT, (sec)	12	13	15
INR	1.0	1.1	1.3
TCT, (sec)	11	12	14
Fibrinogen (mg/dL)	270	250	240

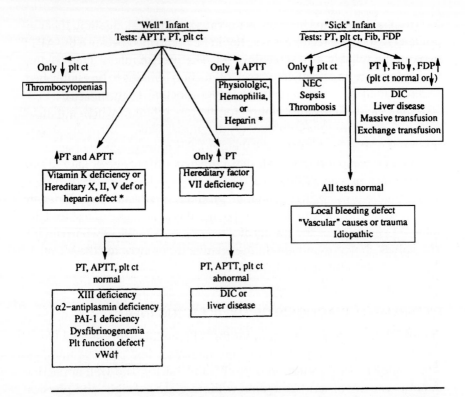

FIGURE 7-1 Differential diagnosis of the bleeding infant.

The basic screening tests (platelet count, APTT, PT) will indicate the following:

- A decreased platelet count as the only abnormality in an infant with petechiae requires the differential diagnosis of thrombocytopenia.
- Prolongation of both the PT (slight) and APTT (marked) with failure of correction of APTT with 1:1 mixing suggests heparin effect (iatrogenic overdose or contamination of catheters); if the PT is corrected in 1:1 mixing, vitamin K deficiency (breastfed infant, no vitamin K at birth) and early severe liver disease are possibilities.
- Prolongation of the APTT alone and correction with 1:1 mixing with normal plasma suggests hemophilia A or B (or a contact factor deficiency [perform factor assays])

- Isolated prolongation of the PT suggests hereditary factor VII deficiency
- If all tests are normal, consider factor XIII, α_2-antiplasmin (α_2-AP), or plasminogen activator inhibitor-1 (PAI-1) deficiency (especially if delayed or persistent umbilical cord stump bleeding, do factor assays) or consider a platelet function defect or von Willebrand disease (plan subsequent tests of primary hemostasis).
- Prolongation of the APTT, PT, and TCT with a normal platelet count and correction with 1:1 mixing with normal plasma suggests hypo or afibrinogenemia or early severe liver disease.
- If all screening studies are abnormal, reevaluate the infant for liver disease or "missed" DIC (do D-dimer test).

In summary, the history, type of bleeding, and results of these tests allow a likely diagnosis to be made that can be confirmed, if needed, at a later date when the neonatal physiologic alterations in clotting tests are no longer present.

The sick-appearing infant who displays evidence of a bleeding tendency is usually either a preterm infant (with respiratory distress, hypoxia, unstable vital signs) or a term infant with evidence of CNS bleeding or sepsis (viral or bacterial). The only sign of bleeding may be shock and pallor (hematoma of liver, adrenal, or kidney, or severe intracranial hemorrhage). Tracheal bleeding in an intubated infant may be due to trauma aggravated by a bleeding tendency. The screening tests (PT, platelet count, fibrinogen, FDP) are usually abnormal. If the most abnormal test is the platelet count, consider sepsis, bowel necrosis (necrotizing enterocolitis), or major vessel thrombosis. Abnormalities in the fibrinogen level and PT with increased FDP confirm the diagnosis of DIC or, less commonly, severe liver disease. In the extremely premature infant, (<32 weeks) the best indicator of DIC is a D-dimer level of >500 ng/mL. Rarely the bleeding and sick infant will have normal screening studies; this combination is particularly seen in intraventricular hemorrhage (IVH) in the premature infant or postoperatively (congenital cardiac lesions) where the bleeding is due to a local lesion or an ill-defined platelet function defect (see following).

GASTROINTESTINAL BLEEDING

Infants with signs of gastrointestinal bleeding (melena or hematemesis), particularly in the first few hours of life, may have swallowed maternal blood during delivery. A gastric aspirate, vomitus, or stool containing gross blood should be tested for adult hemoglobin by the Apt test. The addition of 1% sodium hydroxide to a pink solution containing adult blood will result in a color change from pink to yellow-brown. When the pink color remains, the solution contains mostly fetal hemoglobin and a neonatal origin for the blood must be sought (a hemolyzed sample of the infant's blood is a good control for the test).

INTRACRANIAL HEMORRHAGE

Neonatal intracranial bleeding may result from many etiologies, including birth trauma, hereditary bleeding diatheses, congenital thrombocytopenia, connective tissue disorders (Ehlers-Danlos), hemorrhagic cerebral necrosis due to infection, vascular malformations, and acquired bleeding disorders. The hemorrhagic syndrome of IVH has been studied extensively and remains one of the challenging problems in perinatal medicine. Evidence yielded by many techniques, including ultrasonography, positron emission tomography, and cerebral blood flow studies, led to a reappraisal of the potential etiologies of IVH. The associated parenchymal hemorrhage and the delayed onset of IVH extension of the early subependymal hemorrhage may represent a hemorrhagic component of an initial ischemic lesion. Thus, alterations of the coagulation system may have a more direct etiologic role; that is, an initial ischemic lesion may be due to "microthrombosis" or "infarct," and the hemorrhagic extension may be secondary to a concomitant hemostatic impairment.

From a diagnostic and management viewpoint, it is recommended that all term infants with intracranial hemorrhage have a hemostatic screening battery. If the hemostatic screening tests are all normal, then assay of factor XIII, α_2-antiplasmin, and PAI-1 are indicated; preterm infants (usually <33 weeks' gestation) should have the basic screening tests (PT, fibrinogen, D-dimer, platelet count) to determine whether correctable deficiencies are present.

BIBLIOGRAPHY

Altes A et al: Hereditary macrothrombocytopenia and pregnancy. *Thromb Haemost* 76:29, 1996.

Aronis S et al: Indications of coagulation and/or fibrinolytic system activation in healthy and sick very-low-birth-weight neonates. *Biol Neonate* 74:337, 1998.

Baselga E et al: Purpura in infants and children. *J Am Acad Dermatol* 37:673, 1997.

Carcao MD et al: The platelet function analyzer (PFA-100): a novel in-vitro system for evaluation of primary hemostasis in children. *Br J Haematol* 101:70, 1998.

Dreyfus M et al: Frequency of immune thrombocytopenia in newborns: a prospective study. *Blood* 89:4402, 1997.

Gelman B et al: Impaired mobilization of intracellular calcium in neonatal platelets. *Pediatr Res* 39:692, 1996.

Hathaway WE, Bonnar J: *Hemostatic Disorders of the Pregnant Woman and Newborn Infant,* New York, Elsevier, 1987.

Kulkarni R, Lusher JM: Intracranial and extracranial hemorrhages in newborns with hemophilia: a review of the literature. *J Pediatr Hematol Oncol* 21:289, 1999.

McDonald MM et al: Role of coagulopathy in newborn intracranial hemorrhage. *Pediatrics* 74:26, 1984.

Nuss R, Manco-Johnson M: Hemostasis in Ehlers-Danlos syndrome. Patient report and literature review. *Clin Pediatr* 34:552, 1995.

Rajasekhar D et al: Platelet hyporeactivity in very low birth weight neonates. *Thromb Haemost* 77:1002, 1997.

Ries M et al: The role of α_2-antiplasmin in the inhibition of clot lysis in newborns and adults. *Biol Neonate* 69:298, 1996.

Schmidt BK et al: Do coagulation screening tests detect increased generation of thrombin and plasmin in sick newborns? *Thrombos Haemost* 69:418, 1993.

Seth RD: Trends in incidence and severity of intraventricular hemorrhage. *J Child Neurol* 13:261, 1998.

Shirahata A et al: Diagnosis of DIC in very low birth weight infants. *Semin Thromb Hemost* 24:467, 1998.

Suzuki S et al. (eds): *Perinatal Thrombosis and Hemostasis,* Tokyo, Springer-Verlag, 1991.

Zipursky A: Prevention of vitamin K deficiency bleeding in newborns. *Brit J Haematol* 104:430, 1999.

CHAPTER 8

Thrombocytopenias

Thrombocytopenia (platelet count less than 150,000/µL) can occur at all ages, from the small premature infant to the elderly adult. Etiologic events and associations vary with age and development. The newborn infant is particularly susceptible to decreased platelets; as many as 20 percent of sick premature infants have thrombocytopenia. Pregnancy is associated with several unique causes of thrombocytopenia including preeclampsia and gestational thrombocytopenia; the latter occurs in 5 percent of normal pregnancies. Most cases of non-chemotherapy-induced thrombocytopenia are caused by increased platelet destruction, i.e., immune thrombocytopenic purpura (ITP); decreased production is relatively more prominent in adults.

CAUSES OF THROMBOCYTOPENIA IN THE NEWBORN INFANT

Although the causes of newborn thrombocytopenia are many, the approach to determination of etiology is greatly simplified by division into two broad categories: the "sick" (premature) infant and the "well" (term) infant. In the sick preterm infant, almost any illness will cause at least mild thrombocytopenia. Common etiologies include bacterial or viral sepsis, disseminated intravascular coagulation (DIC), large vessel thrombosis, necrotizing enterocolitis, pulmonary syndromes (respiratory disease syndrome [RDS], meconium and amniotic fluid aspiration, pulmonary hypertension) or asphyxia-hypoxemia. In the full-term infant who appears well, the most likely diagnosis is antibody-mediated (especially alloimmune thrombocytopenia [AIT]) if the platelet count is <50,000/µL, but can also be maternal immune thrombocytopenia (ITP), systemic lupus erythematosis (SLE) (see Chap. 9), viral syndrome, hyperviscosity syndrome, or occult large vessel thrombosis, (i.e., renal vein thrombosis). Overall, infection, including viral syndromes and DIC, with or without asphyxia, are the most common causes of decreased platelets. Bacterial sepsis frequently is associated with acute thrombocytopenia, which may take 6 to 10 days to resolve. Congenital viral infections may produce severe thrombocytopenia by several mechanisms, including megakaryocytic injury, splenic removal, hepatic disease, and platelet-endothelial cell injury. Typically they will manifest the "blueberry muffin" rash, an extramedullary hematopoiesis in the skin, in addition to purpura and abnormal liver tests.

Another mechanism for thrombocytopenia in the newborn is decreased platelet production due to marrow involvement in several disorders (see Table 8-1). Other causes of neonatal thrombocytopenia include infants small for gestational age (which may be a combination of low-grade DIC secondary to polycythemia and hypoxia, and marrow damage), post-exchange transfusion ("wash-out"), neonatal thyrotoxicosis, metabolic disorders (hyperglycinemia, mucolipidosis, propionic acidemia), maternal hypertension (in which neonatal leukopenia is more common), erythroblastosis fetalis, giant hemangioma and placental chorioangioma, and maternal (tolbutamide, hydantoin, azathioprine) and infant (intralipid, tolazoline) drug usage. Hereditary thrombocytopenias (see below) may also present in the neonatal period.

CAUSES OF THROMBOCYTOPENIA IN THE CHILD AND ADULT

Thrombocytopenia in the child and adult may be classified as due to increased destruction, sequestration, or decreased production; these disorders are listed in Table 8-2. The antibody-mediated syndromes are discussed in Chapter 9. Nonimmune causes of increased platelet destruction include the DIC syndromes, Kasabach-Merritt syndrome, hemolytic ure-

---

TABLE 8-1

Bone Marrow Abnormality Associated with Neonatal Thrombocytopenia

Congenital megakaryocytic hypoplasia
Absent radii (TAR) syndrome (leukemoid reaction, absent radius, digits present)
Phocomelia syndrome
Aplastic anemia
Trisomy syndromes (myeloproliferative syndrome)
Osteopetrosis (myeloproliferative syndrome)
Congenital leukemia
Fanconi's pancytopenia (deformed or absent radius and thumb, onset is later in life)

mic syndrome/thrombocytic thrombocytopenic purpura (HUS-TTP), and hypersplenism (see Table 8-2).

TABLE 8-2

Causes of Thrombocytopenia in Children and Adults

Increased platelet destruction and/or sequestration
  Immune thrombocytopenias
    Primary
      ITP, posttransfusion purpura
    Secondary
      Infections: Viral, bacterial, protozoan
      Autoimmune disorders (SLE, Evan's syndrome)
      Lymphoma
      Hodgkin's disease
      Carcinomatosis

Drugs: Heparin	Cimetidine
Gold	Digoxin
Quinidine	Valproic acid
Quinine	α-interferon
Penicillins	

  Nonimmune
    DIC syndromes
    Kasabach-Merritt syndrome
    Hemolytic uremic syndrome
    Thrombotic thrombocytopenic purpura
    Chronic hemolytic anemia and thrombocytopenia
    Congenital or acquired heart disease
    Hypersplenism
    Catheters, protheses, cardiopulmonary bypass
    Familial hemophagocytic reticulosis
Decreased platelet production
  Aplastic anemia, Fanconi's pancytopenia
  Marrow infiltrative processes
    Leukemias
    Metastatic carcinoma
    Myelofibrosis
    Multiple myeloma
    Histiocytoses
    Osteopetrosis
    Infections
  Megakaryocytic thrombocytopenia
    Ethanol abuse
    HIV-1
    Parvovirus infections
    Myelodysplastic syndrome
    Antibody and T-cell suppression
  Nutritional deficiencies
    Iron
    Folate
    B_{12}

TABLE 8-2 CONTINUED
Causes of Thrombocytopenia in Children and Adults

Drug or radiation induced
  Ethanol
  Phenylbutazone
  Chloramphenicol
  Chemotherapeutic agents
Paroxysmal nocturnal hemoglobinuria
Cyclic thrombocytopenia (Garcia's disease)
Hereditary thrombocytopenias (see Table 8-4)
Miscellaneous
  Liver disease
  Uremia, renal diseases, renal transplant rejection
  Exchange transfusion, massive transfusions, extracorporeal circulation
  Heat or cold injury
  Thyroid diseases (hyper-, hypo-)
  Fat embolism
  Allogeneic bone marrow transplantation
  Graft-versus-host disease

DIAGNOSIS OF THROMBOCYTOPENIAS

The clinical context of the occurrence of thrombocytopenia frequently indicates the etiology or mechanism involved (see Fig. 8-1). For example, the HUS/TTP syndrome can be recognized as a distinct cause of reduced platelet count because of its specific systemic manifestations in addition to thrombocytopenia (see Chap. 28).

The first step in diagnosis requires a distinction as to whether the thrombocytopenia is part of a systemic disorder or is an "isolated thrombocytopenia." This is usually made by following a systematic approach using (1) the history (associated illnesses, pharmacologic agents, specific symptoms) and (2) physical examination (anomalies, hepatosplenomegaly, foci of infection, tumor, lymphadenopathy, bleeding) for overall direction, followed by (3) careful interpretation of the complete blood count and examination of the peripheral blood smear for clues to the diagnosis. The complete blood count and blood smear confirm the degree of thrombocytopenia, rule out spuriously decreased platelets, provide clues to associated hematologic disorders, and offer an estimation of platelet size (confirmed by the mean platelet volume). Drugs may need to be changed to exclude their having a role; a database for drug induced thrombocytopenia may be found at *http://moon.ouhsc.edu/jgeorge.*

If the diagnosis is not secure at that point, (4) a bone marrow examination including both needle aspiration and biopsy is indicated. Even in children, the marrow biopsy as well as aspiration should be performed

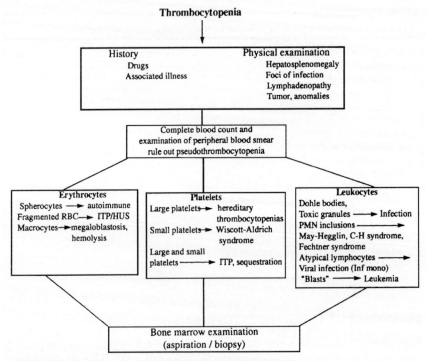

FIGURE 8-1 Evaluation of thrombocytopenia in child or adult with normal hemostatic screening tests and who is not acutely ill. C-H, Chediak Higashi.

(ideally under conscious sedation) to accurately estimate cellularity and look for infiltrative disease (tumor cells). In many instances of suspected childhood ITP, the bone marrow examination is deferred or omitted if there is (1) a typical history (preceding viral infection in an otherwise well child); (2) a normal physical examination except bleeding signs; (3) a normal blood count and blood smear except low platelets; and (4) a decision not to treat with corticosteroids. Watchful waiting with or without treatment will confirm the diagnosis if remission occurs in a few weeks to 2 months. Similarly repeated substantial response to IVIG or to IV anti-D are confirmatory as well. However, if any aspect of the case appears atypical, a marrow examination should be performed in order not to confound the diagnosis of leukemia, early aplasia, or myelodysplasia (MDS).

The use of the bone marrow examination as a guide to the diagnosis is shown in Table 8-3. Although the presence of normal or increased numbers of megakaryocytes may lessen the possibility of decreased platelet production, the conclusion may not be correct in settings where megakaryocytes are present but maturation is impaired.

TABLE 8-3

Bone Marrow Examination as a Guide to the Etiology of Thrombocytopenia

Decreased Megakaryocytes in Normal Marrow	Decreased Megakaryocytes in Abnormal Marrow	Increased or Normal Megakaryocytes in Normal Marrow
Thrombocytopenia with absent radius (TAR)	Aplastic anemia tumor	ITP/SLE
Early Fanconi syndrome or aplastic anemia	Leukemia, myeloma,	Hypersplenism
Idiopathic Amegakaryocytic hypo- plasia	Myelofibrosis, osteopetrosis, myelodysplasia	Infection (AIDS)
Immune-mediated (SLE, AIDS)	Preleukemia	Hereditary thrombo- cytopenia (most cases)
Congenital heart disease	Megaloblastosis	Vascular neoplasms

Figure 8-1 and Table 8-2 suggest that other tests may be required in certain cases to confirm a specific diagnosis or mechanism for the thrombocytopenia; this is in addition to the morphology of blood and bone marrow cells. Useful adjunctive tests are quantitative immunoglobulins, antinuclear antibody (ANA), direct antiglobulin test (Coombs), monospot test, HIV serology, and lupus anticoagulant (LA) test, as well as specific organ-related tests such as thyroid testing. Bone marrow chromosome analysis and flow cytometry may be critical in the diagnosis of refractory thrombocytopenia, i.e., myelodysplastic syndrome, especially in elderly patients. In the future, platelet lifespan estimations such as glycocalicin, platelet reticulocyte counts, and/or thrombopoietin levels, may improve diagnosis and therefore management.

HEREDITARY THROMBOCYTOPENIAS

The familial thrombocytopenias are neither rare nor well-defined. The diagnosis is suspected when a patient with presumed "ITP" has family members with low platelets or a lack of response to "ITP" therapy. Supporting this diagnosis is the onset of thrombocytopenia in infancy or early childhood and the detection of giant or tiny platelets on the blood smear. A classification of hereditary thrombocytopenia is shown in Table 8-4 and is limited to those reported disorders that have characteristic findings allowing differentiation from the others. Platelet size is estimated by both morphologic appearance on blood smears and mean platelet volume since platelet shape-change defects may produce giant platelets during preparation of the smear. For example, the diameter of platelets with severe hereditary giant-platelet syndromes (Bernard-Soulier syndrome, Montreal platelet syndrome) is considerably larger on blood smears than on phase-contrast microscopy of freshly fixed platelets. Overlap between the disorders in Table 8-4 and the hereditary platelet function diseases is known, i.e., Bernard-Soulier syndrome (see Chap. 10).

TABLE 8-4

Hereditary Thrombocytopenias

Disorder	Platelet Inheritance	Function Tests	Other Findings
I. Macrothrombocytes			
Bernard-Soulier syndrome	AR	↓agg to ristocetin, BT markedly increased	Decreased membrane GP Ib-IX (V)
Montreal platelet syndrome	AD	↓agg to thrombin, normal agg to ristocetin, ADP, collagen	Normal to reduced GP Ib
May-Hegglin anomaly	AD	Normal	Dohle bodies in leukocytes
Epstein's syndrome Alport's syndrome	AD	Abnormal agg to ADP, collagen	Renal disease, nerve deafness
(Fechtner variant)		Normal	Leukocyte inclusions
(Sebastian variant)		Normal	Leukocyte inclusions, no associated defect
Gray platelet syndrome	Autosomal	Abnormal agg to ADP, collagen, thrombin	↓alpha granules, pale-staining platelets and agranular megakaryocytes
Genetic thrombo-cytopenia (Najean-Lecompte)	AD	Normal	Normal microscopy and platelet survival
Giant platelets with abnormal glycoproteins	AR	Abnormal to L-epi, AA; normal ristocetin	Membrane GP Ia, Ic, IIa absent; mitral valve defect
II. Normothrombocyte			
Thrombocytopenia with absent radius (TAR)	AR	↓agg to L-epi and collagen	↓megakaryocytes, absent radii, normal thumbs, presenta-tion at birth

TABLE 8-4 CONTINUED

Hereditary Thrombocytopenias

Disorder	Platelet Inheritance	Function Tests	Other Findings
Chediak-Higashi syndrome	AR	↓agg to L-epi and collagen	Oculocutaneous albinism, recurrent infections, large abnormal granules in leukocytes, macrophages
Hereditary intrinsic platelet defect (Murphy)	AD	Normal	↓platelet survival
Familial platelet disorder (Dowton)	AD	Abnormal agg to L-epi and collagen	Hematologic neoplasms, normal GPs
Pseudo-von Willebrand disease	AD	↑agg to ristocetin	↑plt binding of vWf, plt agg with normal plasma, abnormality of GP Ib
III. Microthrombocytes			
Wiskott-Aldrich syndrome	X-linked	Abnormal agg to ADP, collagen thrombin	↓plt survival, eczema, recurrent infections, immune deficiency due to failure of lymphocyte maturation—all due to WASP gene defect

* Classification based on platelet size; bone marrow examination is normal unless noted otherwise. AR, autosomal recessive; AD, autosomal dominant; epi, epinephrine; agg, aggregation; plt, platelet; BT, bleeding time; ADP, adenosine diphosphate; GP, glycoprotein; ↓, decrease; ↑, increase; WASP, Wiskott-Aldrich syndrome protein.

Most of the hereditary thrombocytopenias are characterized by platelet counts of 50 to 100,000/µl, are relatively asymptomatic, and require no management on a day-to-day basis. Exceptions include the following syndromes with more severe bleeding manifestations, which are related at least in part to more severe thrombocytopenia: Wiskott-Aldrich syndrome (see Table 8-4); thrombocytopenia with absent radii (TAR; leukemoid reaction with severe thrombocytopenia in the newborn and a tendency for spontaneous remissions); Chediak-Higashi syndrome (storage pool defect in platelets, abnormal leukocyte function, albinism, increased infections, and predisposition to lymphoma); and Bernard-Soulier syndrome, which has variable thrombocytopenia in addition to errors of measurement because of very large-sized platelets.

RELATIONSHIP OF BLEEDING MANIFESTATIONS TO PLATELET COUNT

The usual manifestations of thrombocytopenic bleeding are petechiae and small ecchymoses. More significant hemorrhage includes mucous membrane bleeding (epistaxis, gastrointestinal, and menorrhagia), intracerebral hemorrhage, and immediate-type bleeding after surgery or trauma. These manifestations are unusual if the platelet count is >50,000/μL unless there is significant platelet dysfunction. The level of platelet count associated with a risk of bleeding in thrombocytopenic patients with randomly aged or "old" platelets circulating in conditions such as leukemia or marrow failure (production deficits) is higher than in patients with disorders such as ITP, who have a population of rapidly turning over young platelets. This concept was first presented by Harker and Slichter in 1972 using the standardized bleeding time as an index of bleeding. As in other conditions, factors other than the level of the platelet count may influence bleeding, such as platelet-function–altering drugs (ASA; NSAIDs, e.g. Motrin), intravascular coagulation syndromes, activation or "exhaustion" of platelets (prosthetic valves), and the coexistence hemostatic defects (i.e., in liver disease or uremia).

Sequestration occurs when the thrombocytopenia of hypersplenism is primarily due to increased platelet pooling in an enlarged spleen. These conditions, in addition to overt or cryptogenic liver disease, include Gaucher's disease, chronic hemolytic disorders, hairy cell leukemia, and, rarely, lymphoproliferative disorders. A massively enlarged spleen can hold up to 90 percent of the total platelet mass (part of the exchangeable pool). The thrombocytopenia is rarely severe and most patients are asymptomatic.

MANAGEMENT

Guidelines for management of the immune thrombocytopenias are discussed in Chapter 9. In general, the management for the other thrombocytopenic disorders is treatment or elimination of the underlying cause, if there is one such as sepsis; management of the ongoing bleeding manifestations with DDAVP, Amicar, or tranexamic acid; local measures for control of bleeding, such as nasal packing and oral contraceptives; and, if needed, platelet transfusion.

For hypersplenism, when thrombocytopenic bleeding is of clinical significance and therapy by medical means (antibiotics, chemotherapy, immunosuppression, i.e., steroids) has been used optimally, splenectomy may be considered. Partial splenectomy, splenic embolism, or radiation therapy may be alternatives but there is little data regarding efficacy. Splenectomy is also effective in raising the platelet count in Wiskott-Aldrich syndrome, but increases the risk of severe infections in these immunocompromised patients; however, this risk is manageable with penicillin prophylaxis and/or monthly IVIG. Marrow transplantation is preferable but requires a suitable donor.

Specific treatment in acquired pure amegakaryocytic thrombocytopenic purpura (AMT) include management of the underlying disorder (HIV-1 or parvovirus infection) or immunosuppression (prednisone, intravenous immunoglobulin, cyclophosphamide, cyclosporine, antithymocyte globulin) in the antibody or T-cell–mediated disorders. Infants with the TAR syndrome can show spontaneous remission after several months so that comprehensive platelet transfusion support should be planned for that interval, as it should for any patient with AMT with platelet counts <10,000/μL.

The management of acute bleeding episodes in nonimmune-mediated thrombocytopenic patients involves the use of intravenous infusions of DDAVP, Amicar (PO or IV), and/or platelet concentrate transfusions. Recent use of infusions suggests a role in this setting as well. If epistaxis is a problem, then antifibrinolytics and a vaporizer/humidifier are used. For vaginal bleeding, estrogen may be useful for acute hemorrhage, followed by oral contraceptives if needed as prophylaxis. For therapy of the immune disorders see Chapter 9. Patients with at least 50,000/μL platelets who display a bleeding tendency (indicating a platelet function disorder) can be treated with DDAVP, except for those hereditary syndromes that have been shown not to respond; for example, Glanzmann's thrombasthenia and Scott syndrome. All patients at risk for bleeding should be advised to avoid platelet-function–inhibiting drugs (ASA, nonsteroidal anti-inflammatory agents, and synthetic penicillins). Patients requiring long-term treatment should be given leukocyte-poor platelet concentrates from limited numbers of donors (apheresis) to decrease alloimmunization (see Chap. 52).

BIBLIOGRAPHY

Ballmaier M et al: Thrombopoietin in patients with congenital thrombocytopenia and absent radii: elevated serum levels, normal receptor expression, but defective reactivity to thrombopoietin. *Blood* 90:612, 1997.

Beardsley DS: Platelet abnormalities in infancy and childhood. Oski FA, Nathan DG (eds.) In: *Hematology of Infancy and Childhood*, 4th edition, Philadelphia, WB Saunders Co., 1993.

Becker PS et al: Giant platelets with abnormal surface glycoproteins: a new familial disorder associated with mitral valve insufficiency. *J Pediat Hematol/Oncol* 20:69, 1998.

Blanchette VS, Rand ML: Platelet disorders in newborn infants: diagnosis and management. *Semin Perinatol* 21:53, 1997.

Breton-Gorius J et al: A new congenital dysmegakaryopoietic thrombocytopenia (Paris-Trousseau) associated with giant platelet alpha-granules and chromosome 11 deletion at 11q23. *Blood* 85:1805, 1997.

Burstein SA: Thrombocytopenia due to decreased platelet production. In Hoffman R et al. (eds.) *Hematology Basic Principles and Practice.* 2nd edition. Churchill Livingstone, 1995, p 1870.

Cahill MR, Lilleyman JS: The rational use of platelet transfusions in children. *Semin Thromb Hemost* 24:567, 1998.

Dowton SB et al: Studies of a familial platelet disorder. *Blood* 65:557, 1985.

George JN et al: Platelets: acute thrombocytopenia. *ASH Education Program Book*, p. 371, 1998.

Hamilton RW et al: Platelet function, ultrastructure, and survival in the May-Hegglin anomaly. *Am J Clin Pathol* 74:663, 1980.

Harker LA, Slichter SJ: The bleeding time as a screening test for evaluation of platelet function. *N Eng J Med* 287:155, 1972.

Hedberg VA, Lipton JM: Thrombocytopenia with absent radii. *Am J Pediatr Hematol Oncol* 10:51, 1988.

Hoffman R: Acquired pure amegakaryocytic thrombocytopenic purpura. *Semin Hematol* 28:303, 1991.

Hofmann WK et al: Memorial lecture. Megakaryocytic growth factors: Is there a new approach for management of thrombocytopenia in patients with malignancies. *Leukemia* 13: S14, 1999.

Milton JG et al: Platelet size and shape in hereditary giant platelet syndromes on blood smear and in suspension: Evidence for two types of abnormalities. *J Lab Clin Med* 106:326, 1985.

Murphy S et al: Hereditary thrombocytopenia with an intrinsic platelet defect. *N Engl J Med* 281:857, 1969.

Najean Y, Lecompte T: Genetic thrombocytopenia with autosomal dominant transmission: A review of 54 cases. *Br J Haematol* 74:203, 1990.

Shcherbina A et al: Pathological events in platelets of Wiskott-Aldrich syndrome platelets. *Brit J Haematol* 106:875, 1999.

Tomer A et al: Autologous platelet kinetics in patients with severe thrombocytopenia: Discrimination between disorders of production and destruction. *J Lab Clin Med* 118:546, 1991.

Warrier I, Lusher JM: Congenital thrombocytopenias. *Curr Opin Hematol* 2:395, 1995.

Young G et al: Sebastian syndrome: case report and review of the literature. *Am J Hematol* 61:62, 1999.

Weiss HJ et al: Pseudo-von Willebrand's disease. An intrinsic platelet defect with aggregation by unmodified human factor VIII/von Willebrand factor and enhanced adsorption of its high-molecular-weight multimers. *N Engl J Med* 306:326, 1982.

CHAPTER 9

Immune Thrombocytopenia

In the 1950s, Harrington transfused plasma from patients with immune thrombocytopenia (ITP) into normal adults and demonstrated thrombocytopenia in the majority of normal recipients. Thus a humoral/immunologic basis, instead of marrow failure to produce platelets, was established as the explanation of thrombocytopenia. These discoveries created the basis for studies of antiplatelet antibodies and the understanding of ITP as an autoimmune disease. Platelet antibodies, both "auto" and "allo," interact with platelet surface antigens resulting in increased platelet destruction by the mononuclear phagocyte system. Immunologic thrombocytopenic purpuras can be either *autoimmune* (ITP) or *alloimmune* (AIT). Autoimmune thrombocytopenia includes primary ITP in adults, children, and pregnant women; and secondary ITP occurring in patients affected by systemic lupus erythematosis (SLE), lymphoproliferative diseases, immunodeficiency, viral infections (including HIV), and drug-related thrombocytopenias. Alloimmune thrombocytopenias include fetal and neonatal alloimmune thrombocytopenia (AIT), post-transfusion purpura, and platelet transfusion refractoriness (see Chap. 52).

PLATELET ANTIGENS AND ANTIBODIES

The platelet membrane components that may serve as targets for auto- and alloantibodies include glycoproteins (GP), single DNA base-change–producing single amino-acid–change polymorphisms (i.e., HPA-1a [PI^{A1}]) blood groups (i.e., group A), and HLA class I molecules. Table 9-1 lists the best-known platelet antigens and indicates their role in the various immune platelet disorders. These can be determined serologically and also, in many cases, by DNA-based typing. The latter is useful when DNA is available but not platelets, i.e., after amniocentesis, or if platelets or antibody reagents are scarce.

Measurement of platelet-associated IgG (PAIgG) for autoantibodies in putative ITP is *not useful* diagnostically primarily because of false positives. More precise estimation of antiplatelet antibody in ITP may be possible in the future by measuring platelet-glycoprotein-specific, platelet-associated antibodies. Determination of anti-platelet antibody to specific platelet alloantigens (i.e., HPA-1A [PL^{A1}]) in AIT is specific in experienced laboratories using appropriate controls.

IMMUNOLOGIC (AUTOIMMUNE) THROMBOCYTOPENIA

Platelet autoantibodies may cause thrombocytopenia in both primary and secondary ITP. Primary ITP is a mild to severe bleeding disorder that can occur at any age after 3 months and is characterized by petechiae, skin and mucous membrane bleeding, menorrhagia, gastrointestinal hemorrhage, and, in as many as 1% of cases, intracranial hemorrhage (ICH). The low platelet count does not always correlate with the bleeding manifestations; platelet function or other factors predisposing to hemorrhage are not well delineated in individual cases. However it is thought that lower platelet counts ($\leq$10–20,000/μl) and more bleeding manifestations may be associated with a greater likelihood of ICH.

Two forms of ITP are recognized: childhood (acute) and adult (chronic). The childhood type commonly follows viral infections and runs a self-limited course, with spontaneous remission in 80 percent of cases within 6 to 12 months. The chronic form is that typically seen in 70 to 80 percent of adults, with the other 20 percent occurring in children; it

TABLE 9-1	
Platelet Antigens in Immune Thrombocytopenias	
Alloimmune thrombocytopenia (AIT)	
PLA1, HPA-1a (Zwa)	Most common cause of AIT in Caucasians
Ko, HPA-2:	Rare cause of AIT
Bak, HPA-3 (Lek):	Infrequent cause of severe AIT
Yuk/Pen, HPA-4:	Most common cause of severe AIT in Asians
Br, HPA-5 (Zav):	Common cause of mild AIT
Autoimmune thrombocytopenia (ITP)	
GPIIb/IIIa	Specific targets not well localized, topographic
GPIb/IX	
GPIa/IIa	
GPV	

may persist indefinitely. The thrombocytopenia in secondary ITP is largely indistinguishable from that of primary ITP although the forms associated with systemic autoimmune disorders, i.e., SLE and Evans syndrome (ITP and autoimmune hemolytic anemia), have a greater tendency to remain chronic or to recur following a transient remission.

The diagnosis of ITP is made by exclusion of secondary and hereditary causes of thrombocytopenia (see Chap. 8). It includes a normal physical examination other than signs of mucocutaneous hemorrhage without hepatosplenomegaly or abnormality of the radial rays, an otherwise normal CBC with review of the blood smear, and a normal bone marrow examination (if performed; see Chap. 8). Although not recommended as part of the diagnostic evaluation, demonstration of platelet autoantibodies (anti-GP IIb-IIIa, Ib-IX, Ia-IIa) may be seen in at least 50 to 75 percent of children and adults with the chronic type of ITP. No prognostic significance has yet been assigned to the presence or absence of any of these antibodies. Testing beyond the CBC is not required in typical cases; additional laboratory investigation depends upon abnormal findings in screening tests and clinical exam. A blood type (and direct antiglobulin test, DAT) is needed for patients in whom anti-D therapy is contemplated (see below).

Immune Thrombocytopenia in Pregnancy

Approximately 5 percent of normal women will develop mild thrombocytopenia during uncomplicated pregnancy, termed gestational thrombocytopenia (GTP). These women do not have a history or other evidence of ITP before becoming pregnant; they may have increased mean platelet size and elevated PAIgG levels. The offspring of women with GTP do *not* have an increased risk of neonatal thrombocytopenia; therefore, no special management considerations are indicated unless the maternal platelet count is low enough to complicate epidural anesthesia. The diagnosis of ITP and gestational thrombocytopenia (GTP) is dependent upon exclusion of other causes of maternal thrombocytopenia, i.e., pre-eclampsia, TTP-HUS, drug-induced thrombocytopenia, DIC, and HIV. The differentiation of ITP from GTP depends upon identification of thrombocytopenia before the current pregnancy (not during a prior pregnancy) and following platelet counts during pregnancy; if the platelet count becomes <50,000/µL, the diagnosis of ITP is much more likely. Maintenance of a platelet count >30,000/µL during gestation and >50,000/µL at delivery appears sufficient to reduce the risk of hemorrhage to the general obstetric population.

Pregnant women who develop ITP during the gestation or who have a history of chronic ITP are at an approximately 10 percent risk for delivering an infant with marked, passively acquired thrombocytopenia. A normal maternal platelet count can be associated with severe neonatal thrombocytopenia when the mother is on treatment or after a splenectomy. Thrombocytopenia may worsen during gestation for uncertain reasons; if so, often the maternal platelet count will return to baseline following delivery (and the end of breastfeeding).

MANAGEMENT

Children

In children, no specific treatment is necessary unless the platelet count is <20,000 to 30,000/μl and/or the patient displays bleeding manifestations beyond scattered petechiae and ecchymoses; special attention must be paid to GI hemorrhages, oral mucosal bleeding ("wet" purpura), or an increased risk of ICH such as following head trauma or with headache. Depending on the urgency of the situation, either oral prednisone (2 to 4 mg/kg/day), intravenous methylprednisolone (5 to 30 mg/kg/day), intravenous immunoglobulin (IVIG) 800 to 1000 mg/kg/day, or IV anti-D at a dose of 75 mcg/kg (in an RH+, DAT− patient) are given daily (except for anti-D) until the platelet count increases substantially. Maintenance therapy with oral prednisone or repeated doses of IV anti-D or IVIG may be used if the platelet count increases but then returns to the previous low level. If oral prednisone is used, the dose is generally tapered and stopped after 3 to 6 weeks regardless of the platelet count; other therapy should be considered at this point if the platelet count is still very reduced.

Impending or established ICH should be treated by immediate platelet transfusion, followed by continuous platelet infusion and intravenous methylprednisolone, followed by IVIG; emergency splenectomy should be reserved for a patient in whom the platelet count cannot be immediately, sufficiently increased. Platelet concentrate transfusions are virtually never indicated except in ICH or life-threatening bleeding since other treatment is usually effective within 24 to 48 hours. The child should avoid platelet-function–inhibiting drugs like ASA, NSAIDs, and glyceryl guaiacolate. Antihistamines, acetaminophen, and the new COX-2 inhibitors (i.e., rofecoxib or celecoxib) are safe to use. The activity of patients with ITP whose platelet counts are >20,000/μL should not be overly restricted; only a small number of contact sports (tackle football, lacrosse, field hockey, and perhaps soccer or basketball) should be avoided in a thrombocytopenic child with a platelet count >30,000/μL.

Chronic ITP in children (persistence after 6 months) with a platelet count <20,000 to 30,000/μL is usually managed by repeated infusions as needed of IV anti-D, IVIG, or low-dose or alternate-day steroids with consideration of splenectomy after at least one year from diagnosis has elapsed in a child over 5 years of age. Because of the increased mortality of post-splenectomy sepsis; pneumococcal, H influenza B, and meningo-coccal vaccines; and prophylactic antibiotics are employed. Other treatments can be used (see below) but usually are reserved for children who fail splenectomy. Unique issues exist in children, i.e., acceleration of bone age with danazol.

Adults

In adults the goal of therapy of ITP in adults is to induce a long-term (i.e., unmaintained by therapy) remission that results in an adequate, but not necessarily normal, platelet count. Similarly to children with ITP, a platelet count ≥20,000 to 30,000/μL is not usually associated with bleeding. Oral prednisone, 1 mg/kg/day, is usually the first treatment; initial IVIG or IV anti-D (75 mcg/kg) may be used concomitantly to increase the count more rapidly. Although 70 percent of patients will respond to steroids initially, only about 30 percent will have a lasting improvement. IVIG and IV anti-D often result in good responses, but relapse in 2 to 4 weeks is usual; refractoriness to repeated infusions may develop in a minority.

Splenectomy is the treatment of choice in adult patients who fail to maintain adequate platelet levels after tapering treatment. No comprehensive long-term data exist, but 60 to 70 percent of patients are thought to achieve a lasting remission after splenectomy. Despite isolated reports, no good correlation has been proven to exist between response to treatment (steroids, IVIG, IV anti-D) and response to subsequent splenectomy.

Refractory patients (those with platelet counts <20,000/μL despite prior splenectomy) who are having bleeding symptoms or who are at risk for bleeding are candidates for treatment after splenectomy. No consensus exists as to the optimal approach for these patients. Single agents such as the attenuated androgen, danazol (400 to 800 mg/day orally if the transaminases allow it), azathioprine (2 mg/kg/day orally), cyclophosphamide (1000 mg/m^2 IV with 2 to 3 monthly infusions or 2 to 4 mg/kg/day orally depending upon leukopenia), and other less well-studied agents may induce treatment-maintained remissions or at least improvement. These agents may require 3 to 4 months for their effects to be seen. However, these drugs typically have undesirable side effects, and limited response rates, and resistance may develop. In practice, we have utilized two oral agents simultaneously. In many instances, if the platelet count is >10,000 to 20,000/µL and no bleeding is present, it may be best to "watch and wait." IVIG can be used (with methyl-prednisolone and/or vincristine) for temporary effect to prevent acute bleeding episodes while awaiting the effect of oral medications. Relapse after a durable unmaintained remission may be related to splenic regrowth; however, accessory splenectomy is substantially less successful than initial splenectomy and should not be automatically undertaken in all patients in whom such splenic tissue is identified.

Pregnancy

A woman with ITP during pregnancy should be treated with oral prednisone or IVIG if the platelet count falls below 20,000 to 30,000/µL or a procedure is contemplated, i.e., amniocentesis or delivery. Intravenous anti-D is being evaluated in clinical trials for use in ITP in pregnancy. Treatment is similar to that given to non-pregnant ITP patients, except that certain side effects of steroids (i.e., tendency to develop diabetes, increased BP, fluid retention, osteoporosis, and depression) are accentuated in pregnancy, making this treatment less desirable. Maintenance therapy can be accomplished with IVIG supplementing low-dose or alternate-day prednisone. Splenectomy is virtually never required and should be used only as a last resort, and then during the second trimester, to control severe bleeding. The maternal platelet count at delivery ideally would be ≥50,000/µL; higher numbers are often required for epidural anesthesia.

The approach to fetal/neonatal thrombocytopenia is controversial because of the low, but not absent, incidence of ICH. A recent review has indicated that of 475 infants born of mothers with ITP, 10 percent were born with moderate thrombocytopenia and 15 percent with severe thrombocytopenia; intracranial hemorrhage occurred in 3 percent and was not affected by mode of delivery. Other studies have shown similar rates of neonatal thrombocytopenia but less intracranial hemorrhage, approximately 1 percent. Fetal blood sampling is almost never warranted because of its 1 percent complication rate. Fetal scalp sampling in early labor may produce falsely low platelet counts because of consistent clumping; review of the smear instead of measuring a count has been advocated. The only clinical predictor of the neonatal platelet count is the platelet count of the previous newborn if the mother's ITP and prior treatment were similar.

A platelet count in the infant at delivery and repeated daily (the platelet count usually decreases after birth) will indicate whether and how severely the infant is affected. Bleeding manifestations are restricted to those infants with low platelet counts. All thrombocytopenic infants should have immediate cranial ultrasonography or CT scan to determine CNS bleeding since ICH can be clinically "silent." The count will achieve normal levels over 1 to 12 weeks. If an ICH is found, treatment should include platelet transfusion (10 ml/kg), IVIG 1 gm/kg/day, and IV methylprednisolone 1 to 2 mg/8h. If the platelets are <20–30,000/μL but there is no serious hemorrhage, treatment may include IVIG with or without steroids.

ASSOCIATION WITH AUTOIMMUNE DISORDERS

Autoimmune hemolytic anemia and ITP may occur together (Evan's syndrome), often with neutropenia, with or without manifestations of an underlying disease such as SLE. Autoimmune thyroid disease may occur in patients with ITP.

ASSOCIATION WITH HIV INFECTION

Individuals infected with HIV may have an immunologic thrombocytopenia that is similar to classical ITP. The thrombocytopenia (HIV-TP) appears to be a combination of HIV infection of megakaryocytes, which decreases platelet production, and antibody (or immune complex)-mediated accelerated platelet destruction. Indications for treatment are similar to those of ITP. Significant thrombocytopenia in HIV-ITP patients may occur "early" in the course of the infection when the viral load is low and the CD4 count high; it is probably best treated with antiretroviral treatment. For platelet-specific treatment, IV anti-D is superior to IVIG for bleeding episodes and for maintenance of the platelet count in patients not given or not responsive to antiviral treatment. Splenectomy is an option for chronic symptomatic thrombocytopenia; prednisone should generally be avoided except for low doses and/or short duration. Management of the end-stage patient with pancytopenia rather than isolated thrombocytopenia is difficult and may require platelet transfusions.

DRUG-INDUCED IMMUNE THROMBOCYTOPENIA

A clinical syndrome resembling ITP can occur in susceptible individuals after ingestion of certain drugs. The offending drug (quinidine, quinine, sulfonamides, valproic acid, heparin, chlorothiazide) binds to antidrug IgG on the platelet surface resulting in platelet destruction or activation and aggregation (Fig. 9-1). One of the most common drugs to cause immune-mediated thrombocytopenia is heparin. (see Chap. 45).

ALLOIMMUNE THROMBOCYTOPENIA

Neonatal and fetal alloimmune thrombocytopenia (AIT) is the platelet equivalent of Rh hemolytic disease of the newborn. Alloantibodies are produced by the mother to specific fetal platelet antigens (lacking in the mother, but present in the fetus and the father). The most commonly involved antigen resulting in serious disease in Caucasians is PL^{A1} (Zw(a), HPA-1a). HLA antigens are probably not a cause of AIT; HLA DR52a is required for anti-PI^{A1} antibody production. The incidence of AIT has been recently reported as 1/1000 deliveries.

The diagnosis of AIT is usually first suspected in a newborn infant with multiple petechiae, skin bleeding, or ICH in 10 to 20 percent of cases. Usually a baby with AIT will be term, may be firstborn, and often does

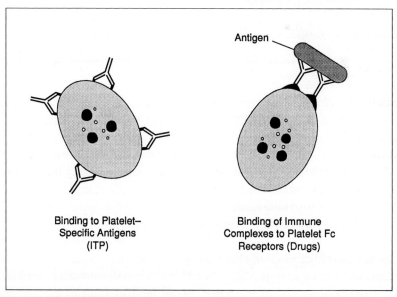

Antigen

Binding to Platelet–
Specific Antigens
(ITP)

Binding of Immune
Complexes to Platelet Fc
Receptors (Drugs)

FIGURE 9-1 Mechanisms for immune thrombocytopenia in ITP and by drugs. IgG molecules are depicted binding to platelet-specific antigens (GP IIb-IIIa, GP Ib-IX) through the Fab segment in ITP. Also depicted are binding of immune complexes (drugs + antibody; viruses + antibody) to platelet Fc receptors through the IgG Fc segment. Both mechanisms lead to clearance of the platelet by the reticuloendothelial system. (Used with permission from Kelton JG: *Hosp Pract* June: 95, 1985.)

TABLE 9-2

Differential Diagnosis of Antibody-Induced Thrombocytopenia in the Newborn Infant: Alloimmune versus Autoimmune

Similarities

1) Unexplained neonatal thrombocytopenia—baby otherwise well;
2) Severe thrombocytopenia (often <50,000/μL within 24 hours of birth);
3) Possibly family history of transient neonatal thrombocytopenia in previous sibling
4) Platelets may fall further after birth
5) Response of platelets to IVIG treatment
6) Significant risk of ICH in severe thrombocytopenia

Mother

■ ITP: moderate or severe thrombocytopenia *or* treatment or s/p splenectomy
■ <15% of all mothers with ITP have neonates with platelet counts <50,000/μL
■ Alloimmune: mother's platelets normal (gestational thrombocytopenia can be confusing—mild thrombocytopenia with no history of ITP or bleeding)

Antibody Studies

■ ITP: mother will have platelet-associated glycoprotein specific antibodies (PAIgG positive in many women without ITP); serum antibody is variable
■ Alloimmune: mother will have strong serum antibody specific to a platelet antigen, i.e., PI^{A1}. Platelet antigen typing will reveal parental incompatibility of the antigen in question, i.e., mother will be PI^{A1} negative and father will be PI^{A1} positive

Response to Platelet Transfusion

■ Both ITP and alloimmune: often transient response to random platelet transfusion
■ Alloimmune: normal response to antigen-negative platelets (concentrated maternal or other)

---

not have obvious causes of thrombocytopenia; the most characteristic finding is a platelet count <50,000/μL within the first 24 hours of life. A clinical diagnosis of AIT should be confirmed by serologic evaluation (see following). An adjunct to clinical diagnosis is the response to platelet transfusions if given. As in autoimmune thrombocytopenia, there may be an excellent response to random donor platelets, but it will be short lived (<24 hours); a normal life span of maternal platelets supports the diagnosis of AIT. The differential diagnosis of AIT versus an infant of a mother with ITP is detailed in Table 9-2. The coincidental association of AIT with maternal thrombocytopenia (i.e., GTP), has been reported.

Optimal serologic evaluation should include determination of platelet alloantigen phenotype of the parents and measurement of platelet antibody in the mother. If maternal serum antiplatelet antibody is detected, confirmation of AIT requires that the antibody be specific for the platelet antigen involved. This evaluation must be performed in an experienced reference laboratory.

Management of the Subsequent Pregnancy in the Family

Since prenatal screening of pregnancies for AIT is not routine, management of fetal AIT is usually in the context of the next pregnancy following the birth of a thrombocytopenic newborn. Because intracranial hemorrhage may occur antenatally in up to 10 percent of cases, considerations of fetal diagnosis in pregnant women, especially those with a previously severely affected child and a homozygous father, will usually require fetal blood sampling at 20 to 24 weeks of gestation to determine the platelet count. Fifty percent of $PI^{A1}+$ fetuses will have a fetal platelet count $\leq20,000/\mu L$ at initial sampling; those with higher counts will have increasing thrombocytopenia without intervention. Intervention includes weekly IVIG and/or prednisone administered to the mother, and *in utero* platelet transfusion at the time of fetal blood sampling to prevent procedure-related hemorrhage. With this approach, >60 to 80 percent of fetal platelet counts will increase; ICH has not been seen in patients whose previous sibling did not have an early hemorrhage in utero.

Post-transfusion Purpura

Another platelet alloimmunization syndrome is the rare disorder called post-transfusion purpura, which presents as severe thrombocytopenic bleeding about 1 week after exposure to a blood product. The incidence of this syndrome may have decreased as a result of leukoreduction of an increasing percentage of blood products. The patient, frequently an elderly woman with a history of pregnancy, becomes sensitized to a platelet alloantigen (usually PL^{A1}) that is lacking on her platelets. The exact mechanism of thrombocytopenia continues to be obscure. The thrombocytopenia is typically very severe and bleeding may be life-threatening. The thrombocytopenia typically persists for days to weeks. The recommended treatment is IVIG and corticosteroids or plasmapheresis. Platelet concentrate transfusions are contraindicated except under extreme circumstances when PL^{A1}-negative platelets should be used.

BIBLIOGRAPHY

Aster RH: Drug-induced immune thrombocytopenia: an overview of pathogenesis. *Semin Hematol* 36:2, 1999.

Beardsley DS, Ertem M: Platelet autoantibodies in immune thrombocytopenic purpura. *Transfus Sci* 19:237, 1998.

Burrows RF, Kelton JG: Incidentally detected thrombocytopenia in healthy mothers and their infants. *N Engl J Med* 319:142, 1988.

Bussel J, Kaplan C: The fetal and neonatal consequences of maternal alloimmune thrombocytopenia. *Baillieres Clin Haematol* 11:391, 1998.

George JN et al: Idiopathic thrombocytopenic purpura: a practice guideline developed by explicit methods for the American Society of Hematology. *Blood* 88:3, 1996.

George JN, Raskob GE: Idiopathic thrombocytopenic purpura: diagnosis and management. *Am J Med Sci* 16:87, 1998.

Lippman SM et al: Genetic factors predisposing to autoimmune diseases. Autoimmune hemolytic anemia, chronic thrombocytopenic purpura, and systemic lupus erythematosus. *Am J Med* 73:827, 1982.

Lucas GF et al: Post-transfusion purpura (PTP) associated with anti-HPA-1a, anti-HPA-2b and anti-HPA-3a antibodies. *Transfus Med* 7:295, 1997.

Kuhne T et al: Current management issues of childhood and adult immune thrombocytopenic purpura (ITP). *Acta Paediatr Suppl* 424:75, 1998.

McCrae KR et al: Pregnancy associated thrombocytopenia: Pathogenesis and management. *Blood* 80:2697, 1992.

McMillan R: Therapy for adults with refractory chronic immune thrombocytopenic purpura. *Ann Intern Med* 126:307, 1997.

Majlufcruz A et al: Usefulness of a low-dose intravenous immunoglobulin regimen for the treatment of thrombocytopenia associated with AIDS. *Am J Hematol* 59:127, 1998.

Nugent DJ: Immune thrombocytopenic purpura: why treat? *J Pediatr* 134:3, 1999.

Pietz J et al: High-dose intravenous gamma globulin for neonatal alloimmune thrombocytopenia in twins. *Acta Pediatr Scand* 80:129, 1991.

Rand ML, Wright JF: Virus-associated idiopathic thrombocytopenic purpura. *Transfus Sci* 19:253, 1998.

Saxon BR et al: Reticulated platelet counts in the diagnosis of acute immune thrombocytopenic purpura. *J Pediatr Hemat Oncol* 20:44, 1998.

Schreiber AD et al: Effect of danazol in immune thrombocytopenic purpura. *N Engl J Med* 316:503, 1987.

Winiarski J: Measurement of platelet antibodies: where do we stand? *Acta Paediatr Suppl* 424:51, 1998.

Wang WC: Evans syndrome in childhood: Pathophysiology, clinical course, and treatment. *Am J Pediatr Hematol Oncol* 10:330, 1988.

CHAPTER 10

Hereditary Platelet Function Defects

A review of the multifunctional role of platelets in primary and secondary hemostasis (Fig. 10-1, Chap. 1), makes it clear that there are many opportunities for hereditary disorders that will result in abnormal platelet plug formation and prolonged bleeding. The nomenclature for classifying specific platelet abnormalities is based on the physiologic defect; namely, (1) adhesion (e.g., Bernard-Soulier syndrome [BSS]), (2) aggregation (e.g., Glanzmann's thrombasthenia), (3) secretion (e.g., storage pool disorders), and (4) disorders of the platelet procoagulant surface (e.g., Scott syndrome) (see Table 10-1). In contrast to von Willebrand disease, hereditary platelet function defects (PFDs) are relatively rare, with platelet secretion disorders being the most common. Platelet secretion disorders include signal-processing defects and storage pool deficiency syndromes due to decreased or absent dense bodies, α-granules, or both; functional defects in secretion or release can also be due to specific abnormalities in the prostaglandin pathway (cyclooxygenase deficiency, thromboxane synthetase deficiency). A few of these genetic defects have been characterized and are associated with specific disorders of platelet function (Table 10-2).

CLINICAL MANIFESTATIONS

Patients with hereditary platelet function defects (PFDs) display hemorrhagic patterns much like thrombocytopenic bleeding; i.e., skin and mucous membrane bleeding (petechiae, ecchymoses), recurrent epistaxis, gastrointestinal hemorrhage, menorrhagia, and immediate-type bleeding after trauma and surgical procedures. Intracranial bleeding is rare. Neonatal purpura may occur, but joint and muscle bleeding is dis-

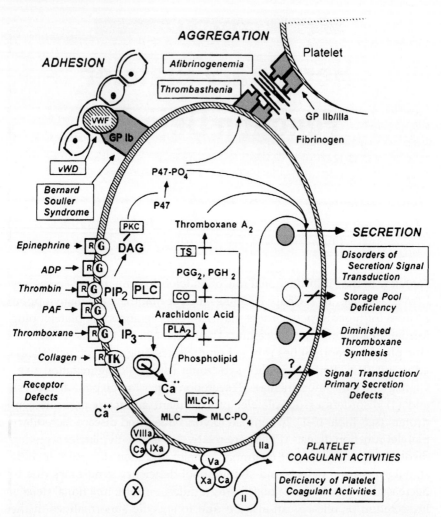

FIGURE 10-1 Schematic representation of normal platelet responses and the congenital disorders of platelet function. Some of the platelet-mediated coagulation protein interactions are also shown. Coagulation proteins are shown by Roman numerals, with the activated forms designated by the letter a. The arrows designate conversions of zymogens to enzymes. CO, cyclooxygenase; DAG, diacylglycerol; G, GTP-binding protein; IP_3, inositol triphosphate; MLC, myosin light chain; MLCK, myosin light-chain kinase; PIP_2, phosphatidylinositol biphosphate; PKC, protein kinase C; PLC, phospholipase C; PLA_2, phospholipase A_2; R, receptor; TK, tyrosine kinase; and TS, thromboxane synthase. (Used with permission from Rao AK and Gabbeta J: Congenital disorders of platelet signal transduction. *Arterioscler Thromb Vasc Biol* 20:285, 2000.)

tinctly uncommon. Bleeding manifestations may be severe or mild depending on the defect. Although exceptions are known, the more severe the specific defect, the worse the bleeding tendency; i.e., severe bleeders with thrombasthenia (type I) have <10 percent platelet glyco-

Hereditary Platelet Function Disorders

	Heredity	Platelet Count	Platelet Size	Platelet Aggregation				
				L-epi	ADP	Collagen	Ristocetin	AA
Abnormalities of Adhesion								
Pseudo VWD	AD	D	N	+	+	+	Increased	+
Bernard-Soulier	AR	D	L	+	+	+	−	+
Abnormalities of primary aggregation								
Glanzmann's Thrombasthenia	AR	N	N	−	−	−	+	−
Abnormalities of secondary aggregation								
Storage Pool Defects								
Dense body deficiency	AR	N	N	−	±	−	±	±
α-granule deficiency (gray platelet syndrome)	AR	D	L	+	±	±	+	+
Mixed α and dense body deficiency	AD			±	±	−	±	±
Factor V Quebec	AD	D	N	−	+	+	+	+
Secretion Defects	Variable	N	N	−	±	−	±	−
Disorder of procoagulation surface								
Scott Syndrome	AR	N	N	+	+	+	+	+

D, decreased; N, normal; L, large; L-epi, L-epinephrine; AA, arachidonic acid; −, absent or decreased; +, present, normal; ±, variable, slight increase; AD, autosomal dominant; AR, autosomal recessive; ADP, adenosine diphosphate; PF, platelet factor; GP, glycoprotein.

TABLE 10-2	
Platelet Secretion Defects	
Storage pool defects:	
a. Dense body deficiency	Decreased thrombin release of ADP and serotonin; decreased dense bodies
b. Gray platelet syndrome	Decreased α-granules and contents, may be associated with myeloproliferative disorders
c. Factor V Quebec	Severe multimerin deficiency; protease degredation of the α-granules
d. Mixed α-granule dense-body deficiency	Decreased α-granules and dense bodies
Signal Processing Defects (failure to release)	Cyclooxygenase deficiency
	Thromboxane synthetase deficiency
	Impaired release of arachidonic acid
	Defects in phosphotidylinositol metabolism
	Defects in calcium mobilization
	Defects in G protein activation
	Impaired response to thromboxane A_2
	Platelet prostaglandin H synthase-1 deficiency
	Defect in phospholipase C activation

protein (GP) IIb/IIIa (integrin $\alpha_{IIb}\beta_3$), whereas type II patients (about 30 percent GP IIb/IIIa) are less severely affected. A similar relationship is observed in BSS in respect to Gp Ib-V-IX complex. A moderately severe bleeding tendency is observed in the Hermansky-Pudlak syndrome (oculocutaneous albinism in association with dense-body deficiency in the platelets). The secretion defect category (storage pool defects and signal-processing defects) have only mild bleeding tendencies.

LABORATORY MANIFESTATIONS

The major laboratory indicator of a PFD is a prolonged bleeding time or other abnormal test of primary hemostasis (the PFA-100 may be abnormal in secretion defects) despite a normal platelet count in patients in whom von Willebrand disease has been excluded. Mild to moderate thrombocytopenia is common in BSS and in the other hereditary thrombocytopenias that may also have associated PFDs (see Chap. 8). Others have characteristically large platelets. Bleeding times may be normal or slightly prolonged in some mild disorders but usually become greatly prolonged after aspirin usage.

Since the mid 1960s, platelet aggregation testing has been the mainstay of the procedures used to diagnose and classify the hereditary PFDs. With careful attention to technical details, the aggregation curves produced by various agonists (L-epinephrine, adenosine diphosphate [ADP], collagen, ristocetin, and arachidonic acid) provide a sensitive method of detection of most disorders. The pattern of the abnormalities in the aggregation curves can be used to tentatively classify the PFD (see Fig. 10-2). More detailed or confirmatory procedures are necessary to identify the specific defect (see Table 10-3).

CLINICAL DISORDERS

Glanzmann's Thrombasthenia

The hallmark of thrombasthenia is abnormal platelet aggregation in response to all agonists (except ristocetin) (Fig. 10-2). Both von Wille-

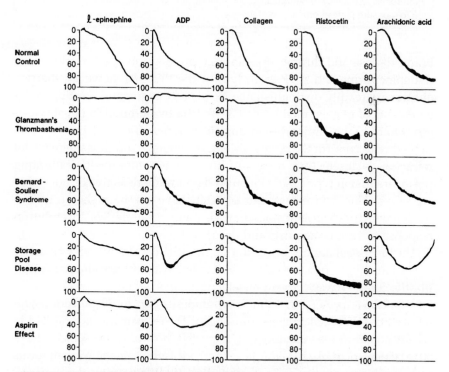

FIGURE 10-2 Platelet aggregation curves for various agonists. Platelet-rich plasma from a normal adult and patients with designated platelet function disorders are shown.

TABLE 10-3

Laboratory Tests Used for Evaluation of Platelet Function

Preliminary Tests

Platelet count and peripheral blood smear (platelet size)

Bleeding time or platelet function analyzer

Platelet aggregation tests (Fig. 10-2)

Clot retraction

Confirmatory Tests

Flow cytometry or Western blotting
    (Glycoprotein Ib-V-IX, IIb-IIIa, annexin V determination)

Electron microscopy (EM) or Immuno-EM
    (Granule morphology and content, cytoskeleton)

Platelet release assays

Thromboxane synthetase, cyclooxygenase determinations

Platelet aggregation tests with ristocetin
    (Distinguishing platelet-type WWD from type IIB VWD)

Prothrombinase assay (prothrombin consumption)
    (To measure platelet procoagulant activity)

---

brand disease and thrombasthenia may prolong the aperture closure of the epinephrine and ADP cartridges of the PFA-100, however, the two entities are readily distinguishable by platelet aggregation testing. Measurements of platelet membrane GP IIb/IIIa by immunochemical (Western blotting) or antibody-binding techniques (flow cytometry) are necessary to confirm the diagnosis of Glanzmann's thrombasthenia. Clot retraction is absent (due to loss of binding receptors for the radi-ating fibrin strands) in type I patients but is only mildly defective or normal in type II patients. Thrombasthenic platelets have also been shown to produce fewer procoagulant microparticles and generate less thrombin in response to various agonists and tissue factor, respectively.

The functional importance of the GP IIb/IIIa receptor is underscored by the fact that type I patients have absent to barely detectable amounts of GP IIb/IIIa complexes and absent platelet fibrinogen, while in type II patients, GP IIb/IIIa is present in subnormal amounts (up to 30 percent), with reduced but detectable platelet fibrinogen. Thrombasthenia is inherited in an autosomal recessive manner; as expected, heterozygous subjects have 50 to 60 percent of IIb/IIIa complexes and are asymptomatic. Variant forms exist in which a qualitative, not quantative, IIb/IIIa receptor defect exists. Deletion and inversions of either the IIb or IIIa gene is population specific.

The laboratory heterogeneity of homozygous disease is illustrated by studies of Iraqi Jews and Arab patients who both have severe disease and marked IIb/IIIa complex deficiency, but can be differentiated by platelet vitronectin receptor expression (normal in the Arab population).

Bernard-Soulier Syndrome

Bernard-Soulier syndrome is an autosomal recessively inherited bleeding disorder characterized by mild thrombocytopenia, giant platelets as visualized on peripheral blood smear, and a defect or deficiency of the platelet GP Ib-V-IX complex. The physiologic defect is exemplified by reduced platelet adhesion to subendothelium via decreased binding of von Willebrand factor. Platelet aggregation is normal except for absent platelet agglutination induced by ristocetin. Dysfunctional variants of BSS, including reduced amounts of sialic acid in the GP Ib-V-IX receptor, have been described. Heterozygotes show intermediate levels of GP Ib-V-IX and some large platelets on the blood smear, but are asymptomatic. Recent studies show that GP V (cleaved by thrombin) is not necessary for GP Ib expression and that GP V deficient platelets are not likely to cause a BSS phenotype.

Storage Pool Defects

Storage pool defects are classified by the type of granular deficiency or secretion defect (see Table 10-2). The study of storage pool organelles by electron microscopy and measurement of platelet nucleotides and serotonin (dense granules) or β-thromboglobulin and platelet factor 4 (α-granules) and their releasability allows confirmation and classification of the storage pool defects. Dense-body storage pool defects have been described in inherited disorders such as Hermansky-Pudlak syndrome, Wiscott-Aldrich syndrome, Chediak-Higashi syndrome, and thrombocytopenia with absent radii (TAR) syndrome. In a few instances storage pool defects have been associated with decreased nucleotide (ADP, ATP) storage or release without producing abnormal platelet aggregation curves.

Other Platelet Function Disorders

Platelet aggregation tests may provide leads to diagnosis of other PFD. A familial impaired aggregation only to L-epinephrine has been associated with decreased α_2-adrenergic receptors (easy bruising and minimally prolonged bleeding time). Isolated impairment in responsiveness to epinephrine can be an inherited defect but is usually associated with few bleeding manifestations. An isolated receptor defect to collagen was associated with abnormal aggregation to collagen but normal responses to

ADP, thrombin, and other agonists; the patient with this defect was a bleeder and had decreased concentrations of platelet GP Ia. Similarly, a congenital PFD was characterized by impairment of platelet responses to ADP that resulted in abnormalities of aggregation like the secretion defect; the defect was due to decreased numbers of ADP receptors.

A platelet secretion defect (normal platelet aggregation to the usual agonists but impaired to thrombin and A23187, a calcium ionophore) has been described in patients with an attention deficit disorder and easy bruising. Since there are many acquired causes of abnormal platelet aggregation in normal individuals (e.g., drugs, infections; see Chap. 11), a final diagnosis of a specific PFD should be reserved until repeat aggregation testing and confirmatory tests can be obtained.

Platelet aggregation tests are abnormal in Scott syndrome, a disorder of platelet coagulant activity. The platelets of these patients have a reduced ability to promote factor X and prothrombin activation that is due to a decreased platelet surface exposure of phosphatidylserine (PS) plus a reduced shedding of microvesicles. The prothrombin consumption test is the only abnormal test.

MANAGEMENT

Acute bleeding episodes in hereditary PFD can usually be managed with DDAVP infusions in all of the defects except thrombasthenia, Scott syndrome, and an occasional severe form of BSS. Recombinant FVIIa has been used successfully in Glanzmann's thrombasthenia patients for surgery and for treatment of epistaxis. For these more severe disorders, platelet concentrate transfusions can be used if local measures do not secure hemostasis. In a few instances, thrombasthenic patients have developed antibodies against the alloantigens that occur on the $\alpha_{IIb}\beta_3$ integrin following transfusion. Alloimmunization against HLA or platelet-specific antigens (e.g., PLA-1) also occurs and may be decreased by use of platelet compatable donors when feasible. Adjunctive therapy with ε-aminocaproic acid is worth trying in mucous membrane bleeding.

BIBLIOGRAPHY

Cattaneo M, Gachet C: ADP receptors and clinical bleeding disorders. *Arterioscler Thromb Vasc Biol* 19:2281, 1999.

Coller BS et al: Glanzmann thrombasthenia: new insights from an historical perspective. *Semin Hematol* 31:301, 1994.

Dachary-Prignet J et al: Aminophospholipid exposure, microvesiculation and abnormal protein tyrosine phosphorylation in the platelets of a patient with Scott syndrome: a study using physiologic agonists and local anaesthetics. *Br J Haematol* 99:959, 1997.

Hardisty R et al: A defect of platelet aggregation associated with an abnormal distribution of glycoprotein IIb-IIIa complexed within the platelet: The cause of a life-long bleeding disorder. *Blood* 80:696, 1992.

Harrison P et al: Performance of the platelet function analyser PFA-100 in testing abnormalities of primary haemostasis. *Blood Coagul Fibrinolysis* 10:25, 1999.

Hayward CP et al: An autosomal dominent, qualitative platelet disorder associated with multimerin deficiency, abnormalities in platelet factor V, thrombospondin, von Willebrand factor, and fibrinogen and an epinephrine aggregation defect. *Blood* 87:4967, 1996.

Kahn ML et al: Glycoprotein V-deficient platelets have undiminished thrombin responsiveness and do not exhibit a Bernard-Soulier phenotype. *Blood* 94:4112, 1999.

Lopez JA et al: Bernard-Soulier syndrome. *Blood* 91:4397, 1998.

Matijevic-Aleksic N et al: Bleeding disorder due to platelet prostaglandin H synthase-1 (PGHS-1) deficiency. *Br J Haematol* 92:212, 1996.

Miller JL: Platelet-type von Willebrand disease. *Thromb Haemost* 75:865, 1996.

Nurden AT: Inherited abnormalities of platelets. *Thromb Haemost* 82:468, 1999.

Poon MC: Recombinant factor VIIa is effective for bleeding and surgery in patients with Glanzmann thrombasthenia. *Blood* 94:3951, 1999.

Rao AK, Gabbeta J: Congenital disorders of platelet signal transduction. *Arterioscler Thromb Vasc Biol* 20:285, 2000.

Rao AK et al: Differential requirements for platelet aggregation and inhibition of adenylate cyclase by epinephrine. Studies of a familial platelet alpha 2-adrenergic receptor defect. *Blood* 71:494, 1988.

Rao AK et al: Mechanisms of platelet dysfunction and response to DDAVP in patients with congenital platelet function defects. A double-blind placebo-controlled trial. *Thromb Haemost* 74:1071, 1995.

Sims PJ et al: Assembly of the platelet prothrombinase complex is linked to vesiculation of the platelet plasma membrane. Studies in Scott syndrome: An isolated defect in platelet procoagulant activity. *J Biol Chem* 264:17049, 1989.

Solum NO: Procoagulant expression in platelets and defects leading to clinical disorders. *Arterioscler Thromb Vasc Biol* 19:2841, 1999.

Weiss HJ et al: Heterogeneous abnormalities of platelet dense granule ultrastructure in 20 patients with congenital storage pool deficiency. *Br J Haematol* 83:282, 1993.

White JG: Use of the electron microscope for diagnosis of platelet disorders. *Semin Thromb Hemost* 24:163, 1998.

CHAPTER 11

Acquired Platelet Function Disorders

Acquired abnormalities in platelets, blood vessels, the plasma milieu, and blood flow may produce deranged platelet-vessel interactions and defective platelet plug formation resulting in prolonged bleeding and/or excessive platelet consumption with microthrombosis. The platelet function disorders (PFD) that are primarily associated with a hemorrhagic tendency are discussed here and are listed in Table 11-1.

In general, an apparent underlying disease or a drug is responsible for the acquired abnormality of platelet function. Patients may be asymptomatic or have characteristic platelet-type bleeding (mucosal, petechiae, or postoperative). The bleeding time is variable with the exception of aspirin effects (see below). New platelet function analyzers that examine platelet function under flow conditions are increasingly being used as an alternative to the bleeding time. These tests may have greater sensitivity to drug effects on platelets.

DRUG-INDUCED PLATELET DYSFUNCTION

The major classes of drugs associated with abnormal platelet function are anti-inflammatory agents, antibiotics, cardiovascular drugs, psychotropic drugs, and anticoagulants (Table 11-2). The cyclooxygenase inhibitors, of which ASA is the major example, interfere with the formation of thromboxane A_2 (a potent aggregator of platelets and vasoconstrictor) in the prostaglandin pathway of the platelet (Chap. 1) and inhibit the release reaction induced by ADP and collagen. Aspirin acts by irreversibly acetylating a serine residue at the active site of cyclooxygenase.

TABLE 11-1
Acquired Platelet Function Disorders* by Proposed Mechanism or Cause

Drug induced
Uremia
Liver disease
Exhausted platelets (storage pool deficiency platelets)
Activated platelets
   Coronary artery disease
   Peripheral vascular disease
   Stroke
Abnormal proteins and antibodies (IgG, IgM)
   Autoimmune disorders (ITP, SLE, connective tissue disorders)
   Multiple myeloma, Waldenstrom's macroglobulinemia
   Dyproteinemias
   Acquired dysfunction with eosinophilia
Hematologic
   Myeloproliferative/myelodysplastic disorders
   Leukemia
   Thalassemmias
Infection
   Infectious mononucleosis
   HIV
   Septicemia
DIC
Other
   Deficiency states (B_{12}, vitamin E, zinc)
   Agammaglobulinemia
   Glycogen storage diseases

* Defined as conditions with abnormal platelet aggregations (usually with prolonged bleeding time and/or clinical bleeding).
DIC, disseminated intravascular coagulation; HIV, human immunodeficiency virus; ITP, immune thrombocytopenic purpura; SLE, systemic lupus erythematosus.

In contrast, other nonsteroidal anti-inflammatory drugs are reversible inhibitors of the enzyme.

Aspirin prolongs the bleeding time in normal subjects by a mean of 4 min, but has a much greater effect in subjects who already have a bleeding tendency such as von Willebrand disease, PFD, or a coagulation disorder such as hemophilia. The effect on the bleeding time in normal subjects of as little as 1 to 2 mg/kg of ASA is noted 2 h after oral ingestion and lasts for 2 to 4 days (bleeding time prolongation) or up to 10 days for platelet aggregation tests. A few subjects are "hyperresponders," with a prolonged bleeding time up to 11 min and showing an increased bleeding tendency. The duration of effect is much less with the reversible inhibitors (6 to 24 h). In contrast, the β-lactam antibiotics are dose dependent in vivo and require high and sustained doses (up to 48 h) to achieve maximal effect on bleeding time and platelet aggregation, which can also

---

TABLE 11-2

Pharmacologic and Other Substances Affecting Platelet Function (Abnormal Platelet Aggregation, Increased Bleeding Time, and/or Clinical Bleeding)

Agent	Mechanism	Result
Acetylsalicylic acid (aspirin)	Cyclooxygenase inhibitor	Bleeding time prolonged, clinical bleeding
Nonsteroid anti-inflammatory agents: (Ibuprofen, indomethacin, Naproxen, Diclofenac)	Prostaglandin synthesis inhibition	Bleeding time prolonged, clinical bleeding uncommon
IIb-IIIa Inhibitors Abciximab integrilin tirofiban	Blocks fibrinogen receptor	Bleeding time prolonged, clinical bleeding
β-Lactam antibiotics: (penicillin G, ampicillin, nafcillin, carbenicillin, ticarcillin, cephalosporins)	Platelet membrane binding; alteration of agonist receptors	Bleeding time prolonged, clinical bleeding
Cardiovascular Verapamil, Nifedipine, Quinidine	Calcium channel blockers Antagonist to a adrenergic receptor	Decreased aggregation with epinephrine, bleeding time prolonged
Psychotropic amytriptyline, nortriptyline, imipramine		Decreased aggregation with ADP, no clinical bleeding
Hemostatics, antithrombotics: (ε-aminocaproic acid, dextran, ticlopidine)	Membrane binding Decreased GP IIb-IIIa receptor function	Clinical bleeding, increased bleeding time
Others: (Halothane, propranolol, nitroglycerin, quinidine, ethanol, sodium valproate)		Increased bleeding time

Epi, epinephrine; ADP, adenosine diphosphate

last 7 to 10 days. Clinical bleeding (easy bruising, epistaxis, hematomas, postsurgical hemorrhage) is seen most often in patients with underlying bleeding disorders who are given these major drugs (ASA, anti-inflammatory agents, antibiotics, anticoagulants), but an occasional "hyperresponder" (with no known underlying defect) will display clinical bleeding.

Many drugs, such as antihistamines, local anesthetics, beta-blockers, and antihypertensive agents, may have an effect on in vitro platelet aggregation tests without significant effects on the bleeding time. The platelet function analyzer (e.g., PFA-100 ®) may have an abnormal closure time with the epinephrine/collagen card (uncommonly with the ADP collagen card) in patients taking many of the medications outlined in Table 11-2. Of the commonly used drugs such as glyceryl guaiacolate, diphenhydramine, chlorpromazine, pseudoephedrine, and acetaminophen, only indomethacin and aspirin have an effect on bleeding time after oral administration. Nevertheless, when diagnostic platelet function tests are performed, the subject should be off all medications (including over-the-counter drugs such as Alka Seltzer™, which contains aspirin) and free of recent viral infections for at least 7 to 10 days (viral infections like Epstein-Barr virus may have a longer effect on platelet function).

UREMIA

A prolonged bleeding time and a tendency to clinical bleeding are frequently noted in chronic renal failure patients with uremia. Although the bleeding time prolongation correlates with the severity of renal failure, the bleeding time is a poor predictor of hemorrhage. Patients with severe anemia of chronic renal failure frequently show a prolonged bleeding time, which improves on correction of the anemia. The PFA-100 is sensitive to anemia and often corrects or improves with modest increases in the hematocrit. Platelet aggregation defects are variably present and persist in patients who are no longer anemic. The cause of the platelet dysfunction is probably multifactorial; possible mechanisms are noted in Chapter 27. Improvement in platelet function after dialysis suggests removal of a "toxic" material (such as guanidinosuccinic acid). The clinical significance of the platelet function deficit is unclear; invasive procedures (e.g., renal biopsies) are usually not associated with excess bleeding.

EXHAUSTED PLATELETS

In many PFD, disturbed platelet–vessel interactions occur, causing platelet activation, perturbation of membrane, and release of storage pool material, and frequently loss of the platelet from the circulation. These disorders, which are a form of acquired storage pool deficiency, are sometimes associated with evidence for changes in soluble clotting factors (fibrinogen, von Willebrand factor) and may result in prolonged bleeding time and abnormal platelet aggregation tests. Common examples include hairy cell leukemia, valvular heart disease (congenital and acquired), vascular malformations, foreign-surface interactions (cardiopulmonary bypass), abnormal small vessels (renal diseases), and small vessel thrombosis (hemolytic uremic syndrome, thrombotic thrombocytopenic purpura).

Evidence for activated platelets in various clinical syndromes has been provided by three general methods. The first is platelet aggregation studies using subthreshold doses of agonists to detect activated platelets in hypercoagulable vascular disorders (increased platelet aggregation) or standard dose agonists to detect exhausted platelets (decreased platelet aggregation of the storage pool deficit pattern). The second is measurement of plasma levels of substances such as β-thromboglobulin, platelet factor 4 (PF4), thromboxane B_2, or thrombospondin to indirectly indicate platelet activation and release. Typically, following in vivo activation, there is a substantial increase in plasma β-thromboglobulin with a small increase in plasma PF4 resulting in an increased β-thromboglobulin/PF4 ratio. The final method is detection of activation-induced platelet-surface changes (expression of P-selectin, thrombospondin, factor Va) or platelet microparticles in a flow cytometry system.

LIVER DISEASE

Patients with liver disease may have bleeding complications for a variety of reasons including qualitative platelet defects (reviewed in Chap. 23). Platelet functional defects are often related to the severity of the liver disease.

ABNORMAL PROTEIN BINDING AND ANTIBODIES

Other acquired abnormalities are due to abnormal proteins binding to the platelets (IgM or IgG antibodies, myeloma proteins, Waldenstrom's macroglobulins, fibrin degradation products [FDP]). Specific functional abnormalities produced by these proteins can involve membrane GP receptors such as GP Ib-V-IX or GP IIb-IIIa, reminiscent of hereditary defects (Bernard-Soulier syndrome, Glanzmann's thrombasthenia). For example, a few patients have developed autoantibodies to GP IIIa that block binding of fibrinogen to the IIb/IIIa complex, but without causing thrombocytopenia. This acquired form of thrombasthenia is associated with severe bleeding (McMillan ref). Abnormalities of platelet function occur in infections (viral and bacterial), systemic lupus erythematosus, and hemophilia, and may be related to direct platelet damage or platelet interaction with IgG or antigen–antibody complexes.

OTHER SYSTEMIC DISORDERS

Glycogen storage diseases types Ia and Ib are associated with a mild bleeding tendency (epistaxis, mucosal bleeding) and abnormal platelet function (increased bleeding time and decreased aggregation to collagen and adenosine diphosphate; low von Willebrand factor in some patients). The defect is acquired since effective therapy with hyperalimentation or portacaval shunt results in correction of the platelet dysfunction.

The bleeding in the myeloproliferative and myelodysplastic disorders can be associated with hypoaggregability and a prolonged bleeding time (see Chap. 33). Qualitative platelet abnormalities include abnormal morphology, acquired storage pool defects, platelet glycoprotein abnormalities, receptor defects (α-adrenergic, Fc, prostaglandin D_2 receptors), and abnormal arachidonic acid metabolism.

MANAGEMENT

The management of the bleeding diathesis associated with acquired PFD is generally related to treatment of the underlying disorder. In most instances the bleeding disorder is mild and rarely requires specific treatment or prophylaxis with platelet transfusions or DDAVP. Removal of the offending drug is usually all that is necessary in drug-related PFD. Recombinant erythropoietin or red cell transfusions frequently correct the anemia and the coexisting bleeding-time defect in uremia (see Chap. 27). Additional treatment modalities used in uremia (usually to decrease the bleeding time) are dialysis, DDAVP, recombinant VIIa, or conjugated estrogens. DDAVP infusions have been used to correct the bleeding time or bleeding tendency in glycogen storage disease and myeloproliferative disorders.

BIBLIOGRAPHY

Abrams C, Shattil SJ: Immunologic detection of activated platelets in clinical disorders. *Thromb Haemost* 65:467, 1991.

Escolar G et al: Evaluation of acquired platelet dysfunctions in uremic and cirrhotic patients using the platelet function analyzer (PFA-100): influence of hematocrit elevation. *Haematologica* 84: 614, 1999.

Fiore LD et al: The bleeding time response to aspirin. *Am J Clin Pathol* 94:292, 1990.

George JN, Shattil SJ: The clinical importance of acquired abnormalities of platelet function. *N Engl J Med* 324:27, 1991.

Harrison P et al: Performance of the platelet function analyser PFA-100 in testing abnormalities of primary haemostasis. *Blood Coag Fibrinol* 10:25, 1999.

Hedner U et al: Clinical experience with recombinant factor VIIa. *Blood Coag Fibrinol* 9:119, 1998.

Mammen EF et al: PFA-100 system: a new method for assessment of platelet dysfunction. *Semin Thromb Hemost* 24: 195, 1998.

Mannucci PM: Desmopressin (DDAVP) in the treatment of bleeding disorders: the first 20 years. *Blood* 90: 2515, 1997.

Mannucci PM: Hemostatic drugs. *N Engl J Med* 339:245, 1998.

McLeod LJ et al: The effects of different doses of some acetylsalicylic acid formulations on platelet function and bleeding times in healthy subjects. *Scand J Haematol* 36:379, 1986.

Pareti FI et al: Acquired dysfunction due to the circulation of "exhausted" platelets. *Am J Med* 69:235, 1980.

McMillan R et al: A non-thrombocytopenic bleeding disorder due to an IgG4-kappa anti-GPIIb/IIIa autoantibody. *Br J Haematol* 957:47, 1996.

Peterson P et al: The preoperative bleeding time test lacks clinical benefit. *Arch Surg* 133:134, 1998.

Robinson MS et al: Flow cytometric analysis of reticulated platelets: evidence for a large proportion of non-specific labelling of dense granules by fluorescent dyes. *Br J Haematol* 100: 351, 1998.

Rodgers GM: Overview of platelet physiology and laboratory evaluation of platelet function. *Clin Obstet Gynecol* 42:349, 1999.

Schafer AI: Bleeding and thrombosis in the myeloproliferative disorders. *Blood* 64:1, 1984.

Schafer AI: Effects of nonsteroidal anti-inflammatory therapy on platelets. *Am J Med* 106:25S, 1999.

Stricker RB et al: Acquired Bernard-Soulier syndrome. Evidence for the role of a 210,000-molecular weight protein in the interaction of platelets with von Willebrand factor. *J Clin Invest* 76:1274, 1985.

Wenger RK et al: Loss of platelet fibrinogen receptors during clinical cardiopulmonary bypass. *J Thorac Cardiovasc Surg* 97:235, 1989.

von Willebrand Disease

In 1926 Erik von Willebrand reported an autosomal bleeding disorder in individuals living on the Åland Islands, an archipelago between Sweden and Finland. von Willebrand disease is characterized by mucocutaneous bleeding (ecchymosis, epistaxis, gastrointestinal bleeding, and menorrhagia) of varying severity in both males and females. This common genetic disorder (up to 1–2 percent of the general population) is comprised of a variety of mutations in the von Willebrand factor gene that results in a quantitative or qualitative deficiency of von Willebrand factor (vWF).

vWF is synthesized in endothelial cells and megakaryocytes, where the protein is stored in Weibel-Palade bodies and platelet α granules, respectively. vWF is initially synthesized within the endoplasmic reticulum as C-terminal link dimers containing two 230 kD pro-vWF monomers. Following glycosylation the C-terminal dimers are then N-terminal multimerized into multimers of 0.6 kD to 20 million daltons. The vWF propolypeptide, also known as vW AgII, plays a pivotal role in the late Golgi acidic compartment to cause N-terminal multimerization and direct the storage of vWF into storage granules (platelets and endothelial cells). von Willebrand factor serves two important biologic functions: 1) it serves as the carrier protein for plasma factor VIII (FVIII), and 2) it serves as the ligand that binds to the glycoprotein Ib receptor on platelets to initiate platelet adhesion to damaged blood vessel walls. While it is still controversial as to where vWF and factor VIII first meet, most evidence suggests that when vWF is synthesized in a cell producing factor VIII, trafficking is altered so that factor VIII is brought into storage granules by vWF. This event occurs after propolypeptide cleavage since persistence of the propeptide prevents factor VIII storage. In patients with absent von Willebrand factor (type 3 vWD), FVIII survival is drastically reduced, resulting in the secondary deficiency of factor VIII.

Figure 12-1 demonstrates the genetic and biochemical structure of the propeptide-mature vWF monomer. The factor VIII binding site is in the D3 domain located on the N-terminus of the mature vWF monomer.

The vWF interaction with platelet GPIb is through the A1 disulfide loop, while the interaction with platelet GPIIb–IIIa is through the C1-domain. Collagen binding is through the A3 and possibly the A1 domain. Physiologically, circulating vWF adheres to damaged, exposed subendothelium under conditions of increased shear. Then, vWF undergoes a structural modification so that it spontaneously binds to circulating platelets and initiates platelet adhesion. During this process, factor VIII is also released from von Willebrand factor, enabling FVIII to bind to activated platelets, where it serves as a primary regulatory cofactor in the plasma coagulation process. Factor VIII that is bound to vWF is protected from inactivation by activated protein C.

Most commonly, von Willebrand disease is caused by the heterozygous defect of the vWF gene resulting in reduced plasma levels of von

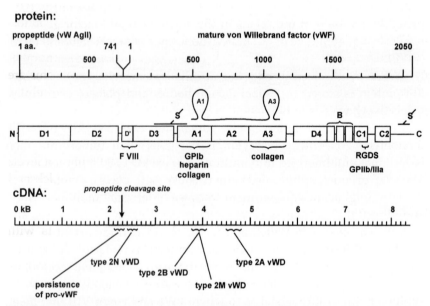

FIGURE 12-1 The relationship between the cDNA and protein structure of human pro-von Willebrand factor. The protein structure and the A, B, C, and D repeats are provided in relationship to the known functional domains of vWF. At the bottom the types of vWD variants and their relative clustering of mutations is illustrated—including types 2A, 2B, 2M, 2N and the persistence of pro-vWF. Each of these lines up with the predicted domain based on the known structure and function of vWF.

Willebrand factor. This heterozygous deficiency (type 1 vWD) is sufficiently common that homozygous patients (type 3 vWD) can occur. Type 3 vWD results in the absence or near absence of vWF, together with a marked secondary reduction in plasma factor VIII (<5 U/dL). von Willebrand disease may also be caused by dysfunctional alterations of the various regions in the vWF molecule as shown in Figure 12-1 including platelet binding (type 2B or type 2M), factor VIII binding (type 2N), or vWF multimerization (type 2A). Understanding the functional classification of von Willebrand disease is important to directing the appropriate treatment of the underlying disorder.

MOLECULAR VARIANTS

Type 1 vWD, the most common type of vWD, affects 1–2 percent of the general population. It accounts for approximately 80 percent of patients with von Willebrand disease and is caused by the heterozygous or partial quantitative deficiency of vWF. While gene deletions and missense or nonsense mutations all can cause reduced levels of von Willebrand factor, the genetic defect causing the vWF mutation in the majority of patients with type 1 vWD is not known. Clinically, these patients range from having mild symptoms to being clinically asymptomatic. The genetic abnormality in one of the vWF alleles accounts for a 50 percent reduction in vWF and a milder secondary deficiency in factor VIII. Since their endothelial cells and platelets contain normal, but reduced, vWF, symptoms are mild and pharmacologic agents such as DDAVP (see below) can release the stored vWF.

Type 3 vWD results from the homozygous deficiency of vWF with absent or profound deficiency in levels of plasma vWF. In the absence of vWF, factor VIII has a markedly accelerated clearance, with plasma levels below 5–10 percent of normal. While patients with type 3 von Willebrand disease are usually not as severely affected as patients with severe hemophilia A, they can have spontaneous bleeding involving central nervous system, GI tract, and mucocutaneous surfaces. Unlike patients with hemophilia, joint bleeding is rarely encountered. Type 3 vWD is the least common variant; it occurs in approximately 1 in 300,000–500,000 individuals. If large gene deletions on both alleles cause absent vWF, alloantibodies to transfused vWF may occur. Patients with point mutations do not usually develop such sensitization.

Type 2A vWD is caused by the abnormal synthesis or proteolysis of vWF multimers, resulting in the presence of only the smaller vWF multimers in plasma. The smaller vWF multimers have reduced binding to platelets; patients exhibit moderate to severe mucocutaneous bleeding. Mutations causing 2A vWD have most commonly been identified in the A2 region of vWF. The abnormal vWF multimers are due to cleavage at the same site on vWF that has been implicated in recurrent thrombotic thrombocytopenic purpura (TTP).

Type 2B vWD is caused by "gain of function" mutations in the A1 region of vWF, causing spontaneous binding to platelets and rapid clearance of both platelets and high-molecular-weight vWF multimers (see Kroner 1992 ref). Thus these patients present with thrombocytopenia, reduced vWF, and absence of high-molecular-weight multimers. This defect is inherited in an autosomal dominant manner. Releasing this abnormal vWF by DDAVP may cause increased thrombocytopenia and inadequate clinical response.

Type 2N vWD, also referred to as "autosomal hemophilia" or the "Normandy" variant, is caused by genetic mutations in the factor VIII binding region of vWF, which results in the rapid turnover of the unbound FVIII and a reduced plasma FVIII level. In order for a person to have symptomatic type 2N vWD, both vWF alleles need to be abnormal. Either both alleles have type 2N mutations (rare) or a 2N mutation is inherited from one parent and type 1 vWD from the other. Since inheriting type 2N together with type 1 will result in only the affected 2N allele being expressed, these patients have low vWF:Ag and an even greater reduction of plasma FVIII. If a patient has homozygous type 2N vWD, the vWF:Ag levels may be normal, but the FVIII levels are between 10 to 20 percent. A true "carrier" of type 2N (only abnormality being a single mutation of one vWF allele) is not symptomatic and is only detected with specific assays of FVIII binding to vWF. Platelet binding of type 2N vWF is usually normal. Thus, patients with type 2N vWD will have normal bleeding times and/or PFA-100 closure times.

Type 2M vWD is caused by the autosomal inheritance of a vWF gene defect that produces decreased or absent binding to platelet GPIb. While dominant inheritance of type 2M vWD has been reported, other patients have milder defects of one allele, which are only clinically apparent when type 1 vWD is inherited on the other allele. This may account for clinical variability within a single family. Plasma vWF binding to FVIII is normal in type 2M vWD.

Platelet-type, pseudo-von Willebrand disease is not a genetic defect of vWF, but presents with similar symptoms and the initial laboratory findings are suggestive of type 2B vWD. The defect is caused by a mutation in the vWF receptor on platelets, glycoprotein Ib (GPIb), which results in spontaneous binding to plasma vWF and clearance of large multimers and platelets from the blood. Since the defect is in the platelet, standard approaches to treating vWD are not helpful. Treatment with normal platelets is usually effective. Subsequent administration of a vWF concentrate may be needed for severe bleeding.

DIAGNOSIS OF VON WILLEBRAND DISEASE

von Willebrand disease is typically suspected in a patient with clinical evidence of mucocutaneous bleeding (ecchymosis, epistaxis, gastrointestinal hemorrhage, and menorrhagia) or postsurgical bleeding. While patients with von Willebrand disease have traditionally been described as having long bleeding times and long APTTs, patients with mild von Willebrand disease often have both a normal bleeding time and normal PTT. Thus, these tests are inadequate for screening. Newer tests of whole blood subjected to sheer-induced agglutination of platelets (PFA-100—see Chap. 4) may improve vWD screening. However, such testing will not identify type 2N vWD. Thus, in the presence of clinical symptoms, most clinicians perform specific vWD testing involving measures of vWF antigen (quantitative), vWF ristocetin cofactor, vWF R:Co (vWF function), plasma levels of factor VIII, and vWF multimers.

Figure 12-2 summarizes the laboratory observations in patients with vWD variants. Characterization of vWF requires quantification (vWF:Ag), function (vWF R:Co), and structural analysis. The vWF R:Co is a pharmacologic assay of the ability of vWF to bind platelet GPIb in the presence of the antibiotic ristocetin. It uses formalin-fixed test platelets and thus is an agglutination, and not an aggregation, of platelets. The vWF R:Co is reduced in parallel with vWF:Ag except in type 2A and type 2M vWD in which the vWF R:Co is more significantly reduced. The adhesive function of vWF can also be measured by the collagen binding assay (vWF:CBA), in which microtiter wells are coated with collagen and utilized to preferentially bind the large vWF multimers. The standard dose ristocetin-induced platelet aggregation (RIPA) using platelet-rich plasma is not very sensitive to reduced vWF and is not abnormal unless the vWD is severe (type 3). Another test requiring further description is the LD-RIPA (low-dose ristocetin-induced platelet aggregation). If low doses of ristocetin are used that do not aggregate normal platelets, the platelet-rich plasma from patients with either type 2B vWD or platelet-type vWD will aggregate. Thus, LD-RIPA is usually performed if the vWF multimers are abnormal in order to detect these variants. Differentiating type 2B from platelet-type vWD requires demonstrating whether the defect is in vWF (type 2B) or platelets (platelet-type vWD) using a test of one component or the other (see Scott ref).

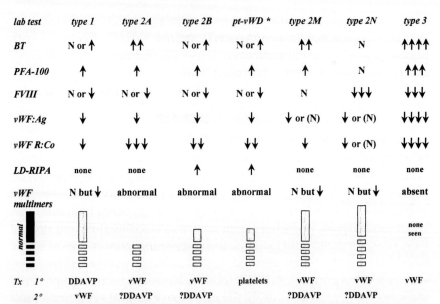

lab test	type 1	type 2A	type 2B	pt-vWD *	type 2M	type 2N	type 3
BT	N or ↑	↑↑	N or ↑	N or ↑	↑↑	N	↑↑↑↑
PFA-100	↑	↑	↑	↑	↑	N	↑↑↑
FVIII	N or ↓	N or ↓	N or ↓	N or ↓	N	↓↓↓	↓↓↓
vWF:Ag	↓	↓	↓	↓	↓ or (N)	↓ or (N)	↓↓↓↓
vWF R:Co	↓	↓↓↓	↓↓	↓↓	↓	↓ or (N)	↓↓↓↓
LD-RIPA	none	none	↑	↑	none	none	none
vWF multimers	N but ↓	abnormal	abnormal	abnormal	N but ↓	N but ↓	absent
Tx 1°	DDAVP	vWF	vWF	platelets	vWF	vWF	vWF
2°	vWF	?DDAVP	?DDAVP		?DDAVP	?DDAVP	

FIGURE 12-2 This chart illustrates the expected laboratory results in patients with various known variants of von Willebrand disease. At the bottom of this figure, the primary (1°) and alternative (2°) treatment (Tx) is provided. The designation of "?DDAVP" is used because DDAVP is sometimes not useful when the released vWF is functionally abnormal. In type 2B vWD, DDAVP may also exacerbate the thrombocytopenia, In type 2M vWD the vWF released may not support platelet adhesion normally and in type 2N vWD, the released FVIII may have an abbreviated survival. The "*" denotes platelet-type vWD, an abnormality of platelet glycoprotein Ib that should be included in the differential diagnosis of variant vWD.

In type 2A vWD, the presence of only small vWF multimers causes a much greater reduction in vWF R:Co than vWF:Ag. Similarly in type 2M vWD there will be a marked discrepancy between vWF antigen and vWF R:Co. In type 2N vWD the FVIII is more reduced that the vWF:Ag.

The blood group of an individual was demonstrated to significantly affect the plasma concentration of vWF, with plasma vWF being lower in group O individuals (see Gill and Montgomery reference). Since this difference is observed in plasma vWF but not platelet vWF, the current hypothesis is that "group O" vWF has increased plasma turnover, which results in reduced plasma vWF concentration. Since this reduced plasma level of vWF may result in a more profound reduction of plasma vWF in patients with mild vWD, it has been recently proposed as a vWD "modifying gene" (a gene that increases the likelihood of clinical symptoms in vWD). Within a family, individuals with the identical inheritance of vWF alleles may have different levels of plasma vWF because they have different blood types. The response of vWF to DDAVP will be similar to patients with mild type 1 vWD.

von Willebrand disease has been reported to occur in individuals who also have factor XI or XII deficiency. In patients with prolongation of the PTT greater than expected for the level of factor VIII, consider the co-deficiency of either factor XI or XII. A recent study indicates that the coexistence of type 1 vWD and factor XII deficiency results in less bleeding that type 1 alone.

MANAGEMENT

The most important step in the management of the patient suspected to have von Willebrand disease is to confirm the diagnosis and determine the correct subtype. As noted in Figure 12-2 the choice of therapeutic agent to treat hemorrhage depends upon the classification. In type 2 variants of vWD, the DDAVP response may be ineffective or insufficient. In type 1 vWD the clinical response to DDAVP may vary from patient to patient; a clinical trial of DDAVP soon after the diagnosis is often performed to determine if the response to DDAVP is adequate. Since patients with type 3 vWD are unresponsive, such clinical trials are not indicated. A clinical trial includes a factor VIII and vWF R:Co level (not bleeding times) before and one hour after a standard dose of DDAVP (IV or nasal). In patients with type 2A, 2B, 2M, or 2N, DDAVP may sometimes be adequate for mild bleeding, but the duration of the response may be reduced, and in some patients with type 2B, thrombocytopenia may worsen. Thus, treatment with vWF concentrate may be required, especially for severe bleeding or for surgical procedures.

Treatment with DDAVP.   Patients with von Willebrand disease do not usually bleed as frequently as patients with hemophilia. vWF and factor VIII that are released by DDAVP usually have the same survival as infusion of plasma-derived vWF and factor VIII in patients with type 1 vWD. The standard intravenous dose for DDAVP is 0.3 µg/kg administered in 30–50 mL of normal saline over 30 min. The vWF and factor VIII level is usually increased 3 to 5 fold and is within the normal range. The plasma half-life of both vWF and FVIII is approximately 12 hours. DDAVP can also be administered intranasally (Stimate, 1.5 mg/mL). The dose is one "puff" (150 µg/puff) for children under 50 kg and two "puffs" (300 µg), one in each nostril, for children over 50 kg and adults.

Treatment with vWF Concentrates.
For patients in whom DDAVP is not indicated or not demonstrated to be efficacious, the use of a "viral-attenuated" vWF (and factor VIII) concentrate is recommended. Humate-P, a plasma-derived concentrate of vWF

and factor VIII, is currently licensed in the United States to treat von Willebrand disease. Other concentrates are undergoing clinical trials. Although the gene for factor VIII is normal in individuals with vWD, administering purified vWF (without factor VIII) does not produce a normal factor VIII level until 12 to 24 hours after administration. For this reason purified vWF or recombinant vWF may have limited clinical utility unless co-administered with recombinant factor VIII. *In the absence of normal vWF, recombinant or monoclonal purified factor VIII preparations have markedly reduced survival and should not be used to treat bleeding in patients with vWD.* Since there is currently no method of rendering cryoprecipitate virus-free (neither heat treatment or solvent-detergent treatment), cryoprecipitate is not recommended unless other concentrates are unavailable. The vWF in solvent-detergent treated plasma (SD-plasma) is abnormal and not recommended for the treatment of vWD. In patients with type 3 severe vWD, administration of 50–60 U/kg of vWF will increase the plasma level of vWF to 100 U/dL (100 percent). The plasma levels of vWF required for surgery or severe bleeding are similar to those required for factor VIII in patients with hemophilia A.

ACQUIRED ABNORMALITIES OF VON WILLEBRAND FACTOR

Alterations in the amount and function of vWF have been identified in many physiologic or pharmacologic states. As noted in Chapter 3, vWF is an acute phase protein and its concentration is increased by inflammation (e.g., vasculitis) and stress (e.g., pregnancy, surgery, exercise, fever). Increased plasma levels of vWF have been suggested as a risk factor for myocardial infarction. The presence of "ultra-large" vWF multimers have been identified in patients with recurrent TTP (see Chap. 28). These larger-than-normal multimers are also released by DDAVP and are present in the plasma of newborn infants, but the half-life of these large multimers appears to be brief and not associated with platelet clumping, in contrast to affects in patients with TTP and some patients with HUS. In such clinical states, the diagnosis of hereditary vWD becomes more difficult. The stress of surgery or newborn delivery may sufficiently increase the plasma concentration of vWF so that a patient with von Willebrand disease has normal plasma levels of vWF.

Acquired vWD Secondary to Autoantibodies. Acquired von Willebrand disease may be seen in a variety of clinical states. Various pathogenic mechanisms have been described, including the development of anti-vWF antibodies. Unlike the antibodies found in patients with hemophilia, the antibodies in acquired vWD do not inhibit vWF function except in rare cases. The binding of antibody to vWF, however, causes the immune complex to be more rapidly removed by the reticuloendothelial system and results in moderate to severe deficiency of vWF. These autoantibodies are associated with autoimmune disorders (SLE or scleroderma), lymphoma, leukemia, multiple myeloma, and monoclonal gammopathies. Antibodies may follow acute infections in childhood or be idiopathic in elderly persons. Usually the vWF:Ag and vWF R:Co are reduced in parallel and appear similar to type 1 or type 3 vWD. While the factor VIII may be reduced, it is not usually as reduced as much as the vWF. Multimeric analysis may be normal or appear similar to type 2 vWD variants. Since the gene for vWF is intact, the synthesis of vWF is normal but its survival is markedly decreased. Administration of DDAVP and determination of the plasma half-life of vWF demonstrates the rapid disappearance of vWF. Specialized laboratory testing can demonstrate that the vWF propolypeptide (vW AgII) is normal or increased in contrast to hereditary vWD, in which the level of vWF and vW AgII are similarly reduced. Some laboratories have developed a diagnostic solid-phase assay for antibodies to vWF. Mixing studies to evaluate inhibition of platelet vWF binding, similar to testing done for factor VIII inhibitors, is often negative because these antibodies are usually non-inhibitory (discussed earlier).

Wilms Tumor. Patients with Wilms tumors occasionally may have markedly reduced vWF levels associated with severe bleeding. While some patients have low vWF assays in the clinical laboratory because of the abnormal presence of hyaluronic acid, others have significant reductions that are associated with major hemorrhage and require replacement therapy. The synthesis of vWF by endothelial cells has been reported in one patient to be normal as demonstrated by immunostaining of kidney section. Whether administration of DDAVP would be beneficial is not known. If a patient with Wilms tumor has excessive bleeding symptoms, vWF testing should be performed and if low levels of vWF are identified, treatment with vWF concentrate should be considered.

Hypothyroidism. Congenital and acquired hypothyroidism is associated with low levels of vWF protein. No autoantibodies are demonstrated and there is a parallel reduction in both vWF and vW AgII, suggesting decreased protein synthesis. Correction of the thyroid deficiency will correct the acquired deficiency. Acute hemorrhage can be managed by DDAVP or vWF replacement. Hyperthyroidism is associated with increased levels of vWF and may mask the diagnosis of true vWD. In patients with thyroid abnormalities, it is important that patients are euthyroid when testing for the presence of vWD.

Abnormal vWF in Congenital Heart Disease. The loss of the normal large vWF multimers has been identified in patients with ventriculoseptal defects, aortic stenosis, and even pulmonary hypertension. These abnormalities may mimic type 2 vWD. Correction of the underlying cardiac defect is usually followed by a normalization of vWF.

Mesenchymal Dysplasias and Other Disorders. Vascular disorders such as mitral valve prolapse, connective tissue disorder, angiodysplasia, giant hemangiomas, and telangiectasia have been associated with low vWF and abnormal vWF multimers. Abnormal synthesis or clearance may be responsible for these findings.

Laboratory Evaluation of Acquired vWD. Laboratory evaluation for a patient with suspected acquired vWD includes assays of vWF:Ag; vWF R:Co; FVIII; vWF multimers; and, if available, the vWF propeptide, vW AgII. If the vWF is reduced, administration of DDAVP followed by assays for vWF will demonstrate a normal release of vWF but a markedly reduced half-life. If available, a solid-phase assay for antibodies to vWF can be diagnostic.

Treatment of Acquired vWD. Bleeding symptoms from acquired vWD may be mild (hypothyroidism) or severe (especially those with intestinal angiodysplasia). If bleeding is mild, DDAVP should be tried. With severe bleeding in the presence of a high-titer antibody to vWF, continuous administration of a vWF concentrate may overcome the antibody-induced accelerated clearance. Administration of IV immunoglobulin or plasmapheresis may be useful. If bleeding is severe or uncontrollable, use of recombinant activated factor VII (rVIIa) concentrate may be effective.

BIBLIOGRAPHY

Alhumood SA et al: Idiopathic immune-mediated acquired von Willebrand's disease in a patient with angiodysplasia: demonstration of an unusual inhibitor causing a functional defect and rapid clearance of von Willebrand factor. *Am J Hematol.*, 60:151, 1999.

Berliner SA et al: A relatively high frequency of severe (type III) von Willebrand's disease in Israel. *Br J Haematol.*, 62:535, 1986.

Erfurth EM et al: Effect of acute desmopressin and of long-term thyroxine replacement on haemostasis in hypothyroidism. *Clin Endocrinol* 42:373, 1995.

Favaloro EJ: Collagen binding assay for von Willebrand factor (VWF:CBA): detection of von Willebrands disease (VWD) and discrimination of VWD subtypes depends on collagen source. *Thromb Haemost* 83:127, 2000.

Federici AB et al: Treatment of acquired von Willebrand syndrome in patients with monoclonal gammopathy of uncertain significance: comparison of three different therapeutic approaches. *Blood* 92:2707, 1998.

Fressinaud E et al: Screening for von Willebrand disease with a new analyzer using high shear stress: a study of 60 cases. *Blood* 91:1325, 1998.

Gill JC et al: The effect of ABO blood group on the diagnosis of von Willebrand disease. *Blood* 69:1691, 1987.

Gill JC et al: Loss of the largest von Willebrand factor multimers from the plasma of patients with congenital cardiac defects. *Blood* 67:758, 1986.

Ginsburg D et al: Molecular basis of human von Willebrand disease: analysis of platelet von Willebrand factor mRNA. *Proc Natl Acad Sci USA* 86:3723, 1989.

Goto S et al: Distinct mechanisms of platelet aggregation as a consequence of different shearing flow conditions. *J Clin Invest* 101:479, 1998.

Hillery CA et al: Type 2M von Willebrand disease: F606I and I662F, mutations in the glycoprotein Ib binding domain selectively impair ristocetin, but not botrocetin-mediated binding of von Willebrand factor to platelets. *Blood* 91:1572, 1998.

Kroner PA et al: The defective interaction between von Willebrand factor and factor VIII in a patient with type 1 von Willebrand disease is caused by substitution of Arg19 and His54 in mature von Willebrand factor. *Blood* 87:1013, 1996.

Kroner PA et al: Expressed full-length von Willebrand factor containing missense mutations linked to type IIB von Willebrand disease shows enhanced binding to platelets. *Blood* 79:2048, 1992.

Mancuso DJ et al: Characterization of partial gene deletions in type III von Willebrand disease with alloantibody inhibitors. *Thromb Haemost* 72:180, 1994.

Mannucci PM: Treatment of von Willebrand disease. *Haemophilia* 4:661, 1998.

Mauz-Korholz C et al: Management of severe chronic thrombocytopenia in von Willebrand's disease type 2B. *Arch Dis Child* 78:257, 1998.

Mohri H et al: Clinical significance of inhibitors in acquired von Willebrand syndrome. *Blood* 91:3623, 1998.

Montgomery RR, Coller BS: von Willebrand disease. In: Colman et al (eds): *Hemostasis and Thrombosis. Basic Principles and Clinical Practice*, J.B. Lippincott, Philadelphia, pp. 134–168, 1994.

Montgomery RR, Scott JP: Hemophilia and von Willebrand disease. In: Nathan DG, Orkin SH (eds): *Hematology of Infancy and Childhood*, W.B. Saunders Co., Philadelphia, pp. 1631–1659, 1998.

Nichols WC, Ginsburg D: von Willebrand disease. *Medicine* 76:1, 1997.

Rosenberg JB et al: Intracellular trafficking of factor VIII to von Willebrand factor storage granules. *J Clin Invest* 101:613, 1998.

Scott JP, Montgomery RR: The rapid differentiation of type IIb von Willebrand's disease from platelet-type (pseudo-) von Willebrand's disease by the "neutral" monoclonal antibody binding assay. *Am J Clin Pathol* 96:723, 1991.

Scott JP et al: Acquired von Willebrand's disease in association with Wilm's tumor: regression following treatment. *Blood* 58:665, 1981.

Tefferi A, Nichols WL: Acquired von Willebrand disease: concise review of occurrence, diagnosis, pathogenesis, and treatment. *Am J Med* 103:536, 1997.

Tsai HM et al: Proteolytic cleavage of recombinant type 2A von Willebrand factor mutants R834W and R834Q: inhibition by doxycycline and by monoclonal antibody VP-1. *Blood* 89:1954, 1997.

von Willebrand EA: Hereditary pseudohaemophilia. *Haemophilia* 5:223, 1999.

Werner EJ et al: Prevalence of von Willebrand disease in children: a multiethnic study. *J Pediatr* 123:893, 1993.

Zeitler P et al: Combination of von Willebrand disease type 1 and partial factor XII deficiency in children: clinical evidence for a diminished bleeding tendency. *Acta Paediatr* 88:1233, 1999.

CHAPTER 13

Hemophilia A (FVIII Deficiency)

Factor VIII (FVIII; antihemophilic factor, AHF) is a 320-kD glycoprotein, synthesized mainly in hepatocytes, which circulates in plasma in a concentration of 0.1–0.2 µg/mL in a stable complex with another glycoprotein, von Willebrand factor. When proteolytically activated by factor Xa or thrombin, VIIIa acts as a cofactor to accelerate the activation of factor X by factor IXa; the coagulant activity is termed FVIII activity; the immunologic quantitation of FVIII is FVIII antigen or VIII:Ag. The genetic deficiency of FVIII is classic hemophilia or hemophilia A, and occurs with an incidence of 1 in 5,000 live male births.

STRUCTURE–FUNCTION RELATIONSHIP

When FVIII is activated by thrombin or Xa in the presence of metal ions on a phospholipid surface (platelets), factor X activation by IXa is enhanced 10,000-fold. This important cofactor activity is derived by limited proteolysis of the native molecule FVIII to VIIIa. The polypeptide structure of the protein is composed of domains in the order A1:A2:B:A3:C1:C2 (see Fig. 20-1). The A domains occur in both the heavy and light chains and have a 30 percent homology with ceruloplasmin and factor V. The second and third A domains are separated by a large connecting region containing most of the N-linked glycosylation sites (the B domain), followed by two C domains of 150 amino acids each, which have a homology with lectin-binding proteins.

Activation of FVIII results in a heterotrimer that consists of a copper-ion–dependent association between the first A domain (50 kD) and a 73-kD fragment containing the third A and two C domains (light chain), as well as a weak ionic association between the first and second subunits. During this activation process the light chain is released from the stabilizing effect of von Willebrand factor, followed by further degradation and inactivation by activated protein C, thrombin, Xa, and possibly plasmin. FVIII activity is dependent on formation of the heterotrimer (VIIIa) and is measured in plasma by three types of assays: one-stage, two-stage, and chromogenic substrate assay. Comparison of these assay techniques is shown in Table 13-1. All three methods give comparable results when

---

TABLE 13-1

Comparison of Factor VIII Assays

One-Stage	Two-Stage	Chromogenic
Methods		
Diluted subject plasma	Diluted subject plasma (adsorbed to remove vitamin K factors)	Diluted subject plasma
+		+
VIII-deficient substrate plasma	+	Regent mixture (IXa, X, Pl, Ca++)
+	Reagent mixture (serum, factor V plasma)	↓
APTT reagent	+	Incubate
		Add to synthetic substrate
↓	Ca++	↓
Add Ca++	↓	Measure color change
↓	Incubate subsample	
Fibrin endpoint	+	
	Ca++, substrate plasma	
	↓	
	Fibrin endpoint	
Advantages		
Simplicity	Precision (especially at low levels)	Precision
Readily automated	Not sensitive to activation	Not sensitive to activation
Widely used for monitoring concentrate usage	No requirement for VIII-deficient plasma	No requirement for VIII-deficient plasma
		Readily automated
Disadvantages		
Need for VIII-deficient plasma	Complex	Requires specific instrumentation
Sensitive to activation	Difficult to standardize reagents	Questionable accuracy in presence of inhibitors
APTT reagent variability	Not easily automated	

Source: Adapted from Brandt JT, Triplett DA: Laboratory assays for factor VIII:C. In: Zimmerman TS, Ruggeri ZM (eds): *Coagulation and Bleeding Disorders. The Role of Factor VIII and von Willebrand Factor,* New York, Marcel Dekker, pp. 343–357, 1989.

assaying normal controls, suspected carriers, and most variants of von Willebrand disease and hemophilia, before and after treatment (if standards used are the same as the treatment product infused, see Lee et al reference).

A subset of mild hemophilia A patients demonstrate normal or minimally prolonged APTTs, as well as significantly lower FVIII levels, when measured by the two-stage and chromogenic assays as compared with the one-stage assay. Recently, the discrepancy in one such mutant ($^{ARG}531^{HIS}$) has been explained by a rapid dissociation of the A_2 subunit from the heterotrimer. Because the two-stage test involves a preincubation phase before actual assay, it is more sensitive to the effect of rapid FVIII inactivation than the one-stage assay. FVIII:Ag is quantitated by immunoradiometric or ELISA assays using human anti-FVIII or monoclonal antibodies.

GENETICS OF HEMOPHILIA A

The gene responsible for hemophilia A is located on the long arm of the X chromosome at Xq28. Females (heterozygotes) with two X chromosomes can carry a mutation on one chromosome and remain unaffected because of the compensating normal gene. A male (hemizygote) will have hemophilia if his X chromosome carries the mutant gene. In a mating between a female carrier and an unaffected male, 50 percent of daughters will be heterozygous for the hemophilia mutation (carriers) and 50 percent of the sons will be hemophiliacs. Conversely, in a mating between a hemophilic male and a normal female, no sons will be affected (paternal Y and maternal X chromosomes), but all daughters will be obligate carriers. Hemophilia A has remained a relatively common bleeding disorder since biblical times because of high sporadic occurrence of the disorder (high mutation rate) and the X-linked inheritance. Consequently, 30 percent of newly diagnosed severe hemophilia A is accompanied by a negative family history for that disease.

Female Hemophilia

Severe hemophilia due to FVIII or factor IX deficiency may rarely be seen in females. The possible causes include homozygosity for the gene (consanguinity in hemophilic family, postzygotic mutation, germ line mutation in a parent marrying into a hemophilic family), chance inactivation of the X chromosome with the normal gene (extreme lyonization), genetic abnormality in a phenotypic female with abnormal gene (Turner's syndrome, testicular feminization, mosaicism), abnormalities involving the

X chromosome (deletion, inversion, translocation) and von Willebrand factor Normandy (see Chap. 12). Family and detailed molecular biologic studies should provide the diagnosis.

Gene Mutation

The FVIII gene was cloned in 1984. At 186 kilobases (kb), it comprises one thousandth of the X chromosome DNA and is one of the largest human genes identified so far. As predicted by the X-linked genetic lethal nature of the disease and size of the gene, 70 percent of families carry different mutations. As of May 1999, 309 single base substitutions, 92 large deletions, 77 small deletions, 28 insertions, as well as one prevalent intron recombinative event (described below), made up the hemophilia A gene mutation database (updated file maintained at *http://europium.csc.mrc .ac.uk*). Genotype–phenotype correlation is ongoing. In families with severe hemophilia A, an intrachromosomal intron–exon recombination, resulting in 3 types of inversions in intron 22 of the FVIII gene, accounts for 50 percent of all affected pedigrees and most of the severe pedigrees with a previously negative history of the disease. Other gene rearrangements, including small and large deletions and insertions, account for most of the other mutations resulting in a severe phenotype. In contrast, almost 100 percent of moderate and mild disease results from single base-pair substitutions, leading largely to a missense message.

Carrier Detection and Prenatal Diagnosis

All newly diagnosed patients and their families should have genetic counseling to include appropriate testing and identification of potential or obligate carriers in the pedigree. Gene-based diagnostic practices used to confirm carrier status and/or perform prenatal diagnosis depend on the type of hemophilia in a particular pedigree. Currently, because of its high frequency in this population, direct gene-mutation analysis for the FVIII intron 22 inversion is recommended for initial carrier detection in severe hemophilia A families. The direct methodology makes it particularly useful when affected and intervening family members are unavailable for testing. When direct analysis for the intron 22 inversion is negative in a severe pedigree, or when gene-based diagnosis in a family with moderate or mild disease is needed, carrier detection is usually performed using linkage analysis of DNA polymorphisms. Techniques using up to 4 intragenic and 4 extragenic restriction length polymorphic markers are informative 97 percent of the time, but only when an affected male patient and intervening family members are available for analysis. In families with more limited pedigrees, direct gene mutation analysis using new conformation-specific gel electrophoresis techniques can be used with similar overall sensitivity. This analysis is expensive, usually research-based, and may take up to 12 weeks to complete, limiting its use in an established pregnancy. Alternatively, carrier detection could be attempted in uninformative cases using determinations of FVIII activity and von Willebrand factor antigen (vWF:Ag). Decreased FVIII activity (0.25 to 0.49 U/ml) with FVIII-vWF:Ag ratios of less than 1.0 identify 91 percent to 99 percent of hemophilia A carriers when multiple well-controlled tests and sophisticated data analysis are used.

When carrier detection is possible, prenatal diagnosis can be performed at most high-risk obstetric centers by either chorionic villus sampling (CVS) at 10 to 12 weeks' gestation or by amniocentesis after 15 weeks' gestation. If DNA markers are not available, fetal blood sampling can be performed at 20 weeks' gestation for direct FVIII plasma activity level measurement. The maternal–fetal combined complication rates for amniocentesis and CVS are 0.5 percent to 1.0 percent and 1.0 percent to 2.0 percent, respectively, and should be discussed in prenatal genetic counseling performed through hemophilia treatment centers. Fetal blood sampling is infrequently available, even in centers for perinatal medicine. The fetal-loss rate for these procedures ranges from 1 percent to 6 percent.

The carrier of hemophilia A may herself have a bleeding disorder. If the factor VIII activity is <40 percent, mild bleeding symptoms (especially with trauma or surgery) may occur and the affected individual should be counseled accordingly.

CLINICAL MANIFESTATIONS OF HEMOPHILIA A

Patients with classical hemophilia display a spectrum of bleeding manifestations [deep muscle and joint hemorrhage, hematomas, easy bruising, posttraumatic deep bleeding, postsurgery and laceration wound bleeding, postoral injury and tooth extraction (molars) oozing, intracranial hemorrhage (ICH), intra- and retroperitoneal bleeding, and gastrointestinal and renal bleeding] (Table 13-2). The propensity to musculoskeletal hemorrhage can lead to recurrent hemarthroses (target joints) and chronic muscle injury and fibrosis. Even the patient with mild disease who is not promptly treated can develop permanent damage to a particular muscle group or joint with a trauma-induced bleed.

The diagnosis of hemophilia A is first suspected in one of several clinical situations: a pregnancy of, or the birth of an infant to, a mother with a family history of hemophilia or a pedigree of X-linked bleeders; in the

TABLE 13-2

Clinical Manifestations in Hemophilia A

Factor VIII Assay	Severe (0–0.01 U/mL)	Moderate (0.02–0.05 U/mL)	Mild (0.06–0.4 U/mL)
Age at onset of bleeding	Within first year	Usually before 2 years	3–14 years or older
Musculoskeletal bleeding	"Spontaneous" joint and muscle bleeding, frequent "target joints"	Joint and muscle bleeding with minor trauma, may have "target joints"	Unusual except with significant trauma
CNS bleeding	Prevalence–3% Mean age 14 years (1 week–53 years)	Less prevalent than severe	Rare; with significant trauma
Postsurgical bleeding	Usually frank bleeding	Wound hematomas and oozing, rarely none	Hematomas and oozing, or none
Inhibitor development	15–20% prevalance	<3%	Very rare
Trauma-induced bleeding	Common with contact sports	Muscle and joint bleeding with contact sports	Significant hematomas; deep bleeding only with significant trauma
Bleeding with tooth extraction	Usual	Common	Often, can be persisitent
Response of level of exercise	None	None	Slight increase (5%)
Response to DDAVP	None	Usually <10%	Usually 2–3 fold
Neonatal manifestations	Postcircumcision bleeding, occasional ICH	Usual post circumcision bleeding. Rare ICH	None
Renal bleeding (hematuria)	Common, may be severe	Not unusual	Can occur, usually mild

* CNS, central nervous system; ICH, intracranial hemorrhage.

absence of a positive family history, the appearance of bleeding in the neonatal period (postcircumcision or puncture wound bleeding, large hematomas, unexplained ICH); or a pattern of easy bruising and deep muscle-joint or posttraumatic bleeding later in life. Severe hemophilia is routinely diagnosed within the first year of life, but mild hemophilia may be unsuspected until a traumatic or surgical challenge in the second or third decade or later. The basic hemostatic screen is usually normal except for a prolonged APTT. The diagnosis is confirmed by a plasma assay for FVIII. In suspected hemophilia without a positive family history, assays for vWF are usually performed to rule out type 3 vWD and consideration is given to vWD Normandy (see Chap. 12). The BT is usually normal in uncomplicated hemophilia A.

TREATMENT OF HEMOPHILIA A

The mainstay of successful hemophilia therapy for either treatment or prevention of acute hemorrhage is prompt and sufficient intravenous replacement of FVIII to hemostatic plasma levels. Treatment performed preventatively or at the first onset of symptoms limits both the amount of the bleeding and the extent of the ensuing tissue damage.

State-of-the-art replacement products are made from either plasma-derived or recombinant FVIII, all of which have similar hemostatic efficacy. The current therapeutic options for hemophilia A are summarized in Chapter 55. Cost continues to be one potential consideration in the choice of FVIII products, but viral safety has been a paramount concern in recent years. Despite the application of double viral inactivation to many plasma-derived products, parvovirus transmission is still possible. Recombinant FVIII has not been linked to transmission of any human viruses, although it currently contains human albumin. In the late 1990s, concern was raised about the potential risk of human or bovine protein-containing products transmitting Creutzfeldt-Jacob disease (CJD) or "new variant" CJD; however, no such cases have occurred to date. These concerns have stimulated the technological advances that will soon produce licensed recombinant factor devoid of all human and animal proteins. Given these considerations, most new patients are treated with monoclonal antibody-purified plasma-derived or recombinant products or, more rarely, directed-donor cryoprecipitate.

The dosing regimen for factor replacement in hemophilia is based on three pharmacologic and therapeutic principles: (1) the volume of the clotting factor's distribution within intravascular or extravascular compartments: this affects in vivo factor recovery in plasma following an infusion; (2) the factor survival, or half-disappearance time, in plasma; and (3) the minimal hemostatic factor level required to control the particular type and extent of the hemorrhage. Clotting factor is dosed in "units" (U) of activity, with 1 unit of factor representing the amount present in 1 mL of normal plasma. Because of its intravascular volume of distribution, one unit of FVIII raises the plasma level by approximately 0.02 U/mL or 2 percent. The half-disappearance time from circulation is biphasic and averages approximately 12 hours. Both recovery and survival may be lower in young children; patients with blood group O may have a shorter factor VIII half-life. Because considerable intrapatient variation in FVIII plasma recovery and survival occurs, presurgical pharmacokinetic studies and frequent laboratory monitoring of FVIII levels during therapy is warranted in situations of potential or ongoing major hemorrhage.

The minimum hemostatic plasma FVIII levels are determined according to the type and extent of bleeding. In general, 30 to 50 percent of normal factor levels are required for most bleeding episodes. Most such therapy is administered at home or in an outpatient setting. However, 50 to 100 percent of normal levels are necessary to treat or prevent life and limb-threatening or postsurgical hemorrhage. In these situations, in-hospital therapy may be required for factor replacement delivered by either bolus or continuous infusion. With bolus therapy, FVIII is infused every 12 hours, using doses designed to maintain a minimum, or trough, factor level of 0.5 U/mL (50 percent). Daily monitoring of factor levels is mandatory. Alternatively, the total daily dose of factor can be delivered by continuous infusion, which results in a constant therapeutic factor level that is not subject to the peaks and troughs observed with bolus injections. Total FVIII usage may decline by as much as 30 percent with this method. Steady-state plasma factor levels also allow for simplified laboratory monitoring. Factor-replacement therapy guidelines for hemorrhage in hemophilia A are outlined in Table 13-3.

DDAVP, 1-deamino 8-D arginine vasopressin, stimulates a 3 to 5 increase in plasma FVIII levels, although its mechanism of action still has not been completely elucidated. Therefore, it provides an effective alternative therapy for minor hemorrhage in most patients with mild hemophilia A (Chapter 58). Antifibrinolytic therapy is used to stabilize a clot by inhibiting the normal process of clot lysis by fibrinolytic system. It provides useful ancillary treatment in patients with hemorrhagic disorders, particularly in the prevention or treatment of oral, nasopharyngeal, or GI hemorrhage. (Chapter 58).

COMPLICATIONS OF HEMOPHILIA

Joint Disease/Prophylaxis

Joint hemorrhage is the most common manifestation of moderate and severe hemophilia. This type of bleeding rarely occurs prior to the child's being ambulatory. By the time they are of preschool age, children can learn to recognize acute joint bleeding by the "tingling" sensation within the

TABLE 13-3

Guidelines for Factor-replacement Therapy for Hemorrhage in Hemophilia A.

Site of Bleed	Hemostatic Factor Level	Factor Dosing Hemophilia A	Comment
Joint	40%–80%	20–40 U/kg qd as needed	Rest/immobilization/ physical therapy rehabilitation following bleed. Several doses may be necessary to prevent or treat target joint.
Muscle	40%–80%	20–40 U/kg qd as needed	Calf/forearm bleed is limb threatening, significant blood loss with femoral/ retroperitoneal bleed.
Oral mucosa	Initially 50%, then antifibrinolyctic coverage usually suffices	25 U/kg	Antifibrinolytic therapy is critical. Do not use with PCCs or APCCs.
Epistaxis	Initially 80%– 100%, then 30% until healing occurs	40–50 U/kg, then 30–40 U/kg qd	Local measures: Pressure/pack/cautery useful for severe or recurrent bleed.
Gastro- intestinal	Initially 100%, then 30% until healing occurs	40–50 U/kg, then 30–40 U/kg qd	Lesion is usually found— endoscopy highly recommended. Antifibrinolytic therapy may be useful.
Genito- urinary	Initially 100%, then 30% until healing occurs	40–50 U/kg, then 30–40 U/kg qd	Evaluate for stones or urinary tract infection. Lesion usually not found. Prednisone 1–2 mg/kg/d × 5–7 days may be useful. Antifibrinolytic contraindicated.
Central nervous system	Initially 100%, then 50%–100% for 10–14 days	50 U/kg, then 25 U/kg q 12 hours or continuous infusion	Anticonvulsants frequently used preventatively. Lumbar puncture requires pro- phylactic factor coverage.
Trauma or surgery	Initially 100%, then 50% until wound healing begins, then 30% until wound healing complete (usually 7–14 days)	50 U/kg, then dose q 12 hours or by continuous infusion	Perioperative and postopera- tive management plan must be in place pre-op; evaluation for inhibitors crucial prior to elective surgery.

joint prior to the development of the overt signs of an acute hemarthrosis, such as pain, swelling, warmth, and decreased range of motion. Ankles, knees, and elbows are affected most commonly. Despite a regimen of prompt factor replacement, rest, ice, and splinting, a cycle of repeated hemorrhage can occur into one or more "target joints." Synovial inflammation from direct exposure to blood causes it to become hyperemic, hyperplastic, and more likely to rebleed. The persistent inflammation can result in a chronic joint effusion, a condition referred to as chronic synovitis. Persistent intraarticular blood also causes progressive degeneration of joint cartilage and bone, known as hemophilic arthropathy.

Chronic arthropathy may lead to severe physical impairment, loss of time from school or work, psychosocial consequences, and increased long-term disability. Therefore, prevention of irreversible joint injury should be a therapeutic goal for patients with hemophilia. Based on earlier observations that individuals with moderate hemophilia rarely develop chronic arthropathy, Swedish physicians theorized that adequate prevention prophylaxis could be accomplished by maintaining minimum (trough) FVIII levels of 1 to 5 percent. They implemented the practice of "primary" prophylactic therapy, the institution of bleeding prevention at age 1 to 2 years, before the onset of significant joint bleeding. Children treated with 25 to 40 U/kg of FVIII three times weekly had fewer than one hemarthrosis per year, and normal joints by standardized orthopedic and radiologic evaluations over 10 years. This outcome required a more than fourfold increase in factor usage compared to the average on-demand regimen. "Secondary" prophylaxis, the same therapy instituted after the onset of significant joint bleeding and early arthropathy, decreases, but does not abolish, joint hemorrhage. Despite improvement in both quality of life and orthopedic scores, joint damage frequently progresses radiographically.

Consequently, in 1994 the Medical and Scientific Advisory Council of the National Hemophilia Foundation recommended that primary prophylaxis begin at age 1 to 2 years for children with severe hemophilia. This practice is slowly being adopted in the pediatric population. Deterrents to its widespread implementation include concerns about the complications associated with the required central venous catheter placement in young children, as well as the current lack of true cost-effectiveness data on primary prophylaxis. Studies are therefore ongoing to determine optimal cost-effective strategies to prevent hemophilic arthropathy. Recently, single-dose prophylaxis with recombinant factor has been advocated for all infants with severe hemophilia as soon after birth as possible in order to prevent ICH.

Hepatitis C, Chronic Liver Disease, and HIV Infection

Between 60 and 95 percent of severe hemophilia patients older than 10 and 12 years of age, respectively, have been infected with hepatitis C virus (HCV). Although 70 to 80 percent of acute HCV infection may be asymptomatic, long-term sequelae are noted in at least 85 percent of exposed persons after an indolent period of up to 20 years. In one study of 155 hemophilia patients who underwent liver biopsy, 70 percent had evidence of chronic active hepatitis, and 15 percent manifested some degree of cirrhosis. Liver failure has been reported in 8 percent of persons with hemophilia who are coinfected with HIV. Furthermore, HIV-positive hemophilic patients who are taking protease inhibitors have an increased frequency of bleeding episodes. In those patients with cirrhosis, hepatocellular carcinoma may occur at a 30-fold increased rate above the baseline.

Treatment with interferon alpha 2b (IFN) has resulted in less than a 25 percent remission rate, defined as a sustained absence of systemic HCV RNA when sensitive PCR detection is used. Among HIV-infected individuals with hemophilia, there have been no long-term remissions. Trials using a combination of interferon alpha and oral ribavirin have demonstrated higher initial and sustained response rates than with interferon alone. Currently, certain genotypes and a low pretherapy HCV RNA titer that becomes undetectable following treatment, may be the best predictors of sustained response to therapy. So far, genotypic variability in HCV strains and lack of protective cross-immunity among different species of HCV have thwarted prospects for a hepatitis C vaccine.

Prognosis: Gene Therapy/The Future

Since the factor VIII gene was cloned, hemophilia has been considered to be one of the genetic diseases most amenable to gene therapy because of: (1) the lack of requirement for tissue-specific expression; (2) the absence of precise regulation of these factor proteins; and (3) the clinical benefit derived from less-than-normal factor expression with, conversely, the lack of known adverse effect from moderate protein overexpression.

With the safe continuous delivery of hemostatically sufficient amounts of factor VIII to prevent hemorrhagic symptoms as the goal, strategies have included both in vivo or ex vivo factor VIII gene addition to target cells (bone marrow stem cells, hepatocytes, fibroblasts) using retrovirus, adenovirus, and adeno-associated virus vectors. Despite the difficulties encountered so far, long-term factor VIII expression in small animal models has been achieved and initial clinical human trials are underway. With cautious optimism, the cure for hemophilia A will soon be a reality.

BIBLIOGRAPHY

Antonarakis SE: Molecular genetics of coagulation factor VIII gene and hemophilis A. *Hemophilia* 4 (Supp 2):1, 1998.

Buchanan GR: Factor concentrate prophylaxis for neonates with hemophilia. *J Pediatr Hemat Oncol* 21:254, 1999.

Connelly S, Kaleko M: Gene therapy for hemophilia A. *Thromb Haemost* 78:31, 1997.

DiMichele DM, Neufeld EJ: Hemophilia: A new approach to an old disease. In: *Hematology/Oncology Clinics of North America*, Neufeld EJ (guest ed) WB Saunders, Philadelphia, pp 1315–1344, 1998.

Eyster ME et al: Natural history of hepatitis C virus infection in multitransfused hemophiliacs: Effect of coinfection with human immunodeficiency virus. The Multicenter Hemophilia Cohort Study. *J Acquir Immune Defic Syndr* 6:602, 1993.

Gordon FH et al: Outcome of orthotopic liver transplantation in patients with haemophilia. *Gut* 42:744, 1998.

Gruppo R: Prophylaxis for hemophilia: State of the art or state of confusion? *J Pediatr* 132:915, 1998.

Herzog RW and High KA: Problems and prospects in gene therapy for hemophilia. *Curr Opin Hematol*, 5:321, 1998.

Kulkarni R, Lusher JM: Intracranial and extracranial hemorrhages in newborns with hemophilia: a review of the literature. *J Pediatr Hemat Oncol* 21:289, 1999.

Lakich D et al: Inversions disrupting the factor VIII gene are a common cause of severe hemophilia A. *Nat Genet* 5:236, 1993.

Lee CA et al: Pharmacokinetics of recombinant factor VIII (Recombinate) using one-stage clotting and chromogenic factor VIII assay. *Thromb Haemost* 82:1644, 1999.

Lenting PJ et al: The lifecycle of coagulation factor VIII in view of its structure and function. *Blood* 92:3983, 1998.

Manco-Johnson MJ et al: A prophylactic program in the United States: Experience and issues. *Semin Hematol* 31:10, 1994.

Mannucci PM, Tuddenham EGD: The hemophilias: progress and problems. *Semin Hematol* 36:104, 1999.

Nilsson IM et al: Twenty-five years' experience of prophylactic treatment in severe haemophilia A and B. *J Intern Med* 232:25, 1992.

Pipe SW et al: Mild hemophilia A caused by increased rate of factor VIII A2 subunit dissociation: Evidence for nonproteolytic inactivation of factor VIIIa in vivo. *Blood* 93:176, 1999.

Racoosin JA, Kessler CM: Bleeding episodes in HIV-positive patients taking protease inhibitors: a case series. *Haemophilia* 5:266, 1999.

Soucie JM et al: The first population-based survey of hemophilia incidence in the United States. *Am J Hematol* 59:288, 1998.

Stuart MJ et al: Bleeding time in hemophilia A: Potential mechanisms for prolongation. *J Pediatr* 108:215, 1986.

Tock B et al: Haemophilia and advanced fibrin sealant technologies. *Haemophilia* 4:449, 1998.

Van den Berg HM et al: Hemophilia prophylaxis in the Netherlands. *Semin Hematol* 31:13, 1994.

Venkateswaran L et al: Mild hemophilia in children: prevalence, complications, and treatment. *Pediatr Hematol Oncol* 20:32, 1998.

Vlot AJ et al: The half-life of infused factor VIII is shorter in hemophilic patients with blood O than in those with blood group A. *Thromb Haemost* 83:65, 2000.

CHAPTER 14

Hemophilia B (Factor IX Deficiency)

The existence of factor IX as a separate clotting factor was recognized over 50 years ago from studies of patients with hemophilic bleeding manifestations. The factor was called plasma thromboplastin component (PTC) or "Christmas" factor in the original reports, which resulted in the synonyms for congenital factor IX deficiency: Christmas disease, PTC deficiency, and hemophilia B. Factor IX, a vitamin K-dependent factor with a molecular weight of 57,000, circulates as a single-chain glycoprotein proenzyme in the concentration of 3 to 5 µg/mL. Factor IX, when activated by factor XIa or factor VIIa-tissue factor in the presence of cofactors (factor VIII, calcium, phospholipid), rapidly converts factor X to Xa. The hereditary deficiency of factor IX results in a bleeding diathesis whose clinical characteristics are indistinguishable from factor VIII-deficient hemophilia.

STRUCTURE–FUNCTION RELATIONSHIP

The gene for factor IX codes for a signal peptide, a propeptide (promoter region), and the mature 415-amino–acid protein that is present in the plasma. The processing steps removing the signal peptide and the leader propeptide occur in the hepatocyte prior to secretion. As shown in Fig. 14-1, the domain structure includes the Gla region containing 12 gamma-carboxyglutamyl residues dependent on the vitamin K carboxylase system. The next two domains, epidermal growth factor-like (EGF), are cysteine-rich, share homology with protein C and factor X, and may function as binding sites for platelet membranes. The next domains are taken by the activation peptide (AP) and its flanking sequences; the AP is formed by peptide bond cleavage at Arg 145-Ala 146 and Arg 180-Val 181. Once cleaved, the AP remains bound to factor IXa, forming disulfide-bonded light and heavy chains. The remainder of the molecule, the "trypsin-like" domain (heavy chain), contains the active center, Ser 365, which is directly involved in cleavage of its substrate, factor X, thus fulfilling its function as a serine protease.

Factor IX is activated by the cleavage of the two bonds by factor XIa or factor VIIa-tissue factor. For physiologic hemostasis, this reaction requires three co-factors: Ca++, phospholipid, and factor VIIIa. The activation of factor IX by factor VIIa-tissue factor complex is more rapid in the presence of factor X. Factor IXa is inactivated by antithrombin (AT), which forms a stable complex at the Asp 359 substrate-binding pocket.

Factor IX coagulant activity is measured by a one-stage APTT assay using factor IX-deficient plasma as substrate; the molecule can be measured quantitatively by immunologic assays using heterologous or monoclonal antibodies (IX:Ag). Activated factor IX can be determined with a chromogenic substrate method (Diapharma Xa based assay, S-2765, or a new FIXa sensitive substrate, CH_3SO_2-D-CHG-Gly-Arg-pNA Pentapharm Ltd, Basel).

GENETICS

Like hemophilia A, factor IX-deficient hemophilia or hemophilia B is an X-linked recessive bleeding disorder. The gene encoding factor IX is located near the terminus of the long arm of the X chromosome. The 34-kb gene contains eight exons and seven introns (Fig. 14-1); the number of exons and splice junction types are highly conserved in homologous vitamin K-dependent proteins.

Hemophilia B is a markedly heterogeneous disorder with a wide range of baseline factor IX and IX:Ag levels and a variety of specific gene defects. Approximately 1 in 30,000 males are affected, with most of the families showing a unique mutation. The ninth edition of the hemophilia database of point mutations and short additions and deletions listed 689 unique molecular events (*http://www.umds.ac.uk/molgen/*). The database included 1918 patient entries, with mutations detected in all regions of the factor IX gene except the poly (A) site. The list contained 425 different amino acid substitutions, and 143 short deletions and/or additions. The database overrepresents defects leading to severe disease, as these are more likely to be analyzed and reported. Founder effects contribute to overrepresentations at some specific sites. Double mutations may be underrepresented due to lack of complete gene screening. Deletions of

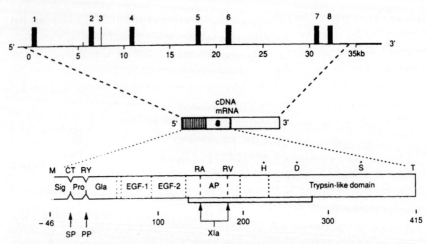

FIGURE 14-1 The factor IX gene and protein. The gene (upper portion) consists of eight exons and the seven intervening sequences totaling 34 kb. Protein is in the lower portion with amino terminus at left and carboxy terminus at right. Sig, signal peptide; the CT (cys-Thr) bond is cleaved by a single peptidase (SP). A second intracellular cleavage by a propeptidase (PP) occurs at RY (Arg-Tyr) removing propeptide (Pro) before secretion. Domains: Gla; EGF (epidermal growth factorlike regions); AP (activation peptide). Factor XIa cleaves RA (Arg-Ala) and RV (Arg-Val) to yield factor IXa. Active site residues for serine protease activity are His221 (H), Asp269 (D), and Ser365 (S). (Used with permission from Thompson AR. Structure and biology of factor IX. In: Hoffman R, et al. (eds). *Hematology Basic Principles and Practice.* New York, Churchill Livingstone, 1991, p 1308.)

the gene and some point mutations may be associated with inhibitor formation (antigen is often negative or absent), which occurs with an incidence of ~3 percent. Point mutations, the most common defect, can be associated with mild and severe hemophilia B.

The Leyden phenotype (severe hemophilia as a child that becomes mild after puberty) has been described in families with defects in the androgen-sensitive promoter region of the gene. If the promoter defect is at the 226 mutation site, disruption of the androgen-sensitive element occurs and the patient fails to recover (hemophilia B Brandenburg). Antigen-positive defects, with clinical severity that is both severe and mild, are also known. These patients have levels of factor IX:Ag that are near normal and discrepantly higher than their factor IX activity levels. Most of these families display point mutations affecting various regions of the gene, ranging from the Gla region to defects in the 180 to 182 and 390 to 397 trypsinlike (catalytic) domain. The latter defects, when associated with a dysfunctional protein that prolongs the PT when ox brain, but not human brain, is used as the source of thromboplastin, are called "BM" phenotype, most of whom have clinically severe disease. The original factor IX-deficient patient, Mr. Christmas, was a severely deficient patient (IX:C, IX:Ag < 0.01 U/mL) whose mutation was Cys206Ser. An Asn346Asp mutation results in a dysfunctional protein with disproportionate bleeding in spite of low-normal FIX activity levels in the carrier (FIX, Denver).

Carrier Detection and Prenatal Diagnosis

Carrier detection using IX activity and IX:Ag assays is possible in only about a third of families because of increased number of mutations with low IX:Ag and the effects of lyonization. At least 50 percent of obligate carriers will have a factor IX activity level < 60 percent; often the level will be in the range where bleeding may occur at time of trauma or surgery (< 30 percent activity). Currently, the most effective method to detect the carrier state is direct sequencing of an amplified DNA fragment to demonstrate heterozygosity (after the defect has been identified in the patient). DNA techniques are able to determine the gene defect in almost all cases, and must be used for attempts at prenatal diagnosis, as levels of IX:Ag and IX activity are not discriminating from the normal fetal levels in most instances (overlap of normal range, contamination by thromboplastic material).

CLINICAL MANIFESTATIONS

The clinical manifestations of mild, moderate, and severe hemophilia B are the same as for hemophilia A. Mild hemophilia B patients may have normal or near-normal APTTs. Therefore, in undiagnosed mild bleeding disorders, a factor IX assay should be performed even if the APTT is reported as normal. Markedly low levels of factor IX are sometimes observed in hemophilia B carriers (extreme lyonization). (See Chap. 13 for other causes of female hemophilia.)

ACQUIRED ALTERATIONS OF FACTOR IX

Physiologically low levels of factor IX are found in the fetus (0.05 to 0.15 U/mL at 20 weeks) and term newborn infant (0.15 to 0.50 U/mL); these levels reach the normal adult range by 6 months of age. Acquired low factor IX has been observed in liver disease, vitamin K deficiency, warfarin therapy, nephrotic syndrome, and acquired factor IX inhibitor states. Factor IX was repeatedly normal in 7 of 7 patients with Gaucher's disease, but factor XI was decreased in 3 of 9 patients tested. Because of the interfering presence of cerebroside levels, caution must be used in interpreting coagulation assays in Gaucher's disease.

Although factor IX has been reported to rise about 1.5 times in normal pregnancy, levels do not change appreciably in women who are carriers; these women may require replacement therapy at delivery. Oral estrogen-progestin agents do not appreciably alter factor IX levels.

TREATMENT AND COMPLICATIONS

The principles of treatment and discussion of complications of hemophilia B are essentially the same as noted for hemophilia A. The specific treatment of hemophilia B consists of the administration of coagulation factor IX concentrates in doses sufficient to raise the factor IX activity level to the therapeutic range. Presently, two coagulation factor IX concentrates manufactured from pooled human plasma (Mononine®, Alphanine SD®) and one that is genetically engineered (BeneFIX®) are licensed. Modern virucidal processes have rendered the newer plasma-based products free of HIV and the hepatitis viruses (see Chap. 55 for further discussion).

Prior to the advent of these coagulation concentrates, prothrombin-complex concentrates (PCC) were utilized. PCC contain the other vitamin K-dependent clotting factors in varying amounts, including activated forms (VIIa, Xa), which cause the products to be thrombogenic during surgery, treatment of crush injuries, major hemorrhages or infected states. Thrombotic complications (deep venous thrombosis, disseminated intravascular coagulation, and myocardial infarction) after use of PCC (prophylaxis, surgery) still occur; therefore, they are no longer the treatment of choice for this disorder. Fresh frozen plasma and solvent-detergent plasma also have been used to replace factor IX. However, therapeutically useful factor IX levels are difficult to obtain without overloading the patient's vascular system, and commonly available FFP is not virally inactivated.

Inhibitors to factor IX develop in approximately 3 percent of hemophilia B patients (see Chap. 20). Point mutations resulting in frameshifts and premature stop codons and gross gene deletions have been documented in association with inhibitor development. Inhibitors usually occur within the first 30 exposure days and in severely deficient patients. Anaphylactoid reactions have been reported to occur in association with inhibitors in factor IX deficiency. These reactions may precede the detection of the inhibitor, may be life threatening, are not product specific, and may necessitate the discontinuation of all factor-IX–containing products. Desensitization to factor IX in patients with anaphylactoid reactions has been successfully performed. Nephrosis has been reported in patients undergoing immune tolerance induction (ITI) to ablate the inhibitor in factor IX deficiency (see Chap. 20). Nephrosis complicating ITI typically occurs after 7 to 9 months of therapy. The etiology of the nephrosis in these patients is poorly defined but may be related to the amount of protein to which these patients are exposed. The nephrosis tends to be steroid resistant but may improve with withdrawal or decrease in the amount of factor IX exposure. Recently, severe hemophilia B has been converted to a milder form of the disease by gene transfer using an adeno- associated viral vector in three adult men.

BIBLIOGRAPHY

Billett HH et al: Coagulation abnormalities in patients with Gaucher's disease: effect of therapy. *Am J Hematol* 51:234, 1996.

Crossley M et al: Recovery from hemophilia B Leyden: An androgen responsive element in the factor IX promoter. *Science* 257:377, 1992.

Dioun AF et al: IgE-mediated allergy and desensitization to factor IX in hemophilia B. *J Allergy Clin Immunol* 102:113, 1998.

Ewenstein BM et al: Nephrotic syndrome as a complication of immune tolerance in hemophilia B. *Blood* 89:1115, 1997.

Green PM et al. Haemophilia B: database of point mutations and short additions and deletions-v9.0. *http://www.umds.ac.uk/molgen*

Guy GP et al: An unusual complication in a gravida with factor IX deficiency: Case report with review of the literature. *Obstet Gynecol* 80:502, 1992.

High KA: Factor IX: Molecular structure, epitopes, and mutations associated with inhibitor formation. In: Aledort LM, et al. (eds): *Inhibitors to Coagulation Factors*, New York, Plenum Press, 1995, pp 79–86.

Kay MA et al: Evidence for gene transfer and expression of factor IX in haemophilia B patients treated with an AAV vector. *Nat Genet* 24:257, 2000.

Ketterling RP et al: The rates and patterns of deletions in the human factor IX gene. *Am J Hum Genet* 54:201, 1994.

Ketterling RP et al: T296-M, a common mutation causing mild hemophilia B in the Amish and others: Founder effect, variability in factor IX activity assays, and rapid carrier detection. *Hum Genet* 87:333, 1991.

Kolkman JA et al: Regions 301–303 and 333–339 in the catalytic domain of blood coagulation factor IX are factor VIII-interactive sites involved in stimulation of enzyme activity. *Biochem J* 339(Part 2):217, 1999.

Lefkowitz J et al: Factor IX Denver: Asn346Asp mutation resulting in a dysfunctional protein with disproportionate bleeding in a carrier female. *Blood* 92:187a, 1998.

Lillicrap D: The molecular basis of haemophilia B. *Haemophilia* 4:350, 1998.

Prasa D, Sturzebecher J: Determination of activated factor IX in factor IX concentrates with a chromogenic substrate. *Thrombos Res* 92:99, 1998.

Spitzer SG et al: Replacement of isoleucine-397 by threonine in the clotting proteinase factor IXa (Los Angeles and Long Beach variants) affects macromolecular catalysis but not L-tosylarginine methyl ester hydrolysis. Lack of correlation between the ox brain prothrombin time and the mutation site in the variant proteins. *Biochem J* 265:219, 1990.

Taylor SAM et al: Characterization of the original Christmas disease mutation (cysteine206serine): From clinical recognition to molecular pathogenesis. *Thromb Haemost* 67:63, 1992.

Warrier I et al: Factor IX: inhibitors and anaphylaxis in hemophilia B. *Jr Ped Hem Oncol* 19:23, 1997.

White G et al: Clinical evaluation of recombinant factor IX. *Sem Hematol* 35:33, 1998.

CHAPTER 15

Hereditary Factor XI Deficiency

Hereditary factor XI (plasma thromboplastin antecedent [PTA]) deficiency was first described by Rosenthal and others in 1955 as a hemophilia-like bleeding disorder that could be treated satisfactorily with plasma. The disorder is inherited in an autosomal manner, with heterozygotes showing a factor XI coagulant activity level of 25 to 60 percent of normal while homozygotes have levels < 15 percent. Both heterozygotes and homozygotes may exhibit bleeding manifestations (usually mucous membrane or postsurgical hemorrhage) of variable severity not necessarily correlated with the plasma factor XI coagulant activity. Over half the reported cases have occurred in Jews; the Ashkenazi Jewish population in Israel has a heterozygote frequency of 1:8.

STRUCTURE–FUNCTION RELATIONSHIP

Factor XI circulates in the plasma as a glycoprotein zymogen (plasma concentration of 4 to 6 µg/mL) of the trypsin group of serine proteases and is complexed to high molecular weight kininogen (HK). The 160-kD molecule is a homodimer composed of two identical 83-kD polypeptides connected by a disulfide bond. The liver and megakaryocyte are sites of factor XI production. Each factor XI monomer is activated by factor XIIa by cleavage at the Arg 369–Ile 370 bond, resulting in a 47-kD heavy chain and a 35-kD light (contains catalytic site) chain. This contact activation of factor XI is not believed to be physiologically important since deficiencies of the contact factors are not associated with a bleeding diathesis. Recent evidence indicates that factor XI may also be cleaved by thrombin and XIa at the same site. This results in the formation of additional thrombin within the clot capable of protecting it from fibrinolytic attack, i.e., by activating a fibrinolytic inhibitor called thrombin activatable fibrinolysis inhibitor, or TAFI. Platelets contain, bind, and promote the activation of factor XI in the presence of HK; factor XIa then activates factor IX in the presence of calcium ions. Under physiologic conditions, factor XIa is inhibited mainly by α_1-antitrypsin but also by antithrombin (AT) and a platelet-specific anti-XIa (see Fig. 15-1).

GENETICS

The gene coding for factor XI is 23 kb and is found on the long arm of chromosome 4 (4q35). Factor XI deficiency is inherited as an autosomal

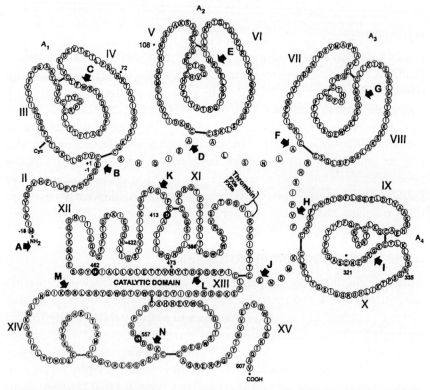

FIGURE 15-1 Amino acid sequence and primary structure of human factor XI. Factor XI circulates in plasma as a homodimer connected by a single disulfide bond linking C321 in both of the apple domains. The 14 introns (A–N) are shown by solid arrows. The exons are denoted by Roman numerals. The four apple domains are labeled A1, A2, A3, and A4. The site of cleavage catalyzed by thrombin, factor XIa, or factor XIIa during the conversion of factor XI to factor XIa is shown with a small arrow. The three members of the catalytic triad are circled in bold. The four N-linked carbohydrate chains are shown by solid diamonds. (Reproduced with permission from Walsh PN: Platelets and factor XI bypass the contact system of blood coagulation. *Thromb Haemost* 82:234, 1999.)

trait. The majority of patients have a parallel reduction in factor XI activity and antigen. Over 15 mutations in the factor XI gene have been identified (see Table 15-1). Most of the cases of factor XI deficiency occur in Ashkenazi Jews and are due to two mutations, designated type II and type III. All types of mutations now identified cause factor XI deficiency by causing a lack of protein in the plasma. Five of eight amino-acid substitutions are in the fourth apple domain of the molecule.

CLINICAL MANIFESTATIONS

The diagnosis of hereditary factor XI deficiency is usually considered in the evaluation of a mild to moderate bleeder or in the evaluation of a prolonged APTT. In addition, it may be prudent to obtain an APTT in Ashke-

TABLE 15-1

Genetic Defects in Factor XI Deficiency

Gene Mutation	Population/Race	Phenotype
Type I - splice junction mutation at exon 14- intron N boundary	Ashkenazi Jewish	Homozygote II/II, (FXI = 0.01 +/– 0.05 U/mL) homozygote III/III, (FXI = 0.09+/–0.08 U/mL)
Type II - stop codon in exon 5	Ashkenazi and Iraqi Jewish	and compound heterozygotes II/III (FXI = 0.03+/–0.016 U/mL) are
Type III - Phe283Leu at exon 9	Ashkenazi Jewish	bleeders. Severity depends on FXI level
Type IV - 14 base pair deletion at exon 14- intron N boundary	Ashkenazi Jewish	II/IV compound heterozygote (FXI = <0.01 U/mL)
Phe442Val Cys128(nonsense codon)	Non-Jewish Non-Jewish	Heterozygote, mild bleeder
Thr386Asp	Arab	Homozygote (FXI = 0.02 U/mL); mild bleeder
Ser248Glu Glu226Arg	African American	Compound heterozygote (FXI = 0.42 U/mL); moderate to severe bleeder
Asp16His Leu302Pro Thr304Ile Glu323Lys Exon 9 - exon 10 splice defect Splice junction defect in exon 5	Non-Jewish Non-Jewish Non-Jewish Non-Jewish Non-Jewish Non-Jewish	Homozygote (FXI = 0.03 U/mL); mild bleeding Heterozygote (FXI = 0.25–0.68 U/mL) trivial bleeding

nazi Jews prior to surgical procedures, especially in children who may not have a positive bleeding history. Hemorrhagic manifestations include prolonged bleeding after surgery or dental extractions, after childbirth or abortion, epistaxis, menorrhagia or easy bruising. Homozygous (0 to 0.15 U/mL) or heterozygous (0.25 to 0.70 U/mL) states can often be separated from the normal adult range by the factor XI activity assay performed on a freshly drawn plasma sample (frozen samples may increase activity). The lower limits of normal used to separate possible heterozygotes may be as high as 0.70 U/mL for factor XI activity. Family studies in Ashkenazi Jews showed a greater overlap between heterozygotes and normal, and suggested the need for molecular studies in borderline cases. When factor XI antigen has been measured, a close correlation with activity assays was seen, with rare exception of a homozygote positive for antigen. The bleeding time is prolonged in some cases, possibly indicating a platelet factor XI defect. As many as 50 percent of heterozygotes may have mildly prolonged bleeding times (personal data).

The frequency and severity of bleeding manifestations have not always correlated with the clotting factor level (heterozygote or homozygote). Some homozygotes do not bleed even after surgical stress, whereas heterozygotes are sometimes severe bleeders. In a detailed study of 45 families (Ashkenazi), bleeding manifestations were documented in 58 percent of 26 homozygous or doubly heterozygous patients, in 20 percent of 46 heterozygotes, and 9 percent of normal family members. Bleeding correlated negatively with factor XI levels, with major factor XI deficiency being a strong predictor of bleeding. In 30 other families (mostly non-Jewish) 48 percent of heterozygotes had a bleeding tendency, including some individuals with factor XI levels between 0.50 and 0.70 U/mL. The possible causes of this variable bleeding tendency that may be associated with, or part of, hereditary factor XI deficiency are listed in Table 15-2. Bleeding tendency is usually, but not always consistent, within a kindred. Associated defects (hemophilia A, platelet function defects, von Willebrand disease) can occur and may be associated with increased bleeding. Noonan's syndrome (dysmorphic facies, short stature, congenital heart disease, easy bruising) is often associated with partial factor XI deficiency. As shown in the patient described in Table 15-3, possible platelet-factor XI interaction defects could result in abnormal bleeding times and a greater hemorrhagic tendency. This example and others in the literature suggest that normal platelet transfusions are sometimes needed to correct the bleeding defect in these patients.

A recent observation that tissue (i.e., platelet)-specific expression of functional factor XI is independent of plasma factor XI expression suggests that patients may exist with marked discrepancies of platelet and

---

TABLE 15-2

Possible Causes of Variation in Severity of Bleeding Tendency in Hereditary Factor XI Deficiency

Inheritance of associated hemostatic defect
  von Willebrand disease
  Platelet function defect (storage pool disease, Bernard-Soulier disease, Glanzmann thrombasthenia)
  Other coagulopathy (factor VIII deficiency)
  Noonan's syndrome

Group O blood type, borderline low vWF activity

Drug ingestion (ASA)

Quantitative/qualitative defect in factor XI molecule

Quantitative/qualitative abnormality in platelet-associated factor XI

Reduced activation of TAFI resulting in clot susceptibility to fibrinolysis.

---

plasma factor XI availability. In addition, factor XI deficiency could result in less TAFI (see Table 15-2) activation and make the clot more susceptible to fibrinolysis. These findings could explain the enigma of homozygotes who do not bleed and heterozygotes who bleed profusely. Interestingly, increased levels of factor XI may be a risk factor for venous thrombosis (see Meijers et al reference).

TABLE 15-3

Hereditary Factor XI Deficiency with Prolonged Bleeding Time*—Effect of Treatment on Hemorrhagic Tendency

Age	Bleeding Episode	Treatment	Response
22	Postpartum hemorrhage	Curettage	Cessation
29	Cervical biopsy	RBC transfusion	Gradual cessation
30	Cone biopsy of cervix	FFP, 15–20 U/kg × 3: RBCs	Minimal effect
		10 packs platelets + DDAVP	Cessation
31	Exploratory laparotomy	5 packs platelets + DDAVP	No response
		10 packs platelets + FFP × 2	Cessation

* Both patient and her son have factor XI levels of 0.25–0.40 U/mL and prolonged bleeding times (often > 20 min); von Willebrand factor and platelet aggregation studies were normal except for decreased response to L-epinephrine.
Note that patient bleeding did not respond to FFP alone in dose that raised factor XI level to 0.6 U/mL.
FFP, fresh frozen plasma; RBC, red blood cells.

TREATMENT

Infusions of fresh frozen plasma or solvent/detergent-treated pooled plasma into hereditary XI-deficient patients have shown the factor XI half-disappearance time to be 45 to 55 h. Frequent infusions (12 to 24 h) are necessary to maintain levels of 40 to 60 percent. A factor XI concentrate available in the UK (Bioproducts Laboratory-BPL) has been used extensively in Europe. Even though the product contains antithrombin, thrombotic events have occurred; viral safety data indicates no transmission of HIV or hepatitis. Since 1993, a factor XI concentrate (Hemoleven) has been used in France (LFB, Lille). The product contains both AT and heparin but has been associated with activation of coagulation and DIC. Both products should be used with caution. Mucous membrane and dental bleeding, frequently seen in factor XI-deficient patients, may respond nicely to adjunctive therapy with antifibrinolytic agents. DDAVP has shown efficacy for surgical hemorrhage in a few patients. An acquired factor XI inhibitor may rarely develop in the transfused patient and may be detected by APTT mixing studies or a Bethesda-type assay (see Chap. 20).

BIBLIOGRAPHY

Asakai R et al: Factor XI deficiency in Ashkenazi Jews in Israel. *N Engl J Med* 325:153, 1991.

Bolton-Maggs PHB et al: Definition of the bleeding tendency in factor XI-deficient kindreds—a clinical and laboratory study. *Thromb Haemost* 73:194, 1995.

Bolton-Maggs PHB et al: The management of factor XI deficiency. *Hemophilia* 4:683, 1998.

Bouma BN, Miejers JCM: Fibrinolysis and the contact system: a role for factor XI in the down-regulation of fibrinolysis. *Thromb Haemost* 82:243, 1999.

Brenner B et al: Bleeding predictors in factor-XI-deficient patients. *Blood Coag Fibrinol* 8:511, 1997.

Cawthern KM et al: Blood coagulation in hemophilia A and hemophilia C. *Blood* 91:4581, 1998.

Castaman G et al: Clinical usefulness of desmopressin for prevention of surgical bleeding in patients with symptomatic heterozygous factor XI deficiency. *Br J Haematol* 94:168, 1996.

Hancock JF et al: A molecular genetic study of factor XI deficiency. *Blood* 77:1942, 1991.

Hu CJ et al: Tissue-specific expression of functional platelet factor XI is independent of plasma factor XI expression. *Blood* 91:3800, 1998.

Imanaka Y et al: Identification of two novel mutations in non-Jewish factor XI deficiency. *Br J Haematol* 90:916, 1995.

Kitchens CS: Factor XI: A review of its biochemistry and deficiency. *Semin Thromb Hemost* 17:55, 1991.

Martincic D et al: Factor XI messenger RNA in human platelets. *Blood* 94:3397, 1999.

Martincic D et al: Identification of mutations and polymorphisms in the factor XI genes of an African American family by dideoxy fingerprinting. *Blood* 92:3309, 1998.

Meijers JCM et al: High levels of coagulation factor XI as a risk factor for venous thrombosis. *N Eng J Med* 342:696, 2000.

Ragni MV et al: Comparison of bleeding tendency, factor XI coagulant activity, and factor XI antigen in 25 factor XI-deficient kindreds. *Blood* 65:719, 1985.

Rosenthal RL et al: Plasma thromboplastin antecedent (PTA) deficiency: Clinical, coagulation, therapeutic and hereditary aspects of a new hemophilia-like disease. *Blood* 10:120, 1955.

Pugh RE et al: Six point mutations that cause factor XI deficiency. *Blood* 85:1509, 1995.

Schnall SF et al: Acquired factor XI inhibitors in congenitally deficient patients. *Am J Hematol* 26:323, 1987.

Sharland M et al: Coagulation-factor deficiencies and abnormal bleeding in Noonan's syndrome. *Lancet* 339:19, 1992.

Shpilberg O et al: One of the two common mutations causing factor XI deficiency in Ashkenazi Jews (type II) is also prevalent in Iraqi Jews, who represent the ancient gene pool of Jews. *Blood* 85:429, 1995.

von dem Borne PA et al: Feedback activation of factor XI by thrombin in plasma results in additional formation of thrombin that protects fibrin clots from fibrinolysis. *Blood* 86:3035, 1995.

Walsh PN: Platelets and factor XI bypass the contact system of blood coagulation. *Thromb Haemost* 82:234, 1999.

Weinstock DJ, Schwartz AD: Factor XI deficiency in an Ashkenazi Jewish child, causing severe postoperative hemorrhage. *J Pediatr Surg* 30:1746, 1995.

Wistinghausen B et al: Severe factor XI deficiency in an Arab family associated with a novel mutation in exon 11. *Br J Haematol* 99:575, 1997.

CHAPTER 16

Contact Factor Deficiencies

Hereditary deficiencies of factor XII (Hageman factor), prekallikrein (PK, Fletcher factor), and high molecular weight kininogen (HK, Fitzgerald, Flaujeac, Williams factors) are coagulation curiosities; all three are associated with a strikingly prolonged APTT without a bleeding diathesis. These coagulation factors, along with factor XI (see Chap. 15), are responsible for the initiation of coagulation through the intrinsic pathway. According to a recently revised hypothesis (see Schmaier reference) circulating complexes of PK-HK assemble on multiprotein receptors on the endothelial cell surface, where factor XII activation is secondary to PK activation. Factor XIIa amplifies PK cleavage to kallikrein and activates factor XI to XIa. Kallikrein cleaves bradykinin from kininogen and is partly responsible for intrinsic plasma fibrinolysis by converting plasminogen to plasmin via activation of urokinase. The biologic consequences and differential diagnosis of the contact factor deficiencies are discussed in the following.

FACTOR XII DEFICIENCY

Factor XII (Hageman factor) is a serine protease glycoprotein with a molecular weight of approximately 84,000 D and a plasma concentration of 30 μg/mL. In vitro surface-mediated (glass, kaolin, silica, dextran sulfate, endotoxin, urates, crude collagen, sulfatides) activation and direct cleavage by kallikrein produce a series of proteolytic cleavages of factor XII that further activates PK and other proenzymes, including factor VII, plasminogen, and complement, C1. With generation of Hageman factor fragments and kallikrein, the contact system is linked to the kinin system, the intrinsic fibrinolytic system, and the complement system. The major inhibitor of factor XIIa is C1 inhibitor; other inhibitors are antithrombin, plasminogen activator inhibitor (PAI), and α_2-macroglobulin.

Factor XII is produced by a single gene located on chromosome 5. Hageman factor deficiency is inherited in an autosomal recessive manner with homozygotes (or double heterozygotes) having <0.01 U/mL factor XII. Heterozygotes show plasma levels ranging from 0.17 to 0.83 U/mL in various studies. The prevalence of severe and mild factor XII deficiency in the normal population has been estimated to be 1.5 to 3 percent. In our experience the most common cause of an isolated prolongation of the APTT in a nonbleeding child or adult (without a lupus anticoagulant) is mild factor XII deficiency. This rather common prevalence of low fac-tor XII levels, as well as the lower levels observed in Asians, may be explained by a recently reported genetic polymorphism (46 C-T substitution) in the 5'-untranslated region of the gene that is associated with low factor XII coagulant activity and antigen. Most of homozygous factor XII subjects are antigen negative; only 2 of 81 cases tested showed factor XII:Ag levels of 0.39 and 0.80 U/mL. Hageman factor deficiency is not associated with a bleeding tendency even at major surgery or pregnancy; however, some individuals with factor XII deficiency have had a thrombotic tendency. In a series of 103 patients with recurrent thromboembolic disease, 15 percent had low factor XII levels in the heterozygous range. Some authors have suggested including factor XII assays in routine thrombophilia screening programs, but a recent study of 350 unselected deep vein thrombosis patients found no increased factor XII deficiency as compared to controls. Activation of the contact system and plasminogen activation after DDAVP infusion occurred in healthy volunteers and was absent in factor-XII–deficient subjects.

Acquired alterations (both increased or decreased levels of factor XIIa, PK, HK, and C-1 INH, as well as the occurrence of kallikrein-inhibitor complexes) of the contact system have been noted in many disorders. These disorders include meningococcal septic shock, other septicemias, coronary artery heart disease, unstable angina pectoris, cardiopulmonary bypass, pharmacological thrombolysis, and both hereditary and acquired angioedema. Spontaneous increase in factor VII activity after cold storage of plasma (cold-promoted activation) depends on factor XII and increased kallikrein activity, and is seen in pregnancy and oral contraceptive users with elevated levels of factor XII.

PREKALLIKREIN (FLETCHER FACTOR) DEFICIENCY

Prekallikrein is a fast-migrating gamma globulin with two forms having molecular weights of 85,000 and 88,000; it circulates in a concentration of

35 to 45 μg/mL as an equimolar complex with HK activation of PK (Fig. 16-1) producing a heavy chain that binds to HK and a light chain with the enzymatic active site. As a protease, kallikrein liberates kinins from kininogens, activates factor XII, activates plasminogen, converts prorenin to renin, interacts with human leukocytes, and destroys C1 components. The major circulating inhibitor of kallikrein is C1 inhibitor plus α_2-macroglobulin and AT. PK may be measured in plasma by amidolytic (substrate PPAN, S-2302), esterolytic, coagulation, and immunochemical assays; the coagulation assay using Fletcher-factor–deficient plasma has limited accuracy due to the need for high plasma dilutions and critical incubation times.

PK, which shares a 58% homology with factor XI, is produced by a single gene that is mapped to chromosome 4. The hereditary deficiency of

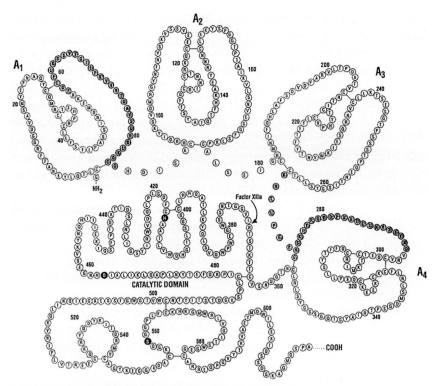

FIGURE 16-1 The structure of prekallikrein. The letters A1 through A4 represent the apple domains of the heavy chain. The arrow at Arg371 represents the factor XII activation site. A circle with a shaded background represents the regions involved in binding to high molecular weight kininogen. (Reproduced with permission from Coleman RW, Schmaier AH: Contact system: a vascular biology modulator with anticoagulant, profibrinolytic, antiadhesive, and proinflammatory attributes. *Blood* 90:3819, 1997.)

PK, or Fletcher factor deficiency, is a rare disorder with few clinical or laboratory consequences except a markedly prolonged APTT without a bleeding tendency. Inheritance is autosomal recessive with the heterozygotes displaying intermediate to normal levels of prekallikrein. Evidence that 5 of 18 homozygotes are antigen positive has been reported. Although the homozygotes' plasma may show in vitro impaired intrinsic fibrinolysis, decreased chemotactic activity, and decreased kinin generation, physiologic observations in humans have failed to reveal any significant impairment in hemostasis, fibrinolysis, or inflammatory responses. Reported clinical associations with the homozygous condition include myocardial infarction, cerebral thrombosis, hyperthyroidism (two cases), and systemic lupus erythematosus (SLE). A patient has been reported with an acquired autoantibody to PK (prolonged APTT, PK of 0.02U/mL), which inhibited the activation of the contact system.

Gestationally dependent decreased levels of PK as well as factor XII have been observed in preterm and term infants and are known to rise to adult levels by 6 months of age. Moderately low levels of PK (15 to 75 percent) are seen in most homozygous HK-deficient subjects. Decreased PK occurs in hereditary angioedema (C1 inhibitor deficiency), infections (bacterial sepsis, typhoid fever, Rocky Mountain spotted fever, dengue), DIC, liver disease, nephrosis, sickle cell disease, chronic renal failure, type II hyperlipoproteinemia, renal allograft rejection, and adult and infant respiratory distress syndrome. These alterations of PK are usually interpreted to mean activation of the contact system.

HIGH MOLECULAR WEIGHT KININOGEN DEFICIENCY

Kininogens occur in human plasma in two forms: HK (120 kD) and a low molecular weight form, LK (68 kD). Both are the products of a single gene that on proteolytic cleavage give rise to bradykinin, a mediator of vasodilation, smooth muscle contraction, and increased vascular permeability; in addition, both are potent inhibitors of cysteine proteases (cathepsins, calpain). HK, but not LK, also plays an important role in the contact phase of coagulation as a carrier and cell surface receptor for factor XI and PK; as a cofactor, HK facilitates enzyme–substrate interactions on the surface since neither factor XI nor PK binds directly to the surface. Other functions ascribed to HK include inhibition of thrombin-induced platelet aggregation, participation in fibrinolysis, and an antiadhesive property (fibrinogen, vitronectin) These structure–function relationships are shown in Fig. 16-2.

When prekallikrein binds to HK on the cell surface (endothelial cells, platelets, neutrophils) in the presence of zinc ions and a membrane-

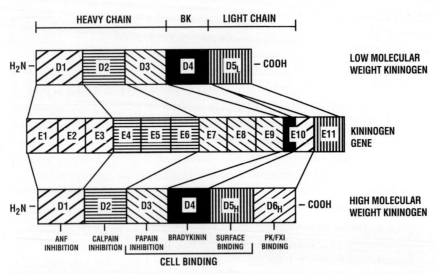

FIGURE 16-2 The domain structure of the kininogens. (Reproduced with permission from Coleman RW, Schmaier AH: Contact system: a vascular biology modulator with anticoagulant, profibrinolytic, antiadhesive, and proinflammatory attributes. *Blood* 90:3819, 1997.)

associated thiolprotease, PK can be activated to kallikrein independently of factor XII and an artificial surface. The amount of HK present regulates the production of kallikrein and, subsequently, factor XIIa. Therefore, deficiency of HK interferes with optimal activation of the contact factor pathway and results in deficient intrinsic activation of factor XI and, subsequently, factor IX, as well as deficient intrinsic fibrinolysis and decreased kinin system functions. These deficiencies have been demonstrated in the plasma of the rare individuals with hereditary deficiencies of HK (Fitzgerald, Williams, Flaujeac traits); since both HK and LK are the result of alternative mRNA splicing of the same gene, most of the dozen or so reported individuals have deficiencies of both the kininogens. Nevertheless, no clinical evidence of hemostatic or other defect has been noted in either the homozygotes (HK usually < 0.01 U/mL) or heterozygotes (HK approximately 0.5 U/mL).

DIAGNOSIS OF CONTACT FACTOR DISORDERS

The diagnosis of a hereditary deficiency of factor XII, PK, or HK is usually considered when evaluating a prolonged APTT in situations where the other screening tests and the clinical history are noncontributory, that is, the diagnosis of the "isolated" prolonged APTT in a nonbleeder. Consideration of Table 16-1 and Fig. 16-3 allow several generalizations to be made.

TABLE 16-1

TABLE 16-1

Coagulation Studies in Hereditary Deficiencies of Contact System

Deficiency	Genotype	Usual Factor Assay* U/mL	Screening APTT(s)	Percent NP corrects PTT	Correction of KPTT, 10 min inc at 37°C
Factor XII	Ho	<0.01	Greatly↑	50	No
(Hageman)	He	0.25–0.55	Slight↑		Yes
Prekallikrein	Ho	<0.01	Greatly↑	>2	Yes
(Fletcher)	He	≈0.5	Normal		
HMWK	Ho	<0.01	Greatly↑	>12.5	No
(Flaujeac, Fitzgerald, Williams)	He	0.3–0.6	Normal		

Some heterozygotes will have factor levels in the normal range and normal screening APTT. He, heterozygote; Ho, homozygote; KPTT, kaolin PPT; NP, normal plasma; inc, incubation.

If the APTT is greatly prolonged (usually greater than twofold the APTT of a severe factor-VIII–deficient hemophiliac) and corrects to the normal range with 1:1 mixing with normal plasma, the homozygous deficiency state (factor XII, PK, or HK) is suspect (factor XII deficiency is more common). If a 10 minute incubation of the patient's plasma (as compared to the usual 3 minutes) "corrects" to near normal (using kaolin or micronized silica as the activator in an APTT), the deficiency state is due to PK; this is the so-called "Fletcher factor" screening test, which is only applicable to possible homozygotes. Specific coagulation factor activity assays using congenitally deficient plasmas and the APTT system are necessary for confirmation and differentiation of factor XII from HK deficiency. The use of potent activators like ellagic acid in the APTT system of or long incubation times, may not allow these differentiations to be made precisely.

Heterozygous Deficiency States

In our own and other laboratories the cause of an "isolated" mildly prolonged APTT (if due to contact factor deficiency and not a LA) is almost always moderate to mild factor XII deficiency. Note that in Fig. 16-3 only factor-XII–deficient plasma corrects into the normal range on 10 minute incubation. The APTT in heterozygotes of PK and HK is usually normal; plasmas contain much greater levels of PK (over 2 percent) and HMWK (over 12.5 percent) than are necessary for the normalization of the APTT. Remember that HK-deficient plasmas usually have a low levels of PK as well. A rare patient may have mild deficiencies of all three factors. Family

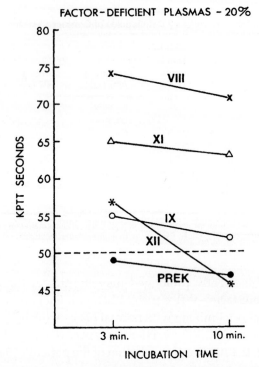

FACTOR–DEFICIENT PLASMAS – 20%

FIGURE 16-3 The results of kaolin PTTs are shown for hereditary deficiencies of various clotting factors (severely deficient plasmas mixed with normal plasma to yield a 0.20 U/mL factor level) at 3 minute and 10 minute incubation times.

members (potential heterozygotes) of a diagnosed homozygous contact-factor–deficiency patient should be identified to prevent future expensive evaluations of a possible mildly prolonged APTT (see Chap. 4).

Plasma samples from some patients with the lupus anticoagulant may give falsely low levels for factor XII in APTT-based clotting assays. If a LA is confirmed, factor XII measurements by a chromogenic or immunologic method should be performed to document a "true" factor XII deficiency.

BIBLIOGRAPHY

Colman RW, Schmaier AH: Contact system: A vascular biology modulator with anticoagulant, profibrinolytic, antiadhesive, and proinflammatory attributes. *Blood* 90:3819, 1997.

Cugno M et al: Activation of the coagulation cascade in C1-inhibitor deficiencies. *Blood* 89:3213, 1997.

DeLa Cadena RA: Fletcher factor deficiency in a 9-year-old girl: mechanisms of the contact pathway of blood coagulation. *Am J Hematol* 48:273, 1995.

Ewald GA, Eisenberg PR: Plasmin-mediated activation of contact system in response to pharmacological thrombolysis. *Circulation* 91:28, 1995

Gallimore MJ et al: Factor XII determinations in the presence and absence of phospholipid antibodies. *Thromb Haemost* 79:87, 1998.

Gordon EM et al: Reduced titers of Hageman factor (factor XII) in Orientals. *Ann Intern Med* 95:697, 1981.

Halbmayer WM et al: The prevalence of factor XII deficiency in 103 orally anticoagulated outpatients suffering from recurrent venous and/or arterial thromboembolism. *Thromb Haemost* 68:285, 1992.

Hathaway WE et al: Clinical and physiologic studies of two siblings with prekallikrein (Fletcher factor) deficiency. *Am J Med* 60:654, 1976.

Hoffmeister HM et al: Alterations of coagulation and fibrinolytic and kallikrein-kinin systems in the acute and postacute phases in patients with unstable angina pectoris. *Circulation* 91:2520, 1995.

Kanaji T et al: A common genetic polymorphism (46 C to T substitution) in the 5' untranslated region of the coagulation factor XII gene is associated with low translation efficiency and decrease in plasma factor XII level. *Blood* 91:2010, 1998.

Kondo S et al: Factor XII Tenri, a novel cross-reacting material negative Factor XII deficiency, occurs through a proteasome-mediated degradation. *Blood* 93:4300, 1999.

Koster T et al: John Hageman's factor and deep-vein thrombosis: Leiden thrombophilia study. *Br J Haematol* 87:422, 1994.

Lammle B et al: Thromboembolism and bleeding tendency in congenital factor XII deficiency—a study on 74 subjects from 14 Swiss families. *Thromb Haemost* 65:117, 1991.

Levi M et al: Reduction of contact activation related fibrinolytic activity in factor XII deficient patients. Further evidence for the role of the contact system in fibrinolysis in vivo. *J Clin Invest* 88:1155, 1991.

Mitropoulos KA et al: Activation of factors XII and VII induced in citrated plasma in the presence of contact surface. *Thromb Res* 78:67, 1995.

Page JD et al: An autoantibody to human prekallikrein blocks activation of the contact system. *Br J Haematol* 87:81, 1994.

Schmaier AH et al: Activation of the plasma kallikrein/kinin system on cells: a revised hypothesis. *Thromb Haemost* 82:226, 1999.

Stormorken H et al: A new case of total kininogen deficiency. *Thromb Res* 60:457, 1990.

Wuillemin WA et al: Activation of the intrinsic pathway of coagulation in children with meningococcal septic shock. *Thromb Haemost* 74:1436, 1995.

CHAPTER 17

Prothrombin, Factor V, Factor VII, Factor X, and Combined Factor Defects

Quantitative and qualitative deficiencies of factor II (prothrombin), factor V (proaccelerin, labile factor), factor VII (proconvertin), and factor X (Stuart-Prower factor) can result in bleeding disorders of varying severity. All of these factor deficiencies are inherited as an autosomal recessive trait (bleeding is noted primarily in the homozygote or double heterozygotes). These disorders are rare: factor II deficiency, fewer than 30 families reported; factor V deficiency, one person per million; factor VII deficiency, 1/500,000; factor X deficiency, 1/500,000. Combined coagulation factor deficiencies will also be discussed below.

PROTHROMBIN DEFICIENCY

Prothrombin (factor II) is a vitamin K-dependent single chain glycoprotein of 579 amino acids with a molecular weight of 72,000 D and a plasma concentration of about 100 µg/mL. Prothrombin is converted to thrombin by factor Xa in the presence of Ca^{++}, factor Va, and phospholipids, a complex is called prothrombinase (Fig. 17-1). The activation of prothrombin results in several well-defined products: Xa cleavage at Arg 271–Thr 272 yields fragment 1–2 (used as a marker of intravascular coagulation) and prethrombin 2, which produces alpha-thrombin. In addition, prothrombinase or the venom of *Echis carinatus* cleaves Arg 320–Ile 321 to produce a two-chain thrombin precursor (meizothrombin) that autocatalyzes to thrombin. Physiologically, the primary enzymatic product is termed alpha-thrombin and is generated via meizothrombin or prethrombin 2. The autolysis products of alpha-thrombin, which have

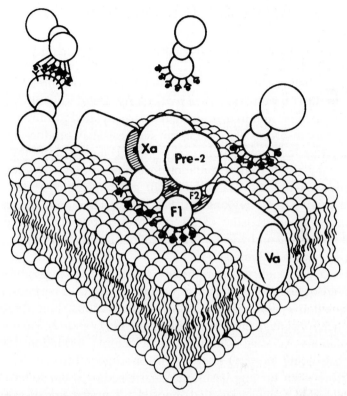

FIGURE 17-1 The prothrombinase complex. Factor Va is shown as a relatively hydrophobic protein binding to the phospholipid bilayer and forming the receptor for one molecule of factor Xa. Factor Xa is shown represented to interact both with factor Va; and, through its γ-carboxyglutamic acid-containing region, with the phospholipid surface itself. A molecule of prothrombin with its three domains, prothrombin fragment 1, fragment 2, and prethrombin 2, is shown associated with factor Va, factor Xa, and the phospholipid surface. Calcium ions are represented by small black dots. Prothrombin molecules are represented in solution both as dimers and monomers and also binding directly to the phospholipid membrane. [From Nesheim et al. In: Mann KG, Taylor FB (eds): *The Regulation of Coagulation,* New York, Elsevier, 1980, p. 145.]

little fibrinogen-clotting activity, are called beta-thrombin and gamma-thrombin.

Several types of assays are available for determination of the biologic activity of prothrombin. The two-stage assay incubates plasma sample with "tissue thromboplastin;" calcium; and factors V, VII, X; and subsamples into a fibrinogen mixture to measure maximum thrombin generation. The one-stage assay is performed similarly, but the fibrinogen is present in the initial incubation and the assay measures rate of thrombin evolution. Both prothrombin and noncarboxylated prothrombin can be activated by *E. carinatus* venom in the absence of Ca^{++}, phospholipid, or factor V.

Several chromogenic substrates are available for use in bioassays of prothrombin (S-2238, S-2160, and Chromozym TH). Immunologic assays that do not distinguish between functional and nonfunctional zymogen molecules (total prothrombin) are particularly useful in identifying dys-prothrombinemias and in measuring noncarboxylated prothrombin.

Hereditary disorders of prothrombin synthesis may produce decreased production of the prothrombin polypeptide chain (hypoprothrombine-mia), or may result from a mutation in the gene that codes for a pre-propeptide region, the Gla domain (10 gamma-carboxyglutamic acid residues), two kringle regions (F1, F2), a light chain, and the catalytic domain. The characteristics of the dysprothrombinemic molecule will depend on the site and effect of the mutation. Examples of these genetic defects are shown in Table 17-1.

Hereditary deficiencies of prothrombin include (1) hypoprothrombine-mia (severe or homozygous; mild or heterozygous); (2) dysprothrombine-mias (qualitative abnormalities, either heterozygous, homozygous, or double heterozygous); and (3) combinations of (1) and (2). Hemorrhagic manifestations are easy bruising and hematoma formation, epistaxis, menorrhagia, and bleeding after trauma or surgery. Bleeding symptoms (postcircumcision oozing, gastrointestinal bleeding, hematomas) in the neonatal period may be initially diagnosed as hemorrhagic disease of the newborn. Hemarthroses are rare. Severe deficiencies (< 0.01 U/mL) have not been reported and may be incompatible with life. Heterozygotes show intermediate prothrombin levels and are asymptomatic.

Laboratory manifestations show a normal hemostatic screen except for prolongation of the APTT and PT; *E. carinatus* venom (Ecarin) clotting time is often abnormal. Discordant levels of prothrombin antigen (high) and activity (low) favor a dysprothrombin, but low concordant levels can be seen in both dysprothrombins and severe hypoprothrombins (see Table 17-1).

Acquired deficiencies of prothrombin include vitamin K deficiency (Chap. 22), liver disease (Chap. 23), and prothrombin deficiency associated with the lupus anticoagulant (Chap. 43) and warfarin therapy (Chap. 60).

Therapy of acute bleeding episodes may be accomplished by achieving a plasma level of 25 percent with fresh frozen plasma. Repeat transfusions are usually not necessary because of the long half-life of prothrombin (3 days).

More intense therapy (major surgery) may require prothrombin-complex concentrates (PCCs) that contain adequate prothrombin. Dana-

TABLE 17-1

Genetic Defects in Dysprothrombinemias

Variant Designation	Mutation and impaired function	Activity (U/dL)	Antigen (U/dL)	Clinical
Madrid Barcelona Obihira	Arg271Cys; FXa activation	3–5	100	Homozygote; severe bleeding
Padua Dhahran	Arg271His; FXa activation	5	95	Homozygote; severe bleeding
Himi I Himi II	Met337Thr; Arg388His; Fib binding	9–10	88	Compd heterozygote; no bleeding
Molise I Tokushima	Arg418Trp; Fib binding	12 12	52 40	Hypo[1]-dys; moderate bleeding
Frankfurt Salakta	Glu466Ala; substrate binding site	13 15	91 100	Homozygote; severe bleeding or none (Salakta)
Corpus Christi Quick I	Arg382Cys; Fib binding site	2	25	Hypo[2]-dys; moderate bleeding (Corpus Christi)
Quick II	Gly558Val; "Arg/Lys binding pocket"	<2	37	Quick I + II-compd heterozygote; severe bleeder
Denver I Denver II	Glu300Lys/Glu309Lys Factor Xa activation	5	20	Compd heterozygote; severe bleeding
Undesignated (Poort)	Tyr44Cys; Gla domain defect	2	5	Homozygote; severe bleeding
Undesignated (Poort)	Cys138Tyr, Trp337Cys; Kringle I defect	4	3	Compd heterozygote; severe bleeding
Greenville	Arg517Gln; fibrinogen interaction	51	102	Heterozygote; No bleeding
Undesignated (Tamary)	Arg340Trp; unstable thrombin	8	4	Compd heterozygote; Hypo[3]-dys; moderate bleeding

[1] Reading frame shift exon 6 (Tokushima)
[2] Replacement of Gln541 with premature stop codon
[3] Frame shift, exon 8, termination of translation

zol or corticosteroids has been used to treat the hypoprothrombinemia associated with the lupus anticoagulant.

FACTOR V DEFICIENCY

Factor V is a large glycoprotein with a molecular weight of 330,000; it circulates in a single chain form with a concentration of 7 μg/mL. Factor V is 40 percent identical to factor VIII, with a similar domain structure (A1,A2, B, A3, C1, C2) Factor V is synthesized in megakaryocytes, vascular endothelial cells, and hepatocytes; 25 percent of the circulating factor V is found in the alpha-granules of platelets. Factor V can be activated by thrombin, Xa, and platelet proteases; the activated factor V or Va binds to the phospholipid bilayer of cell membranes (platelets, endothelial cells, monocytes) forming a receptor for factor Xa and prothrombin; this complex (termed prothrombinase) is responsible for the conversion of prothrombin to thrombin and is much more efficient than Xa alone (see Fig. 17-1). Like factor VIIIa, Va is rapidly inactivated by activated protein C (APC) unless the factor V has a single amino acid substitution (R506Q), which can occur in up to 7 percent of the population and is associated with a thrombotic tendency (Factor V Leiden, Chap. 40). Plasmin also produces proteolytic degradation of factor Va after first enhancing the procoagulant effect.

The factor V gene (80kb) has been mapped to chromosome 1q21–q25 and has 25 exons. Hereditary factor V deficiency or parahemophilia is a mild to moderately severe bleeding disorder inherited in an autosomal recessive mode. The bleeding disorder is variable, with some patients showing surgical- and trauma-induced hemorrhage, menorrhagia, postpartum hemorrhage, neonatal intracranial hemorrhage (ICH), epistaxis, and rare deep hematoma or joint bleeding, while other patients with similar factor V levels have little or no bleeding. The platelet content of factor V is sometimes correlated with these observations. The hemorrhagic form of factor V deficiency is rare (one per million) and only a few genetic defects have been described. A factor-V–deficient family carrying a mutant allele containing a Ala221Val substitution (Factor V New Brunswick) is particularly interesting because the children who were bleeders had the abnormal allele from the father plus a missing or nonexpressed allele from the mother. In another family, a 7-year-old girl with mild bleeding was homozygous for a 4 bp deletion in exon 13 resulting in near-absent factor V activity and antigen in both plasma and platelets. Severe hereditary factor V deficiency has been reported with multiple congenital anomalies (three families).

The homozygotes display coagulant activity levels of < 10 percent of normal, usually with comparable factor V antigen levels. A few patients (4 of 14 and 2 of 21 in two series) have increased factor V antigen, indicating a dysproteinemia. Factor V levels are lower in patients' platelets than in normals and an occasional patient will show a prolonged bleeding time. As expected, the APTT and PT will be prolonged. The evaluation of a new patient should include a factor VIII assay because combined deficiencies of factor V and factor VIII can occur. All other hemostatic tests are normal.

Heterozygotes (type 1 quantitative defects) do not have a bleeding tendency; their factor V levels will range from 40 to 60 percent of normal; occasionally the PT will be prolonged by 1 to 2 sec. An interesting family with a severe bleeding disorder and plasma factor V levels of 36 to 40 percent had a qualitative factor V defect in their platelets in association with mild thrombocytopenia and a slightly prolonged bleeding time (factor V Quebec). These patients have recently been shown to have an inherited disorder distinct from other platelet dysfunctions and associated with decreased platelet multimerin (a massive multimeric factor V binding protein), as well as abnormal thrombospondin, vWF, and fibrinogen in platelet lysates. Platelet aggregation was abnormal to epinephrine.

Acquired factor V deficiency has been noted in acute and chronic liver disease, disseminated intravascular coagulation (DIC) syndromes, and due to acquired inhibitors.

Bleeding episodes are treated with infusions of fresh frozen plasma in a dose to raise the level 20 to 25 percent. No concentrated products are available. Successful management of surgical procedures has been accomplished with daily infusions of fresh frozen plasma. Platelet concentrates are effective in therapy but should be reserved for more serious bleeding or inhibitor patients to prevent platelet alloimmunization.

FACTOR VII DEFICIENCY

Factor VII (proconvertin), a vitamin K-dependent and liver-produced single-chain glycoprotein (50 kD), circulates in a concentration of 0.5 µg/mL. Several enzymes may activate (cleavage of Arg152–Ile153 bond) factor VII to the two-chain form VIIa in vitro: thrombin, plasmin, factor XIIa, factor IXa, and factor Xa (factor IXa is probably the most important in vivo). Coagulation is initiated when VII/VIIa binds to tissue factor (TF) exposed on disrupted cells, forming a complex that generates the active forms of Xa and IXa; these enzymes proteolytically activate factor VII to the 40- to 120-fold more active VIIa. Since native factor VII and

VIIa have the same affinity for TF, the excess amount of factor VII that is available competes for the TF and prevents full expression of the VIIa. However, in addition to this feedback mechanism, the pathway is mainly inhibited by a lipoprotein called tissue factor pathway inhibitor (TFPI; see Chap. 1).

An autosomal recessively inherited bleeding diatheses due to a deficiency of factor VII has been recognized since 1951. Heterozygous patients are usually asymptomatic (factor VII:C levels of approximately 40 to 50 percent), but homozygous or double heterozygous patients have a severe bleeding disorder with manifestations like those of classical hemophilia (factor VII:C levels <0.01–0.03 U/mL). Clinical onset is frequently as an infant, with umbilical stump bleeding, cephalohematoma, or ICH. Over all ages, the prevalence of ICH of 16 percent has been observed. A rare individual may have no history of bleeding or even have a thrombotic tendency. Other common hemorrhagic manifestations include oral mucosal bleeding, epistaxis, hemarthroses, gastrointestinal bleeding, severe menstrual bleeding, and postpartum and postsurgical hemorrhage.

The gene for factor VII is on chromosome 13 near the gene for factor X; the factor VII molecule has nine exons that code for the Gla region, two epidermal growth factor domains, an activation peptide region, and a catalytic domain. A recent summary of factor VII gene mutations described 30 different single base-pair substitutions and 4 short deletions (see Cooper reference). Most of these were single defects, were homozygous or double heterozygous, and were antigen positive. In addition, the same gene mutation (Ala244Val) associated with decreased factor VII activity and antigen was documented in 13 homozygotes in Moroccan and Iranian Jews.

Bleeding manifestations vary from asymptomatic to severe with a strong correlation with low activity and antigen levels (type 1 deficiencies). For example, exclusion of the first EGF domain by a splice site mutation was associated with nil FVII activity and antigen in normally developed infants with lethal ICH at birth.

The diagnosis of factor VII deficiency is suspected when the only abnormal screening test is the PT, thus prompting a factor VII activity assay. In severe factor VII deficiency, the PT is prolonged by up to 20 to 30 sec while heterozygotes show only a prolongation of 1 to 3 sec. In fact, the isolated mildly prolonged PT in an asymptomatic patient may represent mild factor VII deficiency. Plasma levels of factor VII vary significantly in the general population and are influenced by sex, age, and blood lipids (see Chap. 3), as well as polymorphisms in the factor VII gene. An

Arg353Gln substitution is associated with a 20 to 25 percent reduction in plasma factor VII activity in about 10 percent of some populations.

The half-life of factor VII is 4 h; therefore, it is difficult to maintain hemostatic levels with fresh frozen plasma alone. However, for single episode bleeding, a level of 15 percent can be achieved by a fresh frozen plasma transfusion of 10 to 15 mL/kg. Most available PCCs contain relatively little factor VII; a concentrate (Immuno) containing only factor VII and a recombinant factor VIIa (Novo Nordisk) have been used successfully for more severe hemorrhagic events and for surgical procedures (see Chap. 55).

FACTOR X DEFICIENCY

Factor X zymogen is a glycoprotein synthesized in the hepatocyte as a single polypeptide chain (488 amino acids); after posttranslational changes including vitamin K-dependent gamma-carboxylation of the first 11 glutamic acid residues, cleavage of the leader sequence, and glycosylation (15 percent carbohydrate), the mature protein is secreted and circulates as a two-chain disulfide-bonded molecule (light chain, Mr 16,200, heavy chain Mr 42,000) in a concentration of 10 µg/mL. The cleavage of Arg194-Ile 195 bond in the heavy chain produces Xa and an activation peptide of Mr 14,000, which has been used as a marker for intravascular coagulation. Factor X may also be activated by Russell viper venom (RVV) and a cancer procoagulant (cysteine protease). Factor Xa is the key serine protease in the prothrombinase complex (see Fig. 17-1).

The gene for factor X is on chromosome 13q34 where it spans 27 kb, consists of seven introns and eight exons, and shows homology with other vitamin K-dependent proteins. A congenital bleeding disorder is inherited as an autosomal recessive trait. Within a few years after the report of the "Stuart clotting defect" in 1957, it was recognized that factor X deficiency was a markedly heterogeneous group of patients who could be classified by measurements of antigen and by activation defects using extrinsic (PT), intrinsic (PTT), and direct (RVV) systems. Definition of the genetic mutations have begun to clarify the structure–function relationships. At least three groups of defects are indicated in Table 17-2. Gene deletions or signal peptide mutations result in a severe factor X deficiency with reduced protein synthesis, secretion, or stability (Stuart, Santo Domingo); missense mutations are often associated with normal amounts of protein that are abnormal in function (Fruili, substrate pocket binding defect; Marseille, cleavage site defect); and reduced protein from a defective allele that is itself dysfunctional (San Antonio).

TABLE 17-2

Examples of Hereditary Factor X Deficiencies

Variant (Mutation)	FX act (%)	FX ant (%)	PT	APTT	RVVT	Phenotype
Santo Domingo (Gly-20Arg)	<1	<5	Inc	Inc	nd	Severe bleeder (homozygote)
Japanese variant (deletion-intron D)	2.5	<5	Inc	Inc	4.5%	Moderate bleeder (homozygote)
Stuart (Val 298Met)	<0.01	<1	Inc	Inc	nd	Severe bleeder (homozygote)
Friuli (Pro343Ser)	7	100	Inc	Inc	N	Moderate bleeder (homozygote)
Roma (Thr318Met)	3	80	Inc	Inc	N	Moderate bleeder (homozygote)
Marseille (Ser334Pro)	21–26	100	Inc	Inc	Inc	No bleeding (homozygote)
San Antonio (Arg326Cys) (micro-deletion codon 272)	14	36	Inc	N	?	Post-op bleeding (double heterozygote)

Inc, incomplete; N, normal; nd, no data.

Clinically the homozygotes or double heterozygotes exhibit moderate to severe bleeding tendencies, which include hemarthroses, deep hematomas, menorrhagia, and postsurgical hemorrhage. Infants have presented with ICH antenatally and in the neonatal period. Most commonly both the PT and APTT are prolonged; however, variant factor X deficiencies have been reported in which only the PT or, rarely, only the APTT, is abnormal (see Table 17-2). The Stypven time (RVV time) is often prolonged; other screening tests, including the bleeding time, are normal. Heterozygotes are usually asymptomatic and have normal laboratory screening tests except for an occasional slightly prolonged PT.

Besides in liver disease and vitamin K deficiency, acquired factor X deficiency may occur in patients with primary amyloidosis and paraproteinemia, multiple myeloma, or in the elderly with no underlying disease (acquired antibody-induced). The bleeding tendency may be life threatening. Evidence for an inhibitory effect with mixing studies using the PT and APTT may be found; inhibitory effect of patient plasma on the factor X assay and crossed immunoelectrophoresis abnormalities can confirm the diagnosis.

Treatment of acute bleeding episodes in hereditary factor X deficiency is effectively achieved by transfusions of fresh frozen plasma. A level of 10 to 20 percent is sufficient for hemostasis except for complicated surgical procedures where the use of PCCs may be needed. The hereditary deficiency can improve during pregnancy and has been amenable to therapy with estrogens at other times. Acquired antibody induced factor X deficiency has responded to high dose corticosteroids, IVIG or plasmapheresis. The treatment of the acquired deficiency in amyloidosis is more complicated and is discussed in Chapter 32.

COMBINED HEREDITARY COAGULATION FACTOR DEFICIENCIES

Hereditary multiple coagulation-factor deficiencies occurring in the same individual are of two general types: those deficiencies with an established association on a genetic basis (factor V and factor VIII deficiency; vitamin K-dependent factor deficiencies, combined factor VIII and IX deficiency, and deletion of chromosome 13 [VII and X deficiency]); and those multiple deficiencies inherited coincidentally (all of the above plus other combinations).

Combined factor V and VIII deficiency is a well-documented autosomal recessively inherited condition reported in over 60 families (particularly around the Mediterranean basin). Homozygotes display excessive mucosal hemorrhage (epistaxis, menorrhagia) and bleeding after surgical trauma, abortions, and childbirth; hemarthroses are rarely seen. Factor VIII and V levels are from 5 to 30 percent of normal. Heterozygotes show intermediate levels of factor V and factor VIII and may have a mild bleeding tendency. Recent studies have identified multiple mutations of a gene for factor V-VIII deficiency on the long arm of chromosome 18; the gene is responsible for a well-described marker of the endoplasmic reticulum— Golgi intermediate compartment (ERGIC-53), which may function as a molecular chaperone for the transport from Golgi to ER of certain secreted proteins, including factors V and VIII. Newly diagnosed sporadic cases of mild or moderate hemophilia A or factor V deficiency should have both factors V and VIII assayed to not overlook the combined disorder. Treatment of bleeding episodes includes use of DDAVP (to increase level of factor VIII), fresh frozen plasma, or both, depending on severity of the bleeding tendency.

Combined deficiencies of factors II, VII, IX, and X have occurred (mild hemorrhagic symptoms with coagulation factor levels of 15 to 20 percent of normal). Parents of affected individuals have often been normal. The defect has been associated with pseudoxanthoma elasticum, as well as the phenotype of warfarin embryopathy. Vitamin K therapy has increased the factor levels temporarily in some cases. A recent report of a kindred with a missense mutation (Arg394Leu) in the gamma-glutamyl carboxylase gene was associated with a deficiency of all vitamin K-dependent coagulation factors and an autosomal recessive pattern of inheritance.

Intermediate levels of factors VII and X (40 to 50 percent) were observed in two patients with chromosome 13 deletion syndrome (mental retardation, craniofacial dysmorphy, hypospadias, congenital heart disease), which suggested hemizygosity for the genetic loci for the clotting factors. Coincidental combinations include various possibilities and have been reviewed in the reference by Soff.

BIBLIOGRAPHY

Brenner B et al: A missense mutation in gamma-glutamyl carboxylase gene causes combined deficiency of all vitamin K-dependent blood coagulation factors. *Blood* 92:4554, 1998.

Chediak J et al: Successful management of bleeding in a patient with factor V inhibitor by platelet transfusions. *Blood* 56:835, 1980.

Cooper DN et al: Inherited factor VII deficiency: Molecular genetics and pathophysiology. *Thromb Haemost* 78:151, 1997.

Cooper DN et al: Inherited factor X deficiency: Molecular genetics and pathophysiology. *Thromb Haemost* 78:161, 1997.

Degen SJF et al: Prothrombin Frankfurt: A dysfunctional prothrombin characterized by substitution of Glu-466 by Ala. *Thromb Haemost* 73:203, 1995.

Girolami A et al: Congenital deficiencies and abnormalities of prothrombin. *Blood Coag Fibrinol* 9:557, 1998.

Guasch JF et al: Severe coagulation factor V deficiency caused by a 4 bp deletion in the factor V gene. *Br J Haematol* 101:32, 1998.

Haber S: Norethynodrel in the treatment of factor X deficiency. *Arch Intern Med* 114:89, 1964.

Hayashi T et al: Molecular abnormality observed in a patient with coagulation factor X (FX) deficiency: a novel three-base-pair (CTT) deletion within the polypyrimidine tract of the intron D. *Br J Haematol* 102:926, 1998.

Hayward CPM et al: An autosomal dominant, qualitative platelet disorder associated with multimerin deficiency, abnormalities in platelet factor V, thrombospondin, von Willebrand factor, and fibrinogen and an epinephrine aggregation defect. *Blood* 87:4967, 1996.

Henriksen RA et al: Prothrombin Greenville, Arg517Gln, identified in an individual heterozygous for dysprothrombinemia. *Blood* 91:2026, 1998.

Hunault M et al: Mechanism underlying factor VII deficiency in Jewish populations with the Ala(244)Val mutation. *Br J Haematol* 105:1101, 1999.

Ingerslev J, Kristensen HL: Clinical picture and treatment strategies in factor VII deficiency. *Hemophilia* 4:689, 1998.

Lefkowitz JB et al: The prothrombin Denver patient has two different prothrombin point mutations resulting in Glu300-Lys and Glu309-Lys substitutions. *Br J Haematol,* 108:182, 2000.

Knight RD et al: Replacement therapy for congenital factor X deficiency. *Transfusion* 25:78, 1985.

Mazzucconi MG et al: Evaluation of the nature of mildly prolonged prothrombin times. *Am J Hematol* 24:37, 1987.

McVey JH et al: Exclusion of the first EGF domain of factor VII by a splice site mutation causes lethal factor VII deficiency. *Blood* 92:920, 1998.

Murray JM et al: Factor V New Brunswick: Ala221-to-Val substitution results in reduced cofactor activity. *Blood* 86:1820, 1995.

Nichols WC, Ginsburg D: Protein biosynthesis '99. From the ER to the Golgi: insights from the study of combined factors V and VIII deficiency. *Am J Hum Genet* 64:1493, 1999.

O'Marcaigh AS et al: Genetic analysis and functional characterization of prothrombin Corpus Christi (Arg382-Cys), Dhahran (Arg271-His), and hypoprothrombinemia. *Blood* 88:2611, 1996.

Peyvandi F et al: Bleeding symptoms in 27 Iranian patients with the combined deficiency of factor V and VIII. *Br J Haematol* 100:773, 1998.

Poort SR et al: Homozygosity for a novel missense mutation in the prothrombin gene causing a severe bleeding disorder. *Thromb Haemost* 72:819, 1994.

Rao LVM et al: Antibody-induced acute factor X deficiency: clinical manifestations and properties of the antibody. *Thromb Haemost* 72:363, 1994.

Reddy SV et al: Molecular characterization of human factor X San Antonio. *Blood* 74:1486, 1989.

Smith SV et al: Successful treatment of transient acquired factor X deficiency by plasmapheresis with concomitant intravenous immunoglobulin and steroid therapy. *Am J Hematol* 57:245, 1998.

Soff GA, Levin J: Familial multiple coagulation factor deficiencies. Review of the literature: Differentiation of single hereditary disorders associated with multiple factor deficiencies from coincidental concurrence of single factor deficiency states. *Semin Thromb Hemost* 7:112, 1981.

Tamary H et al: Ala244Val is a common, probably ancient mutation causing factor VII deficiency in Moroccan and Iranian Jews. *Thromb Haemost* 76:283, 1996.

Tamary H et al: Molecular analysis of a compound heterozygote for hypoprothrombinemia and dysprothrombinemia (-G 7248/7249 and Arg 340 Trp). *Blood Coag Fibrinol* 8:337, 1997.

Totan M, Albayrak D: Intracranial hemorrhage due to factor V deficiency. *Acta Paediatr* 88:342, 1999.

Triplett DA et al: Hereditary factor VII deficiency: Heterogeneity defined by combined functional and immunochemical analysis. *Blood* 66:1284, 1985.

Williams S et al: Acquired hypoprothrombinemia: effects of Danazol treatment. *Am J Hematol* 53:272, 1996.

CHAPTER 18

Abnormalities of Fibrinogen

The hereditary abnormalities of fibrinogen include afibrinogenemia, hypofibrinogenemia, dysfibrinogenemia, and hypodysfibrinogenemia. These disorders result from genetically controlled quantitative or qualitative changes in the fibrinogen molecule and are described below. Acquired abnormalities of fibrinogen are common because the glycoprotein is a major acute-phase reactant and the major substrate of the key enzymes of the coagulation system, thrombin and plasmin. Intravascular coagulation syndromes are discussed in Chapter 24.

STRUCTURE-FUNCTION RELATIONSHIP

Fibrinogen is a 340-kD glycoprotein synthesized in the hepatocyte and megakaryocyte; it circulates in the plasma in a concentration of 200 to 400 mg/dL. Figure 18-1 indicates the structure–function relationships of the fibrinogen molecule. It is composed of six paired polypeptide chains (alpha, beta, gamma) that are held together by disulfide bonds and organized in a symmetrical dimeric form. Cleavage of fibrinopeptide A (FPA, Aα 1–16) by thrombin exposes a site ("A" polymerization site) in the E domain that binds to the carboxy terminal region of the γ-chain ("a" site) and initiates polymerization of the fibrin monomers (see Fig. 18-2). Fibrinopeptide B (FPB, Bβ 1–14) cleavage occurs more slowly and contributes to lateral fibril and fiber association. This soluble fibrin clot is stabilized by the amidolytic action of activated factor XIII, which forms a covalent bond by the condensation of lysine and glutamine side chains to form gamma-gamma dimers and alpha polymers. The formation of a fibrin clot is the principal, but not exclusive, function of the molecule. Early proteolytic alterations of fibrinogen occur physiologically, leading

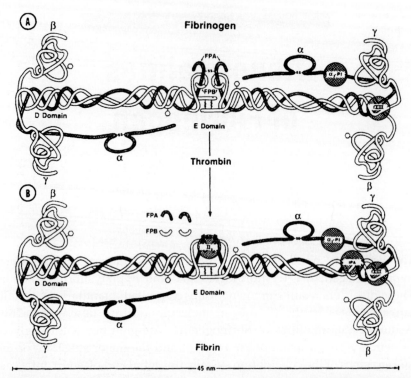

FIGURE 18-1 Fibrinogen consists of three pairs of polypeptide chains, Aα, Bβ, and γ, joined by disulfide bonds to form a symmetric dimeric structure (A). The NH₂-terminal regions of all six chains form the central domain (E domain) of the molecule containing FPA and FPB sequences, which are cleaved by thrombin during enzymatic conversion to fibrin. Carbohydrate moleties (*circles*) are located at one site on each of the γ- and Bβ-chains. Enzymatic conversion of fibrinogen to fibrin (B) by thrombin cleavage results in release of FPA and FPB. A nonsubstrate (secondary) binding site for thrombin (IIa) is present in the central domain of α,β-fibrin, and depends on the presence of the β15 to 42 sequence. Binding sites for IIa, t-PA, factor XIII, and α₂-plasmin inhibitor, respectively, are indicated on the fibrinogen or fibrin molecule. (Used with permission from Mosesson MW: Fibrin polymerization and its regulatory role in hemostasis. *J Lab Clin Med* 116:8, 1990.)

to fibrinogens with lower molecular mass (305 kD and 270 kD). Other later, plasmin cleavage sites, part of the degradation process, include regions between D and E domains in all three chains producing fragments Y, D, and E. These fragments have several biologic functions, including stimulation of human hemopoietic cell lines, vasoactive properties, and bacteria clumping. Many specific binding sites and interactions are known for the fibrinogen molecule, including those with thrombin, calcium, platelet GP IIb–IIIa, fibronectin, factor XIII, plasminogen, tissue plasminogen activator (t-PA), α₂-antiplasmin, collagen, thrombospondin, and other cell interactions (erythrocytes, monocytes).

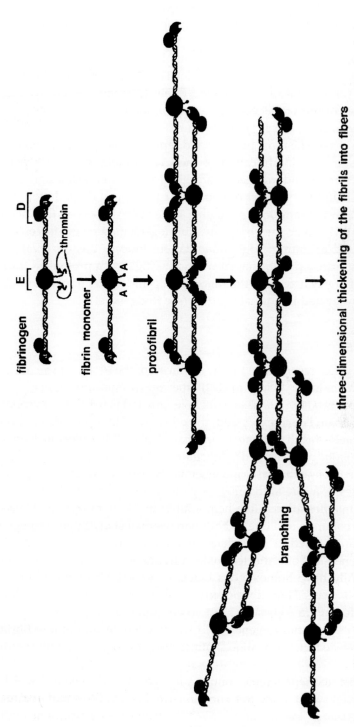

FIGURE 18-2 Schematic representation of formation of a three-dimensional mesh of fibrinogen. After the cleavage of fibrinopeptide A by thrombin, the newly exposed polymerization site "A" binds to the polymerization pocket "a" that is part of the gamma chain of fibrin(ogen). The fibrin monomers thus align in a half-staggered, two-stranded arrangement to form long fibrils. (Adapted with permission from Cote HCF et al: *Blood* 92:2195, 1998.)

Carbohydrate clusters containing sialic acid are present on the Bβ- and γ-chains.

Fibrinogen assay methods are usually based on one of the following principles: (1) coagulation time or velocity (Clauss or thrombin clotting method); (2) amount of coagulable protein (tyrosine content by Biuret colorimeter, or ultraviolet adsorption); (3) amount of precipitable protein (heat to 52 to 58°C, or salt) and (4) immunoreactive protein (antifibrinogen antibodies). The most popular and reproducible method used in the United States is a modification of the Clauss method using a pooled human plasma standard. Because diluted plasma is tested and excess thrombin is used, the effect of heparin or fibrinogen degradation products (FDP) in the sample is negligible. It has been observed that hereditary and physiologic (newborn) dysfibrinogens may give a lower value as compared to immunologic quantitation. Indeed, this observation is used to indicate a dysfibrinogen when investigating a prolonged thrombin time if one realizes that the ratio of antigenic to functional fibrinogen is slightly elevated in normal controls (see Rodgers ref).

GENETICS

The three genes responsible for the synthesis of the α-, β-, and γ-chains of fibrinogen are located close to each other on chromosome 4, band 4q32. Each gene is 6500 to 7500 base pairs in length and is regulated in concert; i.e., if one chain is overexpressed, the other two will upregulate. Several genetic defects result in phenotypes that display either bleeding tendencies, thrombotic complications, difficulties in wound healing, or no known symptoms. Congenital afibrinogenemia, which has been described in 150 families, is a rare autosomal recessively inherited defect with severe bleeding manifestations (like hemophilia) in the homozygote. Consanguinity is common and one or both parents may show hypofibrinogenemia. As anticipated, a gene-deletion mutation has been described in afibrinogenemia. Four affected male individuals in a nonconsanguinous Swiss family have homozygous deletions of ~11 kb of the fibrinogen alpha-chain gene. Hypofibrinogenemia with both recessive and dominant modes of transmission are known. Some of these cases may be examples of a dysfibrinogenemia in which the detection of low fibrinogen was due to functional abnormalities measured by a thrombin clotting assay.

The most frequent genetic abnormality is dysfibrinogenemia, which is usually due to a missense mutation inherited in an autosomal dominant manner. At least half of the nearly 300 families reported are asymptomatic. Table 18-1 lists examples of the over 83 fibrinogens that have had the molecular defect defined. In general, most defects with delayed fibrinopeptide A release have amino acid substitutions at position 16 (arginine) of the chain (thrombin cleaves between 16 and 17). These defects are associated with mild to moderate bleeding symptoms or are asymptomatic. Defects in the Bβ-chain are less frequent and have often been asso-

TABLE 18-1

Examples of Hereditary Dysfibrinogenemias

Designation (Mutation)	Functional Defect	Clinical Manifestations
Mitaka II (AαGlu11Gly)	Impaired binding to thrombin	None
Chapel Hill II (AαArg16His)	Impaired cleavage of FPA	Bleeding and thrombosis
Metz* (AαArg16Cys)	Impaired cleavage of FPA	Bleeding
Naples* (BβAla68Thr)	Impaired cleavage of FPB	Thrombosis
Detroit (AαArg19Ser)	Alteration in "A" site; delayed protofibrin formation	Bleeding
Baltimore I (γGly292Val)	Alteration in "a" site; delayed protofibrin formation	Bleeding and thrombosis
Kurashiki I* (γGly268Glu)	Alteration in D:D self-association site; delayed protofibril formation; abnormal γ-γ cross-linking	None
Lima* (AαArg141Ser; extra oligosaccharide)	Impaired lateral association of protofibrils	Bleeding
Vlissingen I (Delete γAsn319 + γAsp320)	Impaired high-affinity calcium binding site	Thrombosis
Dusart (Paris V) (AαArg554Cys)	Polymerization abnormality; impaired binding with plasminogen	Thrombosis
Paris I (Insertion 15 residues between γ350–γ351)	Altered factor XIIIa crosslinking γ chains	Wound dehiscence

* Homozygous

ciated with a thrombotic tendency. The γ-chain defects are more heterogeneous and result in abnormally delayed fibrin polymerization in association with severe bleeding, thrombosis, or no symptoms. Delayed wound healing due to abnormal XIIIa cross-linking has been described in a few variants (Paris I with elongation of the γ-chain); urea solubility test is abnormal.

CLINICAL MANIFESTATIONS

The most frequent clinical manifestations of bleeding in afibrinogenemia include umbilical cord hemorrhage, deep muscle and joint bleeding, menorrhagia, and other mucous membrane hemorrhage. Table 18-2 shows the clinical and laboratory signs (prolonged thrombin and reptilase times) that lead to the diagnosis of an hereditary disorder of fibrinogen. In a rare dysfibrinogenemic patient the usual laboratory screening tests (TCT, reptilase time) were normal by clot detection end point, but abnormal by a light-scatter optical method (see Lefkowitz ref). The parents of afibrinogenemic patients are either normal or have hypofibrinogenemia. Family members with dysfibrinogenemia may show positive signs (dominant inheritance) or may be asymptomatic; therefore, immediate family members should be screened with the abnormal test (TCT or reptilase time). In complicated or unusual cases, other causes of a prolonged thrombin time should be excluded (see Chap. 4), including heparin effect. Some patients have both qualitative and quantitative defects in fibrinogen with levels ranging from 50 to 120 mg/dL. The TCT is usually marked prolonged and fibrinopeptide release and polymerization abnormalities may be found. Sometimes these hypodysfibrinogenemia patients will show rapid turnover of the abnormal fibrinogen as well as an inhibitory effect on the normal TCT in mixing studies. These patients can have a bleeding disorder and a history of frequent spontaneous abortions (Bethesda III).

ACQUIRED ALTERATIONS IN FIBRINOGEN

Fibrinogen is the prime example of an acute phase reactant protein. As noted above, the synthesis of fibrinogen is keyed to stimulation by interleukins during inflammation, infection, or malignancy. During severe stress or fibrinogen breakdown, the turnover rate (normally 3 to 5 days) may increase 25-fold. In addition to elevations of the fibrinogen level with acute phase reaction, other alterations, such as increased age, gender, race, smoking, and obesity are known. During pregnancy, plasma

TABLE 18-2		
Clinical and Laboratory Manifestations of Congenital Fibrinogen Disorders		
	Clinical	**Laboratory**
Afibrinogenemia	Severe lifelong (often cord bleeding) hemorrhagic diathesis as in moderate to severe hemophilia; splenic rupture	No clotting is seen in all screening tests (APTT, PT, TCT); bleeding time is prolonged; all fibrinogen assays are zero or trace.
Hypofibrinogenemia	Mild bleeding disorder; menorrhagia, recurrent abortions, postsurgery bleeding on occasion, placental abruption	APTT usually normal; PT slightly prolonged or normal*; TCT and reptilase time mildly prolonged; decrease in fibrinogen to < 100–150 mg/dL by thrombin clotting and immunoassay.
Dysfibrinogenemia	Chronic history of bleeding tendency after surgery and trauma; possible poor wound healing. Positive family history (or) Thrombotic tendency (recurrent deep venous thrombosis, pulmonary embolism, etc.) Positive family history (or) Asymptomatic	All screening tests can be normal except prolonged TCT and reptilase time (ranging from a few seconds to > 100 s) with normal fibrinogen level. (APTT and PT may be slightly prolonged); higher fibrinogen level by immunologic test than thrombin clotting method.

* APTT and PT usually are normal until fibrinogen is < 100 mg/dL.

fibrinogen rises as early as the third month and increases gradually to values at term of 350 to 650 mg/dL; a similar estrogen dose-dependent rise is seen during oral contraceptive agent therapy. Hyperfibrinogenemia is a risk factor in stroke and coronary heart disease. Recent data (Brown ref) identify a differential element in Bβ chain regulation that may be one of the factors controlling increased amounts of fibrinogen.

Causes of acquired hypofibrinogenemia include liver disease, ascites, disseminated intravascular coagulation (DIC) states, and L-asparaginase therapy. Other drugs decreasing the plasma fibrinogen level (possibly by affecting monocyte–cytokine interactions) include N-3 fatty acids, ticlopidine, alcohol, fibrates, and pentoxifylline. Posttranslational modifications of the fibrinogen molecule affecting phosphorus or carbohydrate content may occur in the fetus and newborn infant (increased phosphorus and sialic acid) and in liver disease (increased sialic acid). These changes result in a mildly prolonged dilute thrombin time, which can be "corrected" by calcium ions. Therefore, the calcium thrombin time will often fail to detect these changes. Similar thrombin time prolongations may be seen in the nephrotic syndrome (dysfibrinogen).

Other causes of acquired "dysfibrinogenemia" include inhibitor or antibodies (rarely) or incipient or early DIC (commonly). Digital ischemia due to RBC aggregation induced by acquired dysfibrinogenemia was successfully treated by ancrod defibrinogenation. Cold precipitable cryofibrinogen complexed with gamma globulin may be associated with leukocytoclastic vasculitis.

TREATMENT AND COMPLICATIONS

The rare patient with afibrinogenemia requires replacement transfusion therapy for acute bleeding episodes. An adult (plasma volume of 3 L) will require 12 bags of cryoprecipitate to increase the fibrinogen level to 100 mg/dL. The prolonged bleeding time has shortened after DDAVP. A few of these patients may develop antibodies to fibrinogen, which complicates their therapy. Prophylactic cryoprecipitate every 7 to 10 days has been used successfully in children. Patients with bleeding tendencies due to hypo- or dysfibrinogenemias rarely require replacement therapy; when necessary, cryoprecipitate has been useful.

BIBLIOGRAPHY

Abshire TC et al: The prolonged thrombin time of nephrotic syndrome. *J Pediat Hematol/Oncol* 17:156, 1995.

Brown ET, Fuller GM: Detection of a complex that associates with Bβ fibrinogen G-455-A polymorphism. *Blood* 92:3286, 1998.

Cote et al: Gamma-chain dysfibrinogenemias: molecular structure-function relationships of naturally occurring mutations in the gamma chain of human fibrinogen. *Blood* 92:2195, 1998.

Ebert R: *Index of Variant Fibrinogens,* Rockville, MD, RF Ebert, 1990.

Ehmann WC, Al-Mondhiry: Congenital afibrinogenemia and splenic rupture. *Am J Med* 96:92, 1994.

Euler HH et al: Monoclonal cryo-fibrinogenemia. *Arth Rheum* 39:1066, 1996.

Huber P et al: Human beta-fibrinogen gene expression: Upstream sequences involved in its tissue specific expression and its dexamethasone and interleukin 6 stimulation. *J Biol Chem* 265:5695, 1990.

Kwaan HC et al: Digital ischemia and gangrene due to red blood cell aggregation induced by acquired dysfibrinogenemia. *J Vasc Surg* 26:1061, 1997.

Lak M et al: Bleeding and thrombosis in 55 patients with inherited afibrinogenemia. *Br J Haematol* 107:204, 1999.

Lefkowitz JB et al: Fibrinogen Longmont: a dysfibrinogenemia causing prolonged clot-based test results only when using an optical detection method. *Am J Hematol,* 63:149, 2000.

Martinez J: Congenital dysfibrinogenemia. *Curr Opin Hematol* 4:357, 1997.

Matsuda M: The structure-function relationship of hereditary dysfibrinogens. *Int J Hematol* 64:167, 1996.

Mosesson MW: Fibrinogen structure and fibrin clot assembly. *Sem Thromb Hemost* 24:169, 1998.

Nawarawong W et al: The rate of fibrinopeptide B release modulates the rate of clot formation: A study with an acquired inhibitor to fibrinopeptide B release. *Br J Haematol* 79:296, 1991.

Neerman-Arbez M et al: Deletion of the fibrinogen alpha-chain gene (FGA) causes congenital afibrinogenemia. *J Clin Invest* 103:215, 1999.

Reininger A et al: Effect of fibrinogen substitution in afibrinogenemia on hemorheology and platelet function. *Thromb Haemost* 74:853, 1995.

Rodgers GM, Garr SB: Comparison of functional and antigenic fibrinogen values from a normal population. *Thromb Res* 68:207, 1992.

Schorer AE et al: Dysfibrinogenemia: a case with thrombosis (fibrinogen Richfield) and an overview of the clinical and laboratory spectrum. *Am J Hematol* 50:200, 1995.

Factor XIII, α_2-Antiplasmin, and Plasminogen Activator Inhibitor-1 Deficiencies

Hereditary deficiencies of factor XIII (fibrin-stabilizing factor, FSF), α_2-antiplasmin (α_2-AP or α_2-plasmin inhibitor), and plasminogen activator inhibitor-1 (PAI-1) cause a lifelong bleeding diathesis. All three are rare disorders inherited in an autosomal recessive manner. Laboratory hemostatic screening tests, including platelet count, bleeding time, APTT, PT, thrombin time, and fibrinogen levels, are normal. Specific factor assays must be performed to indicate the diagnosis. The mechanism of bleeding in each condition is due to defects occurring after the fibrin clot is formed, that is, lack of cross-linking of the clot by factor XIII and the excessive lysis of the clot due to deficiencies of major physiologic inhibitors of fibrinolysis, α_2-AP and PAI-1 (Fig. 19-1). Additional information regarding these three clotting factors may be found in Chaps. 25 and 41.

FACTOR XIII DEFICIENCY

Factor XIII (plasma transglutaminase, FSF) is a cysteine enzyme that circulates in the plasma (bound to fibrinogen); the plasma zymogen (30 µg/mL) occurs as a tetramer of paired A- and B-chains with a molecular mass of 309,000 D. An intracellular form (found in platelets, megakaryocytes, monocytes, and cells of the placenta, prostate, and uterus) is a dimer of two A chains. Activation of factor XIII is by thrombin in the presence of Ca^{++}, which results in exposure of the active center cysteine. The activation peptide, active center, and calcium binding sites are in the A-chain protein; the B-chain protein serves as a carrier or has a protective function. When activated, XIIIa catalyzes the formation of a covalent

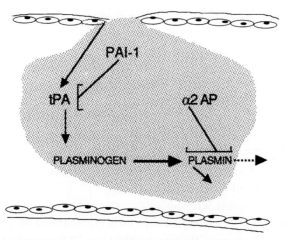

FIGURE 19-1 Excessive plasmin formation in hemostatic plug producing clot lysis and hemorrhage can be due to a deficiency of PAI-1 or α_2-AP.

bond between glutamine and lysine residues thus cross-linking fibrin molecules and α_2-antiplasmin, producing a stable clot with relative resistance to fibrinolysis. Other cross-linked complexes formed by XIIIa are fibrin–fibrin, fibrin–fibrinogen, fibrin–α_2-AP, fibrin–von Willebrand factor, fibrin–thrombospondin, fibrin–fibronectin, and fibronectin–collagen. These substrates have many features in common, such as being adhesive proteins, platelet alpha-granule proteins, and participants in macromolecular complexes on cell or subendothelial surfaces, which suggests they have a role in wound healing, tissue repair, tumor growth, and atherosclerosis.

The factor XIII cross-linking activity may be precisely quantitated by measuring fluorescent dansylcadaverine or labeled putrescine incorporation into casein (a surrogate system) or by a photometric measurement of ammonia released during the cross-linking reaction (Beringwerke reagents). The A and B proteins may be quantitated by immunoassay. A screening test demonstrating that the patient's plasma clot dissolves in 5 M urea or 1 percent monochloroacetic acid is indicative of a severe (< 1 to 2 percent) deficiency of factor XIII. The screening test is clinically useful since usually only severe deficiencies exhibit hemorrhagic tendencies. However, even small amounts of factor XIII appear to protect against severe hemorrhage and complications of pregnancy, as evidenced by a mild phenotype associated with measurable circulating factor XIII (0.35 percent); the A-subunit gene defect was a splicing mutation permitting partial correct splicing of factor XIII mRNA. In addition, a recent survey (Seitz ref) of 60 families indicated that bleeding tendencies do not always correlate with assay levels and that even heterozygotes may occasionally exhibit excessive bleeding.

The gene (160 kb, 15 exons, 14 introns) for the A chain or subunit is located on chromosome 6 and codes for a molecule with four domains: an N-terminal beta sandwich, a core domain containing the catalytic triad residues, and two "barrel domains". The gene for the B chain is located on chromosome 1 and codes for 10 tandem repeats termed "Sushi domains." The most common hereditary deficiency of factor XIII is called type 2 and is due to mutations in the A-subunit gene. The homozygous patient shows no A-subunit protein in the plasma or platelets and the factor XIII activity assay is less than 1 to 2 percent. Plasma B-subunit protein is usually reduced to about 30 percent. Heterozygotes have intermediate values. The over 25 gene defects described are heterogeneous and include a variety of nonsense mutations, missense mutations, small deletions, frameshifts, and splicing abnormalities. The presence of a short tandem repeat (STR) polymorphism in the factor XIII A gene has been used for prenatal diagnosis. Recent reports have indicated that the Val34Leu mutation in the factor XIII A subunit is associated with protection against myocardial infarction and predisposition to ICH (heterozygotes); interestingly, homozygotes for the mutation appear to be protected against venous thrombosis. Mutations in the factor XIII B-subunit gene are extremely rare and result in nil plasma activity in the homozygous state, associated with lack of both B-chain and A-chain antigen (type 1 deficiency) although A subunit may be found in platelets.

About 200 cases of this rare autosomal disorder (frequency of 1 in 2 million) have been reported since 1960. The most common sites of hemorrhage are umbilical cord stump in > 80 percent of cases (1 to 19 days of age) and intracranial (30 percent of cases), which is often spontaneous or after mild trauma. Other sites of bleeding include subcutaneous hematomas, joint bleeding (uncommon), and muscle hematomas. Defective wound healing, delayed bleeding episodes, habitual abortion, and menorrhagia are seen. Treatment of acute bleeding episodes is easily accomplished using plasma or concentrates. The hemostatic level is low (approximately 2 to 3 percent) and the half-disappearance time after infusions is long (9 to 10 days). The availability in Europe of plasma-derived and placenta-derived factor XIII concentrates (Fibrogammin P) have made prophylactic treatment feasible and safe. As illustrated by the following case, prophylaxis can be achieved by single donor plasma.

Case Report—Factor XIII Deficiency, Type 2

A female infant, born at term in 1984, was noted to have persistent bleeding from the umbilical stump. The infant's plasma clot dissolved readily in 5 M urea solution, and the bleeding ceased after an infusion of fresh frozen plasma. Detailed studies revealed:

	Factor XIII (U/mL)	A-subunits (U/mL)	B-subunits (U/mL)
Infant	0.02*	0	0.47
Mother	0.53	0.58	0.80
Father	0.72	0.66	0.7

* Performed 3 weeks after a plasma infusion.

The infant was placed on prophylactic transfusions of fresh frozen plasma (10 mL/kg) every 3 weeks and has remained free of hemorrhage except for a 2-month trial off plasma. At that time increased bruising and a large subcutaneous hematoma appeared, leading to reinstitution of plasma therapy. Growth and development have been normal. A brother born in 1988 also has the disorder. As of 1994, both children remained on prophylaxis, with fresh frozen plasma given every 3 to 4 weeks. An occasional episode of bleeding is seen (hemarthrosis, oral) when the interval is extended to 4 weeks.

Acquired low levels of factor XIII are observed in the following situations: newborn infant (approximately 50 percent of adult), liver diseases, leukemias, disseminated intravascular coagulation (DIC), various malignant diseases, severe falciparum malaria, rheumatoid arthritis, and Henoch-Schönlein purpura. Autoimmune (IgG antibodies) inhibitors of factor XIII activity have been noted as the cause of severe bleeding in adults (abnormal urea solubility tests were noted that did not correct on 1:1 mixing); the majority of reported cases were taking isoniazid or procainamide; one patient had SLE. Successful treatment included cessation of the offending drug, high-dose factor XIII replacement, immunosuppressives, and plasmapheresis. In addition, an eight-year-old female with congenital factor XIII deficiency developed an inhibitor antibody to factor XIII in association with ICH; the inhibitor persisted for several months.

α_2-Antiplasmin Deficiency

α_2-Antiplasmin is a single chain glycoprotein with a molecular weight of 51,000 D and a plasma concentration of 7 mg/dL. α_2-AP is synthesized in the liver and is bound to plasminogen (70 percent) or occurs as a free form, which is a less effective plasmin inhibitor. As noted in the section on fibrinolysis, α_2-AP regulates the system at three levels: (1) α_2-AP blocks the activity of plasmin by forming an instantaneous complex; this fast inhibition is backed up by α_2-macroglobulin; (2) α_2-AP inhibits the adsorption of plasminogen to fibrin; and (3) α_2-AP is cross-linked to fibrin by XIIIa, making the fibrin more resistant to local plasmin. The plasma half-life of the bound form is approximately 2.3 to 2.8 days. The plasma concentration of α_2-AP can be measured by functional assay (usually a chromogenic with the tripeptide S-2251) and by immunologic assays with specific antisera. α_2-AP-plasmin complexes can be measured by sensitive immunologic techniques and are indicators of in vivo activation of the fibrinolytic system.

Inherited α_2-AP deficiency is associated with a severe bleeding disorder (as in hemophilia) in the homozygous state and a mild or asymptomatic disorder in the heterozygous state (Table 19-1). An unusual manifestation of bleeding, intramedullary hematoma of the long bones, has occurred in three sisters with a severe hereditary deficiency (Miyauchi reference). The level of α_2-AP activity ranges from 0.01 to 0.15 U/mL in the homozygote and 0.35 to 0.70 U/mL in the heterozygote. Levels have been known to decrease with advancing age in association with an increased bleeding tendency. In most reported families immunoreactive α_2-AP was reduced in proportion to the functional activity. For instance, a frameshift mutation in the exon coding for the carboxylterminal region of the gene resulted in an elongation of the amino acid sequence and severe protein deficiency in the three sisters noted above. However, normal amounts of immunoreactive α_2-AP have been found in two members of a Dutch family who have activity levels of 0.04 U/mL. The dysfunctional molecule was named α_2-AP Enschede and is due to an alanine insertion adjacent to the reactive site. All hemostatic tests and coagulation assays are normal in 15 families with α_2-AP deficiency reported, except for occasionally shortened euglobulin lysis times. Evidence of a hyperfibrinogenolytic state (increased fragment X or DY) can be detected in patients with acquired, but not hereditary, deficiencies.

Acquired deficiencies of α_2-AP are seen in liver disease (decreased synthesis), nephrotic syndrome (urinary loss), systemic amyloidosis (complex formation and amyloid binding), DIC states and thrombolytic therapy (complex formation with plasmin), cardiopulmonary bypass (hemodilution and consumption), and metastatic cancer (activation of fibrinolytic system). Although many of these disorders have other hemostatic abnormalities in association with low α_2-AP, bleeding manifesta-

TABLE 19-1

Clinical Manifestations of Hereditary α_2-Antiplasmin Deficiency

Disorder	Plasma Levels (Chromogenic Substrate S-2251)	Euglobulin Lysis Time	Bleeding Manifestations
Homozygous deficiency	0.02–0.15 U/mL	Normal or decreased	Umbilical cord stump or postsurgical bleeding Hemarthroses Soft tissue hematomas Prolonged laceration bleeding Muscle bleeding Epistaxis
Heterozygous deficiency	0.35–0.70 U/mL	Normal; occasionally decreased	None (or) Postsurgical bleeding Bleeding after tooth extraction Easy bruising Menorrhagia

tions are apt to be more severe when the level is < 25 to 50 percent of normal.

Fortunately, the bleeding episodes in the hereditary disorder respond well to oral administration of epsilon aminocaproic acid (Amicar) or tranexamic acid. The drug may also be useful in selected cases of acquired deficiency (amyloidosis, cardiopulmonary bypass).

PLASMINOGEN ACTIVATOR INHIBITOR-1 DEFICIENCY

Plasminogen activator inhibitor-1 is a serine protease inhibitor (molecular weight 52,000 D, 379 amino acids) that has a 30 to 50 percent homology with other members of the serpin family. The 12.2 kb gene for PAI-1 is located on chromosome 7, closely linked to the gene for cystic fibrosis. PAI-1 is found in plasma and extracellular sites where it is in complex with vitronectin and in platelets (alpha-granules). PAI-1 is stored or synthesized in the endothelial cells and hepatocytes and is the major fast-acting inhibitor for tissue plasminogen activator (t-PA). Two types of assays have been used for detection of PAI-1 in plasma. An activity assay performed by titration with single-chain t-PA and immunologic assays (ELISA) have indicated a wide normal range of 0.5 to 68 U/mL for activity and 6 to 600 ng/mL for antigen. The wide range is compatible with

PAI-1 as an acute-phase reactant. Since normal individuals may have near-zero plasma levels of PAI-1 on occasion, measurement of PAI-1 activity and antigen in both plasma and serum (for platelet contribution) should be performed in suspected patients.

Nineteen individuals who are heterozygous for a null allele and 7 homozygous patients with PAI-1 deficiency in a single kindred have been reported. The complete deficiency was caused by a frameshift mutation in exon 4 of the PAI-1 gene. Bleeding manifestations included hemarthroses, large hematomas, menorrhagia, easy bruising, and severe postoperative hemorrhage. Only four reports of partial deficiency are known. Fibrinolytic inhibitors, including ε-aminocaproic acid and tranexamic acid, were effective in treating and preventing bleeding episodes. An acquired deficiency of PAI-1 due to an autoantibody in amyloidosis has been associated with a bleeding tendency. Low PAI-1 associated with increased levels of t-PA has resulted in severe postoperative bleeding in at least one patient (Stankiewicz ref).

BIBLIOGRAPHY

Ahmad F et al: Characterization of an acquired IgG inhibitor of coagulation factor XIII in a patient with systemic lupus erythematosus. *Br J Haematol* 93:700, 1996.

Brackmann HH et al: Pharmacokinetics and tolerability of factor XIII concentrates prepared from human placenta or plasma: a crossover randomised study. *Thromb Haemost* 74:622, 1995.

Catto AJ et al: Association of a common polymorphism in the factor XIII gene with venous thrombosis. *Blood* 93:906, 1999.

Dieval J et al: A lifelong bleeding disorder associated with a deficiency of plasminogen activator inhibitor type 1. *Blood* 77:528, 1991.

Egbring R et al: Factor XIII deficiency: pathogenic mechanisms and clinical significance. *Sem Thromb Hemost* 22:419, 1996.

Fay WP et al: Human plasminogen activator inhibitor-1 (PAI-1) deficiency: characterization of a large kindred with a null mutation in the PAI-1 gene. *Blood* 90:204, 1997.

Franco RF et al: Factor XIII Val34Leu is a genetic factor involved in the aetiology of venous thrombosis. *Thromb Haemost* 81:676, 1999.

Holmes WE et al: Alpha-2-antiplasmin Enschede: alanine insertion and abolition of plasmin inhibitory activity. *Science* 238:209, 1987.

Holst FGE et al: Low levels of fibrin-stabilizing factor (factor XIII) in human Plasmodium falciparum malaria: correlation with clinical severity. *Am J Trop Med Hyg* 60:99, 1999.

Ikematsu S et al: Heterozygote for plasmin inhibitor deficiency developing hemorrhagic tendency with advancing age. *Thromb Res* 82:129, 1996.

Killick CJ et al: Prenatal diagnosis in factor XIII-A deficiency. *Arch Dis Child Fetal Neonal Ed* 80:F238, 1999.

Kruithof EKO et al: Plasminogen activator inhibitor 1 and plasminogen activator inhibitor 2 in various disease states. *Thromb Haemost* 59:7, 1988.

Lorand L et al: Autoimmune antibody in a hemorrhagic patient interacts with thrombin-activated factor XIII in a unique manner. *Blood* 93:909, 1999.

Manco-Johnson M et al: Characterization and quantitation on an inhibitor to the A chain of factor XIII (F XIII) in a child with severe factor XIII deficiency. *Blood* 82:596a, 1993.

Mikkola H, Palotie A: Gene defects in congenital factor XIII deficiency. *Sem Thromb Hemost* 22:393, 1996.

Mikkola H et al: Molecular mechanism of a mild phenotype in coagulation factor XIII (FXIII) deficiency: a splicing mutation permitting partial correct splicing of FXIII A-subunit mRNA. *Blood* 89:1279, 1997.

Miura O et al: Molecular basis for congenital deficiency of alpha-2-plasmin inhibitor. A frameshift mutation leading to elongation of the deduced amino acid sequence. *J Clin Invest* 83: 1598, 1998.

Miyauchi Y et al: Operative treatment of intramedullary hematoma associated with congenital deficiency of alpha-2-plasmin inhibitor. A report of three cases. *J Bone Joint Surg* 78:1409, 1996.

Nishida Y et al: A new rapid and simple assay for factor XIII activity using dansylcadaverine incorporation and gel filtration. *Thromb Res* 36:123, 1984.

Okajima K et al: Direct evidence for systemic fibrinogenolysis in patients with acquired alpha-2-plasmin inhibitor deficiency. *Am J Hematol* 45: 16, 1994.

Saito M et al: A familial factor XIII subunit B deficiency. *Br J Haematol* 74:290, 1990.

Seitz R et al: ETRO working party on factor XIII questionnaire on congenital factor XIII deficiency in Europe: status and perspectives. *Sem Thromb Hemost* 22:415, 1996.

Stankiewicz AJ et al: Increased levels of tissue plasminogen activator with a low plasminogen activator inhibitor-1 in a patient with postoperative bleeding. *Am J Hematol* 38:226, 1991.

Takahashi Y et al: Hereditary partial deficiency of plasminogen activator inhibitor-1 associated with a lifelong bleeding tendency. *Intl J Hematol* 64:61, 1996.

Takahashi N et al: Molecular mechanisms of type II factor XIII deficiency: novel Gly562Arg mutation and C-terminal truncation of the A subunit cause factor XIII deficiency as characterized in a mammalian expression system. *Blood* 91:2830, 1998.

CHAPTER 20

Acquired Coagulation Factor Inhibitors

Acquired coagulation factor inhibitors are circulating antibodies that specifically neutralize the procoagulant activity of the various coagulation factors and result in a deficiency state frequently associated with a bleeding tendency. These inhibitors, which are different from the antiphospholipid antibodies or lupus anticoagulant (see Chap. 43), arise as alloantibodies in patients with hereditary factor deficiencies or as autoantibodies in patients with and without an underlying immune disorder. The most common and well-characterized inhibitor is directed against factor VIII (FVIII) and occurs with a prevalence of 15 to 20 percent in severe hemophilia A patients (alloantibody), and much less commonly in postpartum women, elderly individuals, patients with autoimmune disorders, and apparently normal individuals (autoantibodies). Management of these patients is difficult and costly; the attention of an experienced consultant is required.

FVIII INHIBITORS

Nature of the Problem

Based on both prospective and retrospective studies, the cumulative incidence of inhibitor development is 21 to 33 percent in severe hemophilia A patients (Table 20-1).

Among individuals with severe and moderately severe hemophilia A, the question of increased inhibitor incidence associated with exposure to increasingly purer FVIII products has been raised. Although the studies represented in Table 20-1 do not suggest a large increase in inhibitor incidence with increasing product purity, they do demonstrate a downward trend in both the median age at development and the median number of

TABLE 20-1					
Inhibitors/Hemophilia A: Prospective Studies/Inhibitor Development					
Study	**Cumulative Risk**	**Hemophilia Severity**	**Median Age**	**Median Exposure Days**	**Product**
Strauss	21%	S	8 yrs	35	Cryo
Schwartzinger	24%	S/Mod	5 yrs	25	Cryo/IP
Lusher	16%	S/Mod	–	15	Monoclate®
Ehrenforth	33%	S/Mod	2 yrs	12	Cryo/IP/M/R
Bray	31.5%	S/Mod	1.6 yrs	9	Recombinate
Lusher	32.8%	S/Mod	1.6 yrs	9	Kogenate

S, severe; Mod, moderate; Cryo, cryoprecipitate; IP, intermediate purity; M, monoclonal; R, recombinant

factor exposures preceding the time of inhibitor expression. Both observations may have been influenced by more frequent testing in the previously untreated patients (PUP) studies. In both studies of recombinant FVIII therapy in PUP, antibodies were detected after a median of nine exposures at median ages of under 2 years. Alternatively, if not previously detected, new inhibitor development is uncommon after 100 exposures to exogenous clotting factor. Although high-responding inhibitors have historically represented 70 to 80 percent of all inhibitors, both recombinant FVIII PUP studies identified only 30 to 45 percent of the inhibitors as high titer.

High-titer inhibitors can develop in 3 to 13 percent of patients with mild hemophilia A. In the largest series described to date, these inhibitors develop after intensive FVIII replacement therapy, and often result in soft tissue, GI, and GU bleeding manifestations reminiscent of patients with autoantibodies. These antibodies have been found to be associated with a few high-risk FVIII genotypes (Arg593Cys) clustered in the A_2 and C_2 domains (see Fig. 20-1).

It is still not possible to predict inhibitor development in an individual with hemophilia A. The risk factors appear to be multiple and interdependent and involve conditions relating to both the host and the treatment. Host factors include type of hemophilia (A > B) and severity of the defect (i.e., those individuals with no or minimal endogenous factor having a greater tendency toward inhibitor development). HLA and FVIII genotypes are also likely to play a role. Clinically there is a familial clustering of inhibitors. Furthermore, in an analysis of both PUP recombinant FVIII studies, African Americans were found to exhibit an inhibitor incidence that is twice that of Caucasians (50 percent vs. 25 percent). The intron 22 inversion, large deletion, and stop codon FVIII genotypes may be associated with a higher rate of inhibitor development that are smaller

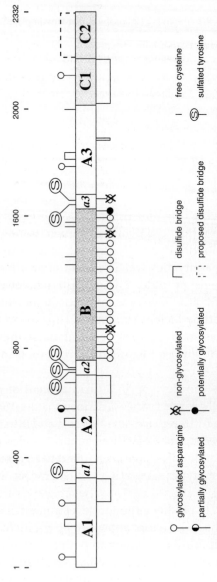

FIGURE 20-1 The factor VIII protein. Mature factor VIII consists of 2332 amino acids that are arranged in a discrete domain structure (A1, A2, B, A3, C1, C2); a1, a2, and a3 denote acidic regions. Disulfide bridges, free cysteine residues, tyrosine sulfation, and glycosylation sites are depicted. (Adapted from Lenting PJ et al: The life cycle of coagulation factor VIII in view of its structure and function. *Blood* 92:3983, 1998.)

deletion and missense mutations. Among HLA genotypes, only a weak association between inhibitor development and class II antigen, DQA 10102, has been observed so far.

The role of replacement therapy in the expression of the inhibitor phenotype is still debated. Issues of clotting-factor product purity have already been discussed. Furthermore, advancing technology applied to both product purification and viral attenuation has been implicated in the creation of FVIII neoantigens. Neoantigen formation has been implicated in several "inhibitor epidemics" among already heavily treated hemophilia A patients, at otherwise low risk for antibody development, who were exposed to such new products.

Much more rarely, FVIII inhibitors may arise spontaneously in "autoimmune" disorders such as rheumatoid arthritis, systemic lupus erythematosus (SLE), Sjögren's syndrome, asthma, inflammatory bowel disease, erythema multiforme, drug reactions (penicillin), and pemphigus. Other underlying conditions include monoclonal gammopathies, malignancies, and pregnancy. However, about half the cases of spontaneous FVIII inhibitors occur in disease-free individuals, in particular, in the first few months postpartum or in elderly individuals. Major bleeding frequently occurs and the mortality rate is high. This phenomenon is extremely rare in children but has occurred in newborn infants from mothers with acquired factor VIII antibodies (transplacental transfer).

FVIII Antibody Characteristics

Although occasional IgM antibodies have been reported, most FVIII antibodies are of the IgG immunoglobulin class. All subclasses are represented; both IgG_1 and IgG_4 are predominant. Light chains have been most frequently of κ or mixed κ and λ type, and less frequently only λ. Taken together, these findings support an oligoclonal origin for the antibodies. Most inhibitors react with a combination of discrete regions of the FVIII light chain (within A_3C_1, C_2, or both) and the A_2 domain of the FVIII heavy chain (Fig. 20-1). Minimal differences in epitope specificity have been observed between alloantibodies developed on either plasma-derived or recombinant FVIII therapy and autoantibodies. However, the high frequency of an otherwise rarely observed single C_2 epitope target has been reported in a new product-associated "inhibitor epidemic".

The reaction between FVIII and its antibody is time dependent and displays two kinetic patterns. The simple or type 1 pattern (in antibody excess) results in complete neutralization of VIII:C; the antibody reacts with FVIII epitopes with great affinity until all antibody is bound. Type 2 or complex kinetics is rapid at first but does not result in irreversible binding (less affinity, more easily dissociated); antibody often coexists with measurable FVIII. The type 1 kinetic pattern is usually seen in congenital hemophilia A patients with inhibitors. When titers of antibody are low, large amounts of FVIII can completely neutralize existing antibody, resulting in hemostatic levels of FVIII. The type 2 pattern is usually observed in spontaneously acquired autoantibody disorders. Measurable levels of FVIII can coexist with antibody available to destroy transfused FVIII.

FACTOR IX INHIBITORS

Factor IX (FIX) inhibitors in hemophilia B occur with an overall incidence of 1 to 6 percent of individuals with severe factor IX deficiency. A subset of FIX inhibitor patients develop severe allergic or anaphylactic reactions upon reexposure to FIX-containing products. The factor IX inhibitor registry includes over 30 such cases. This phenotype can present after as many as 50 previously uncomplicated exposures to plasma-derived or recombinant FIX. Therefore, caution is advised in the transfer of acute care from the clinic to the home setting in predisposed children with severe FIX deficiency.

FIX antibodies are usually of high binding affinity. They are predominately IgG_1 and IgG_4, although a rare IgA inhibitor had been described. Although epitope specificity to both light and heavy chain has been reported, a predominance of IgG_1 and IgG_4 antibodies directed toward the heavy chain have been noted in patients with the allergic phenotype. Complete deletions of the FIX gene are strongly linked to inhibitor development in general, and allergic-type inhibitors in particular. No increase in inhibitor incidence has yet been noted with recombinant FIX in both previously treated and untreated individuals.

Spontaneously acquired FIX autoantibodies are also known (even in children) but are quite rare. These are usually more complex (type II antibodies and occurring most often in patients with an underlying autoimmune disorder). The mainstay of treatment is immunosuppression.

CLINICAL AND LABORATORY MANIFESTATIONS

Hemophilia A and B

The existence of an alloantibody in a hemophiliac patient is suspected when the usual bleeding manifestations of that disease become more severe and/or response to therapy is less than expected. Alternatively it can first be detected by a routine inhibitor screening test. The FVIII or IX assay is usually < 1 percent. The most common and confirmatory test for a FVIII or IX inhibitor is the Bethesda assay (Fig. 20-2). One Bethesda unit (BU) refers to the quantity of antibody that neutralizes 50 percent of the FVIII or IX activity found in normal plasma. The accuracy of the Bethesda assay, particularly for low-titer inhibitors, has been improved by using buffered normal plasma in the incubation step (Nijmegen). A false-positive Bethesda assay may occur from heparin contamination (use Hepzyme, see Manco-Johnson ref) or from the coincidental presence of a lupus anti-coagulant (see Nuss ref). Once an inhibitor is recognized in a hemophiliac patient, serial assays should be done to establish persistence of the inhibitor, severity, and response to antigenic stimulation (transfusion). Inhibitors are classified at "high" or "low responding" based on the historical peak titer and the extent of immune anamnesis upon antigenic rechallenge with FVIII or IX.

Autoimmune Disease

The spontaneous occurrence of an autoantibody type FVIII inhibitor has been noted at any age, but most frequently occurs in postpartum women or in older (55 to 75 years) individuals. New onset major bleeding symptoms, including hemarthroses, melena, deep hematomas, hematuria, and intracranial or retroperitoneal hemorrhage requiring transfusions, occur in over half the patients. Laboratory evaluation reveals normal hemostatic screening tests except for a prolonged APTT, which may show partial to almost complete correction on 1:1 mixing; however, when incubated at 37°C for 1 to 2 h the APTT of the 1:1 mix is prolonged (see Chap. 4). The FVIII assay may indicate decreased but measurable FVIII, despite an increased inhibitor titer by the Bethesda assay. Spontaneous remission may occur at any time; recurrence of the antibody is possible but unusual.

MANAGEMENT GUIDELINES

Inhibitors in Hemophilia A and B

The management of hemorrhage in the presence of inhibitors remains a challenge. Low-responding (minimally anamnestic) inhibitor patients with a history of peak titers < 5 BU can often be successfully treated with larger doses of specific replacement therapy. However, treatment in the presence of a historically high anamnestic response (≥ 5 BU) must bypass the requirement for FVIII or IX. Bypass therapy is most frequently accomplished using prothrombin complex concentrates (PCCs) or activated prothrombin complex concentrates (APCCs), each containing variable

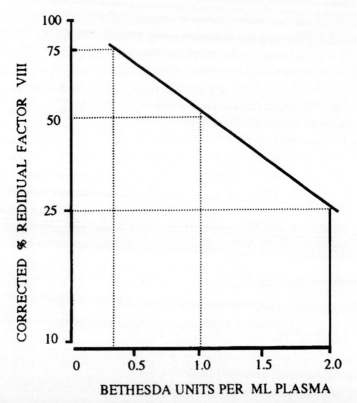

FIGURE 20-2 Graph used to calculate Bethesda units (BU) per mL of plasma. The corrected* percent residual factor VIII in a mixture of equal volumes of patient and normal pooled plasma incubated for 2 h at 37°C is used to indicate the BU. One unit is equal to 50 percent residual or a BU is the amount of antibody that will destroy 0.5 U factor VIII. Plasma is diluted to give a residual between 25 and 75 percent. Type 1 or simple kinetic inhibitors can be determined directly from graph and multiplied by the dilution to obtain final BU. (Adapted from Kasper CK, Ewing NP: J Med Tech 3:431, 1986, with permission.) *The assayed amount in the mixture is corrected for the deterioration of factor VIII in a control (normal plasma and buffer).

amounts of activated factors II, VII, IX, and X (see Chap. 55). Efficacy is limited by the short plasma half-life of activated clotting factors, the potential for DIC and/or thrombosis with frequent or protracted use, and the possibility of stimulating anamnesis due to trace residual FVIII antigen within these concentrates. Concurrent use of antifibrinolytics augments the thrombotic potential of this therapy. Another bypassing agent, recombinant factor VIIA (rFVIIA), has recently been licensed in the United States. Since it is a genetically engineered product containing neither traces of FVIII antigen nor other activated clotting factors, rFVIIA may be particularly useful in the treatment of patients 1) who have never been exposed to plasma-derived products, 2) are already predisposed to DIC or thrombosis, 3) who develop brisk anamnesis with PCC or APCC therapy, or 4) who require concomitant antifibrinolytic therapy. This therapy would also be the treatment of choice for the FIX inhibitor patient with a severe allergic phenotype.

Porcine FVIII has over 75 percent efficacy when used to treat bleeding in hemophilia A inhibitor patients. This product's usefulness relates to its 30 percent homology with human FVIII, allowing both participation in the human coagulation cascade and limited antibody cross-reactivity. Initial dosing is usually between 50 and 150 U/kg. Anamnesis to both human and porcine FVIII can occur with this therapy. Associated allergic reactions can also be severe and limit its use in some individuals. Nonetheless, this product is particularly useful in the treatment of patients who require surgical intervention, who develop major hemorrhage in the presence of a high titer anti-human FVIII inhibitor that precludes treatment with human FVIII replacement, or who require concomitant antifibrinolytic therapy for significant oral hemorrhage.

Plasmapheresis is usually limited to the treatment of life-threatening hemorrhage in the presence of a high-titer inhibitor, when a rapid decrease in the antibody titer can allow for the temporary lifesaving use of a specific factor replacement. A protein A sepharose column, specifically designed for this purpose, was recently made available in the United States by compassionate use protocol.

Recent reports have shown DDAVP may be useful in raising endogenous FVIII levels in inhibitor patients with underlying mild hemophilia A. Its efficacy in these cases suggests that the antibody may be primarily directed toward epitopes present on exogenous FVIII, but not the patient's own protein.

Because none of these therapeutic strategies guarantee the same good outcome as specific factor replacement, the potential for high morbidity and mortality from hemophilic hemorrhage persists. Therefore, inhibitor eradication with immune tolerance therapy (ITT) is currently the best long-term option, particularly for high-responding antibodies. ITT, the regular infusion of specific clotting factor for a period of weeks to years, with or without concomitant immunomodulation therapy, is successful in permanently eradicating the inhibitor in 70 to 85 percent of FVIII inhibitor patients. Dosing regimens in hemophilia A have historically varied and, despite a similar overall success rate, the time to induction of immune tolerance has differed significantly among regimens. Table 20-2

TABLE 20-2

Summary of Immune Tolerance Regimens/Outcomes. References to protocol listed in "Pediatric Issues" reference.

Protocol	Therapeutic Regimen	Success Rate (%)	Median Time on ITT (mos)
Bonn	FVIII: 100 U/kg bid APCC: 40–60 U/kg bid	70%	15
Kasper	FVIII: 50 U/kg qd +/– oral prednisone	73%	3
Dutch	FVIII: 25 U/kg qod→tiw	83%	11.5
Gruppo	FVIII: 100 U/kg q weekly +/– IVIG, cyclophosphamide, prednisone	63%	24
Malmo	Extracorporeal absorption of antibody FVIII: High doses to maintain level >30% +IVIG/ cyclophosphamide	80%	1.3

summarizes the most commonly used ITT protocols for FVIII inhibitors and their outcomes.

Given the intensity and the long-term expense of ITT, optimizing outcome is important. The three major ITT registries for hemophilia A concur that there is a significant correlation between low historical and immediate pre-ITT inhibitors titers and a successful outcome. However, questions about optimal timing, factor dosing, and duration of therapy for high-titer FVIII inhibitors await answers from an international prospective ITT trial due to begin in early 2000. In the meantime, in a child with hemophilia A and a new onset high-titer inhibitor, strong consideration must be given to allowing a natural decline in titer to < 10 BU before beginning ITT in order to optimize outcome. Although the current standard of practice is to treat with daily FVIII doses of at least 100 U/kg/day, both the historical characteristics of the inhibitor as well as ease of venous access should be considered in the design of the ITT dosing regimen.

Due to its much lower frequency, fewer data exist on ITT for FIX inhibitors. Reported overall success rates in this group of patients are as low as 36 percent. Although little is known about good outcome predictors in hemophilia B, almost no successful outcomes have been reported in allergic-type inhibitor patients. Furthermore, the recently reported development of nephrotic syndrome on ITT in this particular group warrants cautious consideration of future attempts at tolerance in these patients. (See Chap. 14.)

Autoimmune Inhibitors

From 60 to 90 percent of patients with autoantibodies to FVIII (uncontrolled reports) benefit from treatment with immunosuppressive drugs (corticosteroids, cyclophosphamides, azathioprine, cyclosporine, vincristine). In an ongoing controlled study over half the patients responded to prednisone therapy alone; some required the addition of cyclophosphamide. A patient with a high-titer postpartum FVIII antibody showed normalization of FVIII after a seven-week course of human interferon-2α, an immune response modifier. Therefore, immunosuppression should be instituted soon after the diagnosis of spontaneous FVIII inhibitors in most patients. Intravenous immunoglobulin, which apparently works by long-term suppression and short-term neutralization (anti-idiotypic antibodies), may have a role in treatment of a limited number of patients.

Since major hemorrhage occurs frequently, hemostasis for acute bleeding remains therapeutically challenging. Low-titer patients occasionally show a hemostatic response to intravenous DDAVP. Measurable levels of FVIII may also be achieved by use of human FVIII concentrates. However, the hemostatic effect of these therapies is often inadequate in moderately-high–titer patients and porcine FVIII is often used to achieve hemostasis. PCCs, APCC's, and rFVIIA have also been used to effectively control hemorrhage in this group of patients. Ultimately, appropriate therapy is selected on the basis of the underlying medical condition, including the likelihood of spontaneous remission, as well as the risk/benefit ratio of the treatment itself.

RARE INHIBITORS

Factor XI Inhibitors

Acquired factor XI inhibitors in hereditary factor XI deficiency are extremely rare, a finding possibly due to the paucity of transfusions in the congenitally deficient patients. A few patients have been reported with antibody titers ranging from 0.75 to 12 BU, and in a patient with a severe thigh hematoma there has been no or occasional postoperative bleeding to 6000 BU. The antibody is usually IgG_4 (when determined), which acts by binding to multiple sites (activation and cleavage), and is frequently time dependent for destruction of factor XI clotting activity. Anamnestic response to transfusion is variable. Bleeding in patients with factor XI inhibitors has responded to increased fresh frozen plasma infusions, plasmapheresis, and bypassing products (prothrombin-complex concentrates and rFVIIa). Screening of previously treated patients for inhibitors prior to elective surgery is recommended.

Spontaneous factor XI inhibitors (autoantibodies) have been reported more commonly; up to 26 cases were known in one report in 1984. Both IgG and IgM antibodies have been described. Most of the patients have underlying autoimmune disorders (rheumatoid arthritis, SLE, or usage of drugs such as chlorpromazine), but rarely show significant hemorrhagic manifestations; most of the patients are diagnosed through evaluation of a prolonged APTT with a normal PT (rule out the LA). In the majority of cases, no specific therapy is necessary; however, immunosuppressive treatment of underlying SLE has been associated with disappearance of the inhibitor.

Acquired Inhibitor of von Willebrand Factor

(See Chapter 12 for a discussion of this inhibitor)

Acquired Factor V Inhibitors

Acquired antibodies in congenital factor V deficiency are exceedingly rare. In one patient, bleeding manifestations worsened and a time-dependent destruction of factor V activity was demonstrated using a factor V assay. Over 30 cases of spontaneous autoantibodies to factor V have occurred in patients in the post-operative period who were previously normal (discussed later in relation to bovine thrombin); most were older adults, except for a 3-year-old child after liver transplantation. Bleeding manifestations have been variable and perhaps related to the accessibility of the patient's platelet factor V to the acquired antibody. The duration of the antibody is relatively short (<10 weeks in most patients) and specific treatment is usually required for acute bleeding episodes. The immunoglobulin class of the antibody may be IgG, IgM, or IgA. The diagnosis is suspected when marked prolongation of the APTT and PT are seen in face of a normal thrombin time and negative tests for lupuslike anticoagulant. (In low-titer inhibitor patients, the platelet neutralization test for lupus anticoagulant may be spuriously positive.) Confirmation is by factor V assay and demonstration of factor V inactivation in plasma mixing tests. Successful treatment of bleeding manifestations has been with platelet concentrates, use of bypassing products or life-saving plasma exchange in one instance of severe intracranial bleeding.

Antithrombin Antibodies

There is an established link between multiple patient exposures to bovine topical thrombin (previous cardiovascular, neurosurgical, or otolaryngologic surgeries) and the development of antithrombin antibodies. Although more frequently described in older patients, several well-documented cases in children have been recently reported. One study detected anti-bovine thrombin antibodies in 10 percent of previously exposed individuals. These patients usually present with no or occasional bleeding symptoms and a markedly prolonged thrombin time (TCT). In particular, the TCT is greatly prolonged when bovine thrombin is used as the reagent; less prolongation of the TCT is seen when human thrombin is used in the TCT. Some studies have indicated a cross-reactivity of the bovine anti-thrombin antibody with human thrombin. Because of the contamination of these preparations with other bovine clotting proteins, antibody development to bovine factors II, VII, V, IX, and X has also been reported. Of these, the anti-bovine factor V antibodies are the most frequent and significant because of the high rate of cross-reactivity with human factor V. Most antibodies develop within the first two weeks following surgery and may persist for weeks to years. No intervention is required for the asymptomatic patient. However, due to the use of bovine proteins in routine clotting factor assays, interference with prothrombin, factor VIII, and anti-Xa activity measurements has been reported. Furthermore, warfarin therapy may be difficult to monitor in the cardiac patient.

Acute and sometimes life-threatening bleeding has been treated with transfusion support, steroids, immunosuppressive therapy, intravenous gamma-globulin, and plasmapheresis. Mortality in such patients is still significant. Avoidance of topical thrombin (bovine) as a hemostatic agent may prevent the occurrence of this clinical syndrome. A recently licensed "fibrin glue" preparation using human instead of bovine thrombin may significantly limit this complication in the future.

Alpha (a) 1-Antitrypsin Pittsburgh

A mutation in the α_1-antitrypsin molecule (Met358Arg) converts the protease to a thrombin and Xa inhibitor that does not require heparin for strong antithrombin activity. The nonimmune mutation designated α_1-AT Pittsburgh has been reported in two unrelated children; the first (age 10 years) had a lifelong history of severe and ultimately fatal soft tissue and postsurgical bleeding; the second patient (age 15 years) was asymptomatic but was noted to have abnormal presurgical screening tests. Both boys displayed marked prolongation of the APTT and thrombin time with moderate prolongation of the PT; 1:1 mixing with normal plasma showed no correction (inhibitory effect). Table 20-3 contains

TABLE 20-3

Rare and Unusual Coagulation Factor Inhibitors

Inhibitor	Antibody Characteristics	Clinical Manifestations	Treatment
Factor VII autoantibody	IgG: progressive destruction of factor VIII activity with incubation at 37°C	Spontaneous occurrence in two older patients; mild to severe bleeding. PT prolonged; other tests normal	No response to IVIG; hemostasis with plasmapheresis and VII concentrate; disappearance with immuno-suppression
Factor II autoantibody	IgG; nonprothrombin activity neutralizing; antibody binds to prothrombin fragment 1	Diffuse bleeding diatheses; PT and APTT abnormal; no evidence for lupus inhibitor factor II level 0.06 U/ml; ↑ to 0.55 with 1:1 mix with normal plasma	Good response to corticosteroids; antibody disappeared in one week
Autoimmune inhibitor of fibrin stabilization	Autoantibody (IgG1 and IgG3) against A and/or B chains of factor XIII	Severe bleeding in adults (one child). Onset related to penicillin allergy and isoniazid usage. Only abnormal test is defective urea solubility of patient and 1:1 1:1 mix with normal plasma	Try immunosuppresive therapy
Heparinlike anticoagulant	Usually not an antibody, but is heparin sulfate proteoglycan: one case with immunoglobulin anticoagulant	Diffuse bleeding diathesis; laboratory tests show marked heparin effect; APTT and TT markedly prolonged; PT slightly prolonged; normal reptilase time. Underlying disorders include acute monoblastic leukemia (infant); multiple myeloma, systemic mastocytosis; neoplastic disease	Protamine sulfate

information on other rare acquired inhibitor syndromes with antibody specificity for coagulation factors; inhibitors are also discussed in appropriate factor deficiency chapters.

BIBLIOGRAPHY

Alumkal J et al: Surgery-associated factor VIII inhibitors without hemophilia. *Am J Med Sci* 318:350, 1999.

Arkin S et al: Activated recombinant human coagulation factor VII therapy for intracranial hemorrhage in patients with hemophilia A or B with inhibitors. *Haemostasis* 28:93, 1998.

Brettler DB et al: The use of porcine FVIII concentrate (Hyate:C) in the treatment of patients with inhibitor antibodies to FVIII: A multicenter US experience. *Arch Intern Med* 149:1381, 1989.

DiMichele DM: Immune tolerance: A synopsis of the international experience. *Haemophilia* 4:568, 1998.

Feinstein DI et al: Diagnosis and management of patients with spontaneously acquired inhibitors of coagulation. *ASH Education Program Book,* p 192, 1999.

Fu YX et al: Multimodality therapy of an acquired factor V inhibitor. *Am J Hematol* 51:315, 1996.

Green D et al: Spontaneous inhibitors of factor VIII: Kinetics of inactivation of human and porcine factor VIII. *J Lab Clin Med* 133:260, 1999

Hilgartner M et al: Pediatric issues in hemophilia. *Hematology 1997-Education Program of the American Society of Hematology,* pp 46–60, 1997.

Horne MK III et al: A heparin-like anticoagulant as part of global abnormalities of plasma glycosaminoglycans in a patient with transitional cell carcinoma. *J Lab Clin Med* 118:250, 1991.

Kreuz W et al: Epidemiology of inhibitor development in hemophilia A patients treated with virus-inactivated plasma-derived clotting factor concentrates. *Vox Sang* 77:3, 1999.

Lawson JH et: Isolation and characterization of an acquired antithrombin antibody. *Blood* 76:2249, 1990.

Manco-Johnson MJ et al: Heparin neutralization is essential for accurate measurement of factor VIII activity and inhibitor assays in blood samples drawn from implanted venous access devices. *J Lab Clin Med* 136:74, 2000.

McMillan C et al: The natural history of FVIII:C inhibitors in patients with hemophilia A: A national cooperative study. II. Observations on the initial development of FVIII:C inhibitors. *Blood* 71:344, 1988.

Negrier C et al: Multicenter retrospective study on the utilization of FEIBA in France in patients with factor VIII and factor IX inhibitors. *Thromb Haemost* 77:1113, 1997.

Nuss R et al: Evidence for antiphospholipid antibodies in hemophilic children with factor VIII inhibitors. *Thromb Haemost* 82:1559, 1999.

Oldenburg J et al. HLA genotype of patients with severe haemophilia A due to intron 22 inversion with and without inhibitors to factor VIII. *Thromb Haemost* 77:238, 1997.

Ortel T et al. Topical thrombin and acquired coagulation factor inhibitors: Clinical spectrum and laboratory diagnosis. *Am J Hematol* 45:128, 1994.

Parquet A et al: Incidence of factor IX inhibitor development in severe haemophilia B patients treated with only one brand of high purity plasma derived factor IX concentrate. *Thromb Haemost* 82:1247, 1999.

Prescott R et al. The inhibitor antibody response is more complex in hemophilia A patients than in most non-hemophiliacs with factor VIII auto-antibodies. *Blood* 89:3663, 1997

Ries M: Severe intracranial hemorrhage in a newborn infant with transplacental transfer of an acquired factor VIII:C inhibitor. *J Pediatr* 127:649, 1995.

Rosendaal FR et al. A sudden increase in FVIII inhibitor development in multi-transfused hemophilia A patients in the Netherlands. *Blood* 81:2180, 1993.

Schnall SF et al: Acquired factor XI inhibitors in congenitally deficient patients. *Am J Hematol* 26:323, 1987.

Schwaab R et al. Haemophilia A: mutation type determines risk of inhibitor formation. *Thromb Haemost* 74:1402, 1995.

Schwartz R et al: A prospective study of treatment of acquired (autoimmune) factor VIII inhibitors with high-dose intravenous gamma-globulin. *Blood* 86:797, 1995.

Solymoss S: Postpartum acquired factor VIII inhibitors—results of a survey. *Am J Hematol* 59:1, 1998.

Tsuchiya H et al: Anaphylactic response to factor VIII preparations in a haemophilic child with an inhibitor of high titre during the tolerance induction. *Eur J Pediatr* 157:85, 1998.

Van den Brink EN et al: Longitudinal analysis of factor VIII inhibitors in a previously untreated mild haemophilia A patient with an Arg(593)-Cys substitution. *Thromb Haemost* 81:723, 1999.

Warrier I et al. Factor IX inhibitors and anaphylaxis in hemophilia B. *Am J Ped Hematol Oncol* 19:23, 1997.

CHAPTER 21

Bleeding Associated with Vascular Disorders

A number of bleeding disorders are associated with abnormalities involving the blood vessels, usually without demonstrable defects in platelets or the coagulation system (exceptions will be noted). These vascular disorders, which are sometimes part of a systemic disease, include the spectrum of vasculitides [Henoch-Schönlein purpura, (HSP)], vascular malformations (hemangiomas, telangiectasias), collagen diseases (Ehlers-Danlos syndrome), and the purpuras (microvascular extravasation of blood into the skin). The hemorrhagic manifestations of these diseases are discussed below.

VASCULITIS

A major cutaneous manifestation of the spectrum of vasculitis (inflammation and necrosis of blood vessels) is raised purpuric lesions (i.e., palpable purpura), which triggers a differential diagnosis of a possible bleeding tendency. Diseases that show such skin lesions include hypersensitivity or leukocytoclastic vasculitis, polyarteritis nodosa, vasculitis associated with malignancy, Wegener's granulomatosis, livedo vasculitis, dysproteinemia (including the cryoglobulinemias), rheumatoid arthritis, and systemic lupus erythematosus (SLE). In most instances, the diagnosis is suggested by the underlying disorder; however, an occasional patient may present with only the cutaneous lesions (skin biopsy is often indicated). With the exception of the petechial-purpuric vasculitic lesions of acute infection (meningococcemia, rickettsial diseases, etc.), which are easily recognized, the most common disorder associated with the differential diagnosis of palpable purpura is hypersensitivity angiitis, or anaphylactoid purpura (HSP) as it is usually called in children, in whom it most commonly occurs.

HSP typically presents in a child (rarely in adults) as a nonthrombocytopenic raised rash occurring over the lower extremities and buttocks, and occasionally involving other parts of the body. The rash is typical in appearance, does not require biopsy, and consists of urticarial wheals and ecchymoses, variable in size (petechiae to confluent spots) and raised to the touch. The purpuric areas evolve in color from red to purple to brown-rust, and then eventually fade; the rash can persist for weeks and recur in crops every few weeks or months. Angioedema of the scalp (20 percent) and extremities (48 percent of cases) may be striking in younger children and is associated with cockade (round papular) purpura on the face and arms as well as lower extremities (called infantile acute hemorrhagic edema).

Other typical manifestations include arthralgia-arthritis, abdominal pain (35 to 85 percent), and signs of nephritis, which may complicate the disease in 20 to 50 percent of cases within 3 months of onset; persistent glomerulonephritis occurs in about 1 percent of cases. Every organ system may be involved in unusual patients, as shown in Table 21-1. Most laboratory tests are helpful only to eliminate other diagnoses or to monitor a particular organ involvement; the diagnosis is based on the clinical manifestations and the typical rash. All hemostatic screening tests are normal except occasional thrombocytosis. Abnormally large multimers of von Willebrand factor have been reported in the plasma of some patients. About half the patients have elevated serum IgA levels. Interestingly, factor XIII levels are decreased (30 to 50 percent) in most patients and are approximately correlated with the activity of the disease. Although hemorrhage may complicate some of the local lesions (gastrointestinal, CNS, pulmonary), a generalized bleeding tendency is not apparent, and surgery and biopsies can be performed without undue risk.

Henoch-Schönlein purpura is considered an immune complex disorder like other hypersensitivity vasculitides and has been associated with a plethora of underlying causes: infection (streptococcus, hepatitis B, cytomegalovirus, Epstein-Barr virus), medications (penicillin, sulfa, phenytoin, iodides, cimetidine, allopurinol), chemicals (insecticides), systemic autoimmune diseases (SLE, rheumatoid arthritis, dermatomyositis), malignancy, and food products (dyes, preservatives). Treatment of HSP is mainly supportive; corticosteroids may slightly decrease the duration of gastrointestinal manifestations but do not appear to alter the course of nephritis. Infusions of a factor XIII concentrate reportedly have benefited severe abdominal crises in HSP. The illness usually lasts 4 to 6 weeks in most cases, but recurrences are frequent, and in rare cases may occur months later; the overall prognosis is excellent with the exception of chronic glomerulonephritis in <1 percent of patients.

TABLE 21-1

Manifestations of Henoch-Schönlein Purpura (Anaphylactoid or Leukocytoclastic Purpura)

Organ	Manifestation
Skin	Palpable purpura, urticaria, petechiae, angioedema
Gastrointestinal tract	Colicky abdominal pain, bleeding, ileus, intussusception, pancreatitis, cholecystitis
Genitourinary	Nephritis, hematuria, nephrosis, scrotal edema, hemorrhage, orchitis
CNS	Apathy, headache, seizures, CNS bleeding (rare), peripheral neuropathy
Cardiac	Myocardial infarction
Musculoskeletal	Arthritis, arthralgia, muscle hematoma
Pulmonary	Hemorrhage, pleural effusion
Laboratory	Positive stool guaiac, hematuria, proteinuria, elevated blood urea, nitrogen, and creatinine; elevated erythrocyte sedimentation rate, leukocytosis, thrombocytosis, occasionally elevated antistreptolysin O and decreased CH50, elevated IgA, decreased factor XIII

ISOLATED PURPURAS

Patients who present with ecchymotic lesions appearing as small to large bruises and whose history reveals only easy bruising with few other bleeding manifestations are candidates for a diagnosis of one of the following causes of isolated purpura, so called because there is no systemic disease and all hemostatic screening tests are normal (see Chap. 5).

Autoerythrocyte Sensitization (Gardner-Diamond Syndrome)

Gardner-Diamond syndrome is a rare disorder characterized by the occurrence of repeated crops of painful erythematous swelling of the skin followed by ecchymoses. In the initial descriptions the lesions could be reproduced by subcutaneous injections of autologous red cells. Most patients are women (>95%), and about half report injuries in the weeks to months prior to the onset of the syndrome. A great many patients have underlying psychological problems, suggesting that this is a form of "psychogenic" purpura. The diagnostic injection of erythrocytes into the skin is no longer used.

Factitious Purpura

Many well-documented examples of secretive self-inflicted injury producing purpuric and petechial lesions have been described. Mechanical maneuvers such as compression or negative suction (mouth, cup, or pinching) may produce lesions that are disturbing to patients or parents

and in whom secondary gain is prominent. The patient may respond to counseling after basic screening tests have proven negative.

Nonaccidental Trauma

A prominent feature of nonaccidental trauma (NAT) due to abuse is ecchymoses; clues to the diagnosis are bruises in several stages of evolution in spite of a report of a single injury, patterns of bruises suggestive of a hand or instrument, and discrepancies between the physical exam and the history. The medical investigation of such cases should include a complete hemostatic screening battery (see Chap. 5) because the diagnosis of a mild bleeding disorder and NAT are not mutually exclusive; several studies of hemostasis in suspected NAT have shown abnormal screening tests leading to diagnoses of von Willebrand disease, platelet function disorders, acquired factor VIII inhibitor, mild hemophilia, and immune thrombocytopenic purpura.

Purpura Simplex

Purpura simplex ("easy bruising") is a frequent complaint of adult women, some men, and active young children. The bruises are typically small (<1 to 2 cm), are not raised, and are found on the proximal extremities or trunk. If the ecchymoses are large (> 2 inches in diameter) or indurated, and not easily explained by trauma, they should be considered abnormal and investigated (see Chap. 5). A few of these subjects will be found to have mild von Willebrand disease or hemophilia. Therapy includes reassurance and a recommendation to avoid aspirin or other antiplatelet agents.

Aging (Senile Purpura)

With aging the subcutaneous tissues atrophy, providing inadequate support for dermal vessels. Purplish-red patches are found over the extensor surfaces of the arms and hands in elderly subjects. The skin is often very thin and tears easily. Treatment includes protection of the skin from avoidable trauma.

Glucocorticoid Excess

Purpura may be seen in Cushing's syndrome and after long-term corticosteroid administration. The cause may be related to reduced collagen synthesis in the skin with atrophy and easy bruising.

Scurvy

Vitamin C is necessary in the final assembly of collagen when proline is converted to hydroxyproline, which stabilizes the helical structure of collagen. The bleeding tendency in scurvy is manifested by perifollicular hemorrhages, ecchymotic purpura, gingival bleeding, and subperiosteal hemorrhage, despite usually normal hemostatic tests. Faulty diet in the chronically or mentally ill, recluse, or diet faddist is the usual cause. The diagnosis is made by the classic skin findings, low concentrations of vitamin C in the plasma, and rapid recovery with vitamin replacement.

VASCULAR MALFORMATIONS

Hemangioma

Juvenile hemangioma or hemangioma of infancy is an angiomatoid malformation caused by abnormal proliferation of capillaries. These tumors grow rapidly in the first year of life and then slowly regress over the next 5 to 8 years or even sooner. More than 90 percent regress completely; however, a few persist into adult life. Most of the tumors are small and remain localized to the skin; a few grow rapidly to an alarming size or proliferate in multiple organs (liver, spleen, bone, lung) causing serious complications such as soft-tissue destruction, endangerment of vital structures (eye, airway), congestive heart failure, and serious bleeding. The bleeding manifestations are due to intratumor hemorrhage (often producing significant anemia) and a generalized bleeding tendency due to acute and chronic DIC, which occurs in a small percentage of cases. The consumption coagulopathy is usually characterized by thrombocytopenia, decreased fibrinogen, increased fibrin degradation products (FDP), and microangiopathic anemia; this is called Kasabach-Merritt syndrome.

Management consists of observation (serial photographs are helpful in following larger lesions) and possibly local compression of the lesion unless life-threatening complications appear (serious thrombocytopenia or DIC, limb or organ endangerment, congestive heart failure). Therapy with oral prednisone (3 to 4 mg/kg/day) is associated with regression in several weeks in about one-third of the cases. Other modalities used with varying success include surgery, arterial embolization, low-dose radiation therapy, cyclophosphamide, and antifibrinolytic agents. The DIC may be controlled temporarily with intravenous heparin or the combination of aspirin and dipyridamole. Recent reports indicate that interferon-α induces regressions of life-threatening corticosteroid-resistant cavernous hemangioma of infancy.

Hereditary Hemorrhagic Telangiectasia

Hereditary hemorrhagic telangiectasia (HHT, Osler-Weber-Rendu disease) is an autosomal disorder manifested by multiple telangiectasia of the skin, gastrointestinal (GI), and respiratory tract. The lesions can be easily injured, leading to epistaxis and GI bleeding. Arteriovenous malformations may be found in the lungs, brain, or other organs. Mutations have been identified in the gene (chromosome 9) for endoglin, which is an endothelial cell receptor for TGF-β, a protein involved in angiogenesis and tissue repair. Similar defects have been localized to chromosome 12.

HHT occurs in one in 2500 to 40,000 individuals. Classically, patients have multiple small red blanching telangiectasia on the lips, tongue, face, and under the fingernails. Pulmonary A-V fistulas are characteristically found in the lower lobes and may require angiography or helical CT scanning to be identified. GI lesions may cause chronic blood loss and profound iron deficiency. CNS lesions may be due to A-V malformations or cerebral abscesses due to pulmonary A-V shunting.

The clinical evaluation should include a careful family history as well as a personal history of epistaxis, GI bleeding, iron deficiency, and pulmonary or neurologic symptoms. Examinations by specialists (e.g., ENT), CT scanning, or angiography may be required. Von Willebrand disease has been linked with HHT; however, this may be a chance association.

Treatment includes direct approaches to bleeding vascular lesions using compression, surgery, or endoscopic laser therapy. GI bleeding may require red cell transfusion and intravenous iron replacement. Catheter-directed embolization may be needed for pulmonary or CNS lesions.

STRUCTURAL DISORDERS

The heritable disorders of connective tissue are those diseases in which the primary defect is due to a molecular alteration in collagen or other structural proteins. A mild bleeding tendency (easy bruising, hematoma formation, poor wound healing) may be present due to defects in procollagen genes, with abnormal collagen formation in the blood vessels and supporting tissues. Because the diagnosis may be first suspected during the evaluation of a possible bleeding diathesis, an awareness of some of these specific defects is necessary.

Enlers-Danlos Syndrome

Most types of Ehlers-Danlos Syndrome (EDS) are associated with easy bruising, but Type IV (ecchymotic or vascular type) is the most clinically important phenotype of this disease (Table 21-2). Type IV is characterized by decreased production of Type III collagen, which stabilizes blood vessels and skin. The defect has been localized to a variety of structural mutations in the COL3A1 gene (chromosome 2), which directs the synthesis of Type III procollagen. This disorder occurs with a frequency of one in 50,000 to 500,000 persons.

Clinically the disorder (Type IV) is heterogeneous; over half of the patients have no family history of the disorder. When severe the skin is very thin (not elastic); there is a prominent venous pattern; and the faces have thin lips, prominent eyes, and a sharp nose. The skin may show "cigarette paper" scarring at old injury sites. Small joint hyperextensibility is observed. Bruising is common; gingival bleeding and hemorrhage after dental extraction can occur. A frequent cause of death is spontaneous arterial rupture or dissection, including stroke. Bowel and uterine rupture (third trimester) have been reported. Some patients have minimal skin findings. A recent report described an association between easy bruising and hyperextensibility of the thumb, which could be due to a mild subtype of EDS.

Diagnosis is accomplished by history and physical examination and laboratory studies of skin biopsies (ultrastructure and immunofluores-

---

TABLE 21-2

Clinical Variants of the Ehlers-Danlos Syndrome

Type	Name	Inheritance	Clinical Features
I	Gravis	AD	Hyperextensible skin, marked bleeding, paper-thin scars, hypermobile joints
II	Mitus	AD	Like I but less severe
III	Benign hypermobility	AD	Soft skin, marked large and small joint hypermobility, minimal bleeding
IV	Arterial, ecchymotic	AR or AD	Thin skin; visible veins; marked bleeding tendency; skin and joints less involved; arterial, bowel, uterine rupture
V	X-linked	XL	Like type II
VI	Ocular	AR	Ocular fragility and keratoconus, soft velvety skin, hypermobile joints, scoliosis
VII	Arthrochalasis multiplex congenita	AD	Congenital hip dislocation, laxity of joints, bruising
VIII	Periodontal	AD	Periodontitis; skin like type II
IX	Cutis laxa (abnormal copper metabolism)	XL	Bladder diverticula and rupture, short arms, occipital horns, no bleeding
X	Fibronectin defect	AR	Like type II; mild bleeding

*AD, autosomal dominant; AR, autosomal recessive; XL, X-linked

cence), along with assessment of collagen synthesis by cultured skin fibroblasts. Hemostatic tests are usually normal, although studies have suggested impaired platelet aggregation that may occur with patient-derived, but not normal, collagen.

Treatment includes protection of the skin from trauma and avoidance of antiplatelet agents. Arterial puncture (e.g., angiography) should be avoided. Surgery may be complicated by wound dehiscence and bleeding.

Osteogenesis Imperfecta

Mutations in the collagen genes (COL1A1 or COL1A2 genes on chromosomes 7 and 17 respectively) produce a change in the structure of type I procollagen and the heterogeneous clinical syndrome of osteogenesis imperfecta. Brittle bones are the main feature of the disorder; both autosomal and recessive forms of the disease are known, ranging in severity from death *in utero* to an occasional fracture and blue sclerae. Some of the patients bruise easily and show a mild platelet functional defect (abnormal aggregation pattern, failure to release) with slightly prolonged bleeding times, although these findings may be coincidental. Treatment is mainly limited to physical therapy and orthopedic surgery, although intravenous diphosphenate has increased bone density and improved clinical outcomes.

Marfan Syndrome

Marfan syndrome is due to a defect in the fibrillin gene (FBN-1 on chromosome 15). Fibrillin is a key component of microfibrils, proteins important in extracellular matrix. This disease, an autosomal dominant condition affecting 1 in 10,000 people, produces multiple skeletal deformities (tall stature, long extremities and digits), ocular lens dislocations, and cardiovascular manifestations (dissecting aortic aneurysm). Connective tissues are often friable and surgical correction of the aortic defect has been associated with severe bleeding, apparently on a vascular basis. Some patients bruise easily, but coagulation and platelet function tests are usually normal.

BIBLIOGRAPHY

Baselga E et al: Purpura in infants and children. *J Am Acad Dermatol* 37: 673, 1997.

Bauman NM et al: Treatment of massive or life-threatening hemangiomas with recombinant alpha(2a)-interferon. *Otolaryngol-Head Neck Surg* 117:99, 1997.

Berg JN et al: Clinical heterogeneity in hereditary hemorrhagic telangiectasia: Are pulmonary arteriovenous malformations more common in families linked to endoglin? *J Med Genet* 33:256, 1996.

Casonata A et al: Abnormally large von Willebrand factor multimers in Henoch-Schönlein purpura. *Am J Hematol* 51:7, 1996.

Frieden IJ: Which hemangiomas to treat—and how? *Arch Dermatol* 133:1593, 1997.

Gibson LE: Cutaneous vasculitis: Approach to diagnosis and systemic associations. *Mayo Clin Proc* 65:221, 1990.

Glorieux FH et al: Cyclic administration of pamidronate in children with severe osteogenesis imperfecta. *N Engl J Med* 339:947, 1998.

Haitjema T et al: Hereditary hemorrhagic telangiectasia (Osler-Weber-Rendu disease): new insights in pathogenesis, complications, and treatment. *Arch Intern Med* 156:714, 1996.

Kaplinsky C et al: Association between hyperflexibility of the thumb and an unexplained bleeding tendency: is it a rule of thumb? *Br J Haematol* 101:260, 1998.

Marini JC: Osteogenesis imperfecta—managing brittle bones. *N Engl J Med* 339:986, 1998.

North KN et al: Cerebrovascular complications in Ehlers-Danlos syndrome type IV. *Ann Neurol* 38:960, 1995.

Pereira L et al: Targeting of the gene encoding fibrillin-1 recapitulates the vascular aspect of Marfan syndrome. *Nature Genetics* 17:218, 1997.

Phillips MD: Stopping bleeding in hereditary telangiectasia. *N Engl J Med,* 330:1822, 1994.

Pope FM et al: Clinical presentations of Ehlers Danlos syndrome type IV. *Arch Dis Child* 63:1016, 1988.

Ratnoff OD: Psychogenic bleeding. In Ratnoff OD, Forbes Cd (eds): *Disorders of Hemostasis,* Philadelphia, W.B. Saunders, 1991, p 550.

Saba HI et al: Treatment of bleeding in hereditary hemorrhagic telangiectasia with aminocaproic acid. *N Engl J Med* 330:1789, 1994.

Scimeca PG et al: Suspicion of child abuse complicating the diagnosis of bleeding disorders. *Pediatr Hematol Oncol* 13:179, 1996.

Shovlin CL et al: Characterization of endoglin and identification of novel mutations in hereditary hemorrhagic telangiectasia. *Am J Hum Genet* 61:68, 1997.

Shulkin BL et al: Kasabach-Merritt syndrome: Treatment with epsilon-aminocaproic acid and assessment by indium 111 platelet scintigraphy. *J Pediat* 117:746, 1990.

Smith LT et al: Mutations in the COL3A1 gene result in the Ehlers-Danlos syndrome type IV and alterations in the size and distribution of the major collagen fibrils of the dermis. *J Invest Dermatol* 108:241, 1997.

Solomon JA et al: GI manifestations of Ehlers-Danlos Syndrome. *Am J Gastro* 91:2282, 1996.

Szer IS: Henoch-Schönlein purpura: When and how to treat. *J Rheumatol* 23:1661, 1996.

Tancrede-Bohin E et al: Schönlein-Henoch purpura in adult patients. *Arch Dermatol* 133:438, 1997.

CHAPTER 22

Vitamin K Deficiency

Soon after the discovery of vitamin K by Henrik Dam in 1929–1935, it was established that the generalized bleeding tendency known as hemorrhagic disease of the newborn (HDN) was due to vitamin K deficiency. It is now known that vitamin K functions as an essential cofactor for the synthesis of the coagulation proteins, factors II, VII, IX, X, protein C, and protein S by promoting a unique posttranslational modification of specific glutamic acid residues to gamma-carboxyglutamic acid (Gla), thus mediating calcium binding to negatively charged phospholipid surfaces. Other proteins dependent on vitamin K for complete synthesis include osteocalcin and protein Z. Protein Z forms a complex with a serine protease inhibitor (protein Z-dependent protease inhibitor, ZPI) on the phospholipid surface and inhibits factor Xa procoagulant activity. Gla-containing proteins have been found in bone, cartilage, dentin, kidney, placenta, pancreas, spleen, lung, testes, and liver tissue.

STRUCTURE AND FUNCTION OF VITAMIN K

Vitamin K is 1,4-naphthoquinone with a methyl group at position 2 and a polyisoprenoid side chain at position 3. Vitamin K_1, phylloquinone, is made by green plants; vitamin K_2 includes a group of compounds made by bacteria and are called menaquinones (MK-n), with n being the number of isoprene units at position 3. The parent compound lacking the side chain is menadione (K_3), which has no vitamin K activity in vitro but can be alkylated to active MK-4 in animal tissues. Intestinal bacteria synthesize MK-7–13 form, which are of relatively small value due to poor adsorption; food sources of menaquinones are limited to animal and soybean products. The major biologic source of vitamin K comes from the ingestion of phylloquinone. The human dietary requirement (RDA) is about 1 microgram per kg and is supplied by green and yellow leafy vegetables, some vegetable oils, and other foods; human milk is low in vitamin K (~2 μg/L) as compared to cow's milk (4 to 18 μg/L). Table 22-1 indicates the major vitamin K analogues. Vitamin K is a lipid-soluble vitamin and is dependent on an intact intestinal fat absorption mechanism for optimal utilization of oral forms of the vitamin. Vitamin K is poorly transported across the placenta; maternal fetal gradients of 18:1 and 30:1 have been reported.

The primary hemostatic function of vitamin K is to mediate the carboxylation of selected 9 to 12 glutamates located near the NH_2 terminus of the protein to Gla residues used to bind calcium to phospholipid membranes, thus allowing formation of critical coagulation complexes ("factor Xase," "prothrombinase," and "protein C-ase"). Figure 22-1 depicts the carboxylation step and the role of vitamin K. The carboxylation process is mediated by a vitamin K-dependent gamma-glutamyl carboxylase, reduced K, carbon dioxide, and oxygen. The cycle is interrupted by warfarin-type compounds that block the epoxide reductase, allowing accumulation of vitamin K epoxide to levels 50 times baseline.

Impairment in carboxylation that occurs in vitamin K deficiency or some types of liver dysfunction (cirrhosis, hepatocellular carcinoma) results in an accumulation of the clotting factor protein with absent or decreased gamma-carboxylation sites and whose half-disappearance time in the circulation is approximately that of the native protein (60 h for noncarboxylated prothrombin). The non- or des-carboxylated protein is also called "protein-induced in vitamin K absence," or PIVKA, and can be used as a marker for vitamin K deficiency or hepatocellular cancer. Even more sensitive markers of vitamin K deficiency are des-carboxylated osteocalcin and decreased Gla excretion in the urine.

TABLE 22-1		
Vitamin K Analogues		
Name	**Source**	**Dosage Form**
Phylloquinone (K1)	Diet; green plants	AquaMEPHYTON Konakion, Konakion MM
Menaquinones-n (K2)	Intestinal bacteria	Kaytwo (MK-4)
Menadione (K3)	Parent compound	Synkayvite

*n = number of isoprene units

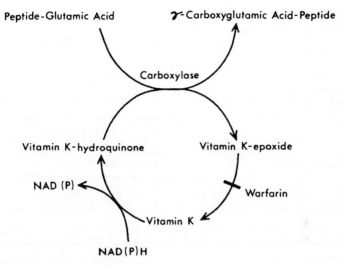

FIGURE 22-1 The vitamin K cycle.

DIAGNOSIS OF VITAMIN K DEFICIENCY

Table 22-2 indicates the progression of the deficiency state and, therefore, the sensitivity of assays used to determine vitamin K status. A bleeding tendency does not occur until the coagulation factor levels are <30 to 35 percent when, therefore, the screening tests (PT, APTT) become abnormal. The more sensitive assays, plasma vitamin K level and noncarboxylated prothrombin assay, as well as the urinary Gla assay (decreased Gla in vitamin K deficiency), are particularly useful in determination of subclinical deficiency states; however, in most clinical situations, the correction of the abnormal coagulation screening tests by vitamin K is the mainstay of diagnosis. With a few possible exceptions such as severe liver disease, hepatocellular carcinoma, and rare cases of multiple vitamin K-dependent coagulation factors, increased noncarboxylated proteins are diagnostic of vitamin K deficiency. All of these exceptions may respond to large doses of vitamin K.

VITAMIN K DEFICIENCY IN INFANCY

Three syndromes of hemorrhagic disease (also called vitamin K deficiency bleeding, VKDB) may be seen in the newborn and young infant; these have been called early, classic, and late HDN, and are described in Table 22-3. Of particular interest are early and late HDN, which raise con-

TABLE 22-2

Markers of Vitamin K Deficiency in Humans

Physiologic Change	Assay or Test
Decreased liver stores of vitamin K	Liver tissue analysis
Altered bone metabolism	Increased serum descarboxylated osteocalcin
Decreased plasma vitamin K	Adult plasma level = 100–1000 pg/mL Cord blood level = <50 pg/mL
Decreased carboxylation of vitamin K dependent proteins	Increased descarboxylated proteins (increased PIVKAs) Decreased urinary excretion of Gla (N = 25–29 µmol/day)
Decreased levels of coagulation factors	Low factors II, VII, IX, X, C, S
Abnormal coagulation screening tests	Prolongation of PT, APTT, Thrombotest

troversial issues regarding management. Early HDN is most likely to occur in newborn infants whose mothers have been on anticonvulsant therapy (phenytoin, phenobarbital, valproic acid, carbamazepine). From 25 to 50 percent of these infants will show biochemical evidence (low vitamin K and increased noncarboxylated prothrombin levels) in cord blood and about 5 percent will have HDN; both can be eliminated by administering 10 mg vitamin K_1 orally daily to the mother 2 weeks before delivery. Vitamin K deficiency embryopathy consisting of radiographic punctate calcifications, nasal hypoplasia, abnormalities of the spine, and other vascular abnormalities with or without a bleeding tendency may be due to maternal vitamin K deficiency (warfarin or malabsorption). Chondroplasia punctate and deficiencies of vitamin K-dependent clotting factors is also associated with a genetic deficiency of epoxide reductase even with vitamin K repletion.

Late HDN occurs mainly in exclusively breastfed infants who have had inadequate amounts of oral vitamin K as neonatal prophylaxis. The estimated prevalence varies from 7 (developed countries) to 20/100,000 (underdeveloped countries) births without neonatal prophylactic vitamin K. Late HDN is frequently associated with intracranial hemorrhage and neurologic residuals. Parenteral vitamin K (IM) at birth or multidose oral vitamin K prevents the syndrome.

Current considerations for prophylaxis are further complicated by a British study in 1992 that showed that intramuscular, but not oral, vitamin K at birth was associated with a 2.3-fold increased relative risk of childhood cancer. Multiple similar studies since that time have refuted these disturbing findings, with exception of one study that indicated that

TABLE 22-3

Vitamin K Deficiency Hemorrhagic Syndromes in Infancy

Syndrome	Age	Common Bleeding Sites	Cause	Frequency (without Vitamin K Prophylaxis)	Prevention
Early HDN	0–24 hours	Cephalohematoma, scalp monitor, intracranial, intra-thoracic, intraabdominal	Maternal drugs: Warfarin, anticonvulsants, antituberculous chemotherapy. Idiopathic	About 5% in high risk pregnancies	Daily oral vitamin K to mother for two weeks before delivery
Classic HDN	1–7 days	Gastrointestinal, skin, nasal, circumcision	Idiopathic, maternal drugs	0.01–1%, varies by population group	Oral or IM vitamin K at birth
Late HDN	2 wks–6 mon	Intracranial, skin, gastrointestinal	Idiopathic Secondary: diarrhea, malabsorption (cystic fibrosis, α_1-antitrypsin deficiency, biliary atresia, hepatitis)	5–20 per 100,000 births	Vitamin K given as IM dose at birth or multiple oral doses (see text)

a small risk of leukemia was not excluded (see Zipursky, von Kries, and the American Academy of Pediatrics references).

A summary of recommendations for prevention of HDN are:

1. Early HDN: Mothers on anticonvulsants, antibiotics, or warfarin (warfarin should be stopped) should receive 10 mg vitamin K_1 orally each day beginning 2 weeks before delivery.
2. Classic HDN: Infants should receive 0.5 to 1 mg vitamin K1 intramuscularly or 2 mg vitamin K_1 orally at birth.
3. Late HDN: Breastfed infants (formula-fed infants receive adequate vitamin K) should receive IM prophylaxis as for classic HDN at birth; repeat oral vitamin K during infancy when diarrhea for more than a few days occurs. IM, but not IV, vitamin K probably acts as depository for sustained effect. Repeat intramuscular dose monthly in infants with hepatitis or malabsorption syndromes.
4. Breastfed infants of mothers on oral anticoagulation should be given a weekly oral supplement of 1 mg of vitamin K.

Multiple oral doses of K_1 or K_2 are necessary to approximate parenteral prophylaxis in breastfed infants in preventing all late HDN. A daily low oral dose of 25 microgram of K_1 for exclusively breast-fed infants has been shown to be as effective as IM prophylaxis. In addition, multiple (2mg at birth, 7 days, and 30 days of life) of a new oral preparation (Konakion MM, a mixed micelle form of vitamin K_1) was equal in effectiveness to IM in a study of infants over the first 8 weeks of life. All other oral regimens used so far have not been as effective in prevention as the intramuscular route. In the United States the standard neonatal prophylaxis with 0.5 to 1.0 mg vitamin K_1 oxide given parenterally (intramuscularly) prevents classic and late HDN.

VITAMIN K DEFICIENCY IN OLDER CHILDREN AND ADULTS

Vitamin K deficiency with or without overt bleeding symptoms may occur at any age and should be suspected in any differential diagnosis of an acquired bleeding tendency. Malabsorption of fat-soluble vitamins (Table 22-4) may be subtle and a clue to a major disorder. Prolonged fasting (3 to 7 or more days) and hyperemesis gravidarum with or without antibiotic therapy may cause a symptomatic deficiency (i.e., elderly patients with poor oral intake or intravenous antibiotic therapy). Warfarin ingestion is an obvious and therapeutically important cause (see Chap. 60); however, surreptitiously or accidental ingestion of short-acting warfarin or long-acting coumarin found in rodenticides (brodifa-

---

TABLE 22-4

Associated Causes of Vitamin K Deficiency

Malabsorption

    α_1-Antitrypsin deficiency
    Abetalipoproteinemia
    Bile duct atresia
    Celiac disease
    Chronic diarrhea
    Cystic fibrosis
    Cholestatic liver disease
    Thermal burn injuries

Fasting

Hyperemesis gravidarum

Alcoholism

Drugs

    Coumarins: warfarin, herbal tea, long-acting rodenticides (brodifacoum)
    Maternal anticonvulsants
    Antibiotics (cephalosporins, NMTT chain)
    Vitamin E megadose
    Salicylates

---

coum) should be considered in bleeding patients with prolonged PT and APTT (sometimes with a poor or no response to usual vitamin K doses). Antibiotics with a N-methyl-thiotetrazole side chain (beta-lactam) and salicylates inhibit vitamin K epoxide reductase and elevate plasma K_1 epoxide levels. Subtle markers of vitamin K deficiency (descarboxylated osteocalcin and urinary Gla excretion) have been noted in osteoporosis and fractures in the elderly.

The pattern of coagulation screening tests shows prolonged (often greatly) PT and APTT with normal thrombin time (ruling out heparin effect) and normal platelet count (unless disseminated intravascular coagulation is also present). The PT is often prolonged early and more severely. When this pattern is seen in a bleeding patient, vitamin K should be given parenterally (subcutaneously or a reduced dose slowly intravenously to avoid reactions) in the following dosage: infant or child 1 to 5 mg; older child 5 to 10 mg; and adult up to 10 mg (see also Chap. 60). The usual response is cessation of bleeding and correction of PT in 4 to 8 h or less. Additional blood product replacement is rarely needed unless the patient is on warfarin and has significant bleeding, at which time fresh frozen plasma should be used. Even though the PT and APTT have returned to normal, a diagnosis of vitamin K deficiency may be confirmed by elevated noncarboxylated prothrombin (which has a half-disappearance time of 60 h); most reference laboratories offer a PIVKA-II determination.

BIBLIOGRAPHY

American Academy of Pediatrics. Vitamin K Ad Hoc Task Force. Controversies concerning vitamin K and the newborn. *Pediatrics* 91:1001, 1993.

Booth SL, Suttie JW: Dietary intake and adequacy of vitamin K. *J Nutr* 128:785, 1998.

Chua JD, Friedenberg WR: Superwarfarin poisoning. *Arch Intern Med* 158:1929, 1998.

Cornelisson M et al: Prevention of vitamin K deficiency bleeding: efficacy of different multiple oral dose schedules of vitamin K. *Eur J Pediatr* 156:126, 1997.

Furie B et al: Vitamin K-dependent biosynthesis of γ-carboxyglutamic acid. *Blood* 93:1797, 1999.

Greer FR: The importance of vitamin K as a nutrient during the first year of life. *Nutr Res* 15:289, 1995.

Greer FR et al: A new mixed micellar preparation for oral vitamin K prophylaxis: randomised controlled comparison with an intramuscular formulation in breast fed infants. *Arch Dis Child* 79:300, 1998.

Golding J et al: Childhood cancer, intramuscular vitamin K, and pethidine given during labour. *BMJ* 305:341, 1992.

Han X et al: The protein Z-dependent protease is a serpin. *Biochemistry* 38:11073, 1999.

Jenkins ME et al: A prospective analysis of serum vitamin K in severely burned pediatric patients. *J Burn Care Rehabil* 19:75, 1998.

Loughnan PM, McDougall PN: Does intramuscular vitamin K1 act as an unintended depot preparation? *J Paediatr Child Health* 32:251, 1996.

Menger H et al: Vitamin K deficiency embryopathy: a phenocopy of the warfarin embryopathy due to a disorder of embryonic vitamin K metabolism. *Am J Med Genet* 72:129, 1997.

Prasad GVR et al: Vitamin K deficiency with hemorrhage after kidney and combined kidney-pancreas transplantation. *Am J Kidney Dis* 33:963, 1999.

Rashid M et al: Prevalence of vitamin K deficiency in cystic fibrosis. *Am J Clin Nutr* 70:378, 1999.

Robinson JN et al: Coagulopathy secondary to vitamin K deficiency in hyperemesis gravidarum. *Obstet Gynec* 92:673, 1998.

Shearer MJ, Seghatchian MJ, editors: *Vitamin K and vitamin K-dependent proteins. Analytical, physiological, and clinical aspects.* London, CRC Press, 1993.

Sutor AH, Hathaway WE, editors: *Vitamin K in infancy. International Symposium.* Stuttgart, Schattauer, 1995.

Sutor AH et al: Vitamin K deficiency bleeding (VKDB) in infancy. ISTH Pediatric/Prenatal Subcommittee. *Thromb Haemost* 81:456, 1999.

von Kries R: Neonatal vitamin K prophylaxis: the Gordian knot still awaits untying. *BMJ* 316:161, 1998.

Zipursky A: Prevention of vitamin K deficiency bleeding in newborns. Review. *Br J Haematol* 104:430, 1999.

CHAPTER 23

Liver Diseases

Bleeding is an all too common clinical problem in patients with acute or chronic liver disease. Sites of gastrointestinal hemorrhage include esophageal or gastric varices, acute gastritis, and peptic ulcer disease. Easy bruising and epistaxis occur frequently. Hemostatic defects are numerous and often pronounced, and include impaired hepatic synthesis of coagulation and fibrinolytic proteins, reduced clearance of activated coagulation factors by the hepatic reticuloendothelial system, and quantitative and qualitative platelet defects (Table 23-1).

PATHOGENESIS

Liver failure can be acute (e.g., fulminant hepatitis, mushroom poisoning, hypoxia, acute fatty liver of pregnancy) or more chronic and progressive (e.g., alcoholic or viral cirrhosis, biliary atresia, primary biliary cirrhosis, amyloidosis, malignancy). Obstructive biliary tract disease can also cause hemostatic abnormalities, such as vitamin K deficiency due to impaired absorption of the vitamins. Although the causes of liver disease are diverse, the coagulopathies associated with liver failure usually fall into one or more of the categories (described later and in Table 23-2).

Impaired Synthesis of Clotting Factors

When the synthetic function of the liver is suppressed by disease, the concentrations of clotting factors in the plasma often fall to levels that promote bleeding. Factor VII and factor V are sensitive indicators of hepatic protein synthesis and may be used as a guide to the severity of the liver

TABLE 23-1	
Hemostatic Defects in Liver Disease	
Defect	**Possible Mechanisms**
Impaired coagulation	
	Decreased hepatic synthesis of clotting/fibrinolytic factors
	Vitamin K deficiency
Thrombocytopenia and platelet function defects	
	Hypersplenism
	Failure to clear platelet inhibitors
	Immune destruction
	Decreased production (e.g., low thrombopoietin production)
Disseminated intravascular coagulation	
	Procoagulants from hepatic cells
	Endotoxins in portal circulation
	Failure to clear activated clotting factors
	Reduced antithrombin and protein C
	Elevated cytokines
	Intercurrent events (e.g., sepsis, peritoneovenous shunts)
Systemic fibrinolysis	
	Reduced α_2-antiplasmin
	Failure to clear fibrinolytic enzymes
	Reduced clearance of tissue plasminogen activator

disease. In fact, the Child-Pugh grading system for liver disease uses the PT as a major criterion for the severity of liver impairment. Abnormal forms of the vitamin K-dependent clotting factors, such as descarboxyl prothrombin, have been identified in patients with acute hepatitis and cirrhosis as well as hepatocellular carcinoma, although the concentrations of these abnormal clotting factors are sufficiently low that they do not contribute to bleeding. Poor nutrition (chronic disease, alcoholism), obstructive biliary tract disease, and malabsorption of fat-soluble vitamins can lead to vitamin K deficiency.

Von Willebrand factor is not synthesized by hepatic parenchymal cells, but is produced by endothelial cells and megakaryocytes; plasma concentrations are markedly increased in patients with hepatic insufficiency. The reason for the elevation is not known, but it could reflect vascular stimulation or damage with release of von Willebrand factor into the blood. Although coagulation factor VIII is synthesized in the liver (liver transplantation brings factor VIII levels to normal in patients with hemophilia A), end-stage liver disease due to hepatitis, alcohol, or other causes

TABLE 23-2

Hemostatic Abnormalities in Hepatic Disease

Condition	PT	APTT	TCT	Fibrinogen	FDP/D-dimer	Euglobulin Clot Lysis Time	Factor V	Factor VIII	Factor VII	Platelets
Acute hepatitis severe	↑↑↑	↑↑	↑↑↑	↓↓↓	↑↑	↓	↓↓	↑↑↑	↓↓	N-↓
Biliary cirrhosis	↑↑↑	↑	N-↑	N-↑	N-↑	N-↓	N-↓	↑	↓↓↓	N-↓
Biliary obstruction	↑↑↑	N-↑	N	N-↑	N	N	N	N-↑	↓↓↓	N
Liver cirrhosis	↑↑↑	N-↑	N-↑	N-↓	N-↑	N-↓	↓↓	N-↑↑	↓↓↓	↓

Fg, fibrinogen; FDP, fibrin(ogen) degradation products; F V (etc), factor V.....; PT, prothrombin time; APTT, partial thromboplastin time; TCT, thrombin clotting time

does not produce a fall in plasma factor VIII activity. Indeed, the concentration of factor VIII rises in the blood parallel with, but somewhat behind, the increase of von Willebrand factor.

Fibrinogen is exclusively synthesized by the liver. Fibrinogen is an acute phase reactant and the liver has a remarkable capacity to conserve fibrinogen synthesis in both acute and chronic liver disease. Profound hypofibrinogenemia is unusual in liver disease but may be associated with end-stage liver failure, disseminated intravascular coagulation (DIC), and acute fulminant hepatitis.

Thrombocytopenia

A mild to moderate reduction in platelet count is common in chronic liver disease and is most often due to hypersplenism with sequestration of platelets within an enlarged spleen. Platelet survival is also reduced in cirrhosis, and has been linked to platelet-associated IgG, especially in hepatitis C and autoimmune hepatitis. Thrombopoietin is produced by the liver and low levels of this growth factor are likely to play a role in the inadequate bone marrow response to thrombocytopenia.

Patients with alcoholic liver disease have additional reasons for thrombocytopenia. Alcohol can reduce platelet production by megakaryocytes and hasten platelet destruction. Folic acid deficiency may contribute to ineffective thrombopoiesis. Fulminant viral hepatitis, either in children or adults, is associated with more dramatic drops in platelet counts. Viral infections inhibit megakaryopoiesis or may lead to accelerated peripheral destruction of platelets that is mediated by immune complexes or acute vascular damage. Occult liver disease with borderline splenomegaly should be considered in the differential diagnosis of mild thrombocytopenia.

Platelet Function Defects

The bleeding time is often prolonged in patients with severe liver disease (up to 40 percent of cirrhotics) and the prolongation is not fully explained by thrombocytopenia alone. The cause of the platelet dysfunction is uncertain, although decreased glycoprotein Ib on the platelet surface and defective platelet signal transduction have been reported. Ex vivo platelet function tests have shown abnormalities in platelet adhesion and platelet aggregation in some patients, but the findings are by no means consistent. It is possible that circulating platelet inhibitors (e.g., fibrin degradation products, dialysable low molecular weight inhibitors) are not adequately cleared by the failing liver. Plasma levels of von Willebrand factor are increased in most patients with liver disease in parallel with the increased levels of factor VIIIC, but the protein appears to have normal multimeric structure.

Disseminated Intravascular Coagulation

Many patients with advanced liver disease show some evidence of chronic low-grade DIC. Fibrinogen survival is reduced, and elevated levels of fibrin degradation products (D-dimer), thrombin–antithrombin (TAT) complexes, and prothrombin activation peptide fragment 1.2 have been identified in the plasma. Infusions of heparin improve these abnormalities, which lends support to the concept that thrombin generation or activation of other clotting factors is involved. The cause of the DIC is not completely understood; hypotheses include the release of procoagulants from degenerating or injured liver cells, low-grade endotoxemia due to portal-systemic shunting, failure of the liver to clear activated clotting factors, and decreases in antithrombin or protein C. In general, however, the DIC is usually mild (in the absence of concurrent sepsis or malignancy).

A diagnostic dilemma is created by the fact that chronic liver disease is accompanied by decreased coagulation/fibrinolytic protein synthesis, decreased clearance of FDP and protease inhibitor complexes, and multifactorial thrombocytopenia. Thus, laboratory assays produce a pattern of results that are consistent with DIC but are primarily due to the multiple defects of chronic liver disease. The conserved nature of hepatic fibrinogen synthesis makes it a useful marker of DIC. Levels of fibrinogen under 100 to 120 mg/dL are rare except in the presence of significant DIC or end-stage chronic liver disease (e.g., transplant candidate). DIC can also be seen in more acute syndromes such as fulminant liver disease (e.g., acute fatty liver of pregnancy, fulminant hepatitis) and following the placement of peritoneovenous shunts in chronic liver disease.

Systemic Fibrinolysis

Many patients with severe liver disease have evidence of low-grade systemic fibrinolysis. The euglobulin lysis time (ELT) is short in up to 40 percent of patients awaiting liver transplantation. Systemic fibrinolysis is most likely caused by reduced hepatic synthesis of α_2-antiplasmin (α_2-AP) and impaired clearance of circulating fibrinolytic enzymes, particularly tissue plasminogen activator, by the diseased liver.

Even though the ELT is shortened in patients with chronic liver disease, it is unlikely that systemic fibrinolysis markedly increases the risk of hemorrhage in stable patients. However, major surgery, in particular liver transplantation and portal-systemic shunt procedures can provoke the release of large amounts of plasminogen activator from injured tissues with limited capacity to clear the activated enzymes. This can temporarily overwhelm protective mechanisms impaired by liver disease and produce severe primary fibrinolysis and bleeding.

Abnormal Fibrinogen Function

Many patients with hepatic insufficiency synthesize an abnormal fibrinogen with increased sialic acid content (similar to fetal fibrinogen). The increased sialic acid appears to inhibit polymerization of fibrin due to a net increase in negative charge. Although the dysfibrinogenemia may prolong the TCT, it is unlikely to be responsible for excessive bleeding. Abnormal fibrinogen and prothrombin (noncarboxylated prothrombin) molecules are also synthesized by patients with primary hepatocellular carcinoma.

Vitamin K Deficiency

Vitamin K deficiency should be considered in conditions that impair bile acid metabolism such as primary biliary cirrhosis and bile duct obstruction. Alcoholism is often associated with poor nutrition and thus may lead to vitamin K deficiency.

LABORATORY SCREENING TESTS

As indicated in Chapter 6, standard screening tests are used to assess possible hemostatic defects in hospitalized patients with liver disease who are actively bleeding or who require invasive diagnostic or therapeutic procedures. Table 23-2 gives the typical patterns of test results for major categories of liver disease. The tests help in the assessment of the severity of the hemostatic defects and provide baseline values for monitoring blood product replacement therapy. PT/INR, APTT, fibrinogen, FDP/D-dimer, and platelet count are all that are necessary for an initial assessment of patients with chronic liver disease who are otherwise stable and not scheduled for surgery. The TCT may be mildly increased in the presence of liver insufficiency, but is markedly prolonged in the presence of very low fibrinogen concentrations. The International Normalized Ratio (INR) method of reporting PT results is probably valid for liver disease within a single institution since it uses a constant conversion factor for a given thromboplastin. However, the INR methodology was created for use in stable warfarin-treated patients and may be misleading when results from two different laboratories are compared (i.e., using different thromboplastin reagents).

MANAGEMENT OF BLEEDING
General

Most of the clinically significant bleeding in patients with advanced liver disease is caused by esophageal varices, peptic ulcer disease, or surgery. Hemostatic defects are often complex but can be divided into several components for purposes of diagnosis and therapy: coagulation defects, platelet function disorders, DIC, and systemic fibrinolysis.

Coagulation Defects

Vitamin K deficiency should be considered early in the management of patients with bleeding due to liver disease. Coagulation screening tests cannot distinguish impaired hepatic synthesis of clotting factors from lack of vitamin K, so that a therapeutic trial of vitamin K is usually indicated if the APTT or PT is prolonged. Doses of 5 to 10 mg/day should be administered orally or subcutaneously for 3 days. Deep intramuscular injections should be avoided in patients with severe coagulopathies because of the possibility of hematoma formation.

Mild coagulation defects will be reflected in a slightly prolonged PT, (INR <1.3) with a normal APTT and fibrinogen concentration. Clotting factor replacement therapy is rarely necessary. If defects are more severe and the patient is bleeding (i.e., the PT and APTT are both moderately increased, but the fibrinogen is >125 mg/dL), then the administration of fresh frozen plasma should be considered; however, volume overload must be considered as well as the short half life of factor VII (~7 hrs). Cryoprecipitate may also be required if the coagulopathy is extremely severe and is associated with markedly low fibrinogen concentrations. Therapy should be monitored with serial coagulation testing.

In a few patients with end-stage liver disease or acute hepatic failure (e.g., fulminant hepatitis B or herpes simplex hepatitis in an infant), the synthesis of clotting factors can be severely impaired. Plasma exchange may be necessary to prepare patients for liver transplantation or to manage refractory bleeding in a patient who is likely to recover spontaneously. Prothrombin-complex concentrates should not be used to replace coagulation factors II, VII, IX, and X because of the risks of thrombosis and their lack of other clotting factors (e.g., factor V).

Platelet Defects

Platelet transfusions are indicated if a patient is actively bleeding and the platelet count is <50,000 to 75,000/μL. The recovery of transfused platelets is impaired in the presence of splenomegaly, but hemostatically effective platelet counts can still be achieved with platelet transfusion in up to 50 percent of patients. Post-infusion platelet counts should be obtained to guide management. The intravenous infusion of DDAVP (see Chap. 58) in doses of 0.3 μg/kg body weight significantly, but transiently, shortens the bleeding time in over 60 percent of patients with liver disease. Although its therapeutic efficacy is unknown, DDAVP is worth a trial in patients with refractory hemorrhage and a prolonged bleeding time. Severe anemia may also impair platelet function and RBC transfusion should be considered for a hematocrit <30 percent.

Disseminated Intravascular Coagulation

Although many patients with advanced liver disease have evidence of chronic low-level DIC, specific therapy is rarely required. Heparin administration is not indicated and is likely to make the bleeding worse. In the rare patient with fulminant liver failure, such as acute fatty liver of pregnancy or severe overwhelming viral hepatitis in children or adults, antithrombin concentrates may be useful. In general, fibrinolytic inhibitors such as ε-aminocaproic acid should be avoided due to a risk of thrombosis.

Systemic Fibrinolysis

Patients with extremely short ELTs who continue to bleed despite optimal clotting factor and platelet replacement therapy may have clinically significant systemic fibrinolysis. Fibrinolysis is of particular concern during or following a major surgical procedure, especially liver transplantation and portal-systemic shunts (see later). Replacement of α_2-AP by the administration of fresh frozen plasma can be attempted. If bleeding continues, the use of antifibrinolytic agents such as ε-aminocaproic acid or tranexamic acid by intravenous infusion should be considered, although DIC must be excluded due to the risk of thrombosis.

SPECIAL PROBLEMS IN LIVER DISEASE

Major Surgery

For elective and semi-elective major surgery the platelet count should be preferably >75,000/μL and the coagulation screening assays should be as close to normalized as feasible (in the face of volume constraints). A recent evaluation of fresh frozen plasma versus solvent/detergent (SD)-treated plasma in liver transplantation concluded that SD plasma was an adequate source of coagulation factors in spite of lower levels of some coagulation proteins (e.g., protein C, protein S, α_2-antiplasmin). Finally, a growing body of experimental work in animal models suggests that fibrin glue may be a useful hemostatic agent in blunt liver trauma.

HELLP/Preeclampsia

The HELLP syndrome (hemolysis, elevated liver enzymes, and low platelets) occurs in association with preeclampsia and has been associated with subcapsular hematoma in 1 percent of cases. Catastrophic hepatic hemorrhage and rupture may occur.

Liver Biopsy

Bleeding following liver biopsy is infrequent (e.g., 0.4 percent) although rates of hemorrhage are substantially increased in patients with malignant disease (up to 14 percent). The bleeding time (BT) has received "mixed reviews" as a predictor of bleeding but a recent prospective study demonstrated a fivefold increased risk of post-biopsy bleeding in patients with an elevated BT. The platelet count should preferably be >50,000/µL prior to liver biopsy. However, mild increases in the PT (e.g., 3 to 4 sec) are probably not a major contraindication to the procedure. With greater prolongations frozen plasma should be administered. The use of DDAVP should be considered in patients with a history of bleeding and a prolonged bleeding time. If the coagulopathy cannot be corrected, the transvenous hepatic vein approach for biopsy has been shown to have fewer bleeding complications. One small (n=51) uncontrolled study demonstrated the efficacy of small-gauge (18G) gel foam plug embolization of the needle track in hemostatically compromised patients.

Liver Transplantation

Bleeding can be extraordinarily severe during the course of orthotopic liver transplantation. Common reasons for excessive bleeding include severe portal hypertension and previous right upper quadrant surgery. In addition, a brisk rise in plasma levels of tissue plasminogen activator (t-PA) and fall in PAI-1 commonly occurs during the anhepatic and reperfusion phases of the surgery and is associated with a reciprocal fall in fibrinogen. A less well-characterized coagulopathy with a sudden prolongation of the APTT occurs immediately after reperfusion of the newly implanted liver and has been attributed to release of a heparin-like substance. Management includes aggressive replacement of red blood cells and clotting factors. The use of antifibrinolytic agents and antithrombin concentrates remains to be determined. The hemostatic defects return to normal over a few days postoperatively if graft function is adequate.

Peritoneal-Venous Shunts for Ascites

After the implantation of peritoneal-venous shunts, DIC is extremely common and is most likely due to the infusion of cellular or fluid-phase procoagulants from the ascitic fluid into the venous circulation. In most instances, the coagulopathy is not sufficiently severe to require removal of the shunt. The DIC can be limited by drainage of the ascitic fluid prior to the placement of the shunt, by temporarily occluding the shunt, or simply by having the patient sit up, which reduces the flow of ascitic fluid within the conduit.

BIBLIOGRAPHY

Bakker CM et al: Disseminated intravascular coagulation in liver cirrhosis. *J Hepatol* 15:330, 1992.

Bathgate AJ, Hayes PC: Acute liver failure: complications and current management (review). *Hosp Med* 59:195, 1998.

Boberg KM et al: Is a prolonged bleeding time associated with an increased risk of hemorrhage after liver biopsy. *Thromb Haemost* 81:378, 1999.

DeLoughery TG: Management of bleeding with uremia and liver disease (review). *Cur Opin Hematol* 6:329, 1999.

Dzik WH et al: Fibrinolysis during liver transplantation in humans: Role of tissue-type plasminogen activator. *Blood* 71:1090, 1988.

Fisher NC, Mutimer DJ: Central venous cannulation in patients with liver disease and coagulopathy—a prospective audit. *Intens Care Med* 25:481 1999.

Freeman JW et al: A randomized trial of solvent/detergent and standard frozen plasma in the treatment of the coagulopathy seen during orthotopic liver transplantation. *Vox Sang* 74(suppl 1):225, 1998.

Gleysteen JJ et al: The cause of coagulopathy after peritoneovenous shunt for malignant ascites. *Arch Surg* 125:474, 1990.

Kajiwara E et al: Evidence for an immunological basis of thrombocytopenia in chronic liver disease. *Am J Gastro* 90:962, 1995.

Kettner SC et al: Endogenous heparin-like substances significantly impair coagulation in patients undergoing orthotopic liver transplantation. *Anesth Analg* 86:691, 1998.

Kovacs MJ et al: Assessment of the validity of the INR system for patients with liver impairment. *Thromb Hemost* 17:727, 1994.

Mannucci PM: Desmopressin (DDAVP) in the treatment of bleeding disorders: the first 20 years. *Blood* 90:2515, 1997.

Martin TG et al: Thrombopoietin levels in patients with cirrhosis before and after orthotopic liver transplantation. *Ann Intern Med* 127:285, 1997.

Patel T: Surgery in the patient with liver disease (review). *Mayo Clinic Proc* 74:593 1999.

Plecha DM et al: Liver biopsy: The effects of needle caliber on bleeding and tissue recovery. *Radiology* 204:101, 1997.

Ratnoff OD: Hemostatic defects in liver disease and biliary tract disease and disorders of vitamin K metabolism. In *Disorders of Hemostasis,* 3rd edition, Ratnoff OD (ed), WB Saunders, Philadelphia, 1996, p422.

Roberts LR, Kamath PS: Pathophysiology and treatment of variceal hemorrhage (review). *Mayo Clinic Proceed* 71:973, 1996.

Segal H et al: Coagulation and fibrinolysis in primary biliary cirrhosis compared with other liver disease and during orthotopic liver transplantation. *Hepatology* 25:683, 1997.

Sheikh RA et al: Spontaneous intrahepatic hemorrhage and hepatic rupture in the HELLP syndrome: four cases and a review. *J Clin Gastro* 28:323, 1999.

Stein SF, Harker LA: Kinetic and functional studies of platelets, fibrinogen, and plasminogen in patients with hepatic cirrhosis. *J Lab Clin Med* 99:217, 1982.

Violi F et al: Prognostic value of clotting and fibrinolytic systems in a follow-up of 165 liver cirrhotic patients, CALC group. *Hepatology* 22:96, 1995.

CHAPTER 24

Disseminated Intravascular Coagulation

Disseminated intravascular coagulation (DIC) is a pathologic process in which a generalized activation of the hemostatic system leads to generation of thrombin. In its most severe form, widespread fibrin formation and subsequent lysis within the vascular system can result in microthrombosis and consumption of platelets and clotting factors. The process may occur rapidly or slowly and with all degrees of magnitude; in its most severe form the result may be organ dysfunction, generalized hemorrhage, and hemolysis due to red blood cell fragmentation in the microvasculature. Other terms synonymous with DIC are consumption coagulopathy and defibrination syndrome. DIC may be acute (uncompensated) with decreased levels of hemostatic components or chronic (compensated) with normal or even elevated levels of clotting factors.

CAUSES

The major triggering mechanism for DIC is the exposure of the blood to a source of tissue factor that initiates coagulation and leads to the production of thrombin. Tissue factor can contact the blood due to mechanical tissue injury (e.g., brain trauma, placental abruption), exposure to malignant cells (e.g., pancreatic cancer, acute promyelocytic leukemia [APL]), or synthesis on the surface of endothelial cells stimulated by endotoxin or cytokines (e.g., sepsis). Thrombin generation in overt DIC is sufficiently intense that anticoagulant mechanisms such as the antithrombin and activated protein C systems are soon overwhelmed. In most cases fibrin forming in the microvasculature undergoes rapid fibrinolysis due to the release of tissue plasminogen activator (t-PA) from adjacent vascular endothelium, leading to generation of the fibrinolytic enzyme, plasmin.

Intravascular coagulation followed by secondary fibrinolysis promotes consumption of clotting factors (particularly fibrinogen, platelets, factor V, and factor VIII) and an increase in the plasma concentration of fibrin split products (e.g., D-dimer) (Fig 24-1).

In most instances the cause of the DIC is quite obvious. In adults the most common causes are acute trauma (especially head injury), severe infections with septicemia, and obstetrical catastrophes such as severe placental abruption, fetal demise, or amniotic fluid embolism. Malignancy (usually disseminated) is a common cause of chronic DIC, often associated with tumor cell emboli in the vasculature and a brisk microangiopathic hemolytic anemia (see Chaps. 29 and 46). Other causes of the syndrome are less common (some are listed in Table 24-1).

The sick newborn infant is particularly prone to DIC because of a decrease in the usual defense mechanisms such as reduced coagulation inhibitors (low protein C, protein S, and antithrombin), low levels of fibronectin, defective fibrinolysis, and an underdeveloped reticuloendothelial system. Infections and trauma (accidents, severe burns) are the

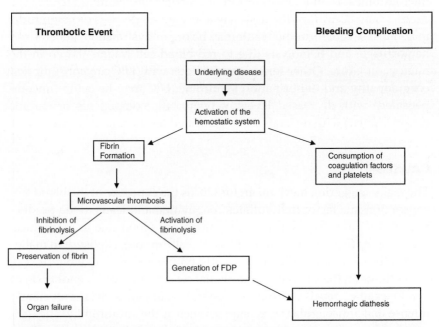

FIGURE 24-1 Sequence of events occurring in disseminated intravascular coagulation. The thrombotic event is characterized by microvascular thrombosis, whereas bleeding complications are caused be consumption of coagulation factors and platelets as well as generation of fibrin degradation products. (Modified and used with permission from Muller-Berghaug G et al., *Thromb Haemost* 82:706, 1999.)

TABLE 24-1

Disorders Associated with Disseminated Intravascular Coagulation, Grouped According to Pathophysiologic Mechanism or Physiologic Status

Tissue damage (release/exposure of tissue factor) or other mediators
    Physical trauma (crushing and penetrating injuries, e.g., brain injury)
    Thermal injuries (burns, cold injury)
    Asphyxia-hypoxia
    Surgery
    Ischemia-infarction
    Rhabdomyolysis
    Fat embolism
    Hypovolemic-hemorrhagic shock
    Hyperthermia (heat stroke)
Malignancies (release of cancer procoagulants, tissue factor, tumor necrosis factor, cell proteases)
    Solid tumors
    Leukemias
Infections (endotoxin release, endothelial cell damage, platelet activation)
    Bacterial (*Meningococcus, Escherichia coli, Salmonella, Pseudomonas, Haemophilus, Pneumococcus,* hemolytic streptococci, *Staphylococcus*)
    Viral (dengue, Lassa, Ebola, Marburg, Hantaan, rubeola, herpes, etc.)
    Protozoan (malaria)
    Other (Rocky Mountain spotted fever, *Candida, Aspergillus, Clostridia, Mycobacterium tuberculosis*)
    Toxic shock syndrome
Vascular and circulatory disorders (abnormal endothelium, foreign surface coagulation, platelet activation)
    Giant hemangioma, vascular tumors
    Aortic aneurysm
    Vascular surgery
    Intracardiac tumor
    Cardiac bypass surgery
    Acute myocardial infarction
    Vasculitis
    Aortic balloon pump
    Malignant hypertension
    Pulmonary embolism
Immunologic disorders (complement activation, tissue factor release)
    Anaphylaxis
    Allergic reactions
    Acute hemolytic transfusion reactions
    Heparin-associated thrombocytopenia
    Renal allograft reaction
    Kawasaki disease
    Drug (quinine, interleukin-1)
Direct enzyme activation
    Pancreatitis
    Snake, spider venoms
Other disorders
    Fulminant hepatic necrosis
    Reye's syndrome

(Continued)

TABLE 24-1 CONTINUED

Disorders Associated with Disseminated Intravascular Coagulation, Grouped According to Pathophysiologic Mechanism or Physiologic Status

Cirrhosis
Le Veen shunt reinfusion
Adult respiratory distress syndrome
Prothrombin-complex concentrate infusion
Hemolytic uremic syndrome
Inflammatory bowel diseases
Sarcoidosis
Amyloidosis
Hemorrhagic shock and encephalopathy syndrome
Homozygous protein C deficiency
Homozygous protein S deficiency
Complications of pregnancy (tissue factor release, ischemia)
    Abruptio placentae
    Amniotic fluid embolism
    Eclampsia and preeclampsia
    Induced (saline) abortion
    Retained dead fetus or missed abortion
    Hydatidiform mole
    Placenta accreta
    Rupture of the uterus
    Chronic tubal pregnancy
    Degenerating fibromyoma
Neonatal DIC
    Infection
    Birth asphyxia
    Hyaline membrane disease
    Aspiration syndromes
    Apneic episodes
    Atelectasis, pneumonia
    Pulmonary hemorrhage
    Cold injury
    Polycythemia
    Abruptio placentae
    Small-for-gestational-age infant
    Maternal hypertensive syndromes
    Dead twin fetus
    Chorangioma of placenta
    Major vessel thrombosis
    Purpura fulminans (protein C, protein S deficiency)
    Necrotizing enterocolitis
    Fetal neoplasms and leukemia
    Brain injury (necrosis and hemorrhage)
    Erythroblastosis fetalis
    Hepatic disease
    Hereditary fructose intolerance
    Giant hemangiomas

major causes of DIC in the older child; mortality from head injury in children is four times greater in those with DIC.

DIAGNOSIS

Clinical Manifestations

The clinical manifestations of DIC are frequently masked by the underlying disorder so that laboratory evidence for the syndrome should be sought in any severely ill patient. The most common sign of severe DIC is bleeding, usually manifested as ecchymoses, petechiae, purpura, trauma-related oozing, and postsurgical hemorrhage. The bleeding diatheses are related to low levels of clotting factors (particularly fibrinogen, factor V, and factor VIII), increased levels of fibrin degradation products (which act as an acquired anticoagulant prolonging the APTT and thrombin time and interfering with platelet function), and thrombocytopenia. Symptoms of vascular thrombosis (in the microvasculature, venous thromboembolism, arterial occlusion) are much less common due to brisk secondary fibrinolysis. However if the fibrinolytic or protein C system is impaired (e.g., in pregnancy, some patients with sepsis or after antifibrinolytic drugs) symptomatic thrombosis may occur, such as renal insufficiency, necrotic skin lesions, or respiratory failure. Purpura fulminans, a lesion more apt to occur with meningococcemia, chicken pox, and Rocky Mountain spotted fever, is usually associated with severe DIC and low levels of protein C. A mild microangiopathic hemolytic anemia is frequently noted (up to 70 percent of cases of DIC), but is seldom severe unless associated with widespread metastatic malignancy.

Laboratory Manifestations

The laboratory tests that are most frequently abnormal in DIC are:

- Reduced platelet count (due to thrombin activation and clearance, destruction in the microvasculature, or endotoxemia in sepsis)
- Increased D-dimer (due to secondary lysis of intravascular fibrin)
- Increased PT (due to reduction of clotting factors, especially factor V)
- Increased APTT (also due to consumption of clotting factors, including factors V and VIII)
- Increased TCT (due to inhibition of fibrin polymerization by fibrin-degradation products)
- Reduced fibrinogen level (due to thrombin-induced conversion to fibrin monomer and fibrin)

- Blood film showing fragmented red cells (formed after injury by fibrin strands, endothelial cell damage or tumor cell emboli)

The laboratory manifestations of DIC vary greatly depending on the specific cause, severity, and chronicity of the disorder. For example, patients with sepsis often have lower platelet counts; subjects with severe brain trauma have marked hypofibrinogenemia; and individuals with malignancy typically have thrombocytopenia and fragmented red cells on blood smear. Most DIC is mild and well compensated; screening tests of hemostasis are normal or only mildly abnormal, but tests of thrombin generation are elevated (thrombin–antithrombin complexes, fibrinopeptide A, prothrombin fragment 1.2) Placental abruption often causes severe disturbances in coagulation, but the abnormalities rapidly resolve following delivery, with prompt regeneration of fibrinogen and clotting factors once delivery is accomplished (e.g., fibrinogen often increases at a rate of 8 to 10 mg/dL/hr). Serial testing is needed to establish the course of the DIC, e.g., progressive, resolving, or chronic).

The diagnosis of DIC is made based on a suggestive clinical presentation (identification of a triggering event) plus laboratory evidence of elevated D-dimer. Reductions in platelets, low fibrinogen concentrations, and prolonged PT or APPT may be found; however, in mild or compensated DIC, these screening tests may be normal. Note that none of these tests are specific for DIC, as other disorders or compensatory mechanisms may modify the results. For example, stress, malignancy, and inflammation are all powerful stimuli for fibrinogen and factor VIII synthesis.

In severe DIC, practically all coagulation factor assays are abnormal, and more specifically, proteases complexed with their inhibitors are frequently elevated. Table 24-2 summarizes some of these test results in DIC. In many instances, assays for individual coagulation factors such as antithrombin and protein C are not very helpful in evaluating consumptive coagulopathies; however, the use of the protease-inhibitor complex or activation peptide assays (thrombin-antithrombin complexes, prothrombin fragment F1.2) has been helpful in clinical studies. In our hands, the major benefit of factor assays has been in complicated and severe coagulopathies to guide replacement therapy, to judge prognosis, or to confirm complicating coagulopathies.

A major clinical challenge is the recognition of primary (systemic) fibrinolysis in patients with DIC. Several diseases are associated with both disorders, notably APL, metastatic prostatic carcinoma, and amniotic fluid embolism. Primary fibrino(geno)lysis is caused by circulating fibri-

TABLE 24-2

Coagulation Assays which May Be Abnormal in Disseminated Intravascular Coagulation

Assay	Normal Value for Adults	Representative Value(s) in DIC Patient*
A. Coagulation Factors		
Prothrombin	0.7–1.5 U/mL	0.2–0.6 U/mL
Factor V activity	0.6–1.5 U/mL	0.05–0.6 U/mL
Factor VIII:C	0.6–1.5 U/mL	0.3–6.0 U/mL
von Willebrand factor	0.6–1.5 U/mL	2.2–10 U/mL
Factor XII activity	0.7–1.3 U/mL	0.3–0.9 U/mL
Prekallikrein (PK) activity	0.75–1.25 U/mL	0.3–0.5 U/mL
C1-inhibitor	0.60–1.40 U/mL	0.64–2.3 U/mL
α_2-Macroglobulin	0.70–1.30 U/mL	0.60–1.20 U/mL
Antithrombin	0.8–1.2 U/mL	0.25–0.7 U/mL
Protein C activity	0.7–1.3 U/mL	<0.06–0.6 U/mL
Protein C inhibitor	0.65–1.3 U/mL	<0.06–0.65 U/mL
Plasminogen	2.2–4.5 CTA U/mL	0.4–3.5 CTA U/mL
α_2-Antiplasmin	0.8–1.2 U/mL	0.2–1.2 U/mL
B. Activation Peptides or Fragments		
Fibrinopeptide A	0.9 ng/mL	13–346 ng/mL
Bβ 1–42 peptide	<1.0 pmol/mL	5–10 pmol/mL
Bβ 15–42 peptide	<1.0 pmol/mL	5–10 pmol/mL
F1.2 fragment	1.97 +/– 0.97 nM	18–56 nM
Factor X activation peptide	66 +/– 20 pmol/L	250–550 pmol/L
C. Enzyme-Inhibitor Complexes		
Thrombin–antithrombin	0.7–2.7 µg/L	3.3–145 µg/L
Plasmin-α_2-antiplasmin complex	0.0–0.5 mg/L	0.3–27 mg/L

* Abnormal values are from patients with severe DIC.

nolytic enzymes (t-PA, plasmin) in the blood, and is recognized clinically by an abnormally short euglobulin clot lysis time (ELT) (see Chap. 25). In general, secondary fibrinolysis in patients with uncomplicated DIC is not associated with circulating fibrinolytic enzymes because local concentrations of fibrinolytic inhibitors (plasminogen activator inhibitor, antiplasmin, liver clearance) is more than sufficient to neutralize them.

Pathologic Manifestations

Detailed necropsy studies of documented clinical DIC show pathologic evidence (disseminated microthrombi) in only 60 to 75 percent of patients. The quantity of fibrin deposited in small vessels may be altered by intense fibrinolysis and severe fibrinogen depletion.

FIBRINOGEN-FIBRIN DEGRADATION PRODUCTS

The sine qua non for the diagnosis of DIC is the presence of elevated levels of FDP. Over 95 percent of all reported instances of DIC have had elevated FDP; although FDP may also be present in many inflammatory (systemic lupus erythematosus, renal disease, hemolytic uremic syndrome, necrotizing enterocolitis) and thrombotic (large vessel thrombosis) conditions without intravascular coagulation. The interaction of three key enzymes (thrombin, plasmin, XIIIa) on fibrinogen produces a series of circulating fragments and complexes called fibrinogen-fibrin degradation products, or FDP (Fig. 24-2). The products formed early in the process are fibrin monomer and complexes of monomer with fibrinolytic fragments X, Y (later D, E) or soluble fibrin I; this material is detected by precipitation from plasma by ethanol or protamine sulfate. This is also the basis for cryofibrinogen. Although the "monomer" test is often positive in DIC, it is not as sensitive as other tests and is not commonly used at present. A more sensitive test is the D-dimer determination, which is performed on citrated plasma samples and detects cross-linked fibrin, but not fibrinogen or the monomer complexes. Performed with monoclonal antibodies against the cross-linked D-dimer site, this procedure has great specificity for fibrin and is positive in DIC, as well as in patients with large-vessel thrombosis. D-dimer tests are now commonly used because of their specificity for fibrin (not fibrinogen) degradation products and widespread availability. Note that two basic types of D-dimer tests are currently available. The latex agglutination test is used in most laboratories and is suitable for the diagnosis of DIC. Highly sensitive ELISA assays for D-dimer are also in use, particularly to exclude deep venous thrombosis or pulmonary embolism (i.e., they have a high negative predictive value) (see Chap. 36).

MANAGEMENT

Although the recognition of DIC is relatively straightforward, the management of the disorder has been controversial. More recent experience, anecdotal reports, and a few controlled studies have led to a general consensus of management, outlined in Fig. 24-3. The most important aspect of management is the recognition and removal or alleviation of the triggering event or underlying cause. When specific therapy and intensive support are successful, DIC is reversed, and unless the consumption process has produced a bleeding tendency, no further treatment for the DIC is necessary. If an invasive procedure or surgery is planned, replacement therapy may be indicated. In this instance or if hemorrhage is on-

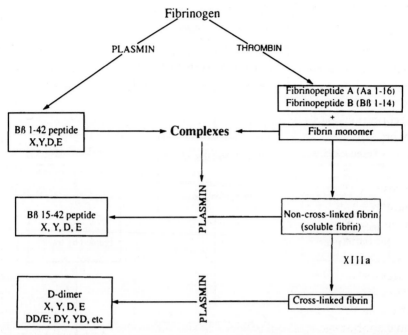

FIGURE 24-2 Action of thrombin and plasmin on fibrinogen and formation of fibrinogen-fibrin degradation products (FDP).

going or worsening, the main therapeutic endeavor should be replacement therapy as guided by the laboratory assessment; that is, administration of frozen plasma, cryoprecipitate, and platelet concentrates to replace clotting factors, fibrinogen, and platelets in doses sufficient to achieve hemostasis. In patients with shock and volume depletion, frozen plasma should be used early for coagulation factor replacement as well as for volume and oncotic effect. Additional therapy includes:

1. Heparin anticoagulation is sometimes indicated if a) the DIC is so brisk that replacement therapy alone fails to provide hemostatic levels of clotting factors and platelets (e.g., APL), b) DIC is complicated by microvascular thrombosis (e.g., renal insufficiency or skin necrosis in sepsis, purpura fulminans), or c) large-vessel thrombosis is found (e.g., venous thromboembolism, aortic aneurism preoperatively). In these instances, the potential benefits of anticoagulation must be tempered by the risks of bleeding; clotting factor and platelet support to or above hemostatic levels is essential. The dose of heparin should be moderate; 5 to 10 U/kg/hr by continuous infusion as needed to interrupt the DIC.

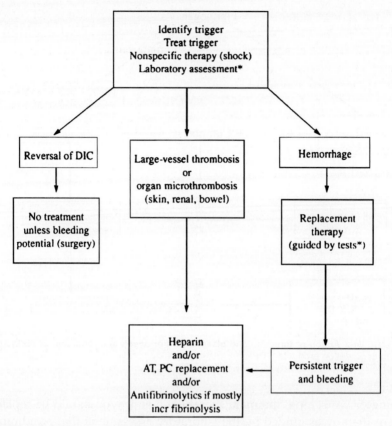

FIGURE 24-3 Guide to management of patient with diagnosis of acute DIC.

2. Specific clotting factor inhibitor concentrates may be helpful in some circumstances. Antithrombin concentrates may provide some measure of benefit in patients with overwhelming sepsis, or acute fatty liver of pregnancy. Protein C or activated protein C concentrates hold promise for treatment of severe DIC in patients with meningococcemia or other severe bacterial sepsis, especially with skin necrosis (Smith ref).

3. Although antifibrinolytic agents are usually contraindicated in DIC, in rare patients, such as those with acute promyelocytic leukemia or prostate cancer, systemic fibrinolysis can coexist. In these patients antifibrinolytic therapy may occasionally be warranted if bleeding has continued despite heparin treatment and replacement therapy, and repeated testing shows the presence of brisk systemic fibrinolysis (e.g., a shortened ELT).

These therapeutic considerations are appropriate for any age. However, fulminate DIC, especially if associated with liver disease (e.g., disseminated herpes simplex virus) in the newborn or young infant, is frequently amenable to exchange transfusion. Purpura fulminans in the neonate is usually associated with homozygous or compound heterozygous protein C (see Chap. 38) or protein S (see Chap. 39) deficiency.

BIBLIOGRAPHY

Baglin T: Disseminated intravascular coagulation: Diagnosis and treatment. *BMJ* 312:683, 1996.

Barbui T et al: The impact of all-trans-retinoic acid on the coagulopathy of acute promyelocytic leukemia. *Blood* 91:3093, 1998.

Bucur SZ et al: Uses of antithrombin III concentrate in congenital and acquired deficiency states. *Transfusion* 38:481, 1998.

Calverley DC, Leibman HA: Disseminated intravascular coagulation. In *Hematology: Basic Principles and Practice,* 3rd ed, Hoffman R (ed), New York, Churchill Livingstone, p 1983, 1999.

Castro MA et al: Disseminated intravascular coagulation and antithrombin III depression in acute fatty liver of pregnancy. *Am J Obstet Gynecol* 174:211, 1996.

Hazelzet JA et al.: Age-related differences in outcome and severity of DIC in children with septic shock and purpura. *Thromb Haemost* 76:932, 1996.

Hulka F et al: Blunt brain injury activates the coagulation process. *Arch Surg* 131:923, 1996.

de Jonge E et al: Current drug treatment strategies for disseminated intravascular coagulation. *Drugs* 55:767, 1998.

Levi M, Ten Cate H: Disseminated intravascular coagulation. *N Engl J Med* 341:586, 1999.

Manco-Johnson MJ: Disseminated intravascular coagulation and other hypercoagulable syndromes. *Intl J Pediat Hem/Onc* 1:1, 1994.

Mesters RM et al.: Factor VIIa and antithrombin III activity during severe sepsis and septic shock in neutropenic patients. *Blood* 88:881, 1996.

Miner ME et al: Disseminated intravascular coagulation fibrinolytic syndrome following head injury in children: frequency and prognostic implications. *J Pediat* 100:687, 1982.

Muller-Berghaus G et al: Disseminated intravascular coagulation: clinical spectrum and established, as well as new, diagnostic approaches. *Thromb Haemost* 82:706, 1999.

Smith OP et al: Infectious purpura fulminans. Diagnosis and treatment. *Br J Haematol* 104:202, 1999.

Tallman MS, Kwaan HC: Reassessing the hemostatic disorder associated with acute promyelocytic leukemia. *Blood* 79:543, 1992.

Wilde JT et al: Association between necropsy evidence of disseminated intravascular coagulation and coagulation variables before death in patients in intensive care units. *J Clin Path* 41:138, 1988.

CHAPTER 25

Systemic Fibrinolysis

Systemic fibrinolysis may be primary or secondary. Primary fibrinolysis is a syndrome of excessive fibrinolysis associated with circulating fibrinolytic enzymes such as plasmin and tissue plasminogen activator (t-PA). Thrombolytic therapy represents the most common and clear-cut example of primary fibrinolysis. Other causes of primary fibrinolysis are quite rare. Secondary fibrinolysis is the compensatory response to disseminated intravascular coagulation, which may be caused by a wide range of underlying disorders (see Chap. 24). The bleeding associated with primary fibrinolysis may be severe, and in some highly selected instances, antifibrinolytic therapy may be beneficial. In contrast, antifibrinolytic therapy in secondary fibrinolytic syndromes can lead to dangerous thrombotic complications.

PATHOPHYSIOLOGY

The fibrinolytic system functions to clear unneeded fibrin from vascular or extravascular sites and is normally highly regulated (see Chap. 1). Following vascular injury, the deposition of fibrin stimulates the release of t-PA from adjacent endothelial cells and perhaps other tissues in the neighborhood of the clot. Plasminogen activator binds to strands of fibrin and converts adsorbed plasminogen to plasmin, with lysis of the fibrin and formation of soluble fibrin degradation products (FDP). Under usual circumstances the fibrinolytic process remains strictly localized to the milieu of the fibrin clot because of the binding of the reactants to fibrin, immediate neutralization of any free plasmin by α_2-antiplasmin (α_2-AP), and inhibition of t-PA by plasminogen activator inhibitor (PAI-1). If fibrinolytic enzymes should escape into the circulation in their active form, they are rapidly inhibited by α_2-AP and cleared by the liver before systemic fibrinolysis can develop. Occasionally, as a result of disease or the administration of thrombolytic agents, fibrinolysis becomes generalized, which can lead to severe bleeding from sites of vascular injury.

In general, systemic fibrinolysis occurs when excessive amounts of plasminogen activator accumulate in the blood or on fibrin surfaces, when fibrinolytic inhibitors are deficient, or when the liver is unable to clear plasminogen activator or plasmin (Table 25-1). Circulating fibrinolytic enzymes attack thrombi present anywhere within the vasculature, destroy fibrinogen and other clotting factors in the blood, and inhibit platelet function (Fig. 25-1). With fibrin-specific thrombolytic agents such as t-PA, the fibrinolytic effect is localized to fibrin surfaces, with reduced amounts of free plasmin in the circulation. Importantly, fibrin-specific agents cannot discriminate pathologic thrombi from hemostatic plugs, so that bleeding with these agents can be as serious as that observed with circulating unbound plasmin.

LABORATORY TESTS

Table 25-2 lists the laboratory tests that are altered in patients with systemic fibrinolysis. The euglobulin lysis time (ELT) provides direct evidence of circulating plasmin or plasminogen activator, the standard

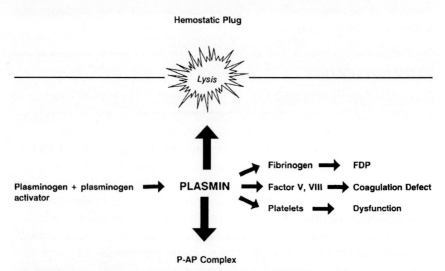

FIGURE 25-1 Hemostatic defects in systemic fibrinolysis. Plasmin destroys circulating clotting factors, impairs platelet function, and lyses hemostatic plugs.

TABLE 25-1

Mechanisms of Systemic Fibrinolysis

Mechanisms	Examples
Circulating plasminogen activators	Thrombolytic agents Malignancy (e.g., acute promyelocytic leukemia) Cardiopulmonary bypass
Decreased inhibitors (α_2-antiplasmin, plasminogen activator inhibitor-1)	Liver disease Amyloidosis Hereditary disorders
Reduced hepatic clearance of plasmin, plasminogen activators	Orthotopic liver transplantation End-stage liver disease with portal hypertension

hemostatic screening tests reflect clotting factor deficiencies and platelet dysfunction, and tests of FDP suggest proteolysis of fibrinogen or fibrin. The ELT is performed by creating a plasma-derived clot free of fibrinolytic inhibitors in a test tube and then observing it closely over the next 60 min for accelerated clot lysis. Because it is quite sensitive, a positive test (i.e., lysis in <60 minutes) does not necessarily indicate that clinical bleeding is a result of systemic fibrinolysis. However, a negative test makes the diagnosis unlikely. Immunoassays are available for plasmin–antiplasmin (PAP) complexes. Levels of PAP have been shown to closely parallel plasmin generation during thrombolytic therapy; however, the assay is not yet being performed in most routine clinical laboratories.

TABLE 25-2

Clinical Laboratory Tests for Systemic Fibrinolysis

Process	Abnormal Tests
Circulating plasminogen activators or plasmin	Euglobulin lysis time t-PA activity Plasmin–antiplasmin complexes
Proteolysis of clotting factors by plasmin	PT APTT Fibrinogen Factors V and VIII
Platelet function defects	Bleeding time
Lysis of fibrin	D-Dimer TCT
Consumption of fibrinolytic reactants	Plasminogen α_2-antiplasmin Plasmin activator inhibitor-1

A low level of α_2-AP is a useful indicator of excessive fibrinolysis. α_2-AP has a very high affinity for plasmin, so the presence of free plasmin only occurs after most of the α_2-AP has been consumed. Plasminogen is present in plasma at 2 μM concentration, versus 1 μM for α_2-AP. Thus, if over half the plasminogen is activated (converted to plasmin), all of the α_2-AP will be consumed and free plasmin will appear in the blood.

The concentration of fibrinogen is a robust and readily available guide to the severity of the fibrinolytic process, assuming other causes of hypofibrinogenemia have been excluded. Severe systemic fibrinolysis is frequently accompanied by a substantial fall in fibrinogen; for example, fibrinogen levels rapidly drop from 350 to 100 mg/dL or even lower following short-term thrombolytic therapy with streptokinase for acute coronary artery thrombosis. One caveat for the measurement of fibrinogen in the setting of active thrombolytic therapy is that the blood collection tubes should contain specific inhibitors of fibrinolytic activity to prevent in vitro fibrinolysis and falsely low fibrinogen levels.

CLINICAL DISORDERS

Bleeding due to brisk systemic fibrinolysis may be extraordinarily severe, particularly in patients undergoing surgery or other invasive procedures. Figure 25-1 illustrates at least three reasons for hemorrhage:

1. Circulating fibrinolytic enzymes rapidly lyse any hemostatic plug in contact with the blood, so that virtually all vascular defects, large or small, begin to bleed.
2. Plasmin destroys fibrinogen, factor V, and factor VIII, producing a major impediment to fibrin formation.
3. Platelet function is seriously impaired due to aggregation defects induced by FDP, and to defects in platelet adhesion as a result of plasmin-induced abnormalities of von Willebrand factor–glycoprotein Ib interactions.

From a clinical perspective, systemic fibrinolysis may be suspected when injuries (e.g., venipuncture sites) that had previously stopped bleeding begin to ooze. Bleeding can occur almost anywhere, but is particularly prominent at sites of trauma or surgery. CNS hemorrhage may be devastating and is more frequent in patients with severe systemic fibrinolysis (e.g., when 150 mg of t-PA was administered in the TIMI II trial) than in those with marked defects in fibrin formation (e.g., hemophilia A) or platelet dysfunction (e.g., thrombocytopenia of <5000/μL).

Thrombolytic Therapy

The infusion of plasminogen activators such as streptokinase, urokinase, or t-PA to produce clot lysis in a coronary artery or other occluded vessel is regularly accompanied by systemic fibrinolysis. As a consequence, the risks of bleeding are increased in patients receiving thrombolytic therapy. In the large Thrombolysis in Myocardial Infarction trial (TIMI), in which intravenous t-PA was administered for treatment of acute coronary artery occlusion, 11 percent of the patients bled, 3 to 4 percent seriously, and 0.5 percent had CNS hemorrhage. Bleeding risk is substantially increased when invasive procedures are performed during fibrinolytic therapy or if patients have associated hemostatic defects. Hemorrhage also occurs following thrombolytic therapy for deep venous thrombosis, pulmonary embolism, or peripheral arterial occlusion.

Liver Disease

As previously mentioned, patients with advanced liver disease develop systemic fibrinolysis caused by a reduction in synthesis of α_2-AP, as well as deficient hepatic clearance of fibrinolytic enzymes. Although many stable patients with end-stage liver disease have some laboratory evidence of fibrinolysis (up to 40 percent have a shortened ELT), fibrinolytic bleeding may be especially pronounced at surgery or after trauma.

Amyloidosis

Rarely, chronic systemic fibrinolysis may occur in patients with generalized amyloidosis. Adsorption of fibrinolytic inhibitors such as α_2-AP to amyloid fibrils, along with elevated levels of plasminogen activator, may be responsible for the hemostatic defects.

Malignancy

A subset of patients with acute promyelocytic leukemia (APL) present with systemic fibrinolysis rather than disseminated intravascular coagulation. The leukemic cells have been shown to produce plasminogen activator (both urokinase and tissue type), which enters the circulation and induces a fibrinolytic state. Studies of APL cells in culture have shown that retinoic-acid–induced differentiation of these cells to more mature myeloid forms decreases leukemic cell tissue factor activity, but cellular elaboration of fibrinolytic enzymes persists. Systemic fibrinolysis also complicates disseminated carcinoma of the prostate or other malignancies.

Cardiopulmonary Bypass

Cardiovascular surgery with extracorporeal circulation increases fibrinolytic activity, particularly of the shed mediastinal blood. However, autotransfusion of this blood does not seem to promote severe systemic fibrinolysis in vivo. Treatment of patients with fibrinolytic inhibitors is associated with decreased blood loss at the time of surgery (see Chap. 31).

Other Surgical Procedures

Local fibrinolysis in the prostatic bed predisposes patients undergoing urologic surgery to both immediate and delayed bleeding. The urine and the tissues of the genitourinary tract are rich in plasminogen activator.

Hereditary Conditions

Rare patients with hereditary defects in α_2-AP or PAI-1 associated with excessive bleeding have been reported (see Chap. 19).

MANAGEMENT

Although not always possible, treatment of an underlying disorder responsible for the coagulopathy is the best approach. For example, therapy of APL eliminates the cells that synthesize plasminogen activators. If bleeding occurs during a course of thrombolytic therapy, the infusion should be stopped because the half-lives of most of the currently available thrombolytic agents are very short (5 to 30 min), and they are rapidly cleared from the circulation.

If systemic fibrinolysis is chronic and mild, then specific antifibrinolytic therapy is not required. An example would be patients with advanced liver disease and short ELTs, but who are not bleeding. However, when fibrinolysis is more severe and bleeding occurs, blood product replacement to correct coagulation and platelet defects is often necessary. Fresh frozen plasma provides clotting factors and α_2-AP, cryoprecipitate contains fibrinogen and factor VIII, and platelet transfusions help correct platelet function defects. Finally, antifibrinolytic therapy using epsilon-aminocaproic acid or tranexamic acid may be needed in some patients (see Chap. 58), but must be approached with caution because of the risk of thrombotic complications. It is often difficult to distinguish primary from secondary fibrinolysis; in the latter condition, fibrinolysis is protective. Even in the setting of thrombolytic therapy with hemorrhagic complications one must carefully weigh the risk of coronary or myocardial rethrombosis versus the severity of the bleeding.

BIBLIOGRAPHY

Bevan DH et al: Cardiac bypass haemostasis: putting blood through the mill. *Br J Haematol* 104:208, 1999.

Bovill EG et al: Hemorrhagic events during therapy with recombinant tissue-type plasminogen activator, heparin, and aspirin for acute myocardial infarction. Results of the thrombolysis in Myocardial Infarction (TIMI) Phase II trial. *Ann Intern Med* 115:256, 1991.

Collen D: The plasminogen (fibrinolytic) system. *Thromb Haemost* 82:259, 1999.

Del Zoppo GJ: Thrombolytic therapy in the treatment of stroke. *Drugs* 54:90, 1997.

Nielsen JD et al: Postoperative blood loss after transurethral prostatectomy is dependent on in situ fibrinolysis. *Br J Urol* 80:889, 1997.

Stump DC et al: Pathologic fibrinolysis as a cause of clinical bleeding. *Semin Thromb Hemost* 16:260, 1990.

Tallman MS: The thrombophilic state in acute promyelocytic leukemia. *Semin Thromb Hemost.* 25:209, 1999.

Tracy RP, Bovill EG: Fibrinolytic parameters and hemostatic monitoring: Identifying and predicting patients at risk for major hemorrhagic events. *Am J Cardiol* 69:52A, 1992.

Williams EC: Plasma α_2-antiplasmin activity. Role in the evaluation and management of fibrinolytic states and other bleeding disorders. *Arch Intern Med* 149:1769, 1989.

CHAPTER 26

Massive
Blood Transfusion

Rapid and exceedingly severe blood loss is now commonplace with the advent of centralized trauma centers, organ transplantation, high-risk obstetrics, complex cardiovascular procedures, and aggressive cancer surgeries. Massive transfusion has been defined as the replacement of more than one blood volume (e.g., 10 U) in <24 h. However, most hemostatic defects occur when more than one blood volume is lost within 2 h. Hemostatic failure is common and results from dilution or consumption of clotting factors, disseminated intravascular coagulation (DIC), systemic fibrinolysis, or acquired platelet dysfunction. The overwhelming sense of urgency that surrounds these patients may be daunting, and optimal treatment demands a practical and simple, yet logical, approach. Making the "right moves" can mean not only the difference between life and death but also allows conservation of valuable blood products.

PATHOPHYSIOLOGY

There are four major categories of hemostatic defects that must be promptly identified and treated in patients with severe bleeding.

Dilution/Consumption

The most common clinical problem is a dilutional coagulopathy resulting from the emergent support of vascular volume by replacement fluids that lack clotting factors or platelets (e.g., crystalloid solutions or packed red blood cells). Dilution is even more profound when packed red cells are administered that are prepared with Adsol, a solution that adds approximately 100 mL normal saline to each unit of blood, with a final hematocrit of about 60 percent. Clotting factors and platelets are virtually absent in Adsol-suspended red blood cells.

An indirect relationship exists between the number of units of blood given during a massive transfusion and the decrease in clotting factors and platelets (Fig. 26-1). The correlation between the two parameters is somewhat variable, possibly due to patient differences in the consumption of platelets and clotting factors at sites of tissue injury. Screening tests of hemostasis in patients with a dilutional coagulopathy typically show prolongation of the PT and APTT, reduced concentrations of fibrinogen, and thrombocytopenia.

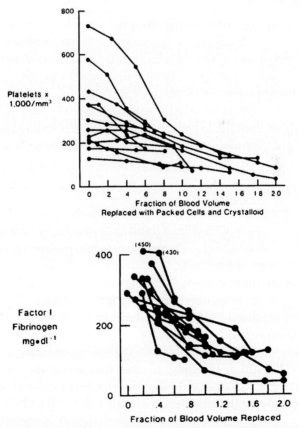

FIGURE 26-1 Decreases in platelet count and fibrinogen as increasing blood volumes are replaced with packed red cells and crystalloid solutions. Each patient is represented by a solid continuous line. (Used with permission from Murray DJ et al: *Anesthesiology* 69:839, 1988.)

Disseminated Intravascular Coagulation

Disseminated intravascular coagulation frequently follows severe head injury with brain tissue trauma. Other causes of DIC associated with massive bleeding are placental abruption, severe hypotension with hypoxia and acidosis, bacterial sepsis, and malignancy. The sudden appearance of DIC following transfusion of red blood cells suggests a major hemolytic transfusion reaction. When DIC complicates the clinical course of patients with trauma or surgical bleeding, consumption of platelets and clotting factors is accelerated, and platelet function can be inhibited by circulating fibrin degradation products (FDP). Most patients with massive bleeding due to trauma usually have only minimal elevations of FDP. Markedly high levels suggest brain trauma or antecedent shock and acidosis.

Systemic Fibrinolysis

Massive hemorrhage, particularly from the gastrointestinal tract, is common in patients with advanced liver disease. These patients can develop systemic fibrinolysis with rapid lysis of thrombi at surgical sites and plasmin-induced destruction of circulating fibrinogen and other clotting factors. Systemic fibrinolysis that occurs during the anhepatic phase of liver transplantation is often associated with hemorrhage (see Chap. 23). The euglobulin lysis time (ELT) should be obtained in bleeding patients with liver disease (or thrombolytic therapy), or in patients who have persistent hemorrhage of unknown cause.

Platelet Dysfunction

Platelet dysfunction is one of the least well-characterized hemostatic defects in the massively bleeding/transfused patient, but is a likely cause of hemorrhage. In addition to thrombocytopenia, platelet function can be impaired by high concentrations of fibrin or fibrinogen degradation products, the premature release of platelet granular contents within the circulation from intravascular platelet trauma ("exhausted" platelets), or dilution by transfused platelets that have been stored for several days before transfusion and require several hours to regain optimal function. Bleeding times are difficult to obtain in the emergency setting and are not likely to predict future bleeding. If other hemostatic defects have been corrected, but hemorrhage continues, platelet dysfunction should be suspected and treated with transfusion of platelets.

LABORATORY TESTS

A practical approach to the management of hemostatic failure in massively transfused patients is to obtain screening laboratory tests both for diagnosis and as a guide to blood product replacement therapy. An initial panel of tests should be obtained, followed by repeated testing at frequent intervals to monitor the impact of continued bleeding and blood product replacement (Table 26-1). The key to effective and efficient administration of blood products in the massively bleeding patient is the availability of frequent assessments of hemostasis. Either point of care testing must be performed or blood must be transported immediately to the laboratory, the assays performed within 30 min, and the results rapidly returned to the emergency room, ICU, or operating suite. A flow sheet is essential to document and analyze results of the laboratory tests, major clinical events, and blood product use.

MANAGEMENT

Ideally, the management of patients with massive bleeding would involve replacement of lost blood with fresh whole blood that contains optimal amounts of platelets and clotting factors. However, fresh blood is rarely available because of limited supplies, rapid outdating, and the current emphasis on blood component therapy. In the past, the transfusion of a fixed ratio of plasma and platelets to units of red blood cells has been advocated. However, this strategy does not always correct all of the hemostatic defects and often wastes blood resources. A third method is to use screening laboratory tests of hemostasis (and hematocrit) to guide blood product replacement therapy (Table 26-2). Blood components used in the management of massively bleeding patients include packed red

---

TABLE 26-1

Laboratory Tests in the Massively Bleeding Patient

INITIAL STUDIES	
Test	**Diagnostic Category**
PT, APTT, fibrinogen, hematocrit	Dilution/consumption
Platelet count	Platelet function
FDP (e.g., D-dimer)	DIC
ELT	Systemic fibrinolysis
FOLLOW-UP TESTS	
Test	**Replacement Therapy**
PT, APTT	Frozen plasma
Fibrinogen	Cryoprecipitate
Platelet count	Platelet concentrates
Hematocrit	Packed red cells

blood cells, fresh frozen plasma, cryoprecipitate, and platelet concentrates.

Red Blood Cells

The selection of red blood cells for transfusion follows standard blood banking practices. Compatible blood groups are outlined below:

Compatible Blood Groups

Patient	Red Cells	Plasma
O	O	Any
A	A (or O)	A(AB)
B	B (or O)	B(AB)
AB	Any	AB

In the majority of patients, blood-group testing to provide type-specific red blood cells can be performed quickly (e.g., 10 min or less) so that the initial use of group O red blood cells is only necessary for short-term support. The full crossmatch takes 30 to 45 min. In emergencies, uncrossmatched group O Rh-negative red blood cells should be administered. If necessary, group O Rh-positive red blood cells can be given to older women and to males. When Rh sensitization is likely to occur (as the result of transfusion of Rh-positive red blood cells to an Rh-negative recipient), Rh immune globulin is usually not effective because of the large quantity of red blood cells infused. However, Rh immune globulin should be considered when an Rh-negative patient has received Rh-positive platelet concentrates.

Fresh Frozen Plasma

The preparation of fresh frozen plasma (FFP) takes 15 to 30 min; its need should be anticipated so that time is allowed for the products to thaw. One unit increases the concentration of each of the clotting factors by

TABLE 26-2

Transfusion "Triggers" for Blood Product Replacement in Patients with Massive Bleeding

Hematocrit < 30%	→	Transfuse red blood cells
Platelet count < 75,000/μL	→	Transfuse platelets
Fibrinogen < 100 mg/dL	→	Transfuse cryoprecipitate (or frozen plasma)
PT and/or APTT > 1.5 × control	→	Transfuse frozen plasma

approximately 5 percent. Alternatives to FFP include plasma frozen within 24 hrs (see Chap. 53). Solvent detergent (SD) plasma has not been compared with frozen plasma for treatment of the hemostatic defects of large volume transfusion. Low levels of α_2-antiplasmin, protein C, and protein S have been reported; clinical studies are needed to assess safety and efficacy of SD plasma in this setting.

Cryoprecipitate

Cryoprecipitate is used to replace fibrinogen and factor VIII and can be given without regard to blood group. Approximately 10 to 15 min is required to thaw and pool the product. The infusion of 8 to 10 bags of cryoprecipitate will increase the fibrinogen concentration in a 70 kg adult by 60 to 100 mg/dL.

Platelet Concentrates

Platelet concentrates are usually available immediately, although 10 to 15 min is required to pool the individual platelet packs. It is important to remember that 10 U random donor platelets contain approximately 500 mL plasma (300 mL for a platelet apheresis product). In the absence of marked dilution or consumption, 8 to 10 bags of platelets should raise the platelet count by approximately 80,000/µL in an adult.

The optimal "triggers" for the transfusion of blood components in the setting of massive bleeding are uncertain. However, studies in these patients have suggested that collapse of hemostasis, as judged by the appearance of generalized microvascular bleeding, commonly occurs when the platelet count falls below 50,000/µL, the concentration of fibrinogen is <50 mg/dL, or the PT/APTT increases to more than 1.5 to 1.8 times that of the control. In an otherwise stable patient, hematocrits as low as 18 to 20 percent are usually well tolerated. However, in a critically ill patient who is supported almost entirely by transfused blood, higher hematocrits are warranted. Criteria for the transfusion of blood products in massively bleeding patients are listed in Table 26-2. Controlled studies will be needed to determine if these values are appropriate as reflected by outcome measures such as salvage of life, expenditure of blood resources, and the transmission of viral disease.

In the most severe bleeding circumstances (and particularly in infants and small children), it is essential to give a mixture of blood products, so that one component does not become excessively diluted by administration of the others. Therefore, at regular intervals (e.g., every 30 to 60 min), appropriate proportions of red blood cells, fresh frozen plasma, cryoprecipitate, and platelets should be administered as indicated by the results of the laboratory tests; immediate correction of all the hemostatic defects may not be possible. For example, the infusion of large amounts of fresh frozen plasma for correction of a markedly prolonged APTT and low fibrinogen could cause the hematocrit to plummet if red blood cells are not administered at the same time.

Special Problems in Management

Uncorrectable APTT

One relatively frequent problem is the inability to correct a prolonged APTT in a patient who has a severe dilutional coagulopathy. The continued administration of frozen plasma only seems to reduce the hematocrit because of dilution and fails to shorten the APTT. If marked systemic fibrinolysis can be excluded, a common cause of this often vexing problem can be the administration of excessive volumes of crystalloid contained in the cell salvage blood (hematocrit of 45 to 50 percent), or even the fluids that are being used by the anesthesiologist. The situation becomes even worse if urine output is low. Several approaches may be tried, including limiting crystalloid infusions, increasing urine volume, switching to packed red blood cells, and (if necessary) treating systemic fibrinolysis.

Long PT and Normal APTT

The PT is frequently minimally to moderately abnormal in patients with trauma, surgery, or sepsis (the mechanism is unknown). However, the APTT may be normal (or even short). In our experience, generalized bleeding tends to correlate with prolongation of the APTT rather than the PT. Therefore, large volumes of fresh frozen plasma should not be used just to correct an isolated prolonged PT.

Citrate Toxicity—Hypocalcemia

Sudden falls in the concentration of ionized calcium are caused by very rapid infusions of citrated plasma. Hypocalcemia is more often observed during surgery in patients with liver injury or during the anhepatic phase of liver transplantation. Most packed red blood cell products do not contain much citrate. However, if large amounts of plasma are being administered, frequent monitoring of the ionized calcium must be performed. Markedly low levels of ionized calcium can result in poor contractility and electrical instability of the heart.

Other Therapeutic Agents

In most instances, the administration of hemostatic agents other than blood products have not proven useful and may be dangerous. The use of DDAVP has not been prospectively studied in patients with massive trauma and bleeding. However, the stress of trauma or surgery would likely maximally stimulate the release of endogenous von Willebrand factor. DDAVP could also lead to hyponatremia or alternations in blood pressure.

Clotting factor concentrates are not usually helpful. Prothrombin-complex concentrates (containing factors II, VII, IX, X) should not be administered because of their thrombogenic potential. Moreover, they cannot correct other clotting factor (e.g., factor V and factor VIII) deficiencies. Because fresh frozen plasma is ordinarily needed for other indications, infusions of purified clotting factors such as factor VIII, factor IX, or antithrombin are rarely warranted. It is not yet known if infusions of recombinant factor VIIa will safely reduce bleeding in severely injured patients.

ε-Aminocaproic acid, tranexamic acid, or aprotinin can be useful in patients with bleeding due to severe systemic fibrinolysis. Most often, the need for antifibrinolytic agents occurs during or following the anhepatic phase in patients undergoing liver transplantation. Even so, it is needed in only a minority of patients. Potential complications include vascular thrombosis and hypotension.

Use of Ancillary Equipment

A rapid infusion device that can quickly deliver large volumes of blood products via a large central intravenous line is extremely important. A blood warmer that is capable of high infusion rates should also be available. The rapid infusion unit should contain a large reservoir into which blood products can be easily added. An intraoperative blood salvage device is useful in many cases of massive bleeding due to trauma or surgery. This equipment may not be appropriate in the presence of bowel injury or malignancy within the surgical field. However, salvage and reinfusion of red blood cells often substantially reduces the need for transfused packed red cells. The use of microaggregate blood filters may sometimes be helpful, although they can become obstructed and slow the infusion of blood. The issue as to whether routine microaggregate filtration of blood products reduces pulmonary vascular injury remains unresolved.

BIBLIOGRAPHY

Ciavarella D, Snyder E: Clinical use of blood transfusion devices. *Transf Med Rev* 2:95, 1988.

Ciavarella D et al: Clotting factor levels and the risk of diffuse microvascular bleeding in the massively transfused patient. *Br J Haematol* 67:365, 1987.

Cosgriff N et al: Predicting life-threatening coagulopathy in the massively transfused trauma patient: Hypothermia and acidoses revisited. *J Trauma* 42:857, 1997.

Counts RB et al: Hemostasis in massively transfused trauma patients. *Ann Surg* 190:91, 1979.

Dzik WH, Kirkley SA: Citrate toxicity during massive blood transfusion. *Transf Med Rev* 2:76, 1988.

Faringer PD et al: Blood component supplementation during massive transfusion of AS-1 red cells in trauma patients. *J Trauma* 34:481, 1993.

Goodnight SH et al: Defibrination following brain tissue destruction. *N Engl J Med* 290:1043, 1974.

Goodnough LT et al: Transfusion medicine. First of two parts—blood transfusion. *N Engl J Med* 340:438, 1999.

Goodnough LT et al: Transfusion medicine. Second of two parts—blood conservation. *N Engl J Med* 340:525, 1999.

Harrigan C et al: The effect of hemorrhagic shock on the clotting cascade in injured patients. *J Trauma* 29:1416, 1989.

Harrigan C et al: Serial changes in primary hemostasis after massive transfusion. *Surgery* 98:836, 1985.

Hippala S: Replacement of massive blood loss. *Vox Sang* 74:399, 1998.

Leslie SD, Toy PT: Laboratory hemostatic abnormalities in massively transfused patients given red blood cells and crystalloid. *Am J Clin Pathol* 96:770, 1991.

Mannucci PM et al: Hemostasis testing during massive blood replacement. A study of 172 cases. *Vox Sang* 42:113, 1982.

Murray DJ et al: Variability of prothrombin time and activated partial thromboplastin time in the diagnosis of increased surgical bleeding. *Transfusion* 39:56, 1999.

Murray DJ et al: Coagulation changes during packed red cell replacement of major blood loss. *Anesthesiology* 69:839, 1988.

Phillips TF et al: Outcome of massive transfusion exceeding two blood volumes in trauma and emergency surgery. *J Trauma* 27:903, 1987.

Velmahos GC et al: Is there a limit to massive blood transfusion after severe trauma? *Arch Surg* 133:947, 1998.

CHAPTER 27

Hemostatic Defects in Renal Disease and Renal Failure

Hemorrhage was a serious and recurring problem for chronic renal failure patients before the routine use of dialysis. However, even with dialysis, up to 50% of patients experience purpura, menorrhagia, epistaxis, or occult gastrointestinal bleeding. Severe hemorrhage is uncommon, except perhaps as a consequence of major trauma or surgery. In contrast, patients with acute renal failure can have gastrointestinal bleeding, which is usually related to anatomic lesions such as peptic ulcer disease or angiodysplasia of the bowel. Thrombosis in renal disease can occur in the settings of nephrotic syndrome (acquired antithrombin deficiency), homocysteinemia, and heparin-associated thrombocytopenia.

PATHOPHYSIOLOGY

Platelet–vascular interactions are consistently impaired in uremic patients, as evidenced by prolonged bleeding-time measurements. Several defects contribute to this abnormality. Guanidinosuccinic acid (GSA) has long been known to accumulate in uremic plasma and to be related in some way to platelet and/or vascular dysfunction. Recent data has suggested that GSA (a derivative of L-arginine) stimulates the release of nitric oxide (NO) from vascular endothelium, which in turn causes impaired platelet adhesion, platelet aggregation, and vascular reactivity. Elevated levels of NO (previously called endothelium-derived relaxing factor) have been identified in uremic plasma and have been shown to increase cyclic GMP in platelets and vascular endothelial cells. Of interest, conjugated estrogens are known both to block production of NO and to shorten the bleeding time (and control bleeding) in uremic patients.

The severe anemia that accompanies uremia also disrupts normal platelet–vascular interactions. Several studies have shown that the prolongation of the bleeding time is inversely proportional to the hematocrit (Fig. 27-1). Correction of the anemia (e.g., raising the hematocrit to approximately 30 percent) not only shortens the bleeding time but also reduces symptoms of bleeding. Improvement in hemostasis may relate to improved diffusion of platelets to the vessel wall in the presence of higher numbers of red cells, and to red cell release of ADP.

Uremic patients have both mildly lowered platelet counts and decreased mean platelet volume (MPV), which results in a reduced platelet mass. The circulating platelet mass is inversely proportional to the bleeding time.

LABORATORY FINDINGS

The bleeding time is frequently abnormal in patients with uremia and can be slightly, moderately, or often severely prolonged (i.e., >30 min). Controversy exists as to whether the bleeding time has the ability to predict clinical bleeding in uremic subjects, particularly since the numbers of patients with significant hemorrhage are substantially fewer than those with long bleeding times. Platelet aggregation abnormalities are variable and do not

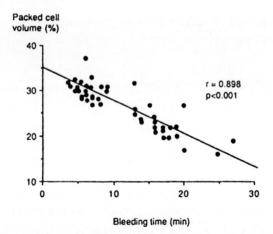

FIGURE 27-1 Correlation between bleeding time and hematocrit (packed cell volume) in patients treated with erythropoietin. (Reprinted with permission from Vignano G et al: *Am J Kid Dis* 18:44, 1991.)

predict bleeding. Screening tests of coagulation (e.g., PT, APTT, TCT, fibrinogen) are generally normal, or may be slightly prolonged due to the presence of ill-defined dialyzable inhibitors in the plasma. Bleeding due to systemic fibrinolysis has not been described in uremic patients.

Patients, particularly children, with the nephrotic syndrome may show abnormalities of the hemostatic screening tests even though they are not uremic. Prolongation of the APTT due to low factor XII and sometimes factor IX is not usually associated with a bleeding tendency. In addition, mild prolongations of the TCT are frequently seen and are probably due to a mild acquired dysfibrinogenemia associated with elevated fibrinogen levels.

MANAGEMENT

Since tests of hemostasis are frequently abnormal in patients with chronic renal failure, yet severe hemorrhage is unusual, therapy must focus on treatment or prevention of bleeding, rather than normalization of laboratory tests such as the bleeding time. An important first step is to review all medications so that aspirin or other drugs that interfere with platelet function can be stopped. Reduction or elimination of heparin for dialysis may be possible in some patients who are at very high risk of bleeding (e.g., following surgery, CNS hemorrhage, hemorrhagic pericarditis).

Listed below are several strategies that can be used for control or prevention of bleeding in patients with chronic renal failure.

Dialysis Alterations

Accelerated schedules of dialysis tend to shorten bleeding times and reduce the severity of bleeding in some, but not all, patients with renal failure. This approach should be tried whenever possible. Peritoneal dialysis was hypothesized to provide improved platelet function compared to hemodialysis, but controlled studies are not available.

Improve Erythroid Mass

Correction of severe anemia produces long-term improvement of platelet function and may also allow other therapeutic measures to be more effective. Both red blood cell transfusions and parenteral erythropoietin are effective, but the latter is preferable because of the risks of chronic transfusion. Hematocrits of 27 to 32 percent have been shown to optimize hemostasis (improved bleeding time, decreased bleeding), whereas higher hematocrits can lead to hypertension or thrombosis.

Improve Platelet Function with DDAVP

Short-term correction of the bleeding time and decreased symptoms of bleeding occur following infusions of DDAVP in 50 to 75 percent of uremic patients (Fig. 27-2). The action of DDAVP is rapid, with effects on the bleeding time observed within minutes, and persisting for at least 4 h. DDAVP may also be administered as a nasal spray. Repeated use results in tachyphylaxis (progressive loss of effect), so DDAVP cannot be used chronically. Transient flushing, headache, and abdominal cramps occur in up to 50 percent of DDAVP-treated patients; water retention and hyponatremia may also occur. Arterial thrombosis has been occasionally reported in elderly patients with advanced atherosclerosis who were treated with DDAVP. Cryoprecipitate has also been used to treat bleeding in uremia, but variability of response, a lag in onset of action (1 to 12 h), and the risks of viral infection have made this approach less attractive.

Improve Platelet Vascular Interactions with Conjugated Estrogens

Large doses of conjugated estrogens (0.6 mg/kg/day for 5 days) can be given intravenously, subcutaneously, or orally, and have been reported to shorten the bleeding time and decrease bleeding in patients with chronic renal failure (Fig. 27-3). Onset of action occurs in about 6 h and persists for 14 days. Maximal benefit is noted in 5 to 7 days. Since the duration of

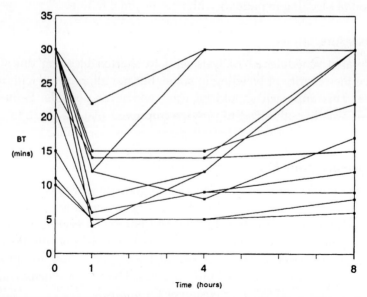

FIGURE 27-2 Bleeding times before and after DDAVP in uremic patients. (Data and permission obtained from Mannucci PM et al: *N Engl J Med* 308:8, 1983.)

effect is substantially longer than that of DDAVP, estrogens have been used to prepare uremic patients for major surgical procedures. A small study showed that low-dose transdermal estradiol shortened the bleeding time and reduced clinical hemorrhage in renal failure patients with prolonged bleeding times. The incidence of adverse effects of chronic estrogen use, such as thrombosis or malignancy, is unknown in the renal failure population.

An often difficult clinical problem is whether to attempt correction of the bleeding time with dialysis or DDAVP prior to percutaneous renal biopsy in patients with renal disease. Study of large series of subjects suggests that rates of hemorrhage are very low with DDAVP or other modalities prior to biopsy.

BIBLIOGRAPHY

Akizawa T et al: Effects of recombinant human erythropoietin and correction of anemia on platelet function in hemodialysis patients. *Nephron* 58:400, 1991.

Castillo R et al: Defective platelet adhesion on vessel subendothelium in uremic patients. *Blood* 68:337, 1986.

DeLoughery TG: Management of bleeding with uremia and liver disease. *Curr Opin Hematol* 6:329, 1999.

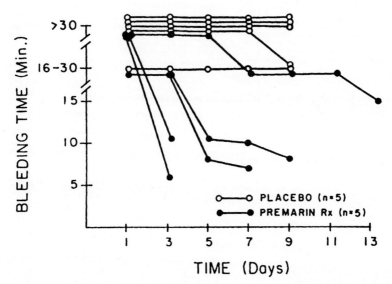

FIGURE 27-3 Patients with abnormal bleeding times and no clinical bleeding treated with conjugated estrogens or placebo. (Reprinted with permission from Shemin et al: *Am J Med* 89:436, 1990.)

Eberst ME et al: Hemostasis in renal disease: pathophysiology and management. *Am J Med* 96:168, 1994.

Gaspari F et al: Aspirin prolongs bleeding time in uremia by a mechanism distinct from platelet cyclooxygenase inhibition. *J Clin Invest* 79:1788, 1987.

Kyrle PA et al: Evidence for an increased generation of prostacyclin in the microvasculature and an impairment of the platelet-granule release in chronic renal failure. *Thromb Haemost* 60:205, 1988.

Livio M et al: Conjugated estrogens for the management of bleeding associated with renal failure. *N Engl J Med* 315:731, 1986.

Mannucci PM et al: Deamino-8-D-arginine vasopressin shortens the bleeding time in uremia. *N Engl J Med* 308:8, 1983.

Michalak E et al: The decreased circulating platelet mass and its relation to bleeding time in chronic renal failure. *Thromb Haemost* 65:11, 1991.

Noris M et al: Uremic bleeding: closing the circle after 30 years of controversies? *Blood* 94:2569, 1999.

Remuzzi G: Bleeding in renal failure. *Lancet* 1:1205, 1988.

Remuzzi G et al: Role of endothelium-derived nitric oxide in the bleeding tendency of uremia. *J Clin Invest* 86:1768, 1990.

Sloand EM et al: Reduction of platelet glycoprotein Ib in uraemia. *Br J Haematol* 77:375, 1991.

Steiner RW et al: Bleeding time in uremia: A useful test to assess clinical bleeding. *Am J Hematol* 7:107, 1979.

Vigano G et al: Recombinant human erythropoietin to correct uremic bleeding. *Am J Kidney Dis* 18:44, 1991.

Weigert et al: Uremic bleeding: pathogenesis and therapy. *Am J Med Sci* 316:94, 1998.

Zwaginga JJ et al: Defects in platelet adhesion and aggregate formation in uremic bleeding disorder can be attributed to factors in plasma. *Arterio Thromb* 11:733, 1991.

CHAPTER 28

Thrombotic Thrombocytopenic Purpura and the Hemolytic Uremic Syndrome

Thrombotic thrombocytopenic purpura (TTP) and the hemolytic uremic syndrome (HUS) are closely related disorders characterized by diffuse microvascular occlusion of the arterioles and capillaries, producing ischemic dysfunction of multiple organs. The microthrombi are primarily composed of platelets; the disorders are presently considered to be due to endothelial cell damage and excessive platelet clumping. TTP is a syndrome (thrombocytopenia, microangiopathic hemolytic anemia, neurologic symptoms, renal disease, fever) that occurs mostly in adults (although Moschcowitz's original patient was a teenager) and may show acute (single episode), intermittent, or chronic-relapsing types.

Hemolytic uremic syndrome (thrombocytopenia, microangiopathic anemia, acute renal failure) occurs mostly in children and is of endemic-epidemic, sporadic, or familial types. Table 28-1 highlights the similarities and differences of the syndromes. Overlapping, but clinically different, syndromes due to vascular damage (thrombocytopenia, microangiopathic hemolysis, diffuse organ involvement) are sometimes seen in disseminated intravascular coagulation (DIC), preeclampsia-eclampsia, HELLP (hemolysis, elevated liver enzymes, low platelet count) syndrome (see Chap. 30), malignant hypertension, acute renal hemograft rejection, systemic lupus erythematosus (SLE), and severe vasculitis.

TABLE 28-1

Comparison of Major Features of Hemolytic Uremic Syndrome and Thrombotic Thrombocytopenic Purpura

Feature	HUS	TTP
Onset and course	Age usually < 3 y Males = females Prodrome (infection, bloody diarrhea) common Recurrence—rare	Peak incidence third decade Females > males Prodrome less common Recurrence—common
Diagnosis	*Triad* Acute renal failure Thrombocytopenia Microangiopathy (CNS involvement unusual) (Fever unusual)	*Pentad* CNS involvement Thrombocytopenia Microangiopathy Renal involvement Fever (Acute renal failure less common)
Etiologic factors	Most often infection (*E. coli, Shigella* gastroenteritis, pneumococcal, etc.) Rare familial and/or recurrent form Adult—postpartum, after mitomycin C, cyclosporin A	Not known in most cases Secondary causes: pregnancy, autoimmune disease, neoplastic, drugs (sulfa, oral contraceptives, iodine, quinine, ticlopidine)
Treatment	Supportive Renal dialysis is mainstay Steroids—no help Heparin—for DIC if present	Steroids Plasma exchange Heparin—No Splenectomy
Prognosis	90% fully recover Rare death	Up to 90% gain remission with plasma exchange Mortality 9–15%

PATHOPHYSIOLOGY

The HUS syndromes may be divided into those with a prodromal diarrheal illness in children (D+ subtype, > 90 percent of cases) and those without the prodrome (often familial occurrence, children and adults, worse prognosis), which has been called D– subtype. The D+ group, or typical HU, is known to be associated with infection with bacteria (*Escherichia coli* 0157: H7; *Shigella dysenteriae*, type 1), producing a renal and other endothelial cell cytotoxin (verocytotoxin, VT) that has been implicated in HUS. VT damages endothelial cells with a loss of antithrombogenic properties and by releasing platelet-clumping substances (ultralarge von Willebrand factor [ULvWF] multimers or other substances) that form microthrombi. Other microorganisms, like pneumococci, and endothelial-altering chemotherapeutic agents, like mitomycin C or cyclosporin A, may operate in a similar manner. In most susceptible individuals the kidney is the major target, but other cells (brain, pancreas) may also be susceptible or, more likely, other organs are damaged by circulating microthrombi. The D– subtype or atypical HUS is a heterogeneous disorder that occurs without the diarrheal or colitic syndrome, although the onset may be associated with other infections. These children have a generally poor outcome (overall mortality of 26 percent in one series) and are more apt to develop recurrences and end-stage renal failure. Patients with familial HUS (up to three generations) are included in this group.

In TTP, after endothelial cells are damaged by toxins, viruses, autoantibodies, or drugs, a platelet-clumping substance is released into the circulation, with subsequent formation of platelet microthrombi. Although other substances such as platelet activating factor, cysteine proteases, arachidonic acid pathway metabolites, and antibodies may have a role in the pathogenesis, much evidence now suggests that the major platelet aggregating agent is ULvWF or fragments thereof. The ULvWF multimers are reduced to smaller multimers by a protease(s) found in normal platelet-poor plasma and cryosupernatant. Thus, the action of these vWF-cleaving proteinases may be critical to the formation of normal vWF and, if their activity is decreased, excessive platelet clumping could occur. A study using a newly developed assay for the vWF-cleaving protease indicated a severe deficiency in acute non-familial TTP either with or without an IgG inhibitor; patients with familial TTP lacked vWF-cleaving protease activity, in contrast to non-familial HUS patients who had normal activity. The benefit of plasma exchange would be both removal of the ULvWF multimers and replacement of the substances necessary for their degradation.

The red blood cell fragmentation (Fig. 28-1) and hemolytic anemia seen in both HUS and TTP are probably due to physical damage to red blood cells by the occlusive effect of the microangiopathy, but the erythrocyte may also be made more susceptible to injury by a reduced antioxidant potential due to a relative deficiency of vitamin E or by antibodies.

CLINICAL MANIFESTATIONS AND DIAGNOSIS

Hemolytic Uremic Syndrome

Approximately 90 percent of cases of childhood HUS (D+ or endemic type) present acutely after a prodromal infectious illness, frequently acute diarrhea or bloody diarrhea (colitislike symptoms); other in-

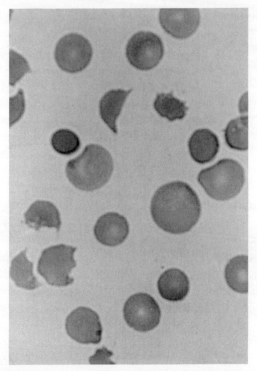

FIGURE 28-1 Oil power view of blood smear of patient with HUS. Note the fragmented red blood cells and microspherocytes. Identical findings are noted in TTP.

fections (mycoplasma, viruses, microtatobiotes, pneumococcus) have also been documented. Neuramidase from pneumococci exposes the Thomsen-Friedenreich receptor (T antigen) on red blood cells, platelets, and endothelium, thus producing IgM antibodies that agglutinate red blood cells and platelets (positive Coombs test); this mechanism has been associated with HUS (normal plasma contains anti-T agglutinins and could aggravate the anemia and thrombocytopenia). By the time the diagnosis is made and acute renal failure is established, an early complication may be excessive fluid administration and hyponatremic seizures.

Thrombocytopenia and anemia are usually present at the onset and last for 1 to 2 weeks and 2 to 4 weeks, respectively; other laboratory tests include leukocytosis and derangements of blood urea nitrogen (BUN), creatine, and electrolytes for degree of renal failure. Abnormal coagulation tests include raised levels of fibrinogen, factor VIII, and von Willebrand factor. The APTT, PT, and thrombin time are usually normal; an occasional patient has shown low antithrombin (AT) or protein C. Other evidence for activation of the coagulation system (in comparison to children with acute renal failure of other etiology) include increase in T-AT complexes, higher D-dimer levels and higher levels of PAI-1 and t-PA with only slight decrease in overall fibrinolytic activity. An occasional patient will display changes compatible with severe DIC and/or a tendency for venous and arterial thrombosis. Complications include CNS involvement (hyponatremic seizures, microthrombosis, cerebral infarction), pancreatic islet cell necrosis and diabetes, hyperglycemia, large bowel infarction, vitamin K deficiency, arterial thrombosis and extremity gangrene, and congestive heart failure.

A rare patient will present with HUS without a prodromal infection and with a tendency to recur. These patients are often older and family occurrence (up to three generations) is known. This group is the atypical or D– type, in which an unknown genetic predisposition is present. Adult HUS may occur with a prodromal illness, in the postpartum period without other illness, secondary to cancer or autoimmune disease, after administration of drugs like mitomycin C or cyclosporine A, or without known cause (primary HUS). The best prognosis is for patients after infection and the worst prognosis occurs in patients with secondary causes.

Thrombotic Thrombocytopenic Purpura

The pentad of neurologic symptoms and signs, hemolytic anemia, thrombocytopenia, renal disease, and fever are present in about 40 to 50 percent of the cases of adult TTP. About 75 percent of patients have hemolytic anemia, thrombocytopenia, and CNS changes. In addition, because of the rarity of the disorder and the confusion with similar diseases (see above), a firm diagnosis may be difficult to make and is dependent on excluding the similar clinical disorders and on the presence of the characteristic red blood cell changes on the blood smear (fragmented cells, schistocytes, microspherocytes; see Fig. 28-1). Laboratory findings include anemia with elevated reticulocytes, thrombocytopenia (worse prognosis when initial count is less that 20,000/µL), leukocytosis, bilirubinemia, and evidence of renal involvement. Although FDP are commonly present (about 60 to 70 percent of patients), most other coagulation tests are normal (APTT, PT, thrombin time, fibrinogen); von Willebrand factor and factor VIII are usually elevated and UL vWF multimers may present. Changes compatible with frank DIC can occur late in the course after extensive organ damage. Lactic dehydrogenase is elevated (1200 to 1400 U/L) and is an indicator of disease activity. The direct antiglobulin test is negative. Bone marrow and gingival biopsies are sometimes helpful by displaying the hyaline microthrombi in small vessels (50 percent of patients). The use of flow cytometry to detect vWF-GP1b positive platelets may become helpful in confirming the diagnosis. When better established, the assay for the vWF-cleaving protease should be helpful in confirming the diagnosis and choosing therapy.

The clinical course of TTP is occasionally acute, but usually differs from HUS in that the onset is more insidious (without a distinct prodromal illness); acute disease activity lasts longer (months rather than weeks) and has a characteristic tendency to relapse. Without intensive treatment the mortality rate approaches 80 percent. TTP has been noted in association with several conditions: pregnancy; Bartonella-like RBC inclusions; drug therapy with ticlopidine, cyclosporine A, mitomycin C, bleomycin, tamoxifen, sulfonamides, penicillamine, rifampin, arsenic, iodine, or oral contraceptives; HIV infection, crack cocaine, autoimmune disorders, bone marrow transplantation, and cancer.

TREATMENT

Hemolytic Uremic Syndrome

Patients with HUS and acute renal failure are provided intensive supportive care (red blood cell transfusions if hemoglobin is < 7 g/dL; fluid and electrolyte balance, nutritional support, treatment of hypertension). Peritoneal dialysis or hemodialysis is instituted on clinical indications (usually a rising BUN or potassium, excessive fluid overload, hyponatremia) and continued until kidney recovery. About three-fourths of patients will require dialysis. Thrombocytopenic bleeding is treated with platelet transfusions only if persistent wound bleeding or a vital site hematoma not responding to local measures occurs; most bleeding observed is mild skin purpura regardless of platelet count levels. No specific pharmacologic therapy (corticosteroids, antiplatelet agents, heparin) is used because most studies have not shown their superiority over no therapy. Heparin is used for thrombotic complications of intravascular catheters as needed. Most patients recover within 1 to 2 weeks, but require long-term follow-up for renal status. A rare patient may develop serious extrarenal progressive organ involvement (brain, pancreas, colon); these patients should have early consideration of plasma exchange with fresh frozen plasma replacement.

Thrombocytic Thrombocytopenic Purpura

Current management of TTP is outlined in Table 28-2. If plasma exchange is not immediately available, FFP (30 mL/kg/day) may be infused until

TABLE 28-2	
Treatment of TTP	

- Daily plasma exchange with FFP, cryosupernatant plasma or solvent detergent plasma 40 ml/kg. Continue daily exchanges until 3 days after complete remission (normal neurologic exam, platelet count >200,000/µL, normal LDH level)
- Intravenous prednisolone, 200 mg/day
- Red cell transfusions as needed
- Platelet transfusions only for life-threatening hemorrhage

the procedure is arranged. The average response time to daily plasma exchanges is 7 to 9 days. Refractory patients may require plasma exchange twice daily and cryoprecipitate-poor or solvent-detergent plasma instead of FFP to more efficiently decrease the abnormal vWF multimers or antibodies. Additional measures in refractory patients include vincristine, a trial of doxycycline (for possible Bartonella-like organisms), intravenous immunoglobulin, and splenectomy. TTP in cancer chemotherapy patients is often refractory and may respond better to immunoadsorption with a staphylococcal A column to remove circulating immune complexes. Some individuals, including two infants, with the chronic relapsing form of TTP have been maintained in a relatively normal state with periodic (every few weeks) administration of FFP or cryosupernant plasma.

PROGNOSIS

With strict attention to supportive care and renal dialysis, the prognosis for immediate survival is excellent in childhood (D+) HUS. Recent data demonstrates that the severity of the gastrointestinal prodrome (watery diarrhea versus bloody diarrhea or prolapse) reflects the severity of the process and resulting long-term outcome. Outcome will be variable in the less common types of HUS (D–, drug induced, postpartum, and familial). Remarkable progress has been made in TTP, from a uniformly fatal disease to complete recovery in >90 percent of patients in one recent series.

BIBLIOGRAPHY

Chintagumpala MM et al: Chronic relapsing thrombotic thrombocytopenic purpura in infants with large von Willebrand factor multimers during remission. *J Pediatr* 120:49, 1992.

Falanga A et al: A cathepsin-like cysteine proteinase proaggregating activity in thrombotic thrombocytopenic purpura. *Br J Haematol* 79:474, 1991.

Furlan M et al: von Willebrand factor-cleaving protease in thrombotic thrombocytopenic purpura and the hemolytic uremic syndrome. *N Engl J Med* 339:1578, 1998.

Galbusera M et al: Increased fragmentation of von Willebrand factor, due to abnormal cleavage of the subunit, parallels disease activity in recurrent hemolytic uremic syndrome and thrombotic thrombocytopenic purpura and discloses predisposition in families. *Blood* 94:610, 1999.

Gerritsen HE et al: Assay of von Willebrand factor (vWF)-cleaving protease based on decreased collagen binding affinity of degraded vWF—a tool for the diagnosis of thrombotic thrombocytopenic purpura (TTP). *Thromb Haemost* 82:1386, 1999.

Gordon LI, Kwaan HC: Cancer- and drug-associated thrombotic thrombocytopenic purpura and hemolytic syndrome. *Sem Hematol* 34: 140, 1997.

Haberle J et al: New strategies in diagnosis and treatment of thrombotic thrombocytopenic purpura: case report and review. *Eur J Pediatr* 158:883, 1999.

Hymes KB, Karpatkin S: Human immunodeficiency virus infection and thrombotic microangiopathy. *Sem Hematol* 34: 117, 1997.

Kwaan HC, Soff GA: Management of thrombotic thrombocytopenic purpura and hemolytic uremic syndrome. *Sem Hematol* 34: 159, 1997.

Lopez EL et al: Association between severity of gastrointestinal prodrome and long-term prognosis in classic hemolytic-uremic syndrome. *J Pediatr* 120:210, 1992.

Mattoo JK et al: Familial, recurrent hemolytic-uremic syndrome. *J Pediatr* 114:814, 1989.

McInyk AMS et al: Adult hemolytic-uremic syndrome. A review of 37 cases. *Arch Intern Med* 155:2077, 1995.

Moake JL: Moschcowitz, multimers, and metalloprotease (editorial). *N Engl J Med* 339:1629, 1998.

Moake JL, Chow TW: Thrombotic thrombocytopenic purpura: understanding a disease no longer rare. *Am J Med Sci* 316:105, 1998.

Muszkat M et al: Ticlopidine-induced thrombotic thrombocytopenic purpura. *Pharmacotherapy* 18:1352, 1998.

Neild GH: Hemolytic uremic syndrome/thrombocytopenic purpura: pathophysiology and treatment. *Kidney Int* 53: Supp 64, S-45, 1998.

Neuhaus TJ et al: Heterogeneity of atypical haemolytic uraemic syndromes. *Arch Dis Child* 76: 518, 1997.

Petermann A et al: Familial hemolytic-uremic syndrome in three generations. *Am J Kid Dis* 32: 1063, 1998.

Raife TJ, Aster RH: von Willebrand proteolysis and doxycycline in thrombotic thrombocytopenic purpura. *Lancet* 352: 324, 1998.

Rock G et al: Laboratory abnormalities in thrombotic thrombocytopenic purpura. *Br J Haematol* 103:1031, 1998.

Tardy B et al: Intravenous prostacyclin in thrombotic thrombocytopenic purpura; case report and review of the literature. *J Intern Med* 230:279, 1991.

Vangeet C et al: Activation of both coagulation and fibrinolysis in childhood hemolytic uremic syndrome. *Kid Int* 54:1324, 1998.

von Vigier RO et al: Positive Coombs test in pneumococcus-associated hemolytic uremic syndrome. A review of the literature. *Nephron* 82:183, 1999.

CHAPTER 29

Bleeding and Cancer

This chapter discusses hemorrhagic disorders that occur in patients with solid tumors, whereas bleeding that complicates hematologic malignancies is discussed in Chapters 32 and 33. The topic of thrombosis and malignancy is considered in Chapter 46. The most common hemostatic defect in cancer patients is thrombocytopenia, which usually develops late in the course of the illness. Less frequently, chronic disseminated intravascular coagulation (DIC); liver failure secondary to metastases; or disorders such as systemic fibrinolysis, circulating anticoagulants, or the synthesis of dysfunctional clotting-factor molecules are seen.

THROMBOCYTOPENIA

Thrombocytopenia in patients with cancer is most often the result of suppression of marrow platelet production by malignancy, chemotherapy, or radiation treatments. Although immune thrombocytopenia (ITP) is classically associated with lymphoid neoplasms, patients with solid tumors also develop ITP. Immune-mediated thrombocytopenia can also be provoked by some of the drugs used in oncology practice, including vancomycin, penicillin, and heparin. The diagnosis and treatment of thrombocytopenia is reviewed in Chapters 8 and 9.

Rarely, cancer patients develop a microangiopathy accompanied by renal failure, anemia, and thrombocytopenia. This occurs most commonly in patients with gastric or breast carcinoma, or following therapy with mitomycin C, cisplatin, bleomycin, or cyclosporin A. The syndrome is strikingly reminiscent of the hemolytic uremic syndrome (HUS) or TTP (Table 29-1), although no specific pathophysiology has been elucidated and no abnormalities of vWF cleaving protease have been identified.

TABLE 29-1
Cancer-Associated Hemolytic Uremic Syndrome*
Adenocarcinoma in 89%   No evident malignancy at time of diagnosis in 35%   Mitomycin C therapy in 98%   Mortality—50% within 8 weeks   Consider therapy with staphylococcal protein A immunopheresis   Avoid transfusion of blood products

* From Lesesne JB et al: *J Clin Oncol* 7:781, 1989.

Cancer-related HUS is often fatal. Treatment with plasmapheresis in this setting is much less effective than in classic TTP/HUS. Any potentially offending drugs should be stopped, and some benefit may be achieved by plasmaphereis, or with staphylococcal protein A immunopheresis of the plasma.

DISSEMINATED INTRAVASCULAR COAGULATION

Pathogenesis

Many tumors can activate coagulation and fibrinolysis in a effort to facilitate the implantation of metastatic cells. The release of cells from the primary tumor can be augmented by the action of proteolytic or fibrinolytic enzymes on nearby blood vessels, and the growth and proliferation of disseminated tumor cells may be facilitated by the formation of a local fibrin meshwork.

Laboratory evidence of activation of coagulation (e.g., increased fibrinopeptide A) in both the early and late stages of cancer is exceedingly common. When the activation of clotting factors and platelets is mild or moderate, a propensity to thrombosis (e.g., venous, arterial, or involving a heart valve) may be found, but when stimulation of the clotting system is brisk and sustained, full-blown DIC can occur with severe hypofibrinogenemia and diffuse bleeding. Coagulation is instigated by tumor cell activation (e.g., via tissue factor or other cancer procoagulants) of factor VII, factor X, or prothrombin; platelets may also be activated and fibrinolysis can be inhibited as well. Cytokines such as interleukin-1 or tumor necrosis factor produced by tumor cells may stimulate nearby macrophages or endothelial cells to become prothrombotic via the synthesis and expression of cell surface tissue factor.

Hemorrhage as a result of DIC in patients with malignancy usually does not occur unless clotting factor depletion is severe; that is, fibrinogen concentrations of <100 mg/dL, factor V or factor VIII of <30%, or platelet counts of <50,000/uL. High concentrations of fibrin degradation products also impair platelet function. A rather wide spectrum of tumors are associated with DIC and bleeding. Common offenders include mucous-producing adenocarcinomas of the bowel or abdomen (e.g., pancreas, gastric, biliary tract), as well as neoplasms that originate in the lung. In childhood, activation of coagulation is most often found in patients with disseminated neuroblastoma and rarely occurs with other tumors.

The malignancy is often widely disseminated when severe hemostatic defects occur, and tumor cell emboli can be found in the microvasculature of the lung or other organs (Fig. 29-1). The intravascular collections of tumor cells can induce a severe microangiopathic hemolytic anemia with thrombocytopenia and circulating fragmented red blood cells.

Clinical Findings and Laboratory Tests

Most patients with malignancy do not have excessive bleeding and have normal screening tests of hemostasis. Hemorrhage, particularly after surgery or invasive diagnostic procedures, can be severe in patients who develop cancer-related DIC. Spontaneous bruising of the skin, hematoma

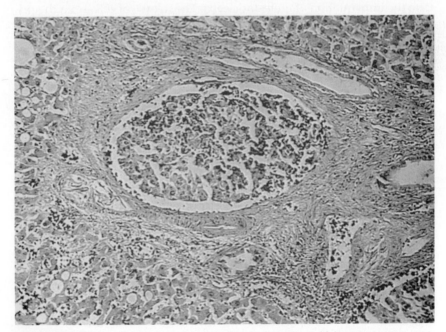

FIGURE 29-1 Tumor cell emboli in microvasculature of a patient with breast cancer.

formation, and bleeding from the mucous membranes or the gastrointestinal tract can occur.

Results of laboratory tests in cancer-related DIC are illustrated in Table 29-2. In addition, sensitive tests that reflect activation of coagulation or fibrinolysis such as circulating thrombin–antithrombin or plasmin–antiplasmin complexes are abnormal in 5 to 10 percent of patients. Fragmented red blood cells are prominent on the peripheral blood smear in patients with disseminated malignancy and DIC. The microangiopathic hemolytic anemia can produce marked elevations of lactic dehydrogenase and indirect hyperbilirubinemia as a result of the red blood cell destruction.

Management

Most patients with mild cancer-related DIC do not require specific therapy such as large volumes of blood products or therapeutic doses of anticoagulants. However, prophylactic antithrombotic measures should be strongly considered for surgical procedures because of the high likelihood of postoperative venous thromboembolism.

Effective chemotherapy or surgery is the best treatment for chronic DIC associated with cancer, but unfortunately is often not possible. When antitumor treatment is effective, tumor cell lysis can expose the blood to even more procoagulant activity, which accelerates the consumption of clotting factors and platelets. In these circumstances, laboratory monitoring to include platelet counts, fibrinogen, and fibrin degradation products is warranted. Temporary anticoagulation with heparin may be necessary during periods of DIC as a consequence of early cycles of chemotherapy.

When cancer-related DIC is severe and associated with bleeding, correction of a prolonged PT and APTT with fresh frozen plasma, hypofibrinogenemia with cryoprecipitate, and thrombocytopenia with platelet

---

TABLE 29-2

Disseminated Intravascular Coagulation in Patients with Cancer

	Mild DIC	Severe DIC	Normal Range
PT	12	18	11–13.5 s
APTT	23	56	25–35 s
Fibrinogen	580	40	175–350 mg/dL
Platelets	650,000	56,000	$175–325 \times 10^3/\mu L$
D-dimer	4	32	< 0.5 µg/mL
ELT	> 60	> 60	> 60 min

concentrates may be required. Although in the past concerns were raised that the administration of blood products would "fuel the fire" and worsen the DIC, this phenomenon rarely occurs. However, if frequent blood-product replacement therapy is needed to balance the accelerated consumption of clotting factors or platelets, then heparin may be needed to inhibit thrombin generation and reduce the intensity of the DIC.

When heparin is used, it should be given together with appropriate blood-product replacement. Heparin should be infused at relatively low rates (e.g., 500 U/h) without a loading dose and increased as needed to maintain hemostatic levels of clotting factors and platelets. Unfortunately, unless effective cancer therapy is available, the prognosis in most of these patients is very poor.

SYSTEMIC FIBRINOLYSIS

Although many tumor cells produce and release fibrinolytic enzymes in culture, systemic fibrinolysis is unusual in cancer patients. Prostate cancer has been reported to be associated with primary fibrinolysis and bleeding, and several other tumors have caused shortened plasma or whole blood clot lysis times. In some instances, systemic fibrinolysis may be found concurrently with DIC; perhaps as an "overflow" of secondary fibrinolysis into the circulating blood because of depletion of fibrinolytic inhibitors or because of the release of both procoagulants and fibrinolytic enzymes from the neoplasm.

The diagnosis of primary fibrinolysis in cancer patients is suggested by the finding of a short euglobulin lysis time (ELT) and a reduced concentration of α_2-antiplasmin (α_2-AP) in the absence of markedly elevated concentrations of D-dimer or other tests sensitive to fibrin degradation products. If D-dimer levels are high, then the constellation of a short ELT and markedly increased D-dimer suggests that both DIC and systemic lysis are present. In those rare patients with primary fibrinolysis without evidence of DIC, the use of antifibrinolytic agents could be considered for temporary control of severe bleeding. However, if DIC is also present, inhibition of secondary fibrinolysis could promote arterial or venous thrombosis including fibrin-induced renal insufficiency.

RARE MALIGNANCY-ASSOCIATED COAGULATION DEFECTS

Several unusual but fascinating coagulopathies have been reported in individual patients with cancer. For example, a man with a bladder carcinoma developed a circulating anticoagulant that was similar to heparin, and another patient with metastatic prostate cancer had a circulating gly-cosaminoglycan that was a direct (i.e., non-antithrombin-dependent) inhibitor of thrombin. Yet another patient with an adrenal carcinoma developed acquired von Willebrand disease due to adsorption of the high molecular weight multimers of von Willebrand factor on the surface of the malignant cells. The multimers reappeared in the plasma following resection of the tumor. Lastly, an acquired dysfibrinogenemia has been associated with primary liver carcinoma. The abnormal fibrinogen can cause prolonged thrombin and Reptilase times and, in some instances, bleeding. Thus when patients with cancer have bleeding with atypical laboratory findings, it is appropriate to screen for inhibitors or for dys-functional clotting factors that may be present.

BIBLIOGRAPHY

Christie DJ et al: Vancomycin-dependent antibodies associated with thrombocyto-penia and refractoriness to platelet transfusion in patients with leukemia. *Blood* 75:518, 1990.

Edwards RL et al: Heparin abolishes the chemotherapy-induced increase in plasma fibrinopeptide A levels. *Am J Med* 89:25, 1990.

Ey FS, Goodnight SH: Bleeding disorders in cancer. *Semin Oncol* 17:187, 1990.

Facon T et al: Acquired type II von Willebrand's disease associated with adrenal cortical carcinoma. *Br J Haematol* 80:488, 1992.

Francis JL et al: Hemostasis and malignancy. *Semin Thromb Hemostas* 24: 93, 1998.

Glassman AB: Hemostatic abnormalities associated with cancer and its therapy. *Ann Clin Lab Sci* 27:391, 1997.

Goad KE, Gralnick HR: Coagulation disorders in cancer. *Hematol Oncol Clin North Am* 10: 457, 1996.

Gordon LI, Kwaan HC: Thrombotic microangiopathy manifesting as thrombotic thrombocytopenic purpura/hemolytic uremic syndrome in the cancer patient. *Semin Thromb Hemostas* 25: 217, 1999.

Hultin MB: Acquired inhibitors in malignant and nonmalignant disease states. *Am J Med* 91:9S, 1991.

Lesesne JB et al: Cancer-associated hemolytic-uremic syndrome: Analysis of 85 cases from a national registry. *J Clin Oncol* 7:781, 1989.

Liebman HA et al: A glycosaminoglycan inhibitor of thrombin: A new mechanism for abnormal hemostatic assays in cancer. *Am J Hematol* 38:24, 1991.

Nakagawa T et al: Clinicopathologic significance of protein induced vitamin K absence or antagonist II and alpha-fetoprotein in hepatocellular carcinoma. *Int J Oncol* 14:281, 1999.

Nand S et al: Hemostatic abnormalities in untreated cancer: Incidence and correlation with thrombotic and hemorrhagic complications. *J Clin Oncol* 5:1998, 1987.

Nanninga PB et al: Low prevalence of coagulation and fibrinolytic activation in patients with primary untreated cancer. *Thromb Haemost* 64:361, 1990.

Ratnoff OD: Hemostatic emergencies in malignancy. *Semin Oncol* 16:561, 1989.

Tefferi A et al: Isolation of a heparin-like anticoagulant from the plasma of a patient with metastatic bladder carcinoma. *Blood* 74:252, 1989.

Van der Plas RM et al: Von Willebrand factor proteolysis is deficient in classic, but not in bone marrow transplantation-associated, thrombotic thrombocytopenic purpura. *Blood* 93: 3798, 1999.

Watson PR et al: Cisplatin-associated hemolytic uremic syndrome. Successful treatment with a staphylococcal protein A column. *Cancer* 64:1400, 1989.

Zurborn KH et al: Investigations of coagulation system and fibrinolysis in patients with disseminated adenocarcinomas and non-Hodgkin's lymphomas. *Oncology* 47:376, 1990.

CHAPTER 30

Hemorrhagic Disorders in Obstetrics

Hemorrhage, either associated with a specific complication of pregnancy and delivery or due to a hereditary or acquired bleeding diathesis, remains an important cause of obstetric morbidity and mortality. Life-threatening bleeding after conception can be due to ectopic gestation, abortion, abruptio placentae, placenta previa, postpartum bleeding (atonic uterus, birth trauma), and defects of the hemostatic system. This chapter will focus on systemic hemostatic defects that contribute to obstetric hemorrhage. However, it should be emphasized that successful management of pregnancy- and parturition-associated bleeding depends on expert obstetrical care and the ready availability of blood products.

HEREDITARY DISORDERS

Most women with obstetric bleeding due to a hereditary defect will have a history of excessive menstrual bleeding. Studies have suggested that up to 17 percent of women with menorrhagia (menstrual blood loss of > 80 mL) will be found to have an inherited defect of hemostasis. Disorders such as von Willebrand disease (vWD) or factor XI deficiency commonly present with menorrhagia at time of menarche (~65 percent) as well as in later life (vWD, 74 percent of patients; factor XI deficiency, 59 percent of patients; as compared with 29 percent in control populations)(see Lee ref). A diagnosis of a hemostatic defect in women with menorrhagia has important implications for future surgery (e.g., hysterectomy) and childbirth (see later). In addition to oral contraceptives, treatment for menorrhagia may include DDAVP (by nasal spray) and antifibrinolytic agents.

Clinically important hereditary disorders of hemostasis in obstetrics are discussed.

von Willebrand Disease

Von Willebrand disease is the most common hereditary bleeding disorder in pregnancy (as well as the general population, see Chap. 12). Fortunately, type 1 vWD is by far the most common subtype (80 to 90 percent of subjects) and is associated with a substantial increase in the vWF complex as pregnancy proceeds (Fig. 30-1). As a consequence, bleeding at time of delivery is very unusual, but can occur following abortion since vWF and factor VIII don't increase significantly until the second trimester. In contrast, type 3 vWD and several of the type 2 variants can cause major hemorrhage and often require treatment. Type 2B and platelet-type vWD are further complicated by progressive thrombocytopenia as pregnancy progresses. Therapeutic modalities (Table 30-1) include DDAVP, a drug that is useful in patients with severe type 1, as well as some with type 2A disease. As discussed in Chapter 58, DDAVP can cause flushing, headache (minor problem), and hyponatremia due to fluid retention (a potentially major problem). Ideally, DDAVP is reserved for postpartum use because of concern about inducing contractions or interfering with the maternal–fetal circulation, although some authorities feel it can safely be given prepartum (e.g., Kadir 1999 ref). A second treatment option is the use of vWF concentrates (that also contain factor VIII) to increases vWF levels to >50 percent in women with type 3 disease and those with type 2 variants that are not treatable with DDAVP. Cryoprecipitate contains vWF and factor VIII, but should be reserved for those instances, due to concerns about viral infection, when vWF concentrates are not available.

Platelet Defects

Platelet-type (or pseudo-) vWD is due to a defect in the glycoprotein lb receptor for vWF that produces increased platelet binding of normal vWF. As a consequence, platelet agglutination and thrombocytopenia occurs. In this disorder, the platelet count often falls as pregnancy progresses, due to an increase in the concentration of normal vWF. DDAVP, vWF concentrates, and cryoprecipitate can all aggravate the thrombocytopenia. Platelet transfusions (sometimes followed by vWF concentrate) may be needed to treat or prevent bleeding.

Women with Glanzmann's thrombasthenia may have no excess bleeding, or may occasionally require blood and platelet transfusions for perinatal hemorrhage. Severe postpartum hemorrhage has also occurred in Bernard-Soulier syndrome. Most of the other platelet function disorders

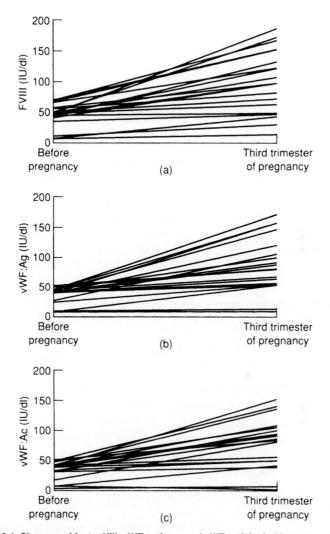

FIGURE 30-1 Changes of factor VIII, vWF antigen, and vWF activity in 22 women with vWD in pregnancy. (Used with permission from Kadir RA et al. *Br J Obstet Gynaecol* **105: 314, 1998.)**

have not been associated with serious bleeding. Hereditary collagen disorders (Marfan, Ehlers-Danlos syndromes) have poor pregnancy outcomes (increased fetal wastage and mechanical complications of labor and delivery related to tissue friability and vessel rupture), but without significant hemorrhage. Anaphylactoid purpura (Henoch-Schoenlin purpura) has occurred during pregnancy but was not associated with excessive bleeding.

TABLE 30-1			
Management of von Willebrand Disease during Pregnancy and the Perinatal Period			
Disease Type	**Pregnancy**	**Delivery**	**Postpartum**
I	Document expected rise in VIII-vWf complex in third trimester	Vaginal: observe. Cesarean section: Concentrate rarely needed	Treat early bleeding with DDAVP + / – concentrate
IIA or IIB	Determine bleeding time and VIII-vWf complex at 36 wks	Vaginal: observe closely, may need concentrate Cesarean section: treat as major surgery	Treat early bleeding with concentrate
III	Expect no rise in VIII-vWf complex: document at 36 wks	Vaginal or cesarean section: treat as major surgery with concentrate	Continue prophylaxis with concentrate until wounds healed

* Concentrate: vWF concentrate. Cryoprecipitate should be reserved for treatment of severe bleeding when concentrates are not available

Coagulation Factor Deficiencies

During normal pregnancy fibrinogen, vWf, and factors II, VII, IX, VIII, X, and XII rise significantly by the third trimester, while factors XI, XIII, and V are stable or fall slightly (see Chap. 3). These physiologic changes tend to ameliorate less severe congenital coagulation factor deficiencies, but will not alter severe defects. The experience with each hereditary disorder is briefly summarized.

Hemophilia A and B

Clinically significant factor VIII or IX deficiency is rare in women (see Chaps. 13 and 14) except for the occasional carrier with low factor levels due to extreme lyonization of the heterozygote. Although factor VIII levels rise in hemophilia A carriers during pregnancy, factor IX levels remain constant or rise only slightly in hemophilia B carriers. Peripartum bleeding has occurred in some factor IX carriers with low factor IX levels. Because minimal hemostatic levels for factor VIII and factor IX is about 0.2 to 0.3 U/mL, carriers should be monitored; if clotting factor levels have not risen significantly, replacement therapy with high-purity factor concentrates should be considered before delivery or for cesarean section (see Chap. 55).

Fibrinogen Abnormalities

Some women with afibrinogenemia have normal menses, but others have severe menorrhagia and recurrent early pregnancy loss. In at least one instance, a rare successful pregnancy and delivery was achieved with weekly fibrinogen infusions. Hypo- and dysfibrinogenemias are also associated with recurrent abortion or abruptio placentae. Dysfibrinogenemic bleeding may worsen over time because the synthesis of abnormal fibrinogen molecules can increase during pregnancy. Bleeding episodes require the use of fibrinogen replacement (e.g., cryoprecipitate, see Chap. 54). A woman weighing 60 kg with severe hypo- or dysfibrinogenemia requires 10 to 15 bags of cryoprecipitate to raise her concentration of normal fibrinogen above 100 mg/dL.

Other Deficiencies

First-trimester spontaneous abortion has been reported in a patient with hereditary dysprothrombinemia. Intrapartum and postpartum hemorrhage may be severe in patients with severe factor V deficiency; adequate hemostasis can be achieved by infusion of 15 mL/kg of frozen or solvent-detergent (SD) plasma in the early puerperium. A woman with severe factor X deficiency showed marked improvement of her bleeding tendency and coagulation tests during pregnancy; she was subsequently treated successfully for many years with exogenous estrogens. Menorrhagia occurs frequently in severe factor VII deficiency; however, only about one-half of reported deliveries have had postpartum bleeding. In two patients postpartum hemorrhage despite fresh frozen plasma infusions was subsequently treated with a factor VII concentrate.

Homozygous factor XIII deficiency causes a severe hemorrhagic tendency but is readily treated with infusions of plasma or cryoprecipitate. One patient had 12 previous pregnancies that were interrupted by severe bleeding and spontaneous abortions; with regular infusions of plasma, the patient's 13th pregnancy proceeded normally without bleeding. Pregnancies in women with severe factor XII deficiency and severe prekallikrein deficiency have been uncomplicated. Some patients with severe factor XI deficiency do not show a clinical bleeding tendency; one such patient known to us experienced a normal pregnancy and delivery without bleeding episodes. If bleeding does occur, frozen or SD plasma or a factor XI concentrate may be needed (see Chap. 55).

ACQUIRED BLEEDING DISORDERS

Thrombocytopenia

The major causes of thrombocytopenia during pregnancy are listed in Table 30-2. The immune thrombocytopenias (ITP) and gestational thrombo-cytopenia are discussed in Chapter 9, and thrombotic thrombocytopenic purpura (TTP) in Chapter 28. The differential diagnosis of low platelets and red blood cell fragmentation in the hypertensive pregnant woman in the third trimester may be particularly difficult, and includes the follow-ing disorders: hypertensive disease of pregnancy (preeclampsia) along with its more severe subtype (in 10 percent), the HELLP syndrome (hemolysis, elevated liver enzymes, low platelets), acute fatty liver of pregnancy (AFLP), TTP, hemolytic uremic syndrome, and abruptio pla-centae with disseminated intravascular coagulation (DIC). A precise diag-nosis is important since therapy varies considerably with each disorder (Table 30-3).

A particularly difficult management problem is whether to use epidural anesthesia in patients with potential bleeding disorders, espe-cially those with thrombocytopenia, platelet function defects, anticoag-

---

TABLE 30-2
Causes of Thrombocytopenia in Pregnancy

Immune
  ITP
  SLE
  Evan's syndrome
  Thyrotoxicosis
  Lymphoproliferative diseases
  Pregnancy-associated thrombocytopenia
Infections
  Bacterial, viral, other
Drugs
  Alcohol, isoniazid, diphenylhydantoin, quinine, sulfonamides, heparin
Other
  TTP
  Preeclampsia/eclampsia, HELLP syndrome
  Chronic hepatitis
  Obstetrical complications with DIC
  Massive blood transfusions
  Bone marrow hypoplasia (toxic, idiopathic)
  Bone marrow malignant disease (cancer, leukemia)
  Megaloblastic anemias

* SLE, systemic lupus erythematosus; ITP, immune thrombocytopenic purpura; DIC, disseminated intravascular coagulation; HELLP, hemolysis, elevated liver enzymes, low platelet counts; TTP, thrombo-cytic thrombocytopenic purpura.

TABLE 30-3					
Differential Diagnosis of Thrombocytopenia in "Preeclampsia"					
Condition					
Manifestation	**HELLP**	**AFLP**	**Abruption**	**TTP**	**HUS**
Onset	Insidious	Acute	Acute	Insidious	Insidious
Thrombocyto-penia	Severe	Mild, early	Mild to severe	Severe	Severe
Abnormal APTT, PT	When liver severely involved	Yes	20% of patients (DIC)	No	No
Elevated FDP	Yes	Yes	Yes	Yes	Yes
Jaundice	Rare	Yes	No	Rare	Rare
Increased liver enzymes	Yes	Yes	No	Occasional	No
Abdominal pain	Yes (epigastric)	Yes (epigastric)	Yes (uterine)	No	No
Renal failure	Rare	Rare	No	No	Yes
Neurologic involvement	Sometimes	Late	No	Yes	Rare

* AFLP, acute fatty liver of pregnancy; HELLP, hemolysis, elevated liver enzymes, low platelets; DIC, disseminated intravascular coagulation; FDP, fibrin degradation products.
SOURCE: Adapted from Martin JN Jr, Stedman CM: *Obstet Gynecol Clin North Amer* 18:181, 1991.

ulants, or antiplatelet agents. Mild prolongation of the bleeding time is seen in patients with the above acquired disorders (microangiopathic thrombocytopenia), but the bleeding time test is a poor predictor of bleeding. Epidural anesthesia is probably contraindicated in most untreated moderate and severe bleeding disorders and in patients on anticoagulants, for fear of inducing cord compression from spinal hematoma.

Obstetric Causes of Disseminated Intravascular Coagulation

Hemorrhage produced or aggravated by DIC is associated with many of the major obstetric complications, including abruptio placentae, amniotic fluid emboli, and dead fetus syndrome. Other triggers are severe sepsis, shock, and acidosis. Diagnosis and management of DIC is discussed in Chapter 24. Important principles of patient management for women with coagulation failure (massive hemorrhage and shock) include correction of the circulating blood volume and tissue perfusion with appropriate volume replacement therapy. In patients who are believed to have major coagulation defects, replacement therapy with plasma, cryoprecipitate, platelet concentrates, and, if needed, packed red cells should be started as soon as possible—guided by laboratory monitoring (PT, APTT, fibrinogen, platelet count, and hematocrit; see Chap. 26).

Vaginal delivery makes less severe demands on the hemostatic mechanism than delivery by cesarean section or hysterotomy, both of which require the same degree of hemostatic competence as other abdominal operations. When a coagulation defect exists, severe bleeding will occur at sites of surgical incisions and may not become apparent until after the operation. In the obstetric patient, extensive bleeding can occur into the abdomen from the uterine incision. It is nearly always advisable in the absence of fetal distress to await spontaneous delivery, avoiding if possible soft tissue damage to the vagina and perineum. After delivery, a contracted myometrium sharply diminishes bleeding from the placental site. Optimal treatment of underlying obstetrical conditions (e.g., placental abruption) is an important component of the management of hemorrhage. In general, prompt delivery facilitates treatment of bleeding. Every effort should be made to correct coagulation failure prior to and following surgical intervention.

Circulating Anticoagulants

Postpartum-acquired factor VIII inhibitors (within several weeks to a year or more after delivery) can cause severe bleeding. In time most of these inhibitors (IgG antibodies) will spontaneously regress. Treatment includes porcine factor VIII, recombinant factor VIIa and immunosuppressive therapy (see Chap. 20).

Acute Fatty Liver of Pregnancy

Acute hepatic failure occurring at term and unrelated to preeclampsia, hepatitis, or hepatotoxic agents is designated acute fatty liver of pregnancy (AFLP). These patients characteristically show biochemical evidence of liver disease (elevated bilirubins, enzymes, and low serum proteins) in association with a severe coagulopathy (low platelets, fibrinogen, and antithrombin [AT], along with elevated fibrin degradation products). The coagulopathy most likely represents failure of hepatic synthesis of clotting factors plus activation of coagulation with DIC. Reports have emphasized the extremely low AT levels seen in AFLP patients (~10 percent of normal) and have suggested a beneficial effect of AT concentrates on the coagulopathy, although it is not yet clear if survival is enhanced (Castro refs). Surviving patients regain normal liver function.

BIBLIOGRAPHY

Castro MA et al: Reversible peripartum liver failure: a new perspective on the diagnosis, treatment, and cause of acute fatty liver of pregnancy, based on 28 consecutive cases. *Am J Obstet Gynecol* 181:389, 1999.

Castro MA et al: Disseminated intravascular coagulation and antithrombin III depression in acute fatty liver of pregnancy. *Am J Obstet Gynecol* 174:211, 1996.

Dashe JS et al: The long-term consequences of thrombotic microangiopathy (thrombotic thrombocytopenic purpura and hemolytic uremic syndrome) in pregnancy. *Obstet Gynecol* 91:662, 1998.

Duerbeck NB et al: Platelet and hemorrhagic disorders associated with pregnancy: a review. Part I. *Obstet Gynecol Survey* 52:575, 1997.

Duerbeck NB et al: Platelet and hemorrhagic disorders associated with pregnancy: a review. Part II. *Obstet Gynecol Survey* 52:585, 1997.

Economides DL et al: Inherited bleeding disorders in obstetrics and gynaecology. *Br J Obstet Gynecol* 106:5, 1999.

Egerman RS, Sibai BM: HELLP syndrome. *Clin Obstet Gynecol* 42:381, 1999.

Esplin MS, Branch DW: Diagnosis and management of thrombotic microangiopathies during pregnancy. *Clin Obstet Gynecol* 42:360, 1999.

Fausett B, Silver RM: Congenital disorders of platelet function. *Clin Obstet Gynecol* 42:390, 1999.

Giles AR et al: Type IIB von Willebrand's disease presenting as thrombocytopenia during pregnancy. *Br J Haematol* 67:349, 1987.

Greer IA et al: Haemorrhagic problems in obstetrics and gynaecology in patients with congenital coagulopathies. *Br J Obstet Gynecol* 98:909, 1991.

Hathaway WE, Bonnar J: Hemorrhagic disorders during pregnancy. In: *Hemostatic Disorders of the Pregnant Women and Newborn Infant*, New York, Elsevier, 1987, pp 76–103.

Isler CM et al: Maternal mortality associated with HELLP (hemolysis, elevated liver enzymes, and low platelets) syndrome. *Am J Obstet Gynecol* 181:924, 1999.

Joseph G et al: Pregnancy in Henoch-Schonlein purpura. *Am J Obstet Gynecol* 157:911, 1987.

Kadir RA: Women and inherited bleeding disorders: pregnancy and delivery. *Semin Hematol* 36:28, 1999.

Kadir RA et al: Pregnancy in women with von Willebrand's disease or factor XI deficiency. *Br J Obstet Gynecol* 105:314, 1998.

Kadir RA et al: Acquired haemophilia, an unusual cause of severe postpartum haemorrhage. *Br J Obstet Gynecol* 104:854, 1997.

Kadir RA et al: The obstetric experience of carriers of haemophilia. *Br J Obstet Gynecol* 104:803, 1997.

Lee CA: Women and inherited bleeding disorders: menstrual issues. *Semin Hematol* 33: 21, 1999.

Locksmith GJ: Amniotic fluid embolism. *Obstet Gynecol Clinics North Amer* 26:435, 1999.

Peaceman AM, Cruikshank DP: Ehlers-Danlos syndrome and pregnancy: association of type IV disease with maternal death. *Obstet Gynecol* 69:428, 1987.

Peaceman AM et al: Bernard-Soulier syndrome complicating pregnancy: a case report. *Obstet Gynecol* 73:457, 1989.

Robertson LE et al: Hereditary factor VII deficiency in pregnancy: peripartum treatment with factor VII concentrate. *Am J Hematol* 40:38, 1992.

Schjetlein R et al: Markers of intravascular coagulation and fibrinolysis in preeclampsia: association with intrauterine growth retardation. *Acta Obstet Gynecol Scand* 76:541, 1997.

Vandermeulen EP et al: Anticoagulants and spinal-epidural anesthesia. *Anesth Analg* 79:1165, 1994.

CHAPTER 31

Bleeding Related to Congenital Heart Disease and Cardiac Surgery

HEMOSTATIC DEFECTS DUE TO CONGENITAL HEART DISEASE

Severe congenital heart disease has been associated with a variety of hemostatic defects. As a consequence, excessive bleeding can become an important clinical problem when patients require cardiac surgery or other major procedures. Fortunately, early and more complete correction of the cardiac abnormalities is now the usual practice, so that bleeding symptoms are much less common than in the past. However, hemostatic defects may still occur in patients who are not candidates for early corrective surgery.

Pathogenesis

A spectrum of hemostatic abnormalities have been described in patients with congenital heart disease, including defects in platelet function, coagulation, and fibrinolysis. In general, cyanotic patients with chronic hypoxia, erythrocytosis, and impaired blood flow have more prominent defects in hemostasis than those with acyanotic heart disease (e.g., ventricular septal defect). In contrast to polycythemia rubra vera, elevated hematocrits in patients with cyanotic congenital heart disease are not usually associated with an increased risk of stroke (Thorne ref).

Platelet Dysfunction

Mild to moderate thrombocytopenia (e.g., 90,000 to 100,000/μL) occurs in some patients with cyanotic congenital heart disease due to shortened platelet survival. Mild defects in platelet aggregation have also been reported and include reduced platelet aggregation with epinephrine, and deaggregation when adenosine diphosphate is used as a stimulus. Bleeding times are occasionally prolonged (up to 8 percent of patients). High-molecular-weight multimers of von Willebrand factor are reduced in some patients with acyanotic congenital heart disease, and in others with severe pulmonary hypertension.

Coagulation

Many cyanotic patients have been assumed to have a coagulopathy because the PT and APTT are frequently prolonged. However, some of these laboratory abnormalities (but not all) return to normal when the volume of anticoagulant is reduced in the collection tube in order to correct for the high hematocrit found in patients with cyanotic congenital heart disease. Some patients have reduced clotting factor synthesis due to chronic passive congestion of the liver. Early reports suggested that low-grade disseminated intravascular coagulation (DIC) occurs, although more recent studies have not substantiated this observation.

Fibrinolysis

About 20 percent of cyanotic patients have a short plasma euglobulin lysis time (ELT), but the origin and significance of this finding is uncertain. Clinically significant systemic fibrinolysis is unlikely because fibrinogen concentrations are not often reduced, and levels of fibrinogen degradation products are usually normal.

Laboratory Tests

Patients with congenital heart disease who have bleeding symptoms or who are candidates for major surgery should undergo screening tests for hemostasis (see Chap. 6). The volume of citrate anticoagulant in the collection tube must be adjusted to avoid spurious coagulation test results in patients with elevated hematocrits (Chap. 2). Laboratory test results compiled from several large series of patients previously reported in the medical literature are listed in Table 31-1. However, at present the frequency of abnormal laboratory test results is undoubtedly lower than anticipated because of early surgical repair of the cardiac lesions.

Clinical Manifestations

Most nonsurgical bleeding in patients with congenital heart disease is mild and limited to recurrent epistaxis and easy bruisability. Hemoptysis may occur and has been noted particularly in patients with pulmonary

TABLE 31-1	
Screening Laboratory Test Results Compiled from Several Reported Series of Patients with Cyanotic Congenital Heart Disease	
Abnormal test results	**Patients**
Platelet count	42%
Bleeding time	8%
ELT	17%
PT	15%
APTT	8%
TT	6%

* From Colon-Otero G et al: *Mayo Clin Proc* 62:379, 1987.

hypertension. Surgical bleeding is unpredictable, although patients with severe hypoxia are at increased risk of hemorrhage. In rare patients, postoperative bleeding is severe, and a few deaths due to hemorrhage have been reported. When surgery is successful, preoperative platelet function defects almost always improve postoperatively, which suggests that the platelet abnormalities were caused by either the cardiac lesions or hypoxia and erythrocytosis.

Management

With modern medical and surgical management, the great majority of patients with congenital heart disease have minimal laboratory abnormalities or bleeding symptoms and do not require treatment. However, a rare individual will have a history of severe bleeding or marked abnormalities in laboratory tests of hemostasis (mainly in association with severe cyanosis) and some require correction of their coagulopathies prior to surgery. One therapeutic approach is to reduce the red blood cell mass by repeated isovolumetric phlebotomy in order to lower hematocrits to <60 to 65 percent. The platelet count, bleeding time, and coagulation factor abnormalities will often improve. However chronic reduction of elevated hematocrits should be limited to patients with marked symptoms of hyperviscosity. Side effects of phlebotomy include dehydration and chronic iron deficiency, which produces more rigid red cells (microcytes) and right shifts in the oxyhemoglobin dissociation curve.

Bleeding following cardiac surgery in infants and children with congenital heart disease is linked to body weight (<8 kg) and duration of cardiopulmonary bypass (CPB). Marked hemodilution is observed in neonates undergoing cardiopulmonary surgery, with a 50% decrease in coagulation factors and a 70% reduction in platelet count. Baseline coagulation tests do not predict postoperative bleeding. Abnormal hemostatic test values and excessive bleeding respond to replacement therapy with platelet concentrates and cryoprecipitate. Fresh frozen plasma is of much less value.

Desmopressin (DDAVP) has been administered prophylactically to increase plasma von Willebrand factor, shorten bleeding times, and reduce blood loss during and following cardiac surgery. However, the benefits remain uncertain. Patients with congenital heart disease have marked elevations in von Willebrand factor and factor VIII activity as a result of surgical stresses, and no further rise is seen after infusions of the drug. DDAVP should be used with caution in the nonsurgical setting because several patients with cyanotic congenital heart disease developed a sudden decrease in peripheral vascular resistance, as well as hypotension, and died following its use.

Aprotinin is a broad spectrum serine protease inhibitor that blocks fibrinolysis as well as kallikrein and other proteolytic enzymes. Several clinical trials in pediatric patients with congenital heart disease suggest that high doses of the drug reduce bleeding in patients with complex cardiac lesions (e.g., transposition of the great vessels) and those requiring reoperation. In contrast, there was little benefit in routine surgeries. Thromboembolic complications did not occur.

HEMOSTATIC DEFECTS CAUSED BY CARDIAC SURGERY AND CARDIOPULMONARY BYPASS

Postoperative bleeding is often a major problem for patients who require cardiac surgery and cardiopulmonary bypass (Table 31-2). In many instances the bleeding is due to local vascular defects that require surgical repair. However, extracorporeal circulation regularly produces hemostatic abnormalities that can contribute to postoperative hemorrhage.

Pathogenesis

Platelet dysfunction is the most common hemostatic defect induced by CPB. In addition to thrombocytopenia, platelet activation with release of alpha and dense granule contents, and inhibition or destruction of platelet receptor proteins have been described. Inhibition of potent *in vivo* platelet agonists such as thrombin by the high doses of heparin used in CPB may be important. The administration of preoperative antiplatelet drugs, prolonged duration of CPB, and hypothermia are also associated, with platelet dysfunction and postoperative hemorrhage.

TABLE 31-2
Causes of Bleeding after Cardiopulmonary Bypass
Common (95–99%) 　Defective surgical hemostasis 　Acquired transient platelet dysfunction Uncommon (1–5%) 　Other platelet dysfunction 　Thrombocytopenia 　Vitamin K deficiency 　DIC 　Inherited hemostatic defects Doubtful significance 　Systemic fibrinolysis 　Heparin 　Protamine excess

* Modified from Woodman RC et al: *Blood* 76:1680, 1990.

Coagulation defects occur during bypass due to dilution, reduced synthesis of clotting factors by the liver due to hepatic insufficiency, and the effects of high doses of heparin. Accelerated fibrinolysis occurs during CPB with marked increases in the concentration of tissue plasminogen activator (t-PA) and a moderate fall in α_2-antiplasmin (α_2-AP). However, these abnormalities are short lived and are not associated with clinically significant systemic fibrinolysis. Plasma fibrinogen falls only to the level expected by hemodilution, and fibrinogen degradation products are not greatly elevated. In contrast, secondary fibrinolysis (presumably including thrombi formed in the surgical field) is brisk, as evidenced by a gradual increase in D-dimer concentrations throughout CPB and for several hours thereafter.

Clinical Manifestations

Excessive and persistent bleeding from chest tubes or wound sites is a common problem in the immediate postoperative period in cardiac surgery patients. The hourly volume of blood that issues from the chest tubes is an excellent indication of the magnitude of bleeding, which frequently exceeds several hundred milliliters per hour. Oozing of blood from venipuncture sites or other areas of trauma (catheters, nasotracheal or nasogastric tubes) suggests a systemic defect of hemostasis.

Laboratory Tests

Preoperative screening tests in cardiac surgery patients seldom predict intraoperative or postoperative bleeding because most excessive bleeding is a result of acquired abnormalities occurring during CPB. Screening tests are warranted in patients with a history of bleeding, pronounced erythrocytosis, or liver insufficiency. The activated clotting time (ACT) is used widely to monitor heparin therapy during bypass, but it should be recognized that hemodilution, platelet counts <50,000/µL, hypothermia, and aprotinin therapy (due to kallikrein inhibition) all also prolong the ACT, leading to suboptimal heparin dosing. For example, studies monitoring heparin concentrations instead of ACTs showed an increase in heparin use, decreased protamine doses, and reduced blood loss and transfusion requirements in those patients followed with the heparin assays.

The combination of rapid turnaround times for laboratory tests (e.g., point of care [POC] instruments or special laboratory protocols), coupled with an algorithm for transfusion of blood products also led to decreased blood loss, transfusion requirements, and operative times. Recently, POC tests that assess platelet function (e.g., platelet activating factor-induced shortening of the clotting time) have proven successful in identifying patients who will respond to DDAVP infusions (see Despotis et al ref. 1999).

Laboratory tests must be obtained in cardiac surgery patients who develop brisk postoperative bleeding and should include the PT, APTT, fibrinogen, bleeding time (or PFA-100), and platelet count. These tests are used to identify defects in hemostatic function and as guides to clotting factor or platelet replacement (see Chap. 6).

Management

Since thrombocytopenia and platelet function defects are so common, platelet concentrates are often given empirically to cardiac surgery patients who have postoperative bleeding. Several studies have documented normalization of platelet counts, bleeding times, and platelet aggregation tests, along with cessation of bleeding following platelet transfusions. Hypothermia magnifies platelet dysfunction, so that rewarming the patient may also be of value. Coagulation abnormalities due to dilution or consumption of clotting factors must also be corrected (e.g., hypofibrinogenemia of <100 mg/dL with cryoprecipitate and markedly prolonged PT and APTT with fresh frozen plasma; see Chap. 26).

Cardiac surgery teams have evaluated prophylactic infusions of DDAVP before or after CPB to improve platelet function and to decrease intraoperative or postoperative bleeding. Early trials were encouraging, but subsequent studies have shown little benefit in terms of decreased blood loss or transfusion requirements in uncomplicated patients who received coronary artery bypass grafts. As previously mentioned, the use of POC platelet function tests during CPB may help identify those patients most likely to benefit from DDAVP. Otherwise, most surgeons and cardiovascular anesthesiologists reserve DDAVP for complex and prolonged surgeries or for patients who develop uncontrolled bleeding.

Antifibrinolytic agents have also been used to decrease bleeding in cardiac surgery patients. Aprotinin (Trasylol), tranexamic acid (TA), and ε-aminocaproic acid (EACA) have been evaluated in clinical trials (Fig 31-1). In almost all of the studies, blood loss during and following surgery was decreased by 30 to 50% and red blood cell transfusions were reduced, so the number of patients who avoided transfusion significantly increased. An increase in thromboembolism, a potential complication of antifibrinolytic therapy, has not been observed in the controlled clinical trials. The antifibrinolytic agents not only inhibit fibrinolysis, but they also preserve platelet function, possibly by the prevention of platelet adhesion defects or by a reduction in circulating levels of fibrin degradation products.

The indications for antifibrinolytic agents in cardiac surgery patients continue to evolve. Most would agree that these drugs are useful when patients are at high risk for bleeding (e.g., reoperation, prolonged CPB, or uremia). Antifibrinolytic agents can also be used as adjunctive therapy in Jehovah's Witnesses in whom blood transfusion is not allowed (see Chap. 58).

Other Hemostatic Problems Relative to Cardiac Surgery

Postoperative Coagulation Factor Inhibitors to Bovine Thrombin

Topical bovine thrombin is used frequently in cardiovascular surgery. Rare patients will produce antibodies either to bovine thrombin or to bovine factor V, which is also present in most preparations of topical thrombin. These antibodies can cross-react in vivo with human thrombin or human factor V and cause bleeding several weeks later. The diagnosis is suggested in postoperative patients with prolonged TCTs, particularly when bovine thrombin is used as the reagent for the thrombin time (see Chap. 20).

Protamine Toxicity

Some patients with diabetes mellitus who are treated with NPH insulin (which contains protamine) may develop IgG or IgE antiprotamine antibodies. When protamine sulfate is given to neutralize the heparin used

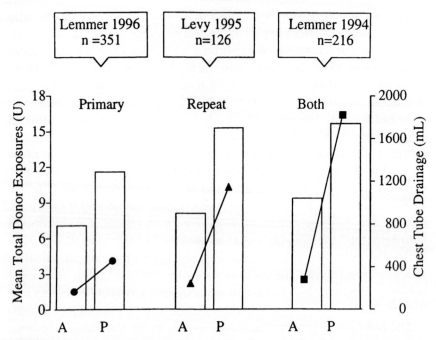

FIGURE 31-1 Effects of full-dose aprotinin on blood loss and transfusion requirements in patients undergoing cardiac surgery involving cardiopulmonary bypass: a summary from 3 large multicenter US trials. A, aprotinin-treated patients; Both, primary and repeat procedures; chest tube drainage, cumulative 24-h chest tube drainage; P, placebo-treated patients; Primary, primary procedures; Repeat, repeat procedures; both, both primary and repeat procedures. (Used with permission from Despotis et al. *Am J Cardiol* 83: 15B, 1999.)

for CPB, sensitized patients can suddenly develop pulmonary hypertension, hypoxia, and occasionally overwhelming DIC. Since protamine contains arginine, one study suggested that arginine conversion to nitric oxide is responsible for the systemic hypotension that has been observed in this syndrome. Reactions can be reduced if protamine is administered slowly and into the systemic rather than the venous circulation.

BIBLIOGRAPHY

Ansell J et al: Does desmopressin acetate prophylaxis reduce blood loss after valvular heart operations? A randomized, double-blind study. *J Thorac Cardiovasc Surg* 104:117, 1992.

Carrel TP et al: Aprotinin in pediatric cardiac operations: a benefit in complex malformations and with high-dose regimen only. *Ann Thorac Surg* 66:153, 1998.

Colon-Otero G et al: Preoperative evaluation of hemostasis in patients with congenital heart disease. *Mayo Clin Proc* 62:379, 1987.

Davies MJ et al: Prospective, randomized, double-blind study of high-dose aprotinin in pediatric cardiac operations. *Ann Thorac Surg* 63:497, 1997.

Despotis GJ, Hogue CW, Jr: Pathophysiology, prevention, and treatment of bleeding after cardiac surgery: A primer for cardiologists and an update for the cardiothoracic team. *Am J Cardiol* 83:15B, 1999.

Despotis GJ et al: Prospective evaluation and clinical utility of on-site monitoring of coagulation in patients undergoing cardiac operation. *J Thorac Cardiovasc Surg* 107:271, 1994.

Despotis GJ et al: The impact of heparin concentration and activated clotting time monitoring on blood conservation. A prospective, randomized evaluation in patients undergoing cardiac operation [see comments]. *J Thorac Cardiovasc Surg* 110:46, 1995.

Despotis GJ et al: Use of point-of-care test in identification of patients who can benefit from desmopressin during cardiac surgery: a randomised controlled trial. *Lancet* 354:106, 1999.

Gill JC et al: Loss of the largest von Willebrand factor multimers from the plasma of patients with congenital cardiac defects. *Blood* 67:758, 1986.

Kern FH et al: Coagulation defects in neonates during cardiopulmonary bypass. *Ann Thorac Surg* 54:541, 1992.

Kestin AS et al: The platelet function defect of cardiopulmonary bypass. *Blood* 82:107, 1993.

Miller BE et al: Hematologic and economic impact of aprotinin in reoperative pediatric cardiac operations. *Ann Thorac Surg* 66:535, 1998.

Miller BE et al: Predicting and treating coagulopathies after cardiopulmonary bypass in children. *Anesth Analg* 85:1196, 1997.

Munoz JJ et al: Is epsilon-aminocaproic acid as effective as aprotinin in reducing bleeding with cardiac surgery?: a meta-analysis. *Circulation* 99:81, 1999.

Perloff JK et al: Risk of stroke in adults with cyanotic congenital heart disease. *Circulation* 87:1954, 1993.

Territo MC et al: Acquired von Willebrand factor abnormalities in adults with congenital heart disease: dependence upon cardiopulmonary pathophysiological subtype. *Clin Appl Thromb/Hemost* 4:257, 1998.

Thorne SA: Management of polycythaemia in adults with cyanotic congenital heart disease. *Heart* 79:315, 1998.

Weiss ME et al: Association of protamine IgE and IgG antibodies with life-threatening reactions to intravenous protamine. *N Engl J Med* 320:886, 1989.

Zehnder JL, Leung LL: Development of antibodies to thrombin and factor V with recurrent bleeding in a patient exposed to topical bovine thrombin. *Blood* 76:2011, 1990.

CHAPTER 32

Lymphoproliferative Disorders

Patients with lymphoproliferative disorders are more often troubled with excessive bleeding than with arterial or venous thrombosis. Causes of hemorrhage are diverse, although thrombocytopenia induced by marrow disease or chemotherapy is the most common problem. However, a wide spectrum of platelet, coagulation, or fibrinolytic abnormalities has been described, often posing diagnostic and therapeutic dilemmas. This chapter covers abnormalities of hemostasis and thrombosis in acute and chronic lymphocytic leukemia; the paraproteinemias, including plasma cell myeloma and macroglobulinemia; and systemic amyloidosis.

ACUTE LYMPHOCYTIC LEUKEMIA

Disseminated intravascular coagulation (DIC) can complicate acute lymphocytic leukemia (ALL) as well as acute promyelocytic or monocytic leukemia (Fig. 32-1). Approximately 5 to 10% of children and adults with ALL will have laboratory evidence of DIC, with greater percentages in patients with T-cell leukemia. Even higher rates of DIC have been reported to occur after initial chemotherapy, although some of these abnormalities may have been secondary to an L-asparaginase induced coagulopathy (see later). Evidence of thrombin activation (increased levels of thrombin–antithrombin complexes, prothrombin activation peptide F1.2) was present in a group of children presenting with ALL, which persisted after treatment (Mitchell ref).

L-asparaginase is commonly used in the treatment of children and adults with ALL and can occasionally produce severe coagulation defects. L-asparaginase inhibits protein synthesis and, as a consequence,

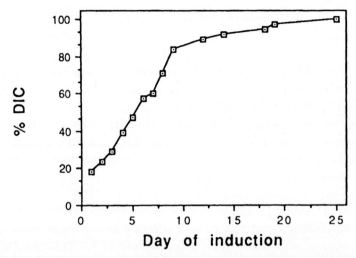

FIGURE 32-1 Cumulative occurrence of all DIC cases during remission induction of adult ALL patients. All cases of DIC occurring before day 1 of induction were plotted on day 1. (Used with permission from Sarris AH et al: *Blood* 79:1305, 1992.)

the formation of several clotting factors (or their inhibitors) by the liver. Bleeding may occur a few days after the completion of a course of therapy and is associated with prolongation of the PT and APTT and a fall in fibrinogen. Thrombosis occurs later, often after 2 to 3 weeks, and has been linked to decreased levels of antithrombin. Of note, both the bleeding and thromboembolic events show a predilection for the CNS, such as intracerebral hemorrhage and cerebral sinus vein thrombosis.

Therapy for the L-asparaginase-induced coagulopathies remains controversial. One study suggested that fresh frozen plasma was ineffective in increasing plasma levels of coagulation factors or their inhibitors such as antithrombin in these patients. Antithrombin concentrates have been used to elevate blood levels of antithrombin, but it is not yet known whether this treatment reduces thrombosis in the cerebral veins or elsewhere.

CHRONIC LYMPHOCYTIC LEUKEMIA/LYMPHOMA

Patients with chronic lymphocytic leukemia (CLL), Hodgkin's disease, and non-Hodgkin's lymphoma occasionally become severely thrombocytopenic by an immune mechanism rather than due to marrow failure. Although less common, acquired von Willebrand disease or platelet function disorders (storage pool disease) have also been described.

Immune Thrombocytopenic Purpura

Immune-mediated thrombocytopenic purpura (ITP) is relatively frequent in patients with CLL (perhaps 10 percent of patients at some point during their illness), and occurs in about 2 percent of patients with Hodgkin's disease. ITP is unusual, but has been occasionally reported, in patients with non-Hodgkin's lymphoma. When associated with Hodgkin's disease, thrombocytopenia is often associated with disease activity, but may also predate the diagnosis or appear long after apparent complete remission. Although not proven, the immune dysregulation that so commonly occurs in the chronic lymphoproliferative disorders may permit the clinical expression of autoimmune phenomena such as ITP.

Standard therapy for ITP is usually successful and includes the use of corticosteroids, splenectomy, or immunosuppressive regimens. Aggressive treatment of the underlying lymphoproliferative disorder does not always correct the immune thrombocytopenia. A search for recurrent lymphoma is warranted when ITP develops in patients who have been previously treated for Hodgkin's disease.

Acquired von Willebrand Disease

In contrast to the hereditary disorder, acquired von Willebrand disease is much less common, but has been reported to occur in association with lymphoproliferative disorders such as CLL, B-cell lymphoma, and plasma cell myeloma (see also Chap. 12). As expected, the bleeding time is prolonged and the components of the von Willebrand factor–factor VIII macromolecular complex are decreased. Von Willebrand antigen and factor VIII levels are often reduced to 5 to 40% of normal, with ristocetin cofactor levels that are even lower or absent. At least two mechanisms are responsible for the reductions in plasma von Willebrand factor. Some patients develop anti-von Willebrand factor antibodies, often IgG, that react with the high-molecular-weight components of the protein. Another mechanism involves the adsorption of plasma von Willebrand factor onto the surfaces of neoplastic lymphoid cells. Bleeding varies from mild to severe.

Treatment of acquired von Willebrand disease includes DDAVP or von Willebrand factor concentrates to transiently elevate von Willebrand factor levels to treat bleeding. Infusions of high doses of intravenous immunoglobulin produced more sustained improvement in several patients with monoclonal gammopathies (Federici ref). Plasmapheresis or plasma exchange is sometimes necessary to remove a high-titer anti-von Willebrand factor antibody. In several instances, splenectomy has been performed to remove a large volume of malignant cells (presumably adsorbing von Willebrand factor) and was followed by increases in von Willebrand factor (see Chap. 12).

HAIRY CELL LEUKEMIA

Thrombocytopenia is often a major clinical problem for patients with hairy cell leukemia and is usually due to a combination of marrow invasion by malignant cells and sequestration of platelets in an enlarged spleen. Platelet function defects, particularly a loss of platelet granules (as visualized by electron microscopy), and reduced platelet aggregation have also been noted in a few patients. It has been suggested that the platelet release reaction occurs in the spleen, where platelets are in contact with large numbers of malignant cells. Splenectomy reportedly normalizes platelet function and increases the platelet count.

PLASMA CELL MYELOMA AND MACROGLOBULINEMIA OF WALDENSTROM

Patients suffering from dysproteinemias such as plasma cell myeloma or macroglobulinemia often have abnormal laboratory tests of hemostasis, although severe bleeding is relatively uncommon. Analyses of large numbers of patients have suggested that patients with IgA paraproteins, κ (rather than γ) light chains, high levels of serum proteins, or markedly increased serum viscosity are more likely to have overt bleeding. A wide array of hemostatic disorders has been described that involve both coagulation and platelet function (Table 32-1). Most of these defects are a consequence of elevated levels of monoclonal proteins. Therapy of these bleeding disorders involves treatment of the underlying disease to reduce or eliminate pathologic immunoglobulins and to reduce plasma viscosity. Intensive plasmapheresis may be necessary to temporarily control bleeding.

TABLE 32-1	
Hemostatic Disorders in Patients with Dysproteinemia	
Coagulation Defects	**Platelet Abnormalities**
Friable clot with increased fibrinolysis	Abnormal clot retraction
Inhibition of factor XIIIa receptor	Inhibition of glycoprotein IIIa
Inhibition of fibrin polymerization	Shortened platelet survival
Heparin-like anticoagulants	Inhibition of platelet adhesion

Recently a patient was reported with plasma cell myeloma that developed a high-titer monoclonal inhibitor to thrombin that prolonged screening tests of coagulation, including the thrombin and reptilase times. The IgG inhibitor had a specific antithrombin effect, but in high concentration also inhibited fibrin polymerization. Plasmapheresis improved the coagulation abnormalities and bleeding symptoms.

Patients with plasma cell myeloma also can develop circulating heparin-like anticoagulants that pose challenging problems in management (Table 32-2). These inhibitors can be differentiated from specific thrombin inhibitors (described previously) by lack of prolongation of the reptilase time and by correction following the addition of polybrene or protamine sulfate. Most of these anticoagulants cause severe and unrelenting bleeding that is often fatal. Chemotherapy to reduce the malignant cell mass, intensive plasmapheresis to remove the circulating anticoagulant, and intravenous protamine sulfate to neutralize the heparin-like glycosaminoglycan have all been tried, unfortunately with only modest success.

AMYLOIDOSIS

In one large series, about 10 percent of patients with systemic amyloidosis had severe bleeding. Easy bruisability is common and usually results from amyloid infiltration of blood vessels in the skin. However, systemic defects of hemostasis also occur. Atrial and inferior vena cava thrombosis have been reported and were thought to be due to marked amyloid infiltration of the heart or vena cava.

TABLE 32-2

Coagulation Studies in Five Patients with Circulating Heparin-like Anticoagulants

Patient	Pro-thrombin Time (17–19 s)	Activated Partial Thrombo-plastin Time (25–40 s)	Thrombin Time (20–23 s)	Reptilase Time (14–16 s)	Fibrin-ogen (190–365) (mg/dL)	Fibrin Split Products (<6 µg/mL)
1	21	48	>600	21	138	5
2	18	46	105	18	626	40
3	25	44	>600	17	432	1
4	28	48	>600	20	883	10
5	27	115	>600	21	371	20

* Used with permission from Tefferi A et al: *Am J Med* 88:184, 1990.

Abnormalities of some laboratory tests, such as a prolonged TCT, are exceedingly frequent in amyloidosis, but are not predictive of bleeding. However, more specific disorders have also been described that are associated with hemorrhage. One of these is factor X deficiency, which is most likely due to adsorption of the clotting factor on amyloid fibrils. Circulating levels of factor X are sometimes as low as 2 to 4 percent of normal and are associated with recurrent hemorrhage. In a few instances, splenectomy was performed to remove a major site of amyloid deposition and was associated with a rise in circulating levels of factor X. However, long-term control of bleeding due to factor X deficiency usually requires a reduction in the amyloid burden with chemotherapy (e.g., melphalan and prednisone).

A second major hemostatic abnormality in amyloidosis is chronic systemic fibrinolysis, which may also produce severe and recurrent bleeding. Primary fibrinolysis can be due to several different mechanisms, including adsorption of α_2-antiplasmin (α_2-AP) on amyloid proteins, a process analogous to the loss of factor X. Elevated plasma levels of the plasminogen activators, t-PA and u-PA, and decreased concentrations of plasminogen activator inhibitor (PAI-1) have also been described. The mechanisms responsible for the increased plasminogen activators or depressed PAI are not known, but could reflect vascular damage produced by amyloid proteins. Antifibrinolytic agents such as ε-aminocaproic acid or tranexamic acid may be useful for symptomatic control of bleeding.

Individual case reports have described other hemostatic defects in patients with amyloidosis. In one report, a patient developed a monoclonal IgA antibody that reacted strongly with factor VIII and was associated with severe bleeding. In another, a monoclonal Benz-Jones protein (i.e., an immunoglobulin light chain) that was bound tightly to fibrinogen produced a severe defect in fibrin polymerization; although the thrombin time was markedly prolonged, excessive bleeding did not occur.

Patients with systemic amyloidosis should have the usual screening tests of hemostasis, which include a euglobulin lysis time and sometimes assays of plasminogen and α_2-AP. Conversely, if a patient with normal liver function is found to have a primary fibrinolytic syndrome, then a diagnosis of systemic amyloidosis should be considered.

The bleeding risk associated with liver biopsy in patients with amyloid has been reported to be about 3 percent, as compared to 0.1 to 0.2 percent in patients with other forms of liver disease. Usually a diagnosis of amyloidosis can be made by biopsy of other sites such as rectal mucosa, skin, or bone marrow with less risk of bleeding.

BIBLIOGRAPHY

Andrew M et al: Acquired antithrombin III deficiency secondary to asparaginase therapy in childhood acute lymphoblastic leukaemia. *Blood Coag Fibrinol* 5:Suppl-36, 1994.

Colwell NS et al: Identification of a monoclonal thrombin inhibitor associated with multiple myeloma and a severe bleeding disorder. *Br J Haematol* 97:219, 1997.

Cools FJ et al: Primary systemic amyloidosis complicated by massive thrombosis. *Chest* 110:282, 1996.

DeLoughery TG, Goodnight SH: Bleeding and thrombosis in hematologic neoplasia. In Wiernik PH, Canellos GP, Dutcher JP, Kyle RA (eds), *Neoplastic Diseases of the Blood*, 3rd ed, New York, Churchill Livingstone, 1995, p 1177.

Dubrey S et al: Atrial thrombi occurring during sinus rhythm in cardiac amyloidosis: evidence for atrial electromechanical dissociation. *Br Heart J* 74:541, 1995.

Federici AB et al: Treatment of acquired von Willebrand syndrome in patients with monoclonal gammopathy of uncertain significance: comparison of three different therapeutic approaches. *Blood* 92:2707, 1998.

Gastineau DA et al: Inhibitor of the thrombin time in systemic amyloidosis: a common coagulation abnormality. *Blood* 77:2637, 1991.

Halton JM et al: Fresh frozen plasma has no beneficial effect on the hemostatic system in children receiving L-asparaginase. *Am J Hematol* 47:157, 1994.

Leibman H: Hemostatic defects associated with dysproteinemias. In Hoffman R, et al., (eds), *Hematology; Basic Principles and Practice*, 3rd ed, New York, Churchill Livingstone, 1999, p 1996.

Mitchell L et al: Increased endogenous thrombin generation in children with acute lymphoblastic leukemia: risk of thrombotic complications in L-asparaginase-induced antithrombin III deficiency. *Blood* 83:386, 1994.

Nur S et al: Disseminated intravascular coagulation in acute leukaemias at first diagnosis. *Eur J Haematol* 55:78, 1995.

Pogliani EM, et al: L-asparaginase in acute lymphoblastic leukemia treatment: the role of human antithrombin III concentrates in regulating the prothrombotic state induced by therapy. *Acta Haematol* 93:5, 1995.

Rosove MH et al: Severe platelet dysfunction in hairy cell leukemia with improvement after splenectomy. *Blood* 55:903, 1980.

Sarris AH et al: High incidence of disseminated intravascular coagulation during remission induction of adult patients with acute lymphoblastic leukemia. *Blood* 79:1305, 1992.

Shapiro AD et al: Thrombosis in children receiving L-asparaginase. Determining patients at risk. *Am J Pediatr Hematol Oncol* 15:400, 1993.

Sletnes KE et al: Disseminated intravascular coagulation (DIC) in adult patients with acute leukaemia. *Eur J Haematol* 54:34, 1995.

Tefferi A et al: Circulating heparin-like anticoagulants: report of five consecutive cases and a review. *Am J Med* 88:184, 1990.

Tornebohm E et al: A retrospective analysis of bleeding complications in 438 patients with acute leukaemia during the years 1972–1991. *Eur J Haematol* 50:160, 1993.

CHAPTER 33

Bleeding in the Myeloid Disorders: Acute Leukemia, Myelodysplasia, and Myeloproliferative Disease

This chapter focuses on bleeding in patients with three types of myeloid disorders: acute myeloid leukemia, myelodysplasia, and chronic myeloproliferative disease (MPD). Although all of these disease processes can be complicated by hemorrhage or thrombosis, bleeding is most prominent in leukemia and myelodysplasia, while thrombosis is more common in MPD (see Chap. 44). Bleeding that occurs in myelodysplasia, polycythemia rubra vera, myeloid metaplasia, and essential thrombocytosis is most commonly attributable to platelet function defects (PFD). In contrast, hemorrhaging in patients with acute leukemia most often occurs because of thrombocytopenia due to decreased platelet production and to consumptive coagulopathies.

ACUTE MYELOID LEUKEMIAS

Thrombocytopenia and Platelet Dysfunction

By far the most common cause of bleeding in patients with acute leukemia is thrombocytopenia. Platelet production is reduced by malignant cells in the marrow at presentation, and is eliminated entirely for 10 days or so by myelotoxic induction therapy. Randomized prospective studies confirm the safety of using 10,000 platelets/μL as a threshold for prophylactic platelet transfusion for patients with acute myeloid leukemia (AML) (but not acute promyelocytic leukemia [APL]). Thrombocytopenic bleeding occurs in about 20 percent of patients during induction therapy, regardless of the transfusion trigger used for prophylactic treatment; additional platelet transfusions should be given for overt bleeding episodes, aiming to raise the platelet count to >50,000/μL.

Although overshadowed by thrombocytopenia, patients with acute myeloid leukemia have intrinsic PFD that may contribute to bleeding. Chemotherapeutic agents, antibiotics, or circulating fibrin degradation products (FDP) can contribute to platelet dysfunction and failure of hemostatic plug formation.

Defibrination Syndrome and Disseminated Intravascular Coagulation

Patients with APL commonly present with severe bleeding and signs of defibrination in addition to thrombocytopenia on laboratory testing (Fig. 33-1). While a similar coagulopathy may occur in other leukemic subsets (especially monocytoid) either at presentation or during treatment, the marked bleeding diathesis and the molecular biology of APL have stimulated research into potential mechanisms for the syndrome. Abnormally high levels of expression of annexin II can be demonstrated on APL cells. This phospholipid-binding protein supports and accelerates t-PA-dependent cleavage of plasminogen to plasmin. APL cells with high concentrations of annexin II support an overproduction of plasmin, which in turn cleaves both fibrinogen and fibrin. Low levels of plasma plasminogen, α_2-plasmin inhibitor, low plasminogen activator inhibitor 1 (PAI-1), and fibrinogen are found in these patients.

The malignant progranulocytes in patients with APL contain tissue factor, which promotes the formation of thrombin via the extrinsic pathway of coagulation. One report has suggested that leukemic cells activate factor X directly via a cysteine proteinase that is analogous to the procoagulant activity described in various solid tumors. Finally, malignant cells can produce large amounts of interleukin-1, a cytokine that stimulates the synthesis and expression of tissue factor by endothelial cells and monocytes. DIC often dramatically worsens following cytoreductive chemotherapy. The process is most likely due to the lysis of leukemic cells and release of preformed tissue factor and other procoagulants into the circulation. In

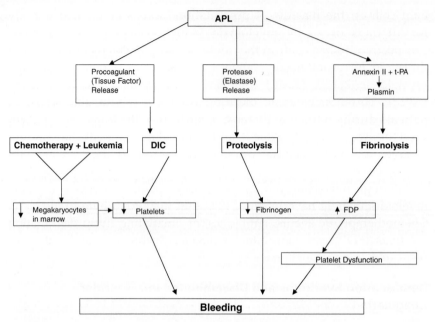

FIGURE 33-1 The coagulopathy in patients with myeloid leukemia, particularly APL, is often complex and consists of classic DIC, systemic fibrinolysis, or hemostatic and vascular defects produced by proteolytic enzymes. (Used with permission from Barbui T, et al: *Blood* 91:3093, 1998.)

contrast, retinoic acid promotes differentiation of malignant promyelocytes to more mature forms with subsequent resolution of the DIC.

Several studies have recently suggested that proteases other than thrombin or plasmin are produced by myeloid cells in patients with acute leukemia. One proteolytic enzyme, elastase, has been identified in leukemia cell cultures. Elastase has a broad spectrum of proteolytic activity and degrades fibrinogen to large and small fibrinogen degradation products. It is not yet clear whether these proteases are responsible for bleeding in patients with acute leukemia.

Recently, the use of all-trans-retinoic acid (ATRA) to promote terminal differentiation of leukemic promyelocytes has raised the complete remission rate to >90%, along with prompt improvement in the coagulopathy associated with the disease. ATRA has been shown to decrease the cellular expression of procoagulants such as tissue factor and cysteine proteinase, an effect that parallels the improvement in fibrinogen concentrations and the fall in D-dimer and thrombin–antithrombin complexes (Fig. 33-2). Fibrinolytic activity and elastase expression do not appear to be altered in APL cells. Cytokine production is increased after ATRA treatment, however, which could be implicated in the thrombotic complications that can accompany the retinoic acid syndrome.

Clinical Findings/Laboratory Tests

Bleeding occurs from diverse sites in patients with acute leukemia, including the skin, mucous membranes, and gastrointestinal tract. However, central nervous system (CNS) hemorrhage is particularly common (and often fatal) in patients with APL. Risk factors for this feared complication include age over 50 years, large numbers of circulating blasts or promyelocytes, severe anemia, and marked thrombocytopenia. The risk of bleeding has been moderately reduced, but not eliminated, in patients with APL following the introduction of ATRA.

When first seen, patients with all forms of myeloid leukemia (not just APL) should have a baseline set of laboratory tests (Table 33-1). In patients with severe coagulopathies, the battery of tests should be repeated at least daily and particularly just before and following chemotherapy, or when the clinical situation changes abruptly (e.g., with sepsis).

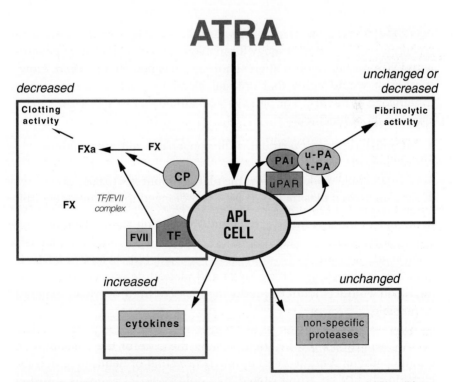

FIGURE 33-2 The effect of all-trans-retinoic acid (ATRA) on the pathways of APL cell interactions with the hemostatic system. TF, tissue factor; CP, cysteine proteinase; PAI, plasminogen activator inhibitor; u-PA and t-PA, urokinase-type or tissue-type plasminogen activator; u-PAR, urokinase-type plasminogen activator receptor. (Used with permission from Barbui T, et al: *Blood* 91:3093, 1998.)

TABLE 33-1	
Baseline Laboratory Tests in Patients with Acute Leukemia	
Tests	**Uses**
PT, APTT, fibrinogen	Reflect severity of the coagulopathy
Platelet count	Bleeding time is not necessary
D-dimer	Measure of secondary fibrinolysis
Euglobulin lysis time	Measure of systemic fibrinolysis
α_2-Antiplasmin	Reflects the intensity of fibrinolysis

If only mild DIC is present, fibrinogen concentrations are usually normal, FDP are only minimally elevated, and the APTT is often short. Occasionally, florid DIC will ensue after chemotherapy, leading to hypofibrinogenemia, prolongation of the PT and APTT, and lowering of antithrombin (AT) and protein C levels. If systemic fibrinolysis is present (common in APL), fibrinogen levels may be very low with normal or only mildly reduced levels of circulating AT or protein C.

Management

A consensus on the best strategy for managing myeloid leukemia patients with DIC or other defibrination syndromes has not been reached. However, most would agree that optimal blood product replacement is a cornerstone of therapy. For patients who are not actively bleeding, management should include:

- Administering cryoprecipitate if fibrinogen concentrations fall to <100 mg/dL.
- Giving platelet concentrates if the platelet count is <10,000/µL.
- Infusing frozen plasma if the APTT is prolonged to >1.5 times control.

Replacement therapy for patients who are bleeding should be more vigorous, with goals of keeping the fibrinogen >125 mg/dL, platelets >50,000/µL, and the APTT more nearly normal. However, if the DIC is quite brisk, correcting clotting factor and platelet defects by administering blood products without producing massive fluid overload may not be possible.

When rapid destruction of fibrinogen and platelets is present, intravenous heparin should be used to slow the pace of the consumption coagulopathy and allow more optimal correction of hemostatic defects. Heparin should be administered by continuous intravenous infusion beginning with a dose of approximately 500 U/h (e.g., 7 U/kg body weight) with a goal of using the lowest dose possible to control DIC and allow effective blood product replacement. When DIC is severe, monitoring heparin therapy is often a problem, particularly if the APTT is markedly prolonged. An anti-Xa inhibition assay (heparin assay) can be used, and although optimal heparin levels for treatment of DIC have not been determined, giving sufficient heparin to maintain the plasma anti-Xa activity from 0.1 to 0.3 U/mL is a reasonable starting point.

In a few patients, bleeding may persist despite optimal heparin therapy and clotting factor replacement. If the ELT is short and α_2-AP levels are markedly reduced (e.g., <30 percent), then consideration should be given to the use of an antifibrinolytic agent such as ε-aminocaproic acid (EACA) or tranexamic acid (TA) in conjunction with heparin and blood products. Although an intriguing possibility, it is not known whether aprotinin, an antifibrinolytic agent with a wider spectrum of antiproteolytic activity, might be more effective than EACA and TA (see Chap. 58).

CHRONIC MYELOID DISORDERS: MYELODYSPLASIA AND MYELOPROLIFERATIVE DISEASE

Myelodysplasia

Bleeding in patients with myelodysplasia is almost always due to thrombocytopenia or intrinsic platelet dysfunction. Platelets often appear abnormal on light and electron microscopy, with variations in shape, size, and granulation. A wide spectrum of PFD has been described including abnormalities in platelet aggregation, the release reaction, and thromboxane synthesis. Some patients, including one child with a major defect in glycoprotein Ib, have defective platelet adhesion. Thrombocytopenia or platelet dysfunction occasionally precedes diagnostic changes in myeloid cells and can provide a clue to the correct diagnosis.

Patients with myelodysplasia who have PFD and bleeding may require transfusion of platelets. DDAVP is sometimes useful, although advanced atherosclerosis could increase the risks of thrombosis in older patients. Antifibrinolytic therapy with EACA or TA is an option for suppression of local fibrinolysis in subjects with refractory oral, nasopharyngeal, or gastrointestinal bleeding.

Chronic Myeloproliferative Disease (Essential Thrombocythemia, Polycythemia Rubra Vera, Myelofibrosis with Myeloid Metaplasia)

Patients with MPD have an increased risk of bleeding due to platelet function defects despite thrombocytosis, or they may develop venous or arterial thrombosis (see Chap. 44). Excessive bleeding has been reported in approximately 15 percent of patients with MPD, most often in patients with myelofibrosis with myeloid metaplasia and essential thrombocythemia. Bleeding is uncommon in patients with chronic granulocytic leukemia during the chronic phase of the disease.

Distorted platelet morphology is commonly observed both on light and electron microscopy. Platelets often appear large, with strange shapes and bizarre granulation (Fig. 33-3). A variety of PFD have been reported, as listed in Table 33-2. Notably, the platelet count, PFD, and the bleeding time often do not correlate with excessive bleeding. It may be safe to withhold treatment and observe younger patients with elevated platelet counts (see Ruggeri ref).

The management of bleeding in patients with uncontrolled MPD and thrombocytosis involves normalization of the platelet count (see Chap. 44). This may require acute lowering of the platelet count by plateletpheresis, followed by chronic suppression of megakaryocytopoiesis with hydroxyurea or anagrelide. If bleeding persists, transfusion of platelets may be necessary. In the rare patient with acquired von Willebrand disease (see Chap. 12), von Willebrand factor concentrates or DDAVP should be considered. Fibrinolytic inhibitors should be used with caution in patients with MPD for fear of producing or potentiating thrombosis.

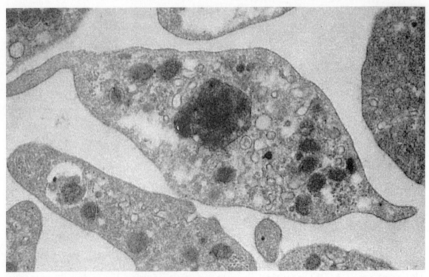

FIGURE 33-3 Giant-size fused granules in a patient with myelofibrosis. (Used with permission from Ramen BKS et al: *Am J Clin Pathol* 91:647, 1989.)

TABLE 33-2
Platelet Function Defects Reported in Patients with Myeloproliferative Disease

Aggregation defects: epinephrine, adenosine diphosphate, collagen
Acquired storage pool disease
Membrane defects
  ■ Glycoprotein IIb/IIIa
  ■ Increased Fc receptor
  ■ Decreased prostaglandin D_2 receptor
  ■ Decreased thromboxane A_2 receptor
  ■ Decreased α-adrenergic receptors
Prostanoid abnormalities
  ■ Decreased thromboxane A_2
  ■ Decreased lipoxygenase
Acquired von Willebrand disease

BIBLIOGRAPHY

Barbui T et al: The impact of all-trans-retinoic acid on the coagulopathy of acute promyelocytic leukemia. *Blood* 91:3093, 1998.

Berndt MC et al: An acquired Bernard-Soulier-like platelet defect associated with juvenile myelodysplastic syndrome. *Br J Haematol* 68:97, 1988.

DeLoughery TG, Goodnight SH: Acute promyelocytic leukemia in the all trans retinoic acid era. *Med Onc* 13:233, 1996.

DeLoughery TG, Goodnight SH: Bleeding and thrombosis in hematologic neoplasia. In: *Neoplastic Diseases of the Blood*, 3rd ed., Wiernik PH, Canellos GP, Dutcher JP, Kyle RA (eds), New York, Churchill Livingstone, 1996, pp 1177–1192.

Feinstein DI: Treatment of disseminated intravascular coagulation. *Semin Thromb Hemost* 14:351, 1988.

Fenaux P et al: Clinical course of essential thrombocythemia in 147 cases. *Cancer* 66:549, 1990.

Landolfi R: Bleeding and thrombosis in myeloproliferative disorders. *Curr Opin Hematol* 5:327, 1998.

Lopez-Pedrera C et al: Tissue factor and urokinase plasminogen activator receptor (uPAR) and bleeding complications in leukemic patients. *Thromb Haemost* 77:62, 1997.

Menell JS et al: Annexin II and bleeding in acute promyelocytic leukemia. *N Engl J Med* 340:994, 1999.

Ramen BKS et al: Platelet function and structure in myeloproliferative disease, myelodysplastic syndrome, and secondary thrombocytosis. *Am J Clin Pathol* 91:647, 1989.

Ravandi-Kashani F, Schafer AI: Microvascular disturbances, thrombosis, and bleeding in thrombocythemia: current concepts and perspectives. *Semin Thromb Hemost* 23:479, 1997.

Rebulla P et al: The threshold for prophylactic platelet transfusions in adults with acute myeloid leukemia. *N Engl J Med* 337:1870, 1997.

Ruggeri M et al: No treatment for low-risk thrombocythaemia: results from a prospective study. *Br J Haematol* 103:772, 1998.

Schwartz BS et al: Epsilon-aminocaproic acid in the treatment of patients with acute promyelocytic leukemia and acquired alpha-2-plasmin inhibitor deficiency. *Ann Intern Med* 105:873, 1986.

Ventura GJ et al: Analysis of risk factors for fatal hemorrhage during induction therapy of patients with acute promyelocytic leukemia. *Hemat Pathol* 3:23, 1989.

Thrombotic Disorders

CHAPTER 34

The Infant
and Child
with Thrombosis

Thrombotic disorders (deep vein thrombosis [DVT], venous thromboembolic disease, arterial thrombosis) are important causes of morbidity in infants and children. Although the overall prevalence and predisposing conditions are different from those in adults, the principles of diagnosis and therapy, with a few exceptions, are similar in the pediatric age group. This chapter emphasizes the differences and presents management guidelines.

Developmental influences are significant in the infant and child and affect use of antithrombotic therapies. The neonate and young infant are particularly prone to thrombosis. Thrombophilic genes and acquired coagulopathies are present in most older infants and children who develop thrombosis, even though the presentation is usually in the context of other underlying medical disorders or trigger factors. Current concepts of thrombosis in infancy, childhood, and adolescence hold that thrombosis in the pediatric population is rarely, if ever, truly idiopathic, (i.e., without any provoking or predisposing factors).

NEONATAL THROMBOTIC DISEASE

Thrombosis in the neonate is characterized by an increased incidence in premature and other high-risk infants, a predilection for major vessels, frequent involvement of the arterial circulation, and relationship to indwelling catheters (umbilical artery catheter [UAC], umbilical venous catheter [UVC]). Unprovoked thromboses do occur and most frequently involve the inferior vena cava; renal veins and cerebral venous sinuses; the aortic, renal, and femoral arteries, as well as the middle cerebral artery.

PATHOPHYSIOLOGY OF NEONATAL THROMBOSIS

The fetus and newborn are more susceptible to thrombosis because their blood exhibits a deficiency of thrombin inhibition and relatively deficient fibrinolysis (see Chap. 3 for details). Cord plasma shows a decreased thrombin generation related to decreased levels of vitamin K-dependent proteins. However, cord whole blood clots with a shorter reaction time and larger clot formation than seen in adults. Except for a brief brisk increase in tissue plasminogen activator (t-PA) at the time of delivery, neonatal plasma contains decreased t-PA, as well as low and altered plasminogen with near normal levels of α_2-antiplasmin (α_2-AP) and plasminogen activator inhibitor (PAI). Therefore, overall fibrinolysis is decreased, except for cord blood where the euglobulin clot lysis time (ELT) is shorter than in the adult, probably due to delayed inactivation of fetal plasmin by fetal α_2-AP. The infant is protected from thrombosis by physiologic depression of factors II, VII, IX, and X, but the balance favors thrombin formation over inhibition, especially in the sick infant. Sick preterm infants with respiratory distress syndrome display a severe plasminogen and AT deficiency that predict a poor outcome. In addition, a large proportion of sick preterm infants exhibit extremely low plasma levels of PC (<0.1 U/mL), so that it is remarkable that spontaneous thrombosis is relatively rare.

Clinically apparent thromboses are usually precipitated by extreme low flow states, severe acidosis, vascular occlusion, and/or damage by catheters. Other acquired risk factors associated with increased thrombosis include infection, hypotension, hypoxia, maternal diabetes mellitus, polycythemia, other causes of disseminated intravascular coagulation (DIC), and, of course, the indwelling catheter.

Diagnosis of Thrombosis in the Neonate

The diagnosis of neonatal thrombosis is suspected based upon clinical observations and confirmed by appropriate imaging studies. Thrombosis often occurs prior to or during labor and delivery. Clinical signs are usually present at delivery or within 24 hours of birth. Observation of a white, pulseless limb at birth suggests a recent occlusion, whereas a black, necrotic extremity reflects a more distant event. Physical inspection may reveal the indentations of circatricial amniotic bands as an occlusive cause. Other thromboses should be excluded with imaging of the head and abdominal vessels. Occasionally combined thromboses of the central nervous system (CNS) have been observed with peripheral arterial thrombosis. Enlarged kidneys secondary to renal vein thrombosis (RVT) may be appreciated in the delivery room or within 24 hours of birth. Term neonates with stroke most often present with seizures within the first 24 hours of life. The middle cerebral artery is most commonly affected. A rapid, efficient evaluation and institution of aggressive therapy may save limbs or organs.

The most common large-vessel thromboses are RVT and aortic thrombosis. RVT often presents in a term or large preterm infant with hematuria, hypertension and a flank mass; hemolytic anemia, thrombocytopenia, and mild DIC may also be present. Massive aortic thrombosis often presents in preterm asphyxiated infants with a UAC in place. Associated symptoms include pallor of lower extremities, poor femoral pulses, upper extremity hypertension or systemic shock, persistent pulmonary hypertension, and evidence for DIC (low platelets and fibrinogen, elevated PT, fibrin-fibrinogen degradation products, and D-dimer).

Non-invasive imaging with high-resolution, pulsed and color flow Doppler ultrasound techniques is the preferred approach for most cases. Magnetic resonance imaging (MRI) with diffusion and flair imaging is the most sensitive study for CNS events because it best detects cerebral infarction (diffusion), as well as early intracranial hemorrhage (flair) that will affect therapeutic decisions. Computerized tomography (CT) is still commonly used to detect and differentiate hemorrhage from CNS thromboses in the neonate. Contrast angiography may be necessary to define the upper venous tree after repeated or prolonged use of central venous access devices, but angiography is contraindicated in infants with renal failure or gut ischemia.

Laboratory Tests in Neonates with Thrombosis

Subtle evidence for activation of coagulation and fibrinolysis is so common in the sick newborn that more sensitive laboratory markers of activation (thrombin–antithrombin, plasmin–antiplasmin, etc.) have not been helpful thus far. Screening coagulation tests with APTT, PT, TCT, fibrinogen, and platelet count are important. A quantitative D-dimer assay may be helpful, as concentrations >500 ng/mL are associated with DIC. The APTT may be prolonged physiologically, especially in the preterm. A long initial value precludes its usefulness as an indicator of heparin effect, should anticoagulation be needed. A neonate with evidence of DIC and thrombosis may show improvement in coagulation tests during heparin therapy due to interruption of coagulation protein and platelet consumption. However, it is important to maintain minimal hemostatic levels during anticoagulant or thrombolytic therapy to prevent bleeding (see Chap. 7).

Severe acquired and/or genetic deficiencies of anticoagulant and/or fibrinolytic proteins may manifest with thrombosis in the neonate and may require replacement therapy for optimal management. The probability of genetic thrombophilia in a neonate with thrombosis is currently under investigation. The occurrence of homozygous, compound heterozygous, and multiple heterozygous thrombophilic traits has been observed in neonates with large vessel thrombosis, purpura fulminans, and/or stroke. Rarely, a maternal lupus anticoagulant (LA) or anticardiolipin antibody (ACA) has resulted in severe perinatal thrombosis from placental transfer to the fetus; testing the mother is helpful to evaluate this possibility.

All neonates with extensive or large vessel thrombosis should be evaluated during the acute event with a panel including AT, PC, free protein S (PS), factor V Leiden, homocysteine, and possibly the prothrombin 20210 mutation and lipoprotein (a) [Lp(a)]. The diagnostic plasma concentration of many coagulation proteins for the adult heterozygote frequently overlaps with the physiologic range of that factor in the newborn period and, therefore, it is difficult to make a causal association of the plasma concentration with thrombotic tendency. Known heterozygotes in the newborn period have levels in or only slightly lower than normal newborn range. Family studies (an affected parent) and follow-up tests are usually necessary to confirm the diagnosis. When abnormal results are determined during an acute thrombotic event, they must be confirmed 3 to 6 months later to exclude consumption due to the acute event and/or physiologic changes. The recent literature emphasizes that the neonatal presentation of genetic thrombophilia is often found in infants carrying two, or even three, distinct thrombophilic mutations.

Treatment of Neonatal Thrombosis

Heparin anticoagulation. Although there are no controlled trials of anticoagulant therapy for neonatal thrombotic lesions, the administration of unfractionated heparin (UH) has been associated with resolution of the vascular occlusion in most instances. Neonatologists and others caring for sick infants are sometimes reluctant to use heparin in clinical situations comparable to when it is used in adults because of the difficulty in monitoring the effect and fear of aggravating intracranial hemorrhage (ICH). Guidelines based on our experience with heparin are shown in Table 34-1.

Newborns show a relative resistance to heparin; however, heparinization can be achieved despite low AT levels. The half-life of heparin is 25 min after intravenous doses of 100 U/kg in term neonates, as compared with 65 min in adults. The APTT is less satisfactory for monitoring because it is already considerably prolonged in sick preterm infants. The direct assay of heparin (heparin anti-Xa level) should be used. The neonate frequently shows resistance to the anticoagulant effects of UH when given in continuous infusions of up to 50 U/kg/hr. The administration of 100 to 200 U/kg of AT concentrate (given as one 500 U vial) will increase heparin sensitivity to unfractionated or low molecular weight heparin, even in babies with near-physiologic baseline levels of AT. The

TABLE 34-1

Anticoagulant Therapy of Neonatal and Pediatric Thrombosis Using Unfractionated and Low Molecular Weight Heparins.

DOSING OF UNFRACTIONATED HEPARIN SODIUM
Unfractionated heparin initial dosage:

Developmental age	Bolus U/kg	Initial infusion U/kg/h
Preterm (<28 weeks):	50	15
Preterm (28–36 weeks):	50	20
Full Term (≥37 weeks):	100	25
Children (>4 weeks):	50	20

Unfractionated dose adjustment:

Heparin assay U/mL	APTT/baseline APTT ratio	Dose adjustment U/kg/h
0.0–0.14	1.00–1.24	Rebolus, increase by 10
0.15–0.29	1.25–1.49	No rebolus, increase by 5
0.30–0.70	1.50–2.49	Continue dose
0.71–0.85	2.50–2.99	Decrease dose by 5
>0.85	≥3.0	Hold for 1 hour, recheck level and restart infusion at decrease of 10

DOSING OF LOW MOLECULAR WEIGHT HEPARIN
Low Molecular Weight Heparin Initial Dosage:

Developmental age	Initial dosage: mg/kg or U/kg (Given subcutaneous every 12 h)	
	Enoxaparin (Lovenox) (mg/kg)	Dalteparin (Fragmin) (U/kg)
Preterm (<28 weeks):	1.0	100
Preterm (28–36 weeks):	1.5	150
Full Term (≥37 weeks):	2.0	200
Children (4 weeks–6 months):	1.2	120
Children (>6 months):	1.0	100

(Continued on next page)

TABLE 34-1 CONTINUED

Anticoagulant Therapy of Neonatal and Pediatric Thrombosis Using Unfractionated and Low Molecular Weight Heparins.

LMWH dose adjustment (U/ml):

Anti-Xa heparin assay	Dose adjustment
0.00–0.24	Increase by 50%
0.25–0.49	Increase by 25%
0.50–1.20	Continue dose
1.21–1.50	Decrease dose by 25%; recheck level two doses later
>1.50	Hold next dose; then decrease dose by 50%; recheck level two doses later.

Specific heparin dosage must be determined by monitoring of anticoagulant effect achieved. These recommendations are general.

- Unfractionated heparin is inhibitory to factors Xa and thrombin. The target therapeutic range using unfractionated heparin is 0.3 to 0.7 U/mL. All therapeutic courses of unfractionated heparin should be initiated by a loading bolus dose. Steady-state levels can be determined after 4 to 6 hours of continuous infusion. Unfractionated heparin should be assayed every 4 to 6 hours until a therapeutic level is achieved and then once a day if there is no reason to suspect a change.
- The APTT ratio shown related to these heparin levels is approximate. Use of the APTT is useful in the neonate only if the baseline value is ≤120% of the adult upper limit of normal. The APTT should not be used in children if the baseline is not within the normal range. The APTT sensitivity to heparin is ideally determined in each laboratory using pooled umbilical cord and adult plasmas. These ratios may not be relevant in other labs. Some neonates require as much as 50 U/kg/hr of UH to maintain a therapeutic plasma level early in the course of treatment.
- Low molecular weight heparins are inhibitory to factor Xa but not thrombin. Therefore, the target anti-Xa level required is higher, 0.5 to 1.2 U/mL. Low molecular weight heparins should be therapeutic 3 to 4 hours after a subQ injection. Anti-Xa assay should be obtained after the second dose of low molecular weight heparin and repeated after each dose until the therapeutic range is achieved. Then the level should be determined after every 2 to 4 doses for the first week of therapy, once a week for a month, then monthly if stable.
- Dose requirements for infants up to 1 year are likely to be intermediate between term newborn and child doses. Currently there is little *ex vivo* data; these recommendations are preliminary and should be adjusted based on level.

infusions of AT may be repeated every 24 to 48 hours and used to maintain therapeutic heparin levels. Low molecular weight heparins (LMWH) are being used in newborn infants with good preliminary results, however, no controlled studies indicating the superiority of LMWH or UH are available. To date it appears that the dose-response of LMWH in the newborn infant may be more predictable owing to less heparin resistance to the product. In addition, LMWH may be administered twice a day subcutaneously and does not require maintenance of a venous line. Initial dosing, dose adjustments, and monitoring are shown on Table 34-1.

Thrombolytic therapy.   Thrombolytic therapy (see Table 34-2) is reserved for recent thrombotic lesions that compromise arterial perfusion (i.e., such as aortic thrombosis or massive RVT) or have occurred in vital areas (intracardiac thrombosis). The most critical complication of thrombolysis is intracranial hemorrhage. A cranial ultrasound to exclude preexisting intracranial hemorrhage is necessary prior to initiating thrombolytic therapy in the neonate. In addition, any abnormal neurologic sign suggestive of stroke or history of profound hypoxia should be fully evaluated, as cranial infarction or hemorrhage within 10 days is a contraindication to thrombolysis. As noted above, the newborn infant has a decreased fibrinolytic response but is able to resolve most clots during heparin therapy alone. The infant is also relatively resistant to urokinase specifically (as opposed to tissue plasminogen activator [t-PA]) and may require two to ten times the dose of urokinase used in adults to achieve thrombolysis. Supplementation of plasminogen (fresh frozen plasma) during fibrinolytic therapy is helpful. Currently, urokinase is not available for clinical use and recombinant tissue plasminogen activator (rt-PA) is being used more frequently. Although rt-PA is effective in newborn infants and children, bleeding complications do occur. Data is being accrued showing that the original dosing of rt-PA in neonates ranging from 0.1 to 0.5 mg/kg/h may be too high. Hopefully, data regarding optimal dosing of rt-PA will soon be available.

Neonates generally do not manifest thrombus recurrence after initial therapy. Therefore, long-term anticoagulation is seldom needed. Infants with severe or multiple thrombophilic traits are the exception and may require life-long anticoagulation beginning in infancy.

Catheter-related Thrombotic Disease

The mechanisms of catheter-related thrombosis include small vascular caliber in relationship to catheter diameter, obstructions of blood flow, low flow, endothelial trauma, and systemic hypercoagulability. Although many serious late complications of UACs and UVCs have been reported, including renal hypertension, aortic thromboatheromata, false aortic aneurysm, paraplegia, endocarditis, organ infarction, and death, these severe sequellae are relatively rare. Heparin "flush" or continuous infusions of low-dose (1 to 2 U/mL) heparin prolong catheter patency safely, but do not appear to be effective in preventing thrombotic lesions. Our impression is that asymptomatic thrombosis related to UACs has been decreased to <5 percent of catheterizations by avoiding repeated attempts at catheter placement; using heparin-bonded catheters; and removing the catheter at the first sign of decreased pulses, "vasospasm," extremity color changes, decreased perfusion, or darkening of the toes ("catheter toes"). If these signs persist despite catheter removal, assume that a thrombus is present, document with ultrasound examination, and treat appropriately with anticoagulation. Other vascular complications may be related to the type of infusate; peripheral gangrene has followed infu-

---

TABLE 34-2

Thrombolytic Therapy of Neonatal and Pediatric Thrombosis Using Recombinant Tissue Plasminogen Activator (rt-PA)

Systemic rt-PA	Local (Site-Directed) rt-PA
Initial Dose:	
0.3 mg/kg/h to a maximum total dose of 3 mg/h without a loading dose	0.03 mg/kg/h up to a maximum total of 0.5 mg/hr total dose for child <30 kg; 1.0 mg/hr total dose for child ≥30 kg;
No concomitant infusion of heparin	Use of concomitant heparin infusion is controversial; heparin, if used, should be 5–10 U/kg/h.
Duration:	
6 to 48 h	6 to 48 h
Dose increase if no effect seen:	
None	May double dose once
Treatment adjuncts:	
Plasminogen may be given in FFP 10 mL/kg if there is poor thrombolysis	

Recommendations for either route of delivery of rt-PA:

Monitoring:
Imaging of thrombus at least q12h (q6h is optimal).

When thrombolysis is documented on imaging study and blood flow is restored, rt-PAinfusions (systemic or local) should be stopped; after one half hour, heparin therapy should commence as described in Table 34-1.

Fibrinogen, TCT, FSP, platelet count. Plasminogen prior to therapy and daily.

Hemostatic levels of fibrinogen (≥100 mg/dL) and platelets (≥50,000/μL) should be maintained transfusing with cryoprecipitate (10 mL/kg) for fibrinogen and/or single-donor platelet concentrates (10 mL/kg) as needed.

If child develops bleeding signs (oozing, hematuria, melena), the rt-PA infusion may be stopped for ½ to 1 h while pressure is applied; the infusion may then be restarted at 0.1 mg/kg/h up to a maximum of 1 mg/h.

Specific rt-PA dosage has not been determined for infants and children. These provisional dosages were proposed by a consensus committee of pediatric interventional radiologists at the Pediatric Thrombolysis Study Group Meeting at the Radiologic Society of North America, Chicago, IL, November 29, 1999.

sion of dopamine. The use of UVC is associated with a 15 percent rate of venous thrombosis, most frequently in the portal vein; these thromboses are usually asymptomatic.

CHILDHOOD THROMBOTIC DISEASE

The incidence of thrombosis in children is about 1 per 100,000 children per year as compared to 1 percent per year in adults. By 6 months of age the infant coagulation system approximates that of the adult, and the developmental deficiencies noted above are no longer present, except for PC, which may not reach the normal adult range until adolescence.

Childhood thrombotic disease is truly multifactorial in etiology; even though thrombophilic defects are prominent, the disorder usually presents in children with underlying medical conditions (Table 34-3). A spontaneous thrombosis in an otherwise healthy child is suggestive of a hereditary deficiency or an antiphospholipid antibody syndrome. Truly idiopathic thrombosis is found in <10 percent of children with DVT, but approximately one-third of children with stroke. During adolescence, additional risk factors, such as athletic-related muscle and joint injury, use of oral contraceptive agents, pregnancy, and smoking add to the predisposition for thrombosis. These risk factors are associated with clinical presentation of hereditary thrombotic disorders in many instances (such as factor V Leiden; prothrombin 20210 mutations; or deficiencies of AT, PC, or PS). Recent data indicates that thrombosis during intensive medical therapy (e.g., for acute leukemia) presents disproportionately in children with underlying thrombophilia; this suggests that coagulation screening may identify children at high risk of thrombosis and may direct efforts at prophylactic anticoagulation in targeted groups of children. The diagnosis and initial management of thrombotic disease in children and adolescents is essentially the same as for adults (see Chap. 36). Children and adolescents who present with thrombosis should be tested for AT, PC, and PS at initial presentation. Severe deficiencies of these proteins, whether genetic or acquired, may require replacement therapy with factor concentrates or fresh frozen plasma for optimal outcome.

Management of Children with Thrombosis

Recommendations for antithrombotic therapy for children are found in Tables 34-1 and 34-2. Children with severe DVT of the lower extremities and those patients with thoracic outlet syndrome, or arterial or pulmonary artery lesions, are candidates for a short course of fibrinolytic therapy to prevent acute infarction or long-term venous valvular damage. Thrombolytic therapy using urokinase infusions (usually 6 to 72 hours) has been given with a continuous infusion of low-dose heparin (10 U/kg/h without a bolus). Currently rt-PA infusions are often limited to 4 to 6 h, and the use of concomitant heparin infusions is controversial. At the end of the thrombolytic infusion, heparin anticoagulant therapy in doses adequate to achieve therapeutic plasma concentrations are given for at least 5 days.

Anticoagulant therapy alone is also adequate for most arterial and venous thromboses in children. Heparin-associated thrombocytopenia and thrombosis is rare in children, but does occur. A plasma sample should be sent to exclude heparin antibodies if the platelet count falls >20 percent on heparin therapy or clinical signs of thrombosis are not

---

TABLE 34-3

Disorders Associated with Deep Venous Thrombosis in Children

Indwelling catheter
Malignancy (especially associated with L-asparaginase therapy)
Congenital heart disease
Infection
After major surgery or trauma
Dehydration
Lupus anticoagulant
Liver disease
Nephrotic syndrome
Inflammatory bowel syndrome
Chronic renal disease
Sickle cell disease
Thalassemia
After prothrombin-complex concentration infusion
Malnutrition
Stroke

---

improving. Heparin is administered for at least 5 to 7 days. Warfarin therapy is begun after 1 to 2 days of heparin therapy, in a single oral dose of 0.2 mg/kg. Ultimate warfarin requirements are age-dependent, with infants requiring an average of 0.3 mg/kg/day to adolescents requiring and average of 0.1 mg/kg/day. Heparin and warfarin are overlapped for 4 to 5 days; when the INR is greater than 2 for two consecutive days, then the heparin is stopped. Any recurrence of thrombotic symptoms temporally associated with warfarin therapy should suggest deficiencies of PC or PS and should be evaluated promptly.

The optimal duration of oral anticoagulation in children is unknown. If the clot is completely resolved on imaging study and the provoking or predisposing factors are resolved, then 3 months may be adequate. All children with residual vascular obstruction should receive oral anticoagulation for at least 6 months. Children with lupus anticoagulants and severe or multiple genetic thrombophilic traits require oral anticoagulation for an indefinite time to prevent recurrence. Children with mechanical prosthetic heart valves are given oral anticoagulation to prolong the INR to 2.5 to 3.5.

PERFORMANCE OF COAGULATION TESTING FOR HEREDITARY DEFECTS

Thromboses due to hereditary deficiencies of coagulation proteins uncommonly present in the infant and child. The late second and third decades of life are the usual time for diagnosis. Nevertheless, heterozygotes for factor V Leiden, AT, PC, PS, plasminogen defects, dysfibrino-genemias, and homocysteinuria have been recognized at all ages, including the newborn infant. Additional mutations, including prothrombin 20210 and methyl tetrahydrofolate reductase C677T (MTHFR), as well as elevations in Lp(a) have been described in pediatric thromboses. Because of the multifactorial aspect of childhood thromboses, children with thrombosis should be tested for all of these traits at the time of presentation (see Table 34-4, level 1 evaluation).

In addition, antiphospholipid antibodies, including LA and ACA, cause thromboses in children. The LA is primarily associated with DVT and PE. It is found in children with malignancy, infection, systemic lupus erythematosus (SLE), and other collagen vascular disorders, as well as the primary antiphospholipid antibody syndrome. The ACA is found in up to one-third of children with stroke. It is less often associated with DVT, PE, or other thromboses. The frequency of genetic thrombophilic traits, including factor V Leiden and the prothrombin 20210 mutation, are also increased in children with stroke. Acquired resistance to activated protein C may result from an antiphospholipid antibody and may be detected on a functional assay. Finally, it is necessary to measure a plasma

---

TABLE 34-4

Laboratory Evaluation of Thrombophilia in the Infant, Child, and Adolescent

Level I Evaluation

Antithrombin
Protein C
Free protein S
Activated protein C resistance
Factor V Leiden mutation
Prothrombin 20210 mutation
Homocysteine
Lp(a)
Lupus anticoagulant (in mother for neonatal thrombosis)
Anticardiolipin antibody (in mother for neonatal thrombosis)

Level II Evaluation

Heparin cofactor II
Thrombomodulin
Tissue factor pathway inhibitor
Plasminogen
PAI-I
TPA
VWF multimers
Platelet aggregations (spontaneous and to low molar agonists)
Viscosity

homocysteine level to detect acquired abnormalities secondary to malabsorption or dietary deficiencies of vitamins B_6, B_{12}, or folate. Unusual abnormalities in procoagulant, anticoagulant, and fibrinolytic proteins, as well as in platelet function, have rarely been described in children with thrombosis. These defects should be investigated in children with unexplained or recurrent thrombosis or a strongly positive family history (level II evaluation, Table 34-4).

PURPURA FULMINANS

Purpura fulminans is the sudden onset of massive microthrombosis and bleeding in the skin associated with skin necrosis and ischemia, systemic DIC, and anemia. It usually occurs in children, but can also be seen in adults. Purpura fulminans is almost always associated with an extreme genetic and/or acquired deficiency of PC or PS. Associated causes for the often rapidly progressing lesions include PC consumption with infection (meningococcemia, group B streptococcal disease, and sepsis secondary to other pathogens), accelerated PS clearance with autoantibodies (varicella), homozygous or compound heterozygous genetic PC or PS deficiency, warfarin-induced skin necrosis in PC and PS-deficient heterozygotes, or (rarely) no known cause. Treatment of this disorder should include assessment of functional PC and PS levels and replacement of the appropriate factors (fresh frozen plasma or concentrate). The use of heparin is controversial. In clinical trials, it has not been possible to prove that heparinization in the setting of purpura fulminans secondary to bacterial sepsis results in greater limb salvage, but persistant DIC and large-vessel thrombosis are indications for heparin therapy. Purpura fulminans with varicella and autoimmune PS deficiency may respond to IVIG. Purpura fulminans in the neonate is secondary to PC or PS deficiency (hereditary or severe acquired) until proven otherwise. Untreated, the lesions result in loss of limb or life. Long-term treatment requires warfarin to keep the INR between 2.5 and 3.5; concentrates (PC deficiency) and plasma (PS deficiency) are given for "break-through" purpura and/or thrombosis.

BIBLIOGRAPHY

Andrew M et al: Arterial thromboembolic complications in paediatric patients. *Thromb Haemost* 78:715, 1997.

Andrew M et al: Venous thromboembolic complications (VTE) in children: first analyses of the Canadian Registry of VTE. *Blood* 83:1251, 1994.

Bonduel M et al: Prothrombotic disorders in children with arterial ischemic stroke and sinovenous thrombosis. *Arch Neurol* 56:967, 1999.

Chalmers EA, Gibson BES: Thrombolytic therapy in the management of paediatric thromboembolic disease. *Brit J Haematol* 104:14, 1999.

De Laet C et al: Plasma homocysteine concentration in a Belgian school-age population. *Am J Clin Nutr* 69:968, 1999.

DeVeber G et al: Prothrombotic disorders in infants and children with cerebral thromboembolism. *Arch Neurol* 55:1539, 1998.

Grotta J: Cerebrovascular disease in young patients. *Thromb Haemost* 78:13, 1997.

Lawson SE, et al: Congenital thrombophilia and thrombosis: a study in cohort of children presenting with symptomatic thromboembolism. *Arch Dis Child* 81:176, 1999.

Manco-Johnson MJ: Antiphospholipid antibodies in children. *Semin Thromb Hemost* 24:591, 1998.

Manco-Johnson MJ: Disorders of hemostasis in childhood: risk factors for venous thromboembolism. *Thromb Haemost* 78:710, 1997.

Manco-Johnson MJ et al: Combined thrombolytic and anticoagulant therapy for venous thrombosis in children. *J Pediatr* 136:446, 2000.

Massicotte P et al: Low-molecular-weight heparin in pediatric patients with thrombotic disease: a dose finding study. *J Pediatr* 128:313, 1996.

McColl M et al: Factor V Leiden, prothrombin 20210 G→A and the MTHFR C677T mutations in childhood stroke. *Thromb Haemost* 81:690, 1999.

Michelson AD et al: Antithrombotic therapy in children. Fifth ACCP Consensus Conference on Antithrombotic Therapy. *Chest* 114:748S, 1998.

Nowak-Göttl U et al: Prospective evaluation of the thrombotic risk in children with acute lymphoblastic leukemia carrying the MTHFR TT 677 genotype, the prothrombin G20210A variant, and further prothrombotic risk factors. *Blood* 93:1595, 1999.

Nowak-Göttl U et al: Increased lipoprotein (a) is an important risk factor for venous thromboembolism in childhood. *Circulation* 100:743, 1999.

Nowak-Göttl U et al: Neonatal symptomatic thromboembolism in Germany: two year survey. *Arch Dis Child Fetal Neonatal Ed* 76:F163, 1998.

Nowak-Göttl U et al: Factor V Leiden, protein C, and lipoprotein (a) in catheter-related thrombosis in childhood: a prospective study. *J Pediatr* 131:608, 1997.

Nuss R et al: Childhood thrombosis. *Pediatrics* 96:291, 1995.

Nuss R et al: Efficacy and safety of heparin anticoagulation for neonatal renal vein thrombosis. *Am J Pediatr Hematol/Oncol* 16:127, 1994.

Randolf AG et al: Benefit of heparin in peripheral venous and arterial catheters: systematic review and meta-analysis of randomized controlled trials. *BMJ* 316:969, 1998.

Ries M et al: The role of a2-antiplasmin in the inhibition of clot lysis in newborns and adults. *Biol Neonate* 69:298, 1996.

Rosendaal FR, et al: Venous thrombosis: a multicausal disease. *Lancet* 353:1167, 1999.

Streif W et al: Analysis of warfarin therapy in pediatric patients: A prospective cohort study of 319 patients. *Blood* 94:3007, 1999.

Trusen B et al: Whole blood clot lysis in newborns and adults after adding different concentrations of recombinant tissue plasminogen activator (rt-PA). *Semin Thromb Hemost* 24:599, 1998.

Van Beynum IM et al: Hyperhomocysteinemia: a risk factor for ischemic stroke in children. *Circulation* 99:2070, 1999.

Zenz W et al: Factor V Leiden and prothrombin gene G20210A variant in children with ischemic stroke. *Thromb Haemost* 80:763, 1998.

Zenz W et al: Intracerebral hemorrhage during fibrinolytic therapy in children: a review of the literature of the last thirty years. *Semin Thromb Hemost* 23:321, 1997.

CHAPTER 35

The Adult
with Thrombosis

Thirty years ago, with the exception of antithrombin (AT) deficiency, little was known about the mechanisms responsible for venous or arterial thromboembolism. Since then, dramatic advances have been made in our understanding of natural anticoagulants, fibrinolytic mechanisms, and platelet reactivity. In just the last several years, some of the most common hereditary thrombophilic states have been identified, such as factor V Leiden and the prothrombin gene mutation, disorders that are found in up to 25 percent of patients with a first DVT (Chap. 40). Many laboratory tests are now available to help identify patients with hereditary and acquired thrombophilia.

Several prothrombotic risk factors often work in concert to produce an overt clinical thrombosis. These risk factors may be hereditary or acquired thrombophilic defects (e.g., resistance to activated protein C [APC] or antiphospholipid antibodies), other disease states (e.g., malignancy, inflammation), physical factors (surgery, inactivity), or hormonal effects (pregnancy, oral contraceptives) (Fig. 35-1). In most patients who have a deep venous thrombosis (DVT) or pulmonary embolism (PE), more than one prothrombotic risk factor can readily be identified. A classic example would be a young woman with factor V Leiden with a prior history of taking oral contraceptives, but who develops a thrombosis after being immobilized during pregnancy (Fig. 35-2). Data is now being generated that will help quantify the relative and absolute likelihood of thromboembolism for both single abnormalities and combinations of defects.

The rationale for using laboratory tests to search for thrombophilic disorders in subjects with thrombosis is strengthened by the need for modifications in clinical care. For example, patients with recurrent venous

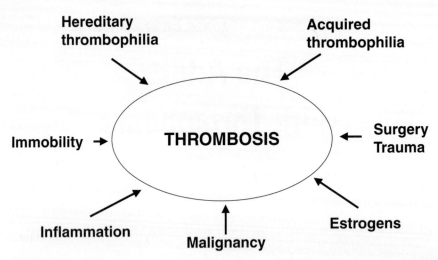

FIGURE 35-1 Common risk factors that promote thrombosis. In most instances more than one abnormality is present.

thrombosis and one or more hereditary or acquired plasma defects may be candidates for long-term therapy with oral anticoagulants, and would benefit from intensive antithrombotic prophylaxis for surgery, pregnancy, or trauma. In some instances, specific treatment is available, such as the use of replacement antithrombin or protein C concentrates during periods of high risk, or supplementation with B vitamins in patients with homocysteinemia (Chap. 42). Counseling can be provided for women with thrombophilia who are considering pregnancy, the use of oral contraceptives, or hormone replacement therapy. When the defect is hereditary, family studies can identify other individuals at risk for thromboembolism. Finally, evaluation of patients with acquired thrombotic abnormalities may lead to the discovery of other diseases, such as malignancy, autoimmune disorders, or myeloproliferative syndromes that might be amenable to treatment.

The diagnostic evaluation of patients with thromboembolism can be approached in several ways, but one option is to determine whether the underlying disorder is hereditary or acquired, and whether the thrombosis involves veins, arteries, or the microvasculature. Although there is often some overlap, these categories provide direction for further evaluation. For example, an adolescent with recurrent deep venous thrombosis with or without a strong family history of venous thromboembolism will likely have one or more of the hereditary thrombophilic states. An elderly man who had previously been well, but who presents to his physician

MODEL OF THROMBOSIS RISK

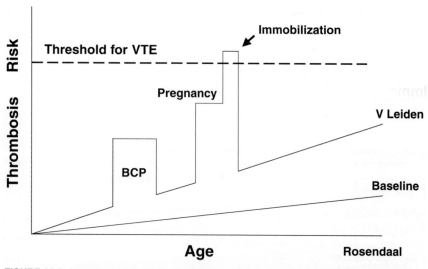

FIGURE 35-2 A concept of thrombosis risk as envisioned by Rosendaal. In this example a young woman with factor V Leiden has an increased risk of thrombosis when she takes birth control pills (BCP) and when she becomes pregnant. However, when a third risk factor is added (in this case immobilization for a pregnancy complication), the threshold for overt thrombosis is exceeded and she develops a deep venous thrombosis in one leg. Note that the likelihood of thrombosis increases progressively with both age and the presence of factor V Leiden. (Adapted with modification from Rosendaal FR: *Lancet* 353:1167, 1999.)

with migratory superficial thrombophlebitis and an embolic stroke should be evaluated for an abdominal or thoracic malignancy.

HISTORY

A thorough history is essential for all patients with a recent or remote history of thrombosis. Detailed information about the circumstances surrounding prior thromboses must be collected, and should include their location, the outcome of diagnostic studies, whether the thrombosis was spontaneous or provoked, and the presence of relevant transient or persistent risk factors. Inquiries should be made about previous antithrombotic therapy, underlying diseases, family history of thrombosis, medications, and habits. A general outline for data collection is included in Table 35-1. This information should help determine whether thromboembolic events are hereditary or acquired, as well as the vascular bed that is involved.

TABLE 35-1

Areas of Emphasis in the History of Patients with Thrombosis

Past History of Thromboembolism

Location (e.g., venous, arterial, microvascular)
Diagnostic studies (e.g., ultrasonography, scans)
Spontaneous or provoked
Predisposing factors (e.g., surgery, trauma, pregnancy)
Prior laboratory tests for thrombophilia
Therapy (e.g., duration, efficacy, complications)

Diseases Associated with Thrombosis

Cancer	Cardiac disease	Hyperlipidemia
Myeloproliferative	Inflammatory	Hemolytic anemia
disorders	disorders	Hereditary thrombotic disorders
Autoimmune	Atherosclerosis	Nephrosis
disorders		

Family History

Pedigree
Thrombosis (location, diagnosis, therapy)
Laboratory studies

Medications and habits

Estrogens, chemotherapy
Tobacco, alcohol, illicit drugs

PHYSICAL EXAMINATION

A complete physical examination is warranted in all patients who present with a new or previous thromboembolism. Special attention should be directed to the vascular system, heart, abdominal organs, extremities, and skin (e.g., livido reticularis). Occasionally, the physical signs of lower extremity deep venous occlusion are extraordinarily subtle; slight dusky discoloration or increased warmth after standing for a few minutes may be the only findings that suggest diversion of blood flow away from the deep veins toward the skin and superficial veins.

LABORATORY EVALUATION

Venous Thrombosis

Data is now available to estimate the frequency of the various hereditary hypercoagulable states in sequential patients presenting with a DVT (Table 35-2). Over 50 percent of individuals will have one or more plasma defects, with even higher rates being observed in subjects with recurrent thromboembolism or a strong family history of thrombosis. Although a

TABLE 35-2			
Estimated Frequency of Hereditary or Acquired Thrombophilia in Sequential Subjects Presenting with DVT.			
Antithrombin deficiency	1%	Prothrombin gene mutation	6%
Protein C deficiency	5%	Elevated factor VIII	16%
Protein S deficiency	3%	Elevated factor XI	11%
Dysfibrinogenemia	0.8%	Homocysteinemia	10%
Factor V Leiden	20%	Antiphospholipid antibodies	10%

thrombosis at a young age suggests thrombophilia, a first event in an older individual by no means excludes the diagnosis. For example, in the Physicians Health Study the risk of idiopathic DVT progressively increased with age in the physicians with factor V Leiden (see Chap. 40). A determination as to whether a thrombosis is spontaneous or provoked does not help to predict the presence of thrombophilia. About 50 percent (+/− 10 percent) are apparently unprovoked, with the remaining half linked to an identifiable injury, surgical procedure, pregnancy, prolonged immobilization, or another event.

Suggested laboratory tests for patients with venous thromboembolism are listed in Table 35-3. Additional information is available in the relevant chapters (e.g., Chap. 40 for the APC-resistance assay). As new thrombophilic disorders are described and validated, additional tests may be added to the panel (see below); candidates include: factor activity assays (XI, IX, X, prothrombin) and genetic tests for defects in thrombomodulin, tissue factor pathway inhibitor, and the endothelial protein C receptor. Testing for fibrinolytic defects (elevated plasminogen activator inhibitor-1 [PAI-1], reduced or defective tissue plasminogen activator [t-PA], or plasminogen), and heparin co-factor II is probably not warranted at present, except in a research setting (e.g., see Chap. 41).

Arterial Thrombosis

Arterial thrombosis most often occurs on a background of atherosclerosis, with a ruptured arterial plaque provoking clot formation. The identification of an underlying hypercoagulable state is more likely in those patients who have acute arterial occlusion in the absence of significant atherosclerosis (Table 35-3). Examples of thrombophilic disorders that provoke arterial thromboembolism include homocysteinemia, antiphospholipid antibody syndrome, myeloproliferative disorders, and malignancy. In some instances a "venous" hypercoagulable state can be associated with an arterial thrombosis. Patients with right-to-left cardiac shunts may develop stroke or other vascular occlusion as a result of diver-

---

TABLE 35-3

Laboratory Evaluation of Patients with Thrombosis (see text for additional tests)

Venous Thrombosis

APC-resistance assay (factor V Leiden)	Homocysteine
Prothrombin gene mutation	Fibrinogen (clottable)
Factor VIII activity	Thrombin time (reptilase time)
Antithrombin activity	Lupus anticoagulant (multiple assays)
Protein S (free antigen or activity)	Anticardiolipin and/or anti-β_2-glycoprotein I
Protein C activity	antibodies
	CBC

Arterial Thrombosis

Antiphospholipid antibodies (see above)	CBC, colony assays (for myeloproliferative
Homocysteine	disorders)
Venous panel (in patients with R to L	Plasma lipids [including Lp(a)]
cardiac shunt, childhood stroke)	High-sensitivity CRP (see text)

Microvascular Thrombosis

CBC, peripheral blood smear	Protein C, protein S (selected patients)
DIC screen	HIT assay (selected patients)
Antiphospholipid antibodies (see above)	

Abbreviations: CBC, complete blood count; APC, activated protein C; Lp(a), lipoprotein(a); CRP, C-reactive protein; HIT, heparin-induced thrombocytopenia.

sion of a venous-side embolus into the arterial circulation. Although controversial, a few patients with hereditary thrombophilic states such as the factor V Leiden or prothrombin gene mutations appear to have an increased risk (OR ~1.5) of arterial occlusive events particularly in the presence of other risk factors for arterial disease, such as smoking, hypertension, diabetes, or obesity (Doggen ref). Childhood stroke has been associated with a high rate of hereditary thrombophilic defects. Finally, sensitive markers of chronic inflammation such as high sensitivity C-reactive protein (using a high-sensitivity assay) or interleukin-6 have been linked to the subsequent development of acute myocardial infarction, although the mechanisms involved are not well understood.

Microvascular Thrombosis

The presence of microvascular thromboses such as dermal necrosis, ischemia of the digits, or microvascular renal disease suggests another set of laboratory tests (Table 35-3). In these patients, a complete blood count and peripheral blood smear to search for evidence of microangiopathic hemolytic anemia (thrombotic thrombocytopenic purpura/hemolytic uremic syndrome) or myeloproliferative disease (erythromelalgia) should be performed. In addition, tests for disseminated intravascular coagulation (DIC), malignancy, endotoxemia, antiphospholipid antibodies, and when appropriate, assays for protein C and protein S (warfarin skin necrosis) and for heparin-associated antiplatelet antibodies should be obtained.

An important consideration in the laboratory evaluation of a patient with thrombosis is the timing of blood tests relative to thrombotic events and antithrombotic therapy. Ideally, the tests should be obtained at least 2 to 3 weeks after stopping oral anticoagulants to minimize the impact of acute thrombosis or anticoagulant therapy on test results. Acute thromboembolism often provokes a rapid fall in AT (and occasionally protein C and protein S) activity. Therapeutic doses of heparin also decrease AT activity, but usually do not affect levels of protein C or protein S. Treatment with warfarin produces a marked drop in protein C and protein S by the inhibition of vitamin K. In general, if levels of AT, protein C, and protein S are normal immediately following a thrombotic event or during heparin therapy, hereditary deficiencies of these proteins are unlikely. Low levels may reflect acquired rather than hereditary deficiencies, so that testing should be repeated at a later date. However, many diagnostic tests are now designed to be informative in the presence of anticoagulants. The assays listed in Table 35-3 are not affected by heparin or warfarin, with the exception of protein C and protein S. Tests such as the second-generation APC-resistance assay and the hexagonal phospholipid neutralization test for the lupus anticoagulant include polybrene, a heparin neutralizer, along with a source of normal clotting factors to correct for warfarin-induced coagulation defects.

OTHER POTENTIAL CAUSES OF THROMBOSIS

Despite the recent advances in our understanding of thrombophilia, a few patients with a strong family or personal history of thrombosis will not have an identifiable hypercoagulable state using standard tests. In some instances new disorders will be discovered to explain the thrombotic diathesis. Others may turn out to have prothrombotic defects in the vessel wall, involving proteins that are not easily measured in the blood. A search for genetic mutations in the genes for these factors may be informative (e.g., thrombomodulin, discussed later). Finally, perturbations in factors that seem very likely to promote thrombosis appear to have only borderline clinical significance at best (e.g., fibrinolytic defects, heparin cofactor II deficiency), may act as a permissive factor in concert with another hypercoagulable state.

Thrombomodulin (TM) is a glycoprotein located on the endothelial surface that binds thrombin and promotes the conversion of protein C to activated protein C. Several mutations in the TM gene have been identified in families with thrombosis. The defects are found scattered throughout the gene and could affect TM function, but do not predictably influence circulating soluble TM levels in the plasma.

Elevated levels of procoagulant clotting factors have also recently been reported to promote thrombosis. In addition to high levels of factor VIII (discussed in Chap. 40), preliminary reports of thrombosis associated with elevations in factors XI, X, and IX have been published. The mechanism underlying these hypercoagulable states has not yet been determined, but could reflect excessive thrombin generation at areas of local vascular injury.

Recently, a mutation in the gene for tissue factor pathway inhibitor (TFPI) has been described that appears to be linked with thrombosis. TFPI is present on the vascular surface, and when combined with factor Xa, is a major inhibitor of tissue-factor–induced thrombin generation (see Chap. 1). Heparin cofactor II is a glycoprotein of the serine protease inhibitor (serpin) family that inhibits thrombin (but unlike antithrombin does not inhibit factor Xa). Several patients with venous thrombosis have been found to have reduced levels (i.e., 50 percent) of heparin cofactor II, but it is not yet clear whether a deficiency of the protein constitutes a true risk factor for thrombosis.

Elevated levels of lipoprotein (a) [Lp(a)] have been linked to premature atherosclerosis, particularly in patients with high concentrations of LDL-cholesterol. The multiple kringle structures of apo-Lp(a) can compete with plasminogen for binding to fibrin or cell surfaces, and has been shown to inhibit fibrinolysis *in vitro*. Increased concentrations of plasma Lp(a) have not been shown to be a risk factor for venous thrombosis in adults, although an association has been reported in children.

Patients with chronic inflammatory disorders (e.g., inflammatory bowel disease) have an increased risk of thrombosis, most likely due to the presence of inflammatory mediators in the blood. Interleukin-1 and tumor necrosis factor have been shown to increase endothelial cell tissue factor expression and to downregulate thrombomodulin, leading to impaired generation of APC. Inflammatory reactions could also promote thrombosis via elevated levels of factor VIII and fibrinogen, or reduced protein S activity.

Finally, current laboratory assays are less than optimal for the identification of heightened platelet reactivity, a process that could play a key role in thrombogenesis. Tests such as measurement of platelet glycopro-tein receptors, platelet aggregation, the circulating platelet aggregate ratio, and plasma levels of platelet-specific proteins lack sufficient pre-dictive value for arterial thrombosis to be clinically useful at present.

BIBLIOGRAPHY

Bertina RM: Molecular risk factors for thrombosis. *Thromb Haemost* 82:601, 1999.

Bovill EG et al: Hereditary thrombophilia as a model for multigenic disease. *Thromb Haemost* 82:662, 1999.

Cattaneo M: Hyperhomocysteinemia, atherosclerosis and thrombosis. *Thromb Haemost* 81:165, 1999.

Doggen CJM et al: Interaction of coagulation defects and cardiovascular risk fac-tors—increased risk of myocardial infarction associated with factor V Leiden or prothrombin 20210A. *Circulation* 97:1037, 1998.

Goodnight SH et al: Hereditary thrombophilia. In: Beutler E, et al. (eds.), *Williams Hematology*, 6th ed., New York, McGraw-Hill, 2001, Chapter 127.

Nowak-Gottl U et al: Increased lipoprotein(a) is an important risk factor for venous thromboembolism in childhood. *Circulation* 100:743, 1999.

O'Donnell J et al: High prevalence of elevated factor VIII levels in patients referred for thrombophilia screening: role of increased synthesis and relationship to the acute phase reaction. *Thromb Haemost* 77:825, 1997.

Ohlin AK, Marlar RA: Thrombomodulin gene defects in families with throm-boembolic disease—a report on four families. *Thromb Haemost* 81:338, 1999.

Prins MH, Hirsh J: A critical review of the evidence supporting a relationship between impaired fibrinolytic activity and venous thromboembolism. *Arch Intern Med* 151:1721, 1991.

Ridker PM, Stampfer MJ: Assessment of genetic markers for coronary thrombosis: promise and precaution. *Lancet* 353:687, 1999.

Ridker PM et al: C-reactive protein adds to the predictive value of total and HDL cholesterol in determining risk of first myocardial infarction. *Circulation* 97:2007, 1998.

Ridker PM et al: Age-specific incidence rates of venous thromboembolism among heterozygous carriers of factor V Leiden mutation. *Ann Intern Med* 126:528, 1997.

Ridker PM et al: Inflammation, aspirin, and the risk of cardiovascular disease in apparently healthy men. *N Engl J Med* 336:973, 1997.

Rosendaal FR: Risk factors for venous thrombotic disease. *Thromb Haemost* 82:610, 1999.

Rosendaal FR: Venous thrombosis: a multicausal disease. *Lancet* 353:1167, 1999.

Salomon O et al: Single and combined prothrombotic factors in patients with idiopathic venous thromboembolism—prevalence and risk assessment. *Arterioscler Thromb Vasc Biol* 19:511, 1999.

Schafer AI: Hypercoagulable states: molecular genetics to clinical practice. *Lancet* 344:1739, 1994.

CHAPTER 36

Deep Venous Thrombosis and Pulmonary Embolism

Venous thromboembolism is a common clinical problem with a reported incidence of over 200,000 episodes per year in the United States. Approximately 1 in 1000 individuals per year are affected. Massive pulmonary embolism (PE) accounts for 5 to 10 percent of all hospital deaths. The mortality rate of untreated PE is about 30 percent, but with optimal therapy this figure can be reduced to 8 percent or even less. Patient survival is significantly reduced in the 3-month period of time following deep venous thrombosis (DVT) and PE.

PATHOGENESIS

Venous thrombi are composed of a fibrin meshwork packed with red blood cells, in contrast to arterial thrombi that usually are white in color due to the incorporation of large numbers of platelets. As demonstrated many years ago, lower extremity venous thrombi tend to originate in areas of sluggish blood flow behind venous valves and then propagate into the lumen of the vein. Based on data from fibrinogen scans, small clots form frequently following stresses such as surgery, but they are ordinarily rapidly destroyed by the fibrinolytic system.

Although venous thrombi often appear to be "spontaneous" in origin, they are associated with one or more predisposing factors in the great majority of instances. Some common situations are hereditary or acquired defects in antithrombotic mechanisms, venous stasis, vascular injury, and circulating activated clotting factors. In many instances, thrombosis occurs as a result of one or more genetic thrombophilic defects (e.g., factor V Leiden) coupled with an acquired thrombogenic stimulus, such as surgery or oral contraceptives (Chap. 35).

Fibrin clots, once formed, remain highly thrombogenic for up to 2 weeks. Functional thrombin molecules are present on the surfaces of fresh thrombi, where they are protected from inactivation. Consequently, in the absence of effective antithrombotic treatment, newly formed clots are likely to propagate, which greatly increases the risk of embolization. In time (e.g., over several months), the thrombi gradually diminish in size or collateral flow develops around sites of venous obstruction.

CLINICAL MANIFESTATIONS

The clinical signs and symptoms of DVT reflect the obstruction by clot of the deep veins in an extremity and are remarkable because of their variability. Massive iliofemoral thrombosis is on the severe end of the spectrum and produces virtually complete obstruction of venous outflow in the leg, a condition termed phlegmasia cerulea dolens (an extremely swollen blue painful leg). Lesser degrees of venous obstruction in the leg produce pain in the calf or thigh, pitting edema of the ankle or lower leg, and a warm dusky reddish-blue discoloration of the skin caused by enhanced superficial venous blood flow. Sometimes these physical signs are very subtle, requiring good light and asking the patient to stand for a few minutes to appreciate differences in size, warmth, color, or edema between normal and involved legs. Finally, at least half the time in infants and children, as well as adults, DVT produces no symptoms whatsoever, particularly when the clots are small or subocclusive.

Some patients with a past history of severe or recurrent venous thrombosis of the legs develop signs of chronic venostasis. Affected extremities are chronically swollen and painful and show dark discoloration of the skin. Ultimately, cutaneous ulcers develop, which are usually located near the malleoli. Recurrent bouts of leg pain and swelling can occur due to intermittent hemodynamic obstruction of blood flow in the absence of the formation of new thrombi.

The classic signs and symptoms of PE are well known and include sudden chest pain, dyspnea, anxiety, and cyanosis. Hemoptysis is uncommon. As in DVT, the clinical presentations of PE vary considerably. Over two-thirds of patients with PE are asymptomatic. Rarely, patients with small but recurrent PE seek medical attention because of chronic pulmonary hypertension with elevated right heart pressures, dyspnea, anxiety, and cyanosis.

DIAGNOSTIC STUDIES

Because the diagnosis of DVT or PE by history and physical examination alone is often misleading (i.e., substantial false positives and false negatives), objective diagnostic studies are required. The venogram remains the gold standard for DVT, but venous ultrasound (US) with compression of the major veins is now the initial diagnostic test of choice.

In the last decade, numerous studies have greatly enhanced our understanding of the natural history of DVT and its diagnosis. Relevant clinical findings include:

- About 25 percent of patients who present with leg symptoms will be found to have DVT.
- Most symptomatic PE are due to embolization from the proximal leg veins (rather than distal [calf] veins).
- About 20 percent of distal DVT will extend up into the proximal veins; most do so within one week.
- Venous US has a high predictive value in patients with symptomatic proximal DVT; the sensitivity and specificity are >95 percent.
- Calculation of the clinical probability of a DVT can be used to enhance the diagnostic value of venous US (Table 36-1).
- Quantitative D-dimer assays (a measure of fibrinolytic activity) have a high *negative* predictive value for DVT; i.e., normal values (<0.5 μg/mL) exclude clinically significant DVT (see later).

Algorithms that incorporate the results of venous US, clinical probability, and D-dimer testing have been developed to aid in the accurate diagnosis of DVT (Fig. 36-1).

Ventilation/perfusion (V/Q) lung scans are the initial diagnostic procedure of choice in patients suspected of PE. Pulmonary angiography is reserved for more difficult diagnostic problems because of its cost, technical difficulty, and side effects. More recently, helical CT (spiral CT) and magnetic resonance imaging (MRI) are becoming more widely used, although clinical trials to document their validity in PE are not yet available. Several clinical principles have emerged that underlie diagnostic testing for PE:

- A normal lung scan excludes PE (a situation that occurs in 10 to 40 percent of patients tested).
- A "high probability" V/Q scan suggests a likelihood of PE in the range of 80 percent. If three or more mismatched defects are found, the likelihood increases to >95 percent.
- Approximately 70 percent of patients with a symptomatic PE will prove to have DVT, the majority of which involve the proximal veins.

TABLE 36-1

Clinical Model for Determining Clinical Suspicion of Deep Vein Thrombosis.

	If present score
Active cancer (treatment ongoing or within previous 6 months or palliative)	1
Paralysis, paresis, or recent plaster immobilization of the lower extremities	1
Recently bedridden >3 days or major surgery within 4 weeks	1
Localized tenderness along the distribution of the deep venous system	1
Entire leg swollen	1
Calf swelling 3 cm > asymptomatic side (measured 10 cm below tibial tuberosity)	1
Pitting edema confined to the symptomatic leg	1
Dilated superficial veins (nonvaricose)	1
Alternative diagnosis as likely or greater than that of DVT	−2

Total Points

Note: In patients with symptoms in both legs, the more symptomatic leg is used. Pretest probability calculated as follows:

	Total points
High	≥3
Moderate	1 or 2
Low	0

Adapted from Wells PS et al: *J Intern Med* 243:15, 1998.

- Clinical models can be used to help determine the pretest probability of PE based on clinical signs/symptoms, the presence of alternative diagnoses, and risk factors (see Wells ref).
- As in DVT, quantitative D-dimer testing has a high negative predictive value for PE.

The above data can be incorporated into a useful clinical algorithm for the diagnoses of PE (see Fig. 36-2).

LABORATORY TESTING

Laboratory tests to identify hereditary or acquired thrombophilic states in patients with venous thromboembolism are discussed in detail in Chapter 35. In brief, candidates for diagnostic laboratory studies are those individuals in whom a specific diagnosis will influence therapy. Examples include duration or intensity of anticoagulants, the use of replacement concentrates (e.g., antithrombin or protein C), specific treatment (e.g., vitamins in homocysteinemia), the use of antithrombotic pro-

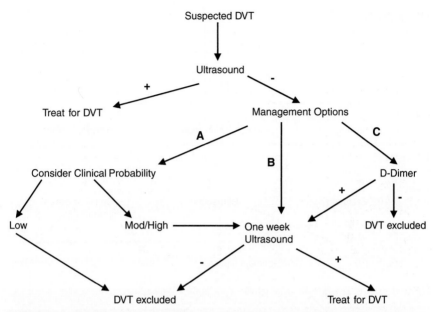

FIGURE 36-1 Algorithm for investigation of patients with first episode of deep vein thrombosis. DVT, deep vein thrombosis; Mod, moderate. (Used with permission from Anderson DR, Wells PS: *Thromb Haemost* 82: 878, 1999.)

phylaxis, estimation of the risks of estrogens, or the need for laboratory studies in family members.

Tests that measure activation of coagulation (e.g., prothrombin activation peptides, F1.2) have been evaluated to determine if they might identify patients with an ongoing prothrombotic state. The most useful of these has proven to be quantitative assays for the fibrin degradation product, D-dimer. Its diagnostic value is highest when it is normal (i.e., <5 μg/mL), with a negative predictive value in both DVT and PE of over 98 percent. Tests for D-dimer are now available using ELISA methods that are rapid (<1 hr) and highly accurate. Whole blood point-of-care tests are also available (e.g., SimpliRED). Other tests, such as the semiquantitative latex agglutination assay for D-dimer (used for the diagnosis of DIC) and tests for the detection of thrombin-antithrombin complexes or F1.2, are not useful for the clinical diagnosis of thromboembolism.

MANAGEMENT

Thrombolytic Therapy

Thrombolytic therapy with streptokinase, urokinase, or recombinant tissue plasminogen activator (t-PA) is considered the treatment of choice

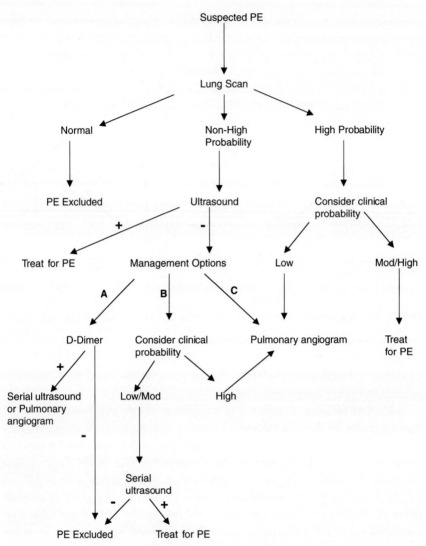

FIGURE 36-2 Algorithm for suspected pulmonary embolism using lung scan as initial investigation. PE, pulmonary embolism; Mod, moderate. (Used with permission from Anderson DR, Wells PS: *Thromb Haemost* 82: 878, 1999.)

for patients who have massive PE with cardiovascular collapse or for those with advanced cardiopulmonary disease in which smaller PE have major clinical consequences. The use of thrombolytic agents remains controversial in patients with less severe PE. The evidence for short- or long-term benefit in relation to the increased risks of bleeding is not yet available.

Fibrinolytic agents reduce the volume of venous clot in the deep veins of the leg as assessed by angiography (e.g., 30 to 40 percent complete clot lysis, 30 percent partial lysis), and several studies have suggested that long-term disability from the postphlebitic syndrome is lessened in treated patients. However, the necessity of 3 or more days of therapy, the 2 to 4 fold increased risk of bleeding (especially CNS), and the fact that the largest clots are less likely to undergo thrombolysis have tempered enthusiasm for thrombolytic therapy in patients with DVT. Thrombolytic agents via administered regional catheters have been advocated and have been successful in relieving symptoms in some patients, but benefits for larger groups of patients have not been verified in controlled clinical trials. Catheter-directed thrombolytic therapy should be reserved for patients with very extensive ileofemoral thrombosis who have low risks of bleeding.

Anticoagulation

Heparin

Unfractionated heparin or low molecular weight heparin (LMWH) should be started as soon as a diagnosis of DVT or PE is made (see Chap. 59). Optimal doses of heparin must be given, as evidenced by APTTs or heparin levels (for unfractionated heparin) in the therapeutic range, to minimize the risk of recurrent thrombosis. Outpatient therapy with LMWH (without laboratory monitoring) for uncomplicated patients with DVT or PE is rapidly gaining acceptance based on numerous studies documenting safety and efficacy (as compared to inpatient intravenous heparin), along with substantial cost savings and increased patient acceptance.

Warfarin

Oral anticoagulation with warfarin should be started shortly after admission in patients with proximal DVT, so that the total duration of heparin therapy will be about 5 days in most patients. The INR should be in the therapeutic range (INR 2–3) for at least 24 hr before heparin or LMWH is discontinued. The optimal duration of oral anticoagulant therapy for patients with DVT or PE is an important but challenging problem. Decisions must be based on the relative risks of morbidity or mortality from recurrent thromboembolism or major hemorrhage. Several principles of treatment have begun to emerge based on clinical trials:

■ Patients with idiopathic thrombosis (i.e., in the absence of identifiable risk factors) have a higher likelihood of recurrence than those whose thrombi were provoked (e.g., by trauma, surgery, etc).

- Subjects with PE (particularly unprovoked) have a much higher risk of recurrent PE and death in the months to years that follow.
- Patients with ongoing (non-reversible) risk factors, such as hereditary thrombophilia or cancer, have a continued increased likelihood of recurrent thrombosis.
- Individuals with a history of thrombosis and persistent antiphospholipid antibodies are very likely to have recurrences.
- If transient risk factors can be removed or treated and the patient is ambulatory, the chances of recurrence are quite low.

Based on clinical trial data and decision analyses, some recommendations for duration of anticoagulants can be made, subject to revision as more data becomes available (Table 36-2).

TABLE 36-2

General Recommendations for Duration of Anticoagulation Therapy

Clinical Scenario	Duration[1]
Provoked VTE; transient risk factor[2]	3 months
Provoked VTE; persistent major risk factor[3]	Indefinite
Idiopathic DVT, single episode[4]	At least 6 months
Idiopathic DVT, recurrent	Indefinite
Idiopathic PE	Indefinite
VTE + thrombophilic state[5] + transient risk factor	At least 6 months after transient RF resolves
VTE + more than one thrombophilic state	Indefinite
Recurrent VTE + thrombophilic state	Indefinite
VTE + persistent antiphospholipid antibodies (APA)	indefinite
Hereditary thrombophilic state or APA—no history of thrombosis	None

Notes:
1. Recommendations must be individualized based on risks of bleeding, co-morbid conditions, family history, and other relevant factors. Future clinical studies may modify or change these recommendations.
2. A provoked VTE includes such conditions as surgery, trauma, prolonged immobilization, pregnancy, or oral contraceptives. A transient risk factor is one that is self-limited (e.g., pregnancy) or can be treated or removed (e.g., oral contraceptives, chronic inflammatory disease).
3. Persistent major risk factor includes entities such as malignancy, prolonged immobilization, chronic inflammatory disease, or unresponsive to treatment. Markedly abnormal venous flow dynamics as a result of a severe post-phlebitic syndrome are considered by some to represent a major ongoing risk for recurrent VTE.
4. Idiopathic VTE are those with no clear identifiable provoking factor.
5. Thrombophilic state: hereditary (e.g., AT deficiency) or acquired (e.g., antiphospholipid antibodies).

Vena Caval Filters

Indications for placement of a filter in the vena cava include patients with proximal DVT who cannot be treated with anticoagulants because of intercurrent bleeding or a very high likelihood of future hemorrhage. Recent data has suggested that filters are effective in reducing fatal and non-fatal PE in the near term (e.g., first several weeks), but that recurrent DVT (likely due to filter thrombosis) is substantially increased in the next two years (Decousus ref). If a filter is used, consideration should be given to long-term oral anticoagulant therapy (if possible) in an attempt to reduce the risks of recurrent DVT.

BIBLIOGRAPHY

Anderson DR, Wells PS: Improvements in the diagnostic approach for patients with suspected deep vein thrombosis or pulmonary function. *Thromb Haemost* 82: 878, 1999.

Brill-Edwards P, Lee A: D-dimer testing in the diagnosis of acute venous thromboembolism. *Thromb Haemost* 82:688, 1999.

Decousus H et al: A clinical trial of vena caval filters in the prevention of pulmonary embolism in patients with proximal deep-vein thrombosis. *N Engl J Med* 338:409, 1998.

Ginsberg JS et al: Sensitivity and specificity of a rapid whole-blood assay for D-dimer in the diagnosis of pulmonary embolism. *Ann Intern Med* 129:1006, 1998.

Ginsberg JS: Management of venous thromboembolism. *N Engl J Med* 335:1816, 1996.

Hirsh J et al: Heparin and low-molecular-weight heparin: Mechanisms of action, pharmacokinetics, dosing considerations, monitoring, efficacy, and safety. *Chest* 114:489S, 1998.

Hyers TM et al: Antithrombotic therapy for venous thromboembolic disease. *Chest* 114:561S, 1998.

Kearon C: Initial treatment of venous thromboembolism. *Thromb Haemost* 82:887, 1999.

Kearon C et al: The role of venous ultrasonography in the diagnosis of suspected deep venous thrombosis and pulmonary embolism. *Ann Intern Med* 129:1044, 1998.

Levine M et al: Hemorrhagic complications of anticoagulant treatment. *Chest* 114:511S, 1998.

Prins MH et al: Long-term treatment of venous thromboembolic disease. *Thromb Haemost* 82:892, 1999.

Wells PS et al: Use of a clinical model for safe management of patients with suspected pulmonary embolism. *Ann Intern Med* 129:997, 1998.

Weitz JI et al: Clot-bound thrombin is protected from inhibition by heparin-antithrombin III but is susceptible to inactivation by antithrombin III-independent inhibitors. *J Clin Invest* 86:385, 1990.

CHAPTER 37

Antithrombin Deficiency

Human antithrombin (AT) is a 58,000 Mr glycoprotein with a plasma concentration of 150 µg/mL. AT or heparin cofactor I is a protease inhibitor belonging to the serpin (serine protease inhibitor) superfamily; it functions by forming a 1:1 stoichiometric complex with activated clotting enzymes (thrombin, Xa, IXa, XIa) via a reactive site (arginine) on AT. The relatively slow complex formation is dramatically accelerated in the presence of heparin or when the AT is activated by cell surface heparan sulfate. The schematic structure of AT and the residues involved in heparin and thrombin interactions are shown in Fig. 37-1. A deficiency (hereditary or acquired) of the protein is associated with a thrombotic tendency as manifested by venous thromboembolism and, rarely, arterial thrombi.

GENETICS

The 19 kb gene (seven exons, six introns) is located on chromosome 1 (1q23-q25). Examples of mutations resulting in either type 1 (quantitative defects) or type 2 (qualitative defects) are shown in Table 37-1. Over 250 mutations have now been reported and are available in a database accessed by the internet: (*http://www.med.ic.ac.uk/dd/ddhc*). The common type 1 defect results in a proportionate decrease in both amount (antigen) and function of AT, and is due to genetic mutations producing silent alleles. The qualitative defects (dysfunctional AT) are associated with point mutations affecting either the serine protease inhibition site for thrombin, Xa, or the heparin-binding site, or both. The heterozygotes for type 1, 2a, and 2b display intermediate levels of antithrombin activity associated with a thrombotic tendency; homozygosity is probably not compatible

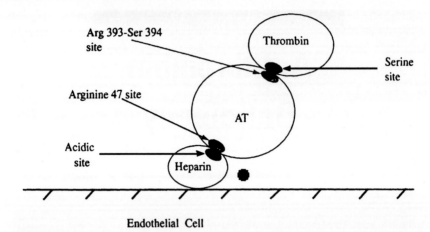

Endothelial Cell

FIGURE 37-1 The scheme for inhibition of thrombin (or other protease, Xa) by antithrombin (AT) when bound to heparin (or heparan sulfate) at the endothelial cell surface. The symbol (●) indicates the proposed site for vitronectin, which acts as a noncompetitive inhibitor forming a ternary complex with heparin-AT and protecting thrombin against rapid inactivation.

with life. In contrast, the heterozygotes for isolated heparin-binding activity (type 2c) rarely have thrombosis. However, homozygotes have shown recurrent venous and arterial thrombi, including massive cardiac thromboses and recurrent thrombophlebitis. Recently, a novel AT defect was reported in an asymptomatic family with only mild reductions in AT antigen and activity (~0.7 U/mL). The defect produced increased amounts of β-antithrombin (very high affinity for heparin due to a defect in glycosylation) (Bayston ref).

Early studies of the prevalence of AT deficiency in the general population suggested an incidence of 1 in 2000 to 5000. Subsequent studies by Tait et al. (1994) estimated type 2C AT deficiency (isolated heparin-binding defects) occurs with a higher frequency of 1 in 350. The prevalence of AT deficiency in consecutive patients being investigated for venous thrombo-embolism is about one percent. The odds ratio for thrombosis is increased 10–20 fold (greater than that for factor V Leiden; see Chap. 40). An age-related incidence of thromboses in affected family members has been noted; the cumulative thrombosis rate ranges from 5 percent at birth through 10 years to 95 percent in AT-deficient subjects by 50 to 60 years of age. Although rare before the second decade, thrombotic complications have been reported in infants. As in other forms of thrombophilia, the chance that an hereditary deficient individual will have thromboembolic complications depends on other risk factors, specifically gene–gene and gene–environment interactions, which increase the risk of thrombosis by

TABLE 37-1
Classification of Hereditary Antithrombin Deficiencies: Examples of Molecular Defects

Type I. Low functional and immunoreactive antithrombin

      1a. Normal molecules synthesized at reduced rate (frameshift, point mutation)
      1b. Decreased amount of abnormal molecules
          Pro407Leu (Utah)
          Arg406Met (Kyoto)

Type II. Low functional but normal immunoreactive antithrombin

      2a. Decreased antithrombin activity and heparin-binding activity
          Pro429Leu (Budapest)
      2b. Decreased antithrombin activity
          Ser394Leu (Denver, Milano 2)
          Ala384Pro (Sudbury, Cambridge, Charleville)
      2c. Isolated low heparin-binding activity
          Arg47Cys (Alger, Tours, Toyama, Paris, Amiens, Barcelona 2)
          Pro41Leu (Basel, Franconville, Clichy)

fivefold and 20-fold, respectively. However, mortality rates are not increased in families with AT deficiency.

CLINICAL MANIFESTATIONS

Measurements of AT include two basic types of clinical laboratory assays: immunologic techniques (rocket immunoelectrophoresis) for the AT antigen, and functional assays using chromogenic substrates (e.g., S-2238) with and without heparin (AT activity; progressive antithrombin and heparin cofactor). The most useful assay utilizes factor Xa as a target; it detects abnormalities of both the active serpin center and the heparin-binding site and is not influenced by levels of heparin cofactor II. A helpful adjunct is the crossed immunoelectrophoretic technique (with heparin in the first dimension), which detects binding to heparin and gross molecular defects. Compared to other coagulation factors, the normal range of AT in adults is rather narrow (i.e., from 0.8 to 1.2 U/mL). With the exception of the fetus and newborn, physiologic alterations of AT levels are infrequently seen. Slightly decreased amounts (to approximately 0.9 U/mL) are noted in men over the age of 50 years and in women of childbearing age; pregnancy and exercise have little effect in most studies.

Profound alterations in AT are seen in the fetus and newborn, where levels range from 0.25 U/mL in the 20-week gestation fetus to 0.5 U/mL in the term infant. Adult levels are reached by 6 months of age. Preterm infants with AT levels of <0.2 U/ml in cord samples have a significantly higher risk of dying of respiratory distress syndrome or cerebral hemorrhage. In most instances, the infant is probably protected against increased thrombotic risk by the physiologically low vitamin K-dependent factors ("warfarin-like effect") and elevated levels of α_2-macroglobulin (inhibits thrombin generation); however, an increased resistance to therapeutic heparin has been observed.

Clinical features of hereditary AT deficiency include first thrombotic episodes at an early age, family history of thrombosis, recurrent venous thromboembolism, thrombosis during pregnancy, occasional resistance to heparin therapy, and idiopathic venous thrombosis. The usual vessels involved are deep veins of the lower extremities, iliofemoral, vena caval, renal, and axillary veins. Cerebral venous thrombosis at all ages, mesenteric venous thromboses, and Budd-Chiari syndrome are all serious clinical problems. Arterial thromboses may rarely occur.

Acquired deficiencies of AT may be significant and are summarized in Table 37-2. The most common and frequently most severe deficiencies of AT occur in conditions such as disseminated intravascular coagulation (DIC; shock, sepsis), acute thrombosis, major surgery and its complications, preeclampsia, and malignancies. AT deficiency associated with failure to synthesize adequate amounts of AT is seen in cirrhosis, severe thalassemia, malnutrition, and in preterm infants. Both loss and failure to synthesize the protein may be observed in acute hepatic failure and the nephrotic syndrome. The acute use of heparin or L-asparaginase, or after prothrombin-complex concentrate infusions or the chronic use of oral contraceptive agents (OCA) (related mainly to the estrogen content), are associated with decreases in circulating AT. The low levels of AT with OCA, L-asparaginase, and after prothrombin-complex concentrate usage have been associated with thrombotic episodes.

MANAGEMENT

In most instances, acute thrombotic episodes in hereditary deficiency of AT are managed in standard fashion by heparin therapy followed by chronic warfarin prophylaxis. Older observations suggested that heparin administration may cause adverse clinical effects in patients with AT deficiency by reducing existing AT levels and aggravating the hypercoagulable state. However, our experience has been that heparin can be used to treat acute thrombosis without replacement with exogenous AT (i.e., AT concentrates), although in clinical situations where bleeding is a risk (parturition or surgery) purified concentrates of AT are very useful. Intravenous heparin decreases plasma AT levels and enhances AT clear-

TABLE 37-2

Acquired Antithrombin Deficiency

Consumption coagulopathy
  Disseminated intravascular coagulation (shock, sepsis)
  Surgery
  Preeclampsia
Liver dysfunction
  Acute hepatic failure
  Cirrhosis
  Polytransfused thalassemia
  Preterm infants
Renal disease
  Nephrotic syndrome
  Hemolytic uremic syndrome
Malignancies
  Leukemia (acute promyelocytic leukemia)
Malnutrition or gastrointestinal loss
  Vascular reconstruction (diabetes, age)
  Protein-calorie deprivation
  Inflammatory bowel disease
Drugs
  Estrogens-progestins
  Heparin
  L-asparaginase
Other
  Vasculitis
  Infection
  Hemodialysis
  Plasmapheresis
  After prothrombin-complex concentrate infusion

ance by increasing uptake in the liver. In patients with acute deep venous thrombosis (DVT), plasma AT levels fall (by about 20 percent) after therapeutic heparin, but the incidence of DVT recurrence is not related to the lower patient AT levels. Even so, extensive thrombus formation with heparin resistance may occasionally be seen in familial AT deficiency.

Warfarin therapy is usually not associated with an appreciable effect on AT levels; however, untreated AT-deficient subjects generate more thrombin than their nondeficient relatives; warfarin inhibits this thrombin formation. Hereditary deficient patients who have had a previous thrombotic episode (DVT) are usually treated with warfarin indefinitely. Rarely, coumarin-induced skin necrosis may be seen in hereditary AT deficiency, although it is seen more often in protein C deficiency. Certain androgenic compounds (danazol, stanozolol, oxymetholone) have been shown to increase AT levels in hereditary deficient patients; however, benefit in prevention of thrombosis has not been established.

Indications for the use of replacement therapy with AT concentrates include thrombosis during pregnancy (delivery, postpartum), refractory thrombosis, and major surgery in hereditary deficiency patients. Other potential indications are posttrauma DIC and hemorrhagic shock, acute nephrotic syndrome, fulminant hepatic failure, and persistent DIC in clinical situations where the measured levels are particularly low. AT concentrate has been used in the sick newborn to prevent thrombotic and hemorrhagic complications. See Chapter 55 for details of concentrate use.

AT concentrates are prepared from normal human plasma by several manufacturers. Recently, a team of researchers have utilized transgenic goats that produce significant quantities of human antithrombin in their milk. It has been estimated that approximately 100 transgenic goats can produce enough AT to meet the world demand for AT replacement therapy.

BIBLIOGRAPHY

Bayston TA et al: Familial overexpression of β antithrombin caused by an Asn135Thr substitution. *Blood* 93:4242, 1999.

Blajchman MA et al: Molecular basis of inherited human antithrombin deficiency. *Blood* 80:2159, 1992.

Buller HR, ten Cate JW: Acquired antithrombin III deficiency: Laboratory diagnosis, incidence, clinical implications, and treatment with antithrombin III concentrate. *Am J Med* 87:44S, 1989.

Demers C et al: An antithrombin III assay based on factor Xa inhibition provides a more reliable test to identify congenital antithrombin III deficiency than an assay based on thrombin inhibition. *Thromb Haemost* 69:231, 1993.

Demers C et al: Thrombosis in antithrombin-III-deficient persons. Report of a large kindred and literature review *Ann Intern Med* 116:754, 1992.

Edmunds T et al: Transgenically produced human antithrombin: structural and functional comparison to human plasma-derived antithrombin. *Blood* 91:4561, 1998.

Egeberg O: Inherited antithrombin deficiency causing thrombophilia. *Thromb Diath Haemorrh* 13:516, 1965.

Gallus AS et al: The relative contributions of antithrombin III during heparin treatment, and of clinically recognizable risk factors, to early recurrence of venous thromboembolism. *Thromb Res* 46:539, 1987.

Goodnight SH, Griffin J: *Hereditary Thrombophilia. Williams Hematology,* 6th ed., Beutler E et al. (eds.), New York, McGraw-Hill, 2001, Chapter 127.

Hathaway WE: Clinical aspects of antithrombin III deficiency. *Semin Hematol* 28:19, 1991.

Lane DA et al: Antithrombin mutation database: 2nd (1997) update for the Plasma Coagulation Inhibitors Subcommittee of the Scientific and Standardization Committee of the International Society on Thrombosis and Haemostasis. *Thromb Haemost* 77:197, 1997.

Manco-Johnson MJ: Neonatal antithrombin III deficiency. *Am J Med* 87:49S, 1989.

Menache D et al: Evaluation of the safety, recovery, half-life, and clinical efficacy of antithrombin III (human) in patients with hereditary antithrombin III deficiency. Cooperative Study Group. *Blood* 75:33, 1990.

Rosenberg RD, Aird WC: Vascular bed specific hemostasis and hypercoagulable states. *N Engl J Med* 340:1555, 1999.

Rosendaal FR: Thrombosis in the young: epidemiology and risk factors. A focus on venous thrombosis. *Thromb Hemost* 78:1, 1997.

Rosendaal FR et al: Mortality in hereditary antithrombin III deficiency—1830 to 1989. *Lancet* 337:260, 1991.

Tait RC et al: Prevalence of antithrombin deficiency in the healthy population. *Br J Haematol* 87:106, 1994.

Van Boven HH et al: Gene-gene and gene-environment interactions determine risk of thrombosis in families with inherited antithrombin deficiency. *Blood* 94:2590, 1999.

Van Boven HH et al: Antithrombin and its inherited deficiency states. *Sem Hematol* 34:188, 1997.

CHAPTER 38

Protein C Deficiency

Over the past two decades numerous clinical, biochemical, and genetic studies have documented protein C (PC) deficiency as a risk factor for hereditary and acquired thromboembolic disease. Protein C is a vitamin K-dependent zymogen for a serine protease that downregulates the coagulation cascade by proteolytic degradation of activated factor V (Va) and activated factor VIII (VIIIa). As with other forms of hereditary thrombophilia, such as protein S and antithrombin deficiencies, the most common sites of venous thrombosis are the deep veins of the legs and the mesenteric veins. Pulmonary embolism occurs in over 40 percent of cases. Cerebral venous and arterial thromboembolic events are rare. In severely affected families, over 50 percent of PC-deficient individuals experience thromboembolic disease by 45 years of age and two-thirds of these individuals will have recurrent thrombosis. Sixty percent of these thrombi occur spontaneously, with the remainder associated with acquired risk factors such as advanced age, immobilization, surgery, malignancy, oral contraceptives, pregnancy, and the antiphospholipid antibody syndrome. Acquired PC deficiencies have been associated with decreased synthesis and increased consumption of the protein due to a wide range of causes.

STRUCTURE AND FUNCTION

Protein C is a vitamin K-dependent glycoprotein with a Mr of 62,000 (462 amino acids) synthesized in the liver and present in plasma at a concentration of 60 nM. Figure 38-1 outlines the structure–function relationships of the PC molecule. Table 38-1 gives the biochemical characteristics of the components of the PC system. The mechanism of regulation of blood coagulation by the PC system is outlined in Fig. 38-2.

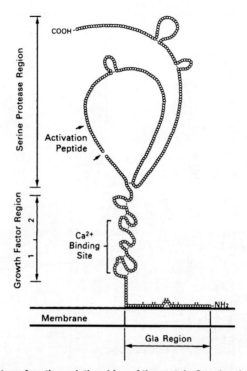

FIGURE 38-1 Structure–function relationships of the protein C molecule. Activation of protein C by thrombin–thrombomodulin complex depends on the presence of divalent cations; calcium is the most effective. A high-affinity binding site for calcium is located in the growth factor region (but probably closer to the heavy chain than depicted in the diagram). The binding of Ca^{++} to the high-affinity site (not the Gla domain) induces a confirmational change in the heavy chain allowing activation to a serine protease (see arrows), which subsequently cleaves activated factor V and factor VIII. (Used with permission of the American Society of Biochemistry and Molecular Biology, Inc. From Esmon CT: *J Biol Chem* 264:4743, 1989.)

HEREDITARY PROTEIN C DEFICIENCY

PC deficiency is autosomally inherited. Homozygous or compound heterozygous individuals may be either severely affected (PC < 0.01U/mL) and develop neonatal purpura fulminans, DIC, and other severe thrombotic complications, or moderately affected (PC level = 0.05 to 0.25U/mL), with recurrent thromboembolic disease later in life. Heterozygous PC, deficiency (plasma levels of PC 0.4 to 0.6 U/mL) has a prevalence of about 1 in 300 in the general population, but most of these individuals, including entire families, do not experience thromboembolic symptoms. In contrast, the incidence of symptomatic disease in PC deficiency is about 1 in 16,000. The clinical expression of thrombosis results from the cosegregation of more than one genetic risk factor and consequent cumu-

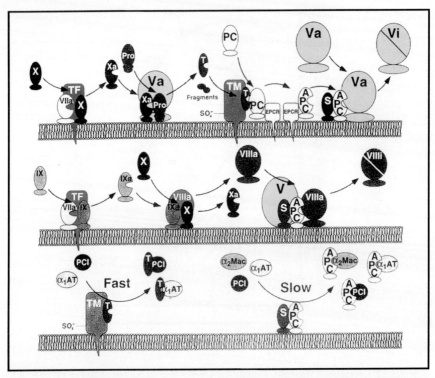

FIGURE 38-2 A simplified view of the regulation of blood coagulation by the protein C pathway. Factor VIIa (VIIa) binds to tissue factor (TF) to activate factor X (X), generating factor Xa (Xa). Factor Xa then binds to factor Va. The complex of factors Xa-V converts prothrombin (pro) to thrombin (T). Thrombin can then either bind to TM or carry out procoagulant reactions like fibrin formation or platelet activation. When bound to TM, thrombin can activate protein C (PC) to activated protein C (APC). This process is enhanced when protein C is bound to the endothelial cell protein C receptor (EPCR). Activated protein C bound to EPCR cleaves substrates other than factor Va. Activated protein C dissociates from EPCR and can then interact with protein S to inactivate factor Va. The middle row shows inactivation of the factor IXa (IXa)-factor VIIIa (VIIIa) complex by APC. In this case, factor V participates with APC and protein S in the inactivation of factor VIIIa. In the bottom row, the plasma proteinase inhibitors that regulate the protein C activation complex and the anticoagulant complex of APC and protein S are illustrated. The following abbreviations were used: α_1-antitrypsin (α_1-AT), α_2-macroglobulin (α_2-Mac), protein C inhibitor (PCI), and antithrombin (AT). For simplicity, the activation of factors VII, V and VIII are not shown. (Used with permission from Esmon CT et al: *Thromb Haemost* 82:251, 1999.)

lative or synergistic effects on thrombotic risk. For example, recent studies have demonstrated that factor V Leiden (Chap. 40) cosegregates with PC deficiency in about 20% of families, with disease penetrance considerably higher in those with two, compared to only one, genetic defect. The list of possible cosegregating risk factors is growing and includes factor V Leiden, hyperhomocysteinemia, high levels of factor VIII, and concurrence of protein S or antithrombin deficiency. Interestingly, the

TABLE 38-1

Proteins of the Protein C System

Protein	Chromosome	Gene (kb)	Exons	Plasma t½ (days)	Concentration (nM)	Molecular weight
Prothrombin	11	21	14	2.5	1400	72,000
Protein C	2q14-21	11	9	0.25	60	62,000
Protein S	3	80	15	1.75	300	75,000
Factor V	1q21-25	80	25	0.5	20	330,000
Factor VIII	Xq28	186	26	0.3–0.5	0.7	330,000
Thrombo-modulin	20p12-cen	3.7	Intronless	Unk	0.3 (soluble)	75,000
EPCR	20q11.2	6	4	Unk	2.5 (soluble)	49,000
PCI	14q32.1	11.5	5	Unk	90	57,000

Abbreviations: EPCR, endothelial protein C receptor; PCI, protein C inhibitor; Unk, unknown.

prothrombin G20210A polymorphism does not appear to confer additional risk of thrombosis in PC deficiency (Bovill 2000 ref). In unselected outpatients with a first thrombotic event, the relative risk of thrombosis related to PC deficiency is increased 6.5-fold. The relative risk of thrombosis is considerably higher in families with thrombophilia; the risk is further compounded by oral contraceptive use, pregnancy, and other acquired risk factors.

The most recent publication from the international database for PC gene mutations documents 160 unique mutations among 334 entries (Reitsma ref). The underlying genetic disorder does not appear different comparing symptomatic and asymptomatic PC-deficient individuals (e.g., asymptomatic parents of symptomatic homozygotes), further supporting the importance of cosegregating risk factors in pathogenesis of thrombophilia.

ACQUIRED DEFECTS

Acquired PC deficiency has been associated with intravascular consumptive processes including disseminated intravascular coagulation (DIC), acquired purpura fulminans (bacterial sepsis, varicella), severe preeclampsia, respiratory distress syndrome, the postoperative state, and IgG paraproteinemia (inhibitor to PC). Decreased synthesis of PC can be due to hepatocellular disease, oral anticoagulant therapy, vitamin K deficiency, L-asparaginase therapy, and methotrexate/cyclophosphamide/5-flourouracil therapy in breast cancer. Uremia has been associated with a dialyzable inhibitor of PC when measured using clotting-based PC assays.

Miscellaneous associations include postoperative liver transplant, hemodialysis, plasmapheresis, and sick newborn infants (respiratory distress syndrome and infants of diabetic mothers).

DIAGNOSIS AND MANAGEMENT

PC deficiency is most commonly identified using immunologic and functional assays on plasma samples. Phenotypically, two distinct subtypes are recognized. Type I deficiency is characterized by equal reduction of both PC antigen and activity levels due to reduced synthesis or stability of the abnormal allelic product. In type II deficiency, activity levels are reduced to a greater extent than antigen due to production and secretion of a dysfunctional protein. Type II deficiency can be further subtyped (II A, low clotting and low amidolytic activity; II B, low clotting but normal amidolytic activity). Table 38-2 gives a classification of PC deficiency based on assay results. For most clinical purposes, a clotting-based functional assay should be used, as this screens for the broadest set of abnormalities. Preterm infants have PC levels around 0.30 U/mL, which rise to 0.5 U/mL by term and reach adult levels (0.65 to 140 U/mL) by about 4 years of age. Protein C levels subsequently increase by 4 percent per decade.

Acquired disorders are identified by performing a PC activity assay in the appropriate clinical setting. Heterozygous PC deficiencies are more complex due to overlap of the normal and abnormal ranges at the lower end of the normal range. Values less than 0.55 U/mL can be confidently interpreted as consistent with heterozygous deficiency. Values between 0.55 and 0.65 U/mL could fit with either a deficiency state or the lower end of the normal range. The latter circumstance requires repeat measures and analysis of disease segregation within the family. As noted above, homozygotes and double heterozygotes have very low levels, which are usually proportionate to the severity of disease.

Patients presenting with symptomatic thromboembolic disease should be studied 2 to 3 weeks after heparin and warfarin therapy have been completed. If patients require long-term warfarin therapy they can be switched to subcutaneous low molecular weight heparin for 3 to 5 days to allow for measurement of PC levels after correction of the warfarin effect. Assays done during an acute illness (including thromboembolism), even if obtained before warfarin therapy is started, may be misleading, with low values due to accelerated consumption of PC. Molecular biologic techniques can define the underlying genetic mutation(s) and allow the design of simple PCR screening assays for specific mutations, a technique particularly useful in the study of family groups.

TABLE 38-2			
Assay Classification of Heterozygous PC Deficiency			
	Activity		
Types	**Clotting**	**Amidolytic**	**Antigen**
I (Common)	Low	Low	Low
II A	Low	Low	Normal
II B	Low	Normal	Normal

The acute management of heterozygous PC-deficient patients during and after a first episode of thrombosis or pulmonary embolism disease does not differ from other patients with thromboembolism. The institution and duration of warfarin therapy in the context of thrombophilia is discussed in Chapter 35.

Neonatal purpura fulminans and, less frequently, massive venous thrombosis in the neonate, although rare, should be considered to be due to homozygous or double-heterozygous PC or PS deficiency until proven otherwise. Left untreated, the condition will almost certainly lead to death due to thrombosis. Heparin alone has not been successful in the treatment of neonatal purpura fulminans, although it has been useful in an acquired form occurring at an older age. Measurements of PC are undetectable in the neonate and are at heterozygous levels in the parents. Symptoms resolve with heparin and FFP (which contains PC) at 10 to 20 mL/kg every 12 hours. Protein C concentrates are preferred to FFP and should be continued while lesions resolve over 6 to 8 weeks, followed by treatment with warfarin. The target INR for warfarin is 3 to 4.5 because of the risk of recurrent purpura fulminans. Patients with homozygous or double-heterozygous PC deficiency and PC levels of 5 to 20 percent in the plasma have been successfully treated with LMW heparin, although supplementation with PC may also be needed. Liver transplantation has also been successful in selected patients. Acquired severe PC deficiency (PC < 0.01 to 0.02 U/mL) secondary to infection (post-varicella, meningococcemia) has been successfully treated with a combination of heparin and PC concentrates. A similar approach may be useful in the acquired purpura fulminans syndrome in the sick neonate with thrombosis.

The occurrence of warfarin-induced skin necrosis has been associated with heterozygous and moderate homozygous (or double-heterozygous) PC deficiency. These progressive, purpuric skin lesions occur during the first few days of oral anticoagulant therapy, particularly following a loading dose of warfarin, due to the early depletion of PC ($t_{1/2}$ = 6 hr) compared to other vitamin K dependent factors, thus producing a relative state of hypercoagulability. The syndrome has been reported almost entirely in individuals treated for acute thromboembolic disease, in contrast to patients given prophylactic warfarin for chronic atrial fibrillation. In known PC-deficient individuals, heparin (or LMWH) should be administered during warfarin initiation. Warfarin should be started at low doses (e.g., 1 to 2 mg/day) and gradually increased after the first 2 to 3 days to slowly attain a therapeutic level. In patients with a history of warfarin skin necrosis, FFP and PC concentrates can be used during the initiation of anticoagulant therapy.

BIBLIOGRAPHY

Andrew M et al: Guidelines for antithrombotic therapy in pediatric patients. *J Pediatr* 132:575, 1998.

Bovill EG et al: The G20210A prothrombin polymorphism is not associated with increased thromboembolic risk in a large protein C deficient kindred. *Thromb Haemost* 83:366, 2000.

Bovill EG et al: Hereditary thrombophilia as a model for multigenic disease. *Thromb Haemost* 82:662, 1999.

De Stefano V et al: Clinical manifestations and management of inherited thrombophilia: retrospective analysis and follow-up after diagnosis of 238 patients with congenital deficiency of antithrombin III, protein C, protein S. *Thromb Haemost* 72:352, 1994.

Esmon C et al: Endothelial protein C receptor. *Thromb Haemost* 82:251, 1999.

Gerson WT et al: Severe acquired PC deficiency in purpura fulminans associated with disseminated intravascular coagulation: treatment with protein C concentrate. *J Pediatr* 9:418, 1993.

Koster T et al: Protein C deficiency in a controlled series of unselected outpatients: an infrequent but clear risk factor for venous thrombosis (Leiden thrombophilia study). *Blood* 85:2756, 1995.

Lane DA et al: Inherited thrombophilia: part I. *Thromb Haemost* 76:651, 1996.

Lane DA et al: Inherited thrombophilia: part II. *Thromb Haemost* 76:824, 1996.

Mann KG et al: Molecular biology, biochemistry, and lifespan of plasma coagulation factors. In Beutler E, et al. (eds.), *Williams Hematology* 5th edition, New York, McGraw-Hill, 1995, p 1206.

Monagle P et al: Homozygous protein C deficiency: description of a new mutation and successful treatment with low molecular weight heparin. *Thromb Haemost* 79:756, 1998.

Nesheim M et al: Thrombin, thrombomodulin and TAFI in the molecular link between coagulation and fibrinolysis. *Thromb Haemost* 78:386, 1997.

Reitsma PH et al: Protein C deficiency: a database of mutations, 1995 update. On behalf of the Subcommittee on Plasma Coagulation Inhibitors of the Scientific and Standardization Committee of the ISTH. *Thromb Haemost* 73:876, 1995.

Rosendaal FR: Risk factors for venous thromboembolic disease. *Thromb Haemost* 82:610, 1999.

Smith OP, White B: Infectious purpura fulminans: diagnosis and treatment. *Br J Haematol* 104:202, 1999.

Suzuki K et al: Protein C inhibitor: structure and function. *Thromb Haemost* 61:337, 1989.

Tait RC et al: Prevalence of protein C deficiency in the healthy population. *Thromb Haemost* 73:87, 1995.

CHAPTER 39

Protein S Deficiency

Protein S (PS) is a vitamin K-dependent plasma glycoprotein that serves as the cofactor for the anticoagulant function of activated protein C (APC) in inactivating factors Va and VIIIa. It also has been shown to directly bind to and inhibit factors Va, VIIIa, and Xa. PS is synthesized in hepatocytes, endothelial cells (EC), and other tissues. Hereditary deficiency of PS is associated with a thrombotic tendency.

STRUCTURE–FUNCTION RELATIONSHIP

Protein S (Mr 69,000) is a vitamin K-dependent, nonenzymatic cofactor to APC; PS and APC form a 1:1 stoichiometric complex on the surface of negatively charged phospholipid membranes (platelet, EC). Protein S, which circulates in plasma in the concentration of 20 to 25 µg/mL, is synthesized by vascular EC; hepatocytes; megakaryocytes; and cells of human testes, kidney, and brain. As shown in Fig. 39-1, PS contains multiple domains: from the NH2 terminus, the Gla-containing domain (phospholipid binding), the thrombin-sensitive region, four epidermal growth factor (EGF)-like domains (calcium binding and cofactor function), followed by a region homologous to a sex hormone binding globulin (binding to C4BP).

Protein S exists in two distinct forms in plasma. Approximately 40 percent occurs as free PS, the remainder being reversibly bound to a high molecular weight (570 kDa) protein, C4b binding protein (C4BP). Only free PS has cofactor activity for APC; however the binding of PS to C4BP does not directly affect the complement regulatory function of C4BP. C4BP is composed of two types of polypeptide chains, an α chain of Mr 72,000 and a β chain of Mr 45,000. C4BP molecules are heterogeneous; the

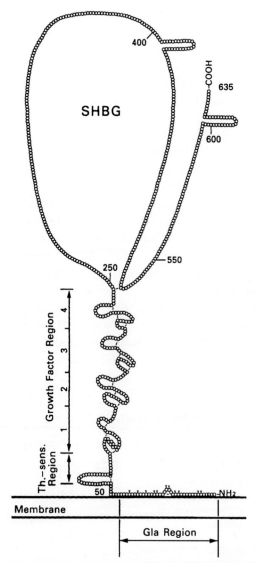

FIGURE 39-1 Molecular model of protein S. Protein S is depicted binding to phospholipids of the cell membrane by means of the Gla (glutamic acid residues) domain at the NH$_2$ terminal portion of the molecule. The EGF (epidermal growth factor) domains are numbered 1, 2, 3, and 4 and represent the calcium-binding cofactor function region. The region homologous to a sex hormone binding globulin (SHBG) functions to bind protein S to C4BP Th-sens, thrombin-sensitive region. (Used with permission of the American Society of Biochemistry and Molecular Biology, Inc. From Esmon CT: *J Biol Chem* 264:4743, 1989.)

common oligomer is a spiderlike structure with seven α chains and a β chain (only the β-chain–containing molecule binds PS). Since C4BP is an acute phase reactant, the total amount of PS bound varies widely according to the total quantity and relative amount of β-chain–containing C4BP present in a given condition; e.g., the level of free PS may be decreased in inflammatory or related conditions (Table 39-1). Elevated levels of free PS, which occur in the rare disorder of familial C4BP deficiency, are not associated with hemorrhagic tendencies.

The existence of two forms of PS in the plasma, free or complexed with C4BP, can complicate laboratory assays. The equilibrium between the two forms depends on the functional integrity of both proteins as well as the concentration of C4BP (especially the β chain molecules). Immunologic assays using treatments to dissociate (dilute plasma, incubation) or remove (polyethylene glycol adsorption) the complexed form allows quantitative measurements of bound PS, free PS, or both (total PS). Functional assays of PS using PS-depleted plasma and clotting time assays can be used to determine the clotting cofactor function (inactivation of factor Va by APC) of free PS. The clotting time assay usually approximates the free PS. In some assay systems for free protein S, the presence of factor V Leiden may yield falsely low levels of functional protein S, although this problem has been reduced with newer assays. Physiologic variations

---

TABLE 39-1

Conditions Associated with Acquired Protein S Deficiency

Conditions with increased C4BP (acute phase reaction, hormonal)
  Pregnancy
  Oral contraceptive agents
  Diabetes mellitus
  Inflammation (inflammatory bowel disease, stasis ulcers)
  Systemic lupus erythematosus
  Male tobacco smokers
  AIDS
  Renal allograft rejection
  Nephrosis (plus selective urinary loss)
Conditions with decreased synthesis (PS, C4BP, or both)
  Preterm and term infants
  Liver disease
  Vitamin K deficiency
  Coumadin therapy
  Chemotherapy for breast cancer
Conditions with increased cell binding of PS
  Polycythemia vera
  Sickle cell disease
  Essential thrombocythemia

include a lower mean free PS level in normal females than normal males, lower free PS in pregnancy and women on oral contraceptives, and lower total and free PS in newborn infants.

GENETICS

The cDNA for human PS has been cloned and fully characterized. There are two copies of the gene, called PS α and PS β; both are located on chromosome 3. On the basis of multiple base changes in PS β (termination codons, frameshifts), it is considered a pseudogene.

Protein S deficiency is inherited in an autosomal dominant manner similar to that of protein C (PC) deficiency. Over 100 different mutations in the protein S gene associated with thrombosis have been identified. The most common heterozygous type I deficiency state is associated with about 50 percent of the normal total PS antigen and decreases of free antigen and functional (clotting assay) PS to about 30 to 40 percent of normal. The usual type II heterozygote (normal level of total PS and free PS antigen but low functional PS) is relatively rare; a more common type has been described with normal total PS, but low free and functional PS, designated as type III. Double heterozygotes with markedly low levels of free and functional PS are known; in addition, data on two infants with (1) homozygous PS deficiency and (2) compound heterozygous PS deficiency who presented with neonatal purpura fulminans and low or undetectable PS antigen or activity (Fig. 39-2) have been described. Screening tests for hereditary PS deficiency include either free protein S antigen or a PS functional (clotting) assay.

CLINICAL MANIFESTATIONS OF PROTEIN S DEFICIENCY

Events including recurrent deep vein thrombosis (DVT), pulmonary embolism, cerebral and mesenteric thrombosis, superficial thrombophlebitis, and arterial thromboses (cerebral and occlusive disease) are seen in many PS heterozygotes before age 40, but rarely before age 15 years. Approximately 3% of unselected consequentive outpatients presenting with venous thromboembolism will be found to have PS deficiency. Reported odds ratios for thrombosis have varied considerably in the literature, from 1.6 to 11.5. The higher odds ratios may reflect concomitant thrombophilic defects such as factor V Leiden. Thrombosis recurrence rates are 3 to 4% per year. Arterial thrombosis seems to occur more frequently in subjects with PS deficiency than in other thrombophilic states, and is often associated with smoking, obesity, or other acquired arterial risk factors. Homozygous and compound heterozygous PS deficiency is associated with neonatal purpura fulminans (Fig. 39-2).

As in PC deficiency, the many causes of acquired PS deficiency (Table 39-1) make the precise diagnosis and classification of hereditary PS defects more difficult. The low levels of free PS in inflammatory conditions such as systemic lupus erythematosis, nephrotic syndrome, thrombophlebitis, or even diabetes mellitus may be associated with the higher C4BP concentrations (increased bound or complexed PS). Unlike PC, PS is less likely to be reduced in disseminated intravascular coagulation (DIC), sepsis, and septic shock. Acquired PS deficiency is seen in patients with a lupus anticoagulant, and has also been reported as a sequela to varicella infections in children.

MANAGEMENT

The heterozygous form of PS deficiency may be discovered at any age; unlike PC deficiency, even newborn infants who have moderately low total PS on a physiologic basis (level about 25 percent) have near normal levels of free or functional PS (levels about 50 percent of adult value). This observation is related to near-absent levels of C4BP in the fetus and newborn; by

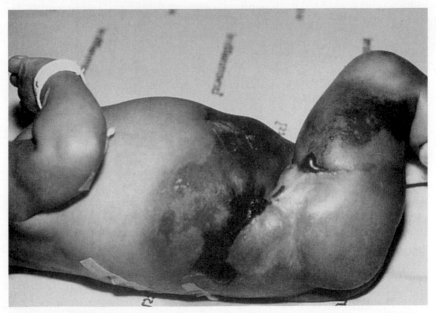

FIGURE 39-2 Homozygous protein S deficiency. Note purpuric and necrotic skin lesions.

6 months of age adult levels are approximated. Thrombotic events are rare in children and begin to occur at adolescence (similar to PC deficiency). Management of PS heterozygotes who have a thrombotic event is essentially the same as that of PC deficiency, i.e., initial heparinization and fibrinolytic therapy if indicated, followed by gradual institution of warfarin therapy. Warfarin-induced skin necrosis has occurred in PS deficiency.

To date, two infants with homozygous or compound heterozygous PS deficiency have been described. Both had purpura fulminans, CNS, and ocular lesions (like severe neonatal PC deficiency) in association with very low to undetectable PS. Both infants were successfully managed by administration of fresh frozen plasma and warfarin therapy. Thrombotic episodes and DIC tend to recur without periodic (at least once weekly fresh frozen plasma infusion) administration of PS-containing material. PS has a half-life of 36 to 60 h.

BIBLIOGRAPHY

Comp PC et al: Familial protein S deficiency is associated with recurrent thrombosis. *J Clin Invest* 74:2082, 1984.

D'Angelo A et al: Autoimmune protein S deficiency in a boy with severe thromboembolic disease. *N Eng J Med* 328:1753, 1993.

Dahlback B: Protein S and C4b-binding protein: Components involved in the regulation of the protein C anticoagulant system. *Thromb Haemost* 66:49, 1991.

De Stefano V et al: Clinical manifestations and management of inherited thrombophilia: Retrospective analysis and follow-up after diagnosis of 238 patients with congenital deficiency of antithrombin III, protein C, protein S. *Thromb Haemost* 72:352, 1994.

Esmon CT: The roles of protein C and the thrombomodulin in the regulation of blood coagulation. *J Biol Chem* 264:4743, 1989.

Faioni EM et al: Free protein S deficiency is a risk factor for venous thrombosis. *Thromb Haemost* 78:1343, 1997.

Gandrille S et al: Protein S deficiency: A database of mutations. For the Plasma Coagulation Inhibitors Subcommittee of the Scientific and Standardization Committee of the International Society on Thrombosis and Haemostasis. *Thromb Haemost* 77:1201, 1997.

Ginsberg JS et al: Acquired free protein S deficiency is associated with antiphospholipid antibodies and increased thrombin generation in patients with systemic lupus erythematosus. *Am J Med* 98:379, 1995.

Gomez E et al: Homozygous protein S deficiency due to a one base pair deletion that leads to a stop codon in exon III of the protein S gene. *Thromb Haemost* 71:723, 1994.

Heeb MJ et al: Protein S binds to and inhibits factor Xa. *Proc Natl Acad Sci USA* 91:2728, 1994.

Koeleman BPC et al: Factor V leiden: an additional risk factor for thrombosis in protein S deficient families? *Thromb Haemost* 74:580, 1995.

Malm J et al: Changes in the plasma levels of vitamin K-dependent proteins C and S and of C4b-binding protein during pregnancy and oral contraception. *Br J Haematol* 68:437, 1988.

Malm J et al: Plasma concentrations of C4b-binding protein and vitamin K-dependent protein S in term and preterm infants: Low levels of protein S-C4b-binding protein complexes. *Br J Haemat* 68:445, 1988.

Manco-Johnson MJ et al: Lupus anticoagulant and protein S deficiency in children with postvaricella purpura fulminans or thrombosis. *J Pediatr* 128:319, 1996.

Pabinger I et al: The risk of thromboembolism in asymptomatic patients with protein C and protein S deficiency. A prospective cohort study. *Thromb Haemost* 71:441, 1994.

Pung-amritt P et al: Compound heterozygosity for one novel and one recurrent mutation in a Thai patient with severe protein S deficiency. *Thromb Haemost* 81:189, 1999.

Simmonds RE et al: Clarification of the risk for venous thrombosis associated with hereditary protein S deficiency by investigation of a large kindred with a characterized gene defect. *Ann Int Med* 128:8, 1998.

Van Wijnen M et al: A plasma coagulation assay for an activated protein C-independent anticoagulant activity of protein S. *Thromb Haemost* 80:930, 1998.

CHAPTER 40

Factor V Leiden, Prothrombin Gene Mutation, and Elevated Factor VIII

In the last seven years three of the most common risk factors for venous thromboembolism (VTE) have been identified: factor V Leiden, the prothrombin gene mutation, and high levels of factor VIII. Each defect confers a mild to moderate increased risk of thrombosis; i.e., an odds ratio of ~4. Because these abnormalities are so frequent, one or more are found in up to one-third of patients presenting with VTE. Moreover, combined disorders (as a result of gene–gene interactions) are seen regularly, and if present, lead to an even greater likelihood of thrombosis. Although the pathologic mechanisms underlying the three disorders are diverse, all most likely promote thrombosis via an increased generation of thrombin at injury sites, shifting the hemostatic balance in a prothrombotic direction.

ETIOLOGY AND PATHOGENESIS

Factor V Leiden

In 1993 Dahlback first described families with thrombosis whose plasma was resistant to the effects of activated protein C. The defect was found to reside in factor V; i.e., glutamine changed to arginine at amino acid 506, due to a G to A transition at nucleotide 1691. The abnormal factor V was named Factor V Leiden. This point mutation makes factor Va resistant to the proteolytic action of activated protein C (APC) so that activated factor V persists, rather than being inactivated by the serine protease (Fig. 40-1).

FACTOR V LEIDEN

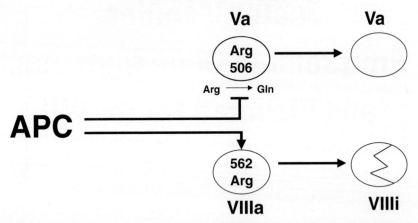

FIGURE 40-1 Diagram of the molecular defect in the factor V Leiden mutation. Normally, activated protein C (APC) cleaves factors Va and VIIIa, which results in the inactivation of the clotting factors, e.g., VIIIi. The factor V Leiden mutation involves a glutamine (Gln) instead of an arginine (Arg) at position 506, which blocks the action of APC and allows persistence of activated factor V.

From 3 to 8 percent of Caucasians are heterozygous for the factor V Leiden defect, 1/1000 are homozygous, and a very few are "pseudo-homozygotes," who have factor V Leiden combined with heterozygous factor V deficiency. The factor V Leiden mutation is thought to have arisen ~30,000 years ago in a single Caucasian progenitor living in Europe. The evolutionary advantage of factor V Leiden is not known with certainty, but could reflect reduced intrapartum blood loss or lessened bleeding after trauma.

It should be noted that >90 percent of subjects who are resistant to the action of APC will have factor V Leiden on genetic testing. Other causes of APC resistance include treatment with oral contraceptives, the presence of a lupus anticoagulant, and other rare genetic defects in factor V. APC-resistance assays are discussed in the section on laboratory diagnosis.

Many clinical studies have shown clearly that the odds ratio (OR) for thrombosis in subjects with factor V Leiden is increased 2 to 8-fold, but because the defect is so common, it accounts for 20 to 25 percent of venous thromboses. In the Physicians Health Study, the relative risk of primary (idiopathic) venous thromboembolism was increased to 3.5, which rose further with age (>60 yr) to 7.0 (Fig. 40-2). However, the baseline risk of thrombosis is rather low at ~0.45 percent/year, as estimated

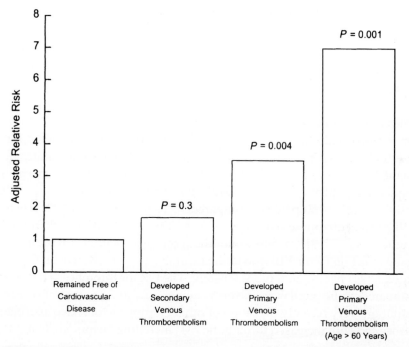

FIGURE 40-2 Adjusted relative risks for future venous thromboembolism among apparently healthy men with the factor V Leiden mutation. Secondary venous thromboembolism includes events associated with cancer, surgery, or trauma. (Adapted with permission from Ridker et al: _N Engl J Med_ 332: 912, 1995.)

from new thrombosis rates in relatives of symptomatic carriers of the defect.

Prothrombin Gene Mutation

In 1996, a genetic defect (nt G20210A) was discovered in the 3' untranslated region of the prothrombin gene that was linked to an increased risk of VTE. The mutation was associated with elevated levels of prothrombin (~130 percent by either antigen or activity assays). The increased concentration of prothrombin could contribute to thrombotic risk by promoting enhanced thrombin generation. Individuals who have increased levels of prothrombin, but without the prothrombin gene mutation, also have an increased risk of thrombosis. The prothrombin gene mutation (heterozygous) is found in about 2 to 3 percent of Caucasians, and has been identified in 4 to 8 percent of subjects presenting with a first VTE. The OR of thromboses is increased 2 to 6-fold. Rare homozygotes have been reported who have an even greater likelihood of thrombosis.

Elevated Levels of Factor VIII

Recently, an association between elevated levels of factor VIII (>150 percent as measured by an activity assay) and venous thrombosis has been recognized. Inflammatory states, ABO blood group (group O), and increased von Willebrand factor are all associated with high factor VIII activity, but the association with thrombosis persists when these variables are factored into the statistical analyses. Moreover, family studies have suggested that high (or low) factor VIII levels are hereditary, although a specific polymorphism in the factor VIII gene that determines factor VIII levels has not yet been identified. As many as 23 percent of sequential patients presenting with thrombosis will have factor VIII activity levels >150 percent, compared to 11 percent of controls. Factor VIII is an acute-phase reactant; however, the factor VIII assays in these studies were obtained many months after presentation, excluding an acute effect on factor VIII due to the thrombosis itself. Moreover, the elevated levels persist on repeated testing. The OR for thromboses has been estimated to be similar to factor V Leiden and the prothrombin gene mutation. Very recently, elevation of other clotting factors have also been associated with increased thrombotic risk, including factors XI, X, and IX.

CLINICAL ASPECTS

Factor V Leiden, the prothrombin gene mutation, and elevated levels of factor VIII are each associated with a mild to moderate increased risk of VTE. Deep venous thrombosis (DVT) is most common, but superficial thrombophlebitis and more unusual thromboses, such as abdominal or cerebral vein thrombosis, have been reported. Of interest, factor V Leiden has been found to have a lower risk of PE than other thrombophilic states. Whether factor V Leiden and the prothrombin gene mutation are linked to arterial thromboses (e.g., myocardial infarction [MI], stroke) is a matter of some controversy. Several studies have shown an increased risk of MI in the presence of the mutations (e.g., OR 1.5), which is substantially increased (up to 3.5 or higher) if other arterial risk factors are present (e.g., smoking, diabetes, hypertension). However, other large studies (e.g., The Physicians Health Study) were unable to demonstrate an association with MI or stroke.

Because these thrombophilic defects are so common, the likelihood of gene–gene interactions (i.e., two or more mutations in the same individual) or gene–environment interactions (e.g., factor V Leiden and oral contraceptives) is exceedingly common. In fact, the great majority of thromboses in affected individuals are likely due to the presence of multiple defects (see Fig. 35-1). In many instances the presence of a second hereditary defect or environmental risk factor multiplies the risk of thrombosis (rather than being simply additive).

Of the many environmental risk factors for thrombosis, estrogens play a prominent role, particularly in patients with factor V Leiden or the prothrombin gene mutation. For example, more than 45 percent of pregnant women with a VTE will be found to have factor V Leiden, and in a study of 40 patients (mostly young women on oral contraceptives) with cerebral vein thrombosis, 20 percent had the prothrombin gene mutation. The use of oral contraceptive agents in women with factor V Leiden increase the OR for thromboses 30 to 80 fold, with the absolute increase in risk rising from 0.8 to 28.5/10,000 women/year. The magnitude of a possible increase in risk for the use of hormone replacement therapy in women with thrombophilia is not yet known, but it is likely to be significantly elevated.

Finally, pregnancy loss and other pregnancy-related complications (e.g., preeclampsia, fetal growth retardation) are associated with the entire spectrum of thrombophilic states, and are most probably due to placental vascular insufficiency as a consequence of thrombosis. Several studies have shown that the OR of pregnancy loss (stillbirth) is increased to ~3.5 in women with factor V Leiden or the prothrombin gene mutation (see Chap. 51).

LABORATORY DIAGNOSIS

The factor V Leiden and prothrombin gene mutations are readily identified using standard DNA diagnostic methods, and are now available in many laboratories. Prothrombin concentrations can be measured by standard activity or antigen assays, but as yet these tests are not sufficiently sensitive or specific to identify subjects with the prothrombin gene mutation. Factor VIII levels are measured in a standard one-stage factor VIII assay or by a chromogenic assay.

The second-generation APC-resistance assay (currently widely used) can be employed as a screening test for factor V Leiden, since the test readily separates heterozygotes, homozygotes, and pseudohomozygotes from normals. In this test, purified APC is added to patient plasma diluted (1/5) in factor-V–deficiency plasma, and the ability of the APC to prolong the APTT or other clotting time test is determined. The test reflects the ability of the APC to cleave factor Va (and VIIIa), which prolongs the APTT. Results are usually expressed as a ratio of the clotting time (in seconds) of patient plasma with APC divided by the clotting time of the plasma without APC. A low ratio (e.g., 1.6) suggests APC-resistance (normal range 2 to 2.6).

The first-generation APC resistance test is performed as described, except that the patient plasma is not diluted in factor-V–deficient plasma. Consequently the assay is sensitive to other disorders that can modify the effects of APC on factors V or VIII (e.g., elevated levels of factor VIII, protein S deficiency), which can shorten the APTT and therefore lower the clotting time ratio. However, abnormal first-generation APC-resistance tests also identify subjects at risk of thrombosis, in addition to those with factor V Leiden. Recently the APC-resistance test has been further modified, in which a dilute tissue factor test system is used, and the quantity of endogenous thrombin generation is estimated by measuring the area under the thrombin-generation curve. This test appears to have increased sensitivity and is able to distinguish the greater APC-resistance produced by third-generation, as compared to second-generation, oral contraceptives (see Chap. 51).

THERAPY

Standard protocols for heparin or LMW heparin followed by oral anticoagulants (INR 2-3) are used for treatment of thrombosis in patients with factor V Leiden, the prothrombin gene mutation, or elevated factor VIII levels. The optimal duration of antithrombotic therapy is not yet clear and must be individualized. In general, patients with a single thrombophilic defect and a first provoked DVT should be treated for six months, presuming the provoking factor was transient or can be removed (e.g., cessation of birth control pills). Patient with recurrent thromboses, particularly if unprovoked ("spontaneous") may require long-term treatment. Additional suggestions for therapy are covered in Chapter 36. The ability of anticoagulant therapy (e.g., SC heparin or LMWH) to prevent recurrent pregnancy loss or other pregnancy-related complications in thrombophilic women is not yet clear. However it seems likely that heparins given in prophylactic (not therapeutic) doses may prove to be safe and effective (see Chap. 51).

BIBLIOGRAPHY

Dahlback B: Inherited thrombophilia: resistance to activated protein C as a pathogenic factor of venous thromboembolism. *Blood* 85:607, 1995.

De Visser MC et al: A reduced sensitivity for activated protein C in the absence of factor V Leiden increases the risk of venous thrombosis. *Blood* 93:1271, 1999.

Gerhardt A et al: Prothrombin and factor V mutations in women with a history of thrombosis during pregnancy and the puerperium. *N Engl J Med* 342:374, 2000.

Hirsh J et al: Duration of anticoagulant therapy after first episode of venous thrombosis in patients with inherited thrombophilia. *Arch Intern Med* 157:2174, 1997.

Kamphuisen PW et al: Increased levels of factor VIII and fibrinogen in patients with venous thrombosis are not caused by acute phase reactions. *Thromb Haemost* 81:680, 1999.

Koster T et al: Role of clotting factor VIII in effect of von Willebrand factor on occurrence of deep-vein thrombosis. *Lancet* 345:152, 1995.

Koster T et al: Venous thrombosis due to poor anticoagulant response to activated protein-C-Leiden Thrombophilia Study. *Lancet* 342:1503, 1993.

Kraaijenhagen RA et al: High plasma concentration of factor VIIIc is a major risk factor for venous thromboembolism. *Thromb Haemost* 83: 5, 2000.

Kupferminc MJ et al: Increased frequency of genetic thrombophilia in women with complications of pregnancy. *N Engl J Med* 340:9, 1999.

Lindmarker P et al: The risk of recurrent venous thromboembolism in carriers and non-carriers of the G1691A allele in the coagulation factor V gene and the G20210A allele in the prothrombin gene. *Thromb Haemost* 81:684, 1999.

Lindqvist PG et al: Factor V Q^{506} mutation (activated protein C resistance) associated with reduced intrapartum blood loss-a possible evolutionary selection mechanism. *Thromb Haemost* 79:69, 1998.

Margaglione M et al: Increased risk for venous thrombosis in carriers of the prothrombin G—>A^{20210} gene variant. *Ann Intern Med* 129:89, 1998.

Martinelli I et al: High risk of cerebral-vein thrombosis in carriers of a prothrombin-gene mutation and in users of oral contraceptives. *N Engl J Med* 338:1793, 1998.

Martinelli I et al: Heightened thrombin generation in individuals with resistance to activated protein C. *Thromb Haemost* 75:703, 1996.

Middeldorp S et al: The incidence of venous thromboembolism in family members of patients with factor V Leiden mutation and venous thrombosis. *Ann Intern Med* 128:15, 1998.

Poort SR et al: A common genetic variation in the 3'-untranslated region of the prothrombin gene is associated with elevated plasma prothrombin levels and an increase in venous thrombosis. *Blood* 88:3698, 1996.

Price DT, Ridker PM: Factor V Leiden mutation and the risks for thromboembolic disease: A clinical perspective. *Ann Intern Med* 127:895, 1997.

Ridker PM et al: G20210A mutation in prothrombin gene and risk of myocardial infarction, stroke, and venous thrombosis in a large cohort of US men. *Circulation* 99:999, 1999.

Rosendaal FR: High levels of factor VIII and venous thrombosis. *Thromb Haemost* 83:1, 2000.

Rosendaal FR: Risk factors for venous thrombotic disease. *Thromb Haemost* 82:610, 1999.

Rosendaal FR: Venous thrombosis: a multicausal disease. *Lancet* 353:1167, 1999.

Rosendaal FR et al: A common prothrombin variant (20210 G to A) increases the risk of myocardial infarction in young women. *Blood* 90:1747, 1997.

Rosendaal FR et al: Factor V Leiden (resistance to activated protein C) increases the risk of myocardial infarction in young women. *Blood* 89:2817, 1997.

Salomon O et al: Single and combined prothrombotic factors in patients with idiopathic venous thromboembolism—prevalence and risk assessment. *Arterioscler Thromb Vasc Biol* 19:511, 1999.

Svensson PJ, Dahlbäck B: Resistance to activated protein C as a basis for venous thrombosis. *N Engl J Med* 330:517, 1994.

Vandenbroucke JP et al: Increased risk of venous thrombosis in oral-contraceptive users who are carriers of factor V Leiden mutation. *Lancet* 344:1453, 1994.

Zivelin A et al: A single genetic origin for a common Caucasian risk factor for venous thrombosis. *Blood* 89:397, 1997.

Chapter 41

Fibrinolytic Defects and Thrombosis

Defects in the fibrinolytic system are attractive candidates as risk factors for venous and arterial thrombosis given the central role of fibrin generation and fibrin lysis in thrombosis. Prins and Hirsh, who reviewed the evidence for a causal role of hypofibrinolysis in symptomatic venous thrombosis in 1991, concluded that there was no evidence for an increased thrombotic risk associated with impaired fibrinolytic activity. However, they did find an association between impaired fibrinolysis and postoperative thrombosis. The latter observation requires confirmation with prospective trials. Clinical reports since 1991 continue to support the conclusion that measuring components of the fibrinolytic system are not useful in the diagnosis and management of venous thrombosis, with the exception of the identification of abnormal fibrinogen molecules (dysfibrinogenemias). On the arterial side of the circulation a weak association has been established between high levels of PAI-1 and recurrent myocardial infarction.

Transgenic mice lacking either the tissue plasminogen activator (t-PA) or urokinase-like plasminogen activator (u-PA) gene are normal at birth and have normal survival, reflecting the complementary nature of these two pathways for plasminogen activation and, in part, explaining the lack of association between fibrinolytic impairment and thrombotic disease in humans. However, the double u-PA/t-PA transgenic knockout and plasminogen knockout mouse models exhibit overt thrombotic disease with shortened life span, further evidence for the importance of redundancy in this system. The recently recognized role for u-PA and plasmin in the activation of matrix metalloproteinases (MMP) may play an important role in the process of arteriosclerosis through modulation of extracellular matrix degradation. Figure 41-1 outlines the expanded role of the fibrinolytic system to include MMP activation.

PATHOGENESIS

Decreased or Dysfunctional Plasminogen

At least 30 families have been reported with hereditary abnormalities of plasminogen synthesis. Half of these individuals had decreases in both plasminogen activity and antigen (type I), and the remainder had dysfunctional proteins caused by a variety of defects that usually involved the active center of the protein (type II). The majority of patients have been heterozygous for the disorder. Most of the studies of plasminogen defects come from Japan, where an autosomal dominant mode of inheri-

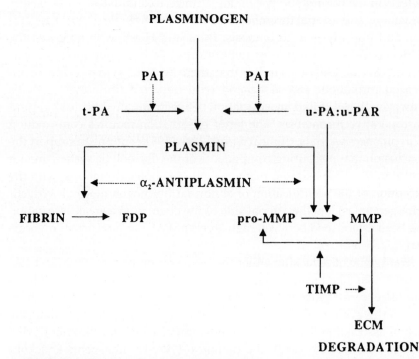

FIGURE 41-1 Schematic representation of the fibrinolytic system. PAI-plasminogen activator inhibitor; t-PA-tissue-type plasminogen activator; u-PA-urokinase-type plasminogen activator; U-PAR-urokinase-type plasminogen activator receptor; MMP-matrix metalloproteinase; ECM-extracellular matrix; TIMP-tissue inhibitor of metalloproteinase. Note that plasmin can convert latent pro-MMPs into the active form of the enzymes which in turn degrade extracellular matrix. Inhibition of the system may occur via PAI, α_2-antiplasmin, or TIMP. (Used with permission from Collen D: *Thromb Haemost* 82:259, 1999.)

tance has been observed with a gene frequency of 0.018. In the Japanese families the propositus was identified because of thromboembolic disease. Surprisingly, although the biochemical defect was genetically transmitted to other family members, it was not associated with manifestations of clinical thromboembolism.

Recently, two unrelated individuals with severe plasminogen deficiency, each homozygosity for a different point mutation in the plasminogen gene were observed to suffer from ligneous conjunctivitis, but not thrombotic disease. The conjunctivitis responded to plasminogen infusions.

Reduced Synthesis of Plasminogen Activators

Rare families have been described with thrombophilia and reduced post-venous occlusion fibrinolytic enhancement, usually due to high levels of PAI-1, but not to decreased levels of t-PA or u-PA. Reevaluation of two of these families revealed no clear relationship of the thrombosis to hypofibrinolysis, but rather to the presence of protein S deficiency. When low levels of t-PA were observed following venous occlusion in families with thrombosis, the laboratory studies only measured t-PA antigen, with no supporting molecular biologic evidence of a genetic defect.

High Resting Levels of Plasma Plasminogen Activator Inhibitor

Because PAI-1 behaves as an acute-phase reactant, elevated concentrations of PAI-1 antigen or activity in the blood are rather common, which complicates their interpretation in patients with thromboembolic disease. Circulating PAI-1 is bound tightly to vitronectin, which protects the inhibitor from inactivation and perhaps helps target the fibrinolytic inhibitor to sites of vascular injury. PAI-1 levels are strongly and positively correlated with triglyceride concentration, which further complicates interpretation of PAI-1 assay results, especially in the presence of cardiovascular disease. A polymorphism in the promoter region of the PAI-1 gene (4G/5G) has been correlated with circulating levels of PAI-1. The 4G allele was associated with enhanced gene expression and decreased fibrinolysis among the DVT patients. The role of this polymorphism in the pathogenesis of venous thromboembolism remains to be determined (Sartori ref).

Dysfibrinogenemias

Hundreds of mutations have been discovered that involve the fibrinogen molecule. Most of the dysfibrinogenemias produce bleeding, but 10 to 15 percent of the defects are associated with thrombosis (see Chap. 18). In a few cases, hemorrhage and thrombosis can both occur if the plasma concentration of the dysfunctional fibrinogen is low.

Some of the dysfibrinogenemias predispose to thrombosis because the abnormal fibrinogen generates fibrin that is resistant to fibrinolysis. One of these abnormal fibrinogens forms plasma clots that fail to lyse when they are placed in a solution containing plasmin. This has been designated fibrinogen Chapel Hill III (Fig. 41-2). Other fibrinogens produce fibrin that is unable to bind t-PA. Yet another fibrinogen (Milano II) cannot bind thrombin, so that higher residual concentrations of thrombin react with normal fibrinogen and accelerate thrombogenesis. Many dysfunctional fibrinogen molecules associated with thrombosis produce fi-

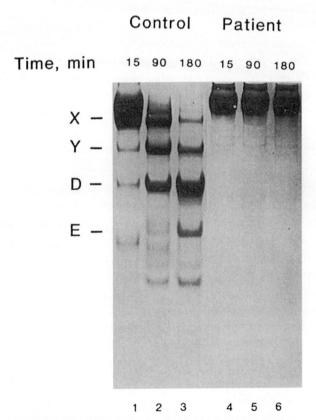

FIGURE 41-2 Sodium dodecyl sulfate polyacrylamide electrophoresis of patient and control fibrin samples treated with plasmin. On the left (lanes 1, 2, and 3) multiple fibrin degradation products are formed from normal fibrin. On the right (lanes 4, 5, and 6), fibrinolysis is absent. The patient was a 16-year-old male with recurrent deep and superficial venous thrombosis and a pulmonary embolism. (Used with permission from Carrell N et al: *Blood* 62:439, 1983.)

brin clots that are physically rigid or appear translucent on visual inspection.

Factor XII Deficiency

Fibrinolysis occurs both on the surface of cells (endothelium or platelets) and in the plasma, where it is stimulated by activation of the intrinsic system. Patients with severe (homozygous) deficiencies of factor XII have deficient fluid-phase fibrinolysis when measured in vitro, and have occasionally been reported to have venous thromboembolism (e.g., Mr. Hageman, the index patient with factor XII deficiency died of a massive pulmonary embolism following a pelvic fracture).

Matrix Metalloproteinases (MMP)

The MMPs (collagenase, elastase, etc.) can produce extracellular matrix proteolysis, thus enabling inflammatory, malignant, endothelial, and smooth muscle cells to migrate through the extracellular matrix, and also cause the release and activation of cytokines, growth factors, and other bound matrix components (Fig. 41-1). Investigation of transgenic mouse models has revealed a role for MMPs in angiogenesis, wound healing, growth and metastasis of malignancies, arteriosclerosis, ischemic myocardial disease, and infection. A more complete understanding of the regulation and actions of MMPs is likely to help elucidate the pathogenesis of arterial atherothrombosis.

LABORATORY STUDIES

Unfortunately, global screening tests are not yet available to detect impairment of the fibrinolytic system. Prolongation of the euglobulin lysis time (ELT) has not proven to be a reliable indicator of defective fibrinolysis. Assays are now available for measuring antigen and activity concentrations of t-PA, u-PA, and PAI-1. These assays can be performed on plasma from individuals who are in a resting state or following stimulation of fibrinolysis (by venous occlusion for 10 to 15 min or an infusion of DDAVP) to measure fibrinolytic "capacity." The value of these assays for clinical study of patients with hereditary or acquired thromboembolic disease remains uncertain. Some of the difficulties inherent in these assays include dietary influences, diurnal variations in fibrinolytic activity, and inconsistent results after DDAVP or venous occlusion.

The identification of the dysfibrinogenemias that are associated with thrombosis relies on tests that reflect the polymerization of fibrinogen.

The TCT, Reptilase time, and fibrinogen assays that include both antigen and activity measurements are used to identify defects in fibrinogen function (Table 41-1). Heterozygous or homozygous factor XII deficiency can be identified with a sensitive APTT and coagulation factor assay. Measurement of plasma PAI-1 necessitates special processing due to the presence of platelet PAI-1 (see Macy et al).

CLINICAL MANIFESTATIONS

Hereditary Disorders

Hereditary abnormalities of the fibrinolytic proteins t-PA, u-PA, or PAI-1 do not appear to be strong risk factors for venous or arterial thromboembolism. However, elevated levels of PAI-1 associated with the 4G polymorphism may contribute to the likelihood of thrombosis when other risk factors are present. Measurement of PAI-1 or analysis of the 4G/5G genotype does not seem warranted in most patients with venous thrombosis, but might be considered if all other thrombophilia studies are negative. Hereditary dysfibrinogenemia is a rare (<1% of patients), but important, cause of thrombosis; screening is inexpensive (TCT, fibrinogen) and should be included in evaluations for thrombophilia. The evidence for factor XII deficiency as a risk factor for venous or arterial thrombosis is equivocal and factor XII assays are not usually performed in patients with thrombosis.

Acquired Abnormalities

Impaired fibrinolysis, as evidenced by elevated resting levels of plasma PAI-1, have been noted in several disorders. Clinical studies have shown that patients with impaired fibrinolysis when measured preoperatively had a higher rate of venous thrombosis after hip surgery. A similar corre-

TABLE 41-1	
Laboratory Values in a 15-Year-Old Girl with Cerebral Sinus Vein Thrombosis	
Fibrinogen (functional assay) (175–325 mg/dL)	52 mg/dL
Fibrinogen (immunologic assay) (165–350 mg/dL)	317 mg/dL
TCT (20–30 s)	>100 s
Reptilase time (12–21 s)	59.4 s

* The patient's mother and maternal grandmother had recurrent thrombosis and similar laboratory findings

lation was found when elevated PAI-1 levels were discovered immediately after surgery. These conclusions are supported by the study of Prins and Hirsh in 1991, and by the observation that intermittent calf compression (known to stimulate fibrinolysis) during surgery protects against postoperative thrombosis. Because these findings could be clinically important, additional research is needed to determine if screening tests and subsequent prophylactic antithrombotic therapy would reduce the risk of postoperative thrombosis.

MANAGEMENT

Patients with acute thrombosis and evidence of impaired fibrinolysis (e.g., decreased plasminogen, dysfibrinogenemia), should be treated as usual with heparin followed by oral anticoagulants. Sufficient data are not yet available to determine if defects in fibrinolysis pose a long-term risk of thrombosis, so that a determination of the duration of anticoagulant therapy must be individualized. If asymptomatic relatives are also found to have laboratory evidence of impaired fibrinolysis, elective anticoagulation is not routinely indicated, given the low rates of thrombosis reported in these patients. Prophylactic antithrombotic therapy for surgery is recommended in both patients and their affected relatives.

Rare patients with ligneous conjunctivitis and homozygous plasminogen deficiency appear to benefit from plasminogen infusions.

Little data are available to help decide whether or not to treat patients with acquired defects of fibrinolysis. Aggressive prophylactic therapy (e.g., anticoagulants, leg compression) prior to orthopedic or general surgery in patients with elevated levels of PAI-1 or who have clinical conditions often linked with impaired fibrinolysis seems appropriate (i.e., the obese, smokers, or diabetics). Whether young patients with myocardial infarction and evidence of impaired fibrinolysis might benefit more from long-term anticoagulants than antiplatelet therapy is not known.

BIBLIOGRAPHY

Carmeliet P, Collen D: Gene manipulation and transfer of the plasminogen and coagulation system in mice. *Semin Thromb Hemost* 22:525, 1996.

Engesser L et al: Elevated plasminogen activator inhibitor (PAI), a cause of thrombophilia? A study in 203 patients with familial or sporadic venous thrombophilia. *Thromb Haemost* 62:673, 1989.

Erickson LA et al: Development of venous occlusions in mice transgenic for the plasminogen activator inhibitor-1 gene. *Nature* 346:74, 1990.

Halbmayer WM et al: The prevalence of factor XII deficiency in 103 orally anticoagulated outpatients suffering from recurrent venous and/or arterial thromboembolism. *Thromb Haemost* 68:285, 1992.

Koster T et al: John Hageman factor and deep vein thrombosis: Leiden Thrombophilia Study. *Br J Haematol* 87:422, 1994.

Levi M et al: Reduction of contact activation related fibrinolytic activity in factor XII deficient patients. Further evidence for the role of the contact system in fibrinolysis in vivo. *J Clin Invest* 88:1155, 1991.

Macy EM et al: Sample preparation for plasma measurement of plasminogen activator inhibitor-1 antigen in large population studies. *Arch Path Lab Med* 117:67, 1993.

Nguyen G et al: Residual plasminogen activator inhibitor activity after venous stasis as a criterion for hypofibrinolysis: a study in 83 patients with confirmed deep vein thrombosis. *Blood* 72:601, 1988.

Prins MH, Hirsh J: A critical review of the evidence supporting a relationship between impaired fibrinolytic activity and venous thromboembolism. *Arch Intern Med* 151:1721, 1991.

Prins MH, Hirsh J: A critical review of the relationship between impaired fibrinolysis and myocardial infarction. *Am Heart J* 122:545, 1991.

Ridker PM et al: Baseline fibrinolytic state and the risk of future venous thrombosis. A prospective study of endogenous tissue-type plasminogen activator and plasminogen activator inhibitor. *Circulation* 85:1822, 1992.

Sartori MT et al: 4G/5G polymorphism of PAI-1 gene promoter and fibrinolytic capacity in patients with deep vein thrombosis. *Thromb Haemost* 80:956, 1998.

Schuster V et al: Homozygous mutations in the plasminogen gene of two unrelated girls with ligneous conjunctivitis. *Blood* 90:958, 1997.

Shigekiyo T et al: Type I congenital plasminogen deficiency is not a risk factor for thrombosis. *Thromb Haemost* 67:189, 1992.

CHAPTER 42

Homocysteinemia

Elevated levels of homocysteine in the blood (homocysteinemia) are strongly associated with premature vascular disease as well as both arterial and venous thromboembolism. The rare homozygous genetic disease homocysteinuria occurs as a result of several different mutations in a key enzyme (cystathionine β-synthase [CβS]) involved in methionine metabolism, which produces markedly elevated levels of homocysteine in the plasma. This severe disorder is noted for neurologic defects, marfanoid features, ectopic lens, premature atherosclerosis, and, importantly, arterial and venous thromboses. In 1969, Dr. Kilmer McCully, a pathologist studying children with homocysteinuria, suggested that mild to moderate homocysteinemia might also be associated with premature coronary disease or stroke in otherwise normal adults.

METHIONINE METABOLISM

Methionine is a by-product of protein catabolism that is metabolized to homocysteine (Fig. 42-1). Two enzymes and three vitamins play key roles in the regulation of circulating homocysteine levels. CBS controls the breakdown of homocysteine to cystathionine in the transsulfuration pathway and, when severely impaired, leads to the inherited metabolic disease homocysteinuria. The second enzyme, methylene tetrahydrofolate reductase (MTHFR), is involved in the remethylation pathway, in which homocysteine is converted to methionine. A mutation at nucleotide 677 (G->T) causes the enzyme to be thermolabile with an associated mild loss of enzymatic activity. As many as 11 percent of the general population is homozygous for this mutation, which can lead to homocysteinemia in the presence of dietary folate depletion. As seen in the figure, deficiencies of

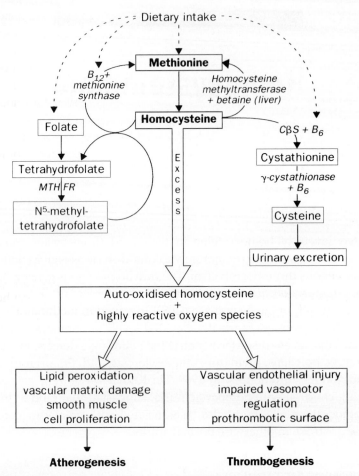

FIGURE 42-1 Homocysteine metabolism and possible mechanism of atherothrombotic disease. (Used with permission from Hankey GJ, Eikelboom JW: *Lancet* 354:407, 1999.)

vitamin B_6, vitamin B_{12}, or folic acid due to deficient diets or disease can produce elevated levels of plasma homocysteine.

MECHANISMS OF VASCULAR DISEASE AND THROMBOSIS

A series of laboratory studies have shown that homocysteine is injurious to blood vessels and converts endothelial cells from an antithrombotic to a prothrombotic phenotype. Effects on the vasculature include smooth muscle cell proliferation and reduced vascular reactivity due to impaired endothelial synthesis of nitric oxide. Acute or chronic elevations of plasma homocysteine concentrations reduce the compliance of blood vessels in primates and man. Endothelial cell effects also include increased expression of tissue factor and factor Va, along with decreased thrombomodulin, protein C activation, and heparan activity (causing impaired antithrombin binding). Blocks in endothelial-cell–mediated fibrinolysis, as well as increased binding of Lp(a), have been described. In vitro activation of platelets is suggested by increased excretion of thromboxane metabolites in the urine of subjects with homocysteinuria. However, it is not yet clear which of these defects are primarily responsible for the vascular disease and thrombosis seen in patients with persistent homocysteinemia.

CLINICAL MANIFESTATIONS

Arterial Disease

Data from a large number of studies strongly suggest that elevated levels of homocysteine are associated with an increased risk of arterial occlusion (Fig. 42-2). In one study, each 5 nmol/ml increase in plasma homocysteine was associated with a 2 to 4-fold increase in the odds ratio (OR)

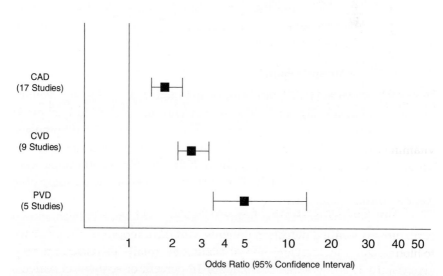

FIGURE 42-2 Summary odds ratios with 95% confidence intervals on a log scale for studies of fasting homocysteine levels and arterial vascular disease. CAD, coronary artery disease; CVD, cerebrovascular disease; PVD, peripheral vascular disease. (Adapted and modified from Boushey C et al: *JAMA* 274:1049, 1995.)

for vascular disease. In the Physicians Health Study (PHS), the relative risk for myocardial infarction (MI) was increased to 3.4 if homocysteine levels were >15.8 nmol/ml. An even higher odds ratio for stroke (7.4) was found in a British study of middle-aged men. A Framingham study showed that homocysteine levels were linked to carotid stenosis in the elderly, most likely due to dietary deficiencies of folic acid or vitamin B_6. Moreover, a large study in nurses showed that women with high dietary intakes of folate and vitamin B_6 had substantially reduced risks of fatal and non-fatal MI, particularly if they chronically ingested small amounts of alcohol. Finally, a Norwegian group showed that the death rate after interventions for coronary heart disease (e.g., grafting, angioplasty, medical therapy) was dramatically increased if homocysteine levels were >14 nmol/mL (Nygard ref). However, not all studies have shown a positive association of homocysteine and vascular disease. The MRFIT and ARIC studies (see refs) did not identify an association between high homocysteine levels and subsequent vascular disease in groups of relatively healthy individuals followed for several years. Interestingly the ARIC and several other studies suggest that low serum levels of vitamin B_6 are associated with cardiovascular disease independently of homocysteine levels.

In summary, the majority of the studies show a strong relationship between arterial disease and elevated levels of homocysteine. However, it is important to point out that it has not yet been shown that lowering homocysteine levels with vitamin therapy (see later) will slow the progression of atherosclerosis or lower the risk of thrombosis.

Venous Thromboembolism

Homocysteinemia is also a well-documented risk factor for venous thromboembolism (Fig. 42-3). The Leiden Thrombophilia Study showed that the OR for thrombosis was significantly increased to 2.5 if homocysteine levels were >18 nmol/mL, with an even more pronounced effect in women (OR=7.0) or in those >50 years (OR 5.5). Similar findings were reported from the PHS, with a relative risk of 3.4 observed for idiopathic venous thromboembolism, which was comparable to the increased risk seen with heterozygosity for factor V Leiden (3.6). As has been shown with other combined defects in patients with thrombophilia, the presence of both factor V Leiden and homocysteinemia greatly increased the relative risk to 21.8 (Fig 42-4). Since about 10 percent of sequential patients presenting with venous thrombosis will have elevated levels of homocysteine, homocysteinemia is one of the more common risk factors for thrombophilia. As in arterial disease, studies have not yet been published

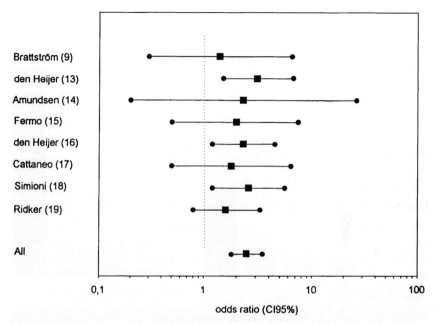

FIGURE 42-3 The odds ratios with 95% confidence intervals for venous thrombosis in subjects with elevated fasting homopcysteine levels from eight controlled studies. (Used with permission from den Heijer M et al: *Thromb Haemost* 80:847, 1998.)

to show that lowering homocysteine levels in affected subjects will reduce the risk of future thrombosis.

OTHER CLINICAL SETTINGS

End-stage renal disease, renal transplantation, and cyclosporin therapy are all associated with high levels of homocysteine. The mechanisms are complex and appear to be due to multiple metabolic defects as well as reduced excretion of homocysteine by the kidney. High levels of homocysteine have been associated with accelerated vascular disease in patients with renal failure. Reducing elevated homocysteine levels to normal is much more difficult in these patients, often requiring higher doses of folic acid and the addition of vitamin B_6.

About 40 percent of women with systemic lupus erythematosus (SLE) have homocysteinemia, which has been linked to arterial and venous thrombosis (Petrie ref). Finally, as has been shown with other forms of thrombophilia (e.g., factor V Leiden), homocysteinemia has been implicated in placental dysfunction syndromes and pregnancy loss (see Chap. 51).

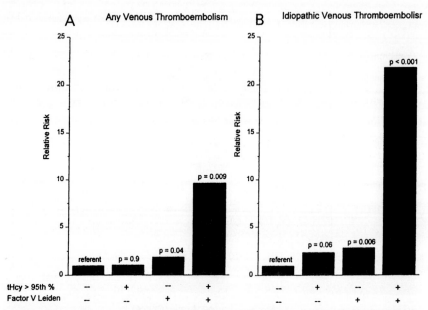

FIGURE 42-4 Relative risks of developing venous thrombosis associated with homocysteinemia and factor V Leiden. Data are shown for any venous thrombosis (A), and idiopathic venous thrombosis (B), stratified by the presence (+) or the absence (−) of the risk factor. (Used with permission from Ridker PM et al: *Circulation* 95:1777, 1997.)

DIAGNOSIS AND THERAPY

A diagnosis of homocysteinemia is based on measuring plasma levels of homocysteine using high performance liquid chromatography (HPLC) or immunoassay. Recently, data is emerging that immunoassay may be the preferable method because of improved accuracy with reduced variability and cost. Morning fasting blood samples are required because high protein meals can elevate homocysteine levels. The blood should be centrifuged immediately to remove cellular elements that can generate homocysteine at rates up to 10 to 15 percent/h. Plasma levels remain stable over at least a month's time, suggesting that a single sample reflects the ambient state. Methionine loading tests are usually not clinically indicated unless minor defects in the transsulfuration pathway are being sought. Identification of the thermolabile variant of MTHFR is readily accomplished using DNA technology. However, the great majority of clinical studies have shown that this heterozygous or homozygous defect in the enzyme is not a major risk factor for arterial or venous disease (see Brattstrom ref). A chronic dietary deficiency of folic acid is usually required before a homozygous MTHFR defect is associated with homocysteinemia.

The mainstay of treatment for homocysteinemia is an increased intake of folic acid, which is readily available in the diet. For example, one cup of orange juice provides 100 µg of folate. Other common sources of the vitamin are beans, spinach, and cereals. Flour has recently been fortified with folic acid in the United States. Over-the-counter vitamin supplements contain 400 to 800 µg of folic acid. For most patients, a good diet plus a daily multivitamin will lower homocysteine levels to the normal range within several weeks. Subsets of patients with elevated homocysteine levels may require higher doses of folic acid; e.g., up to 5 mg daily for two weeks followed by 1 to 2 mg/day thereafter. Before beginning folate therapy, vitamin B_{12} deficiency (e.g., pernicious anemia, PA) should be excluded by measuring plasma methylmalonic acid or vitamin B_{12} levels. High doses of folic acid in patients with PA could allow progression of neurologic disease in spite of correction of the anemia. Consideration should also be given to vitamin B_6 (pyridoxine) supplementation (e.g., 50 mg/day), based on the studies suggesting that high intakes of this B vitamin may lower the risks of cardiovascular disease, independent of its effect on homocysteine levels.

BIBLIOGRAPHY

Bostom AG et al: Nonfasting plasma total homocysteine levels and stroke incidence in elderly persons: The Framingham Study. *Ann Intern Med* 131:352, 1999.

Bostom AG et al: Nonfasting plasma total homocysteine levels and all-cause and cardiovascular disease mortality in elderly Framingham men and women. *Arch Intern Med* 159:1077, 1999.

Boushey CJ et al: A quantitative assessment of plasma homocysteine as a risk factor for vascular disease. Probable benefits of increasing folic acid intakes. *JAMA* 274:1049, 1995.

Brattstrom L et al: Common methylenetetrahydrofolate reductase gene mutation leads to hyperhomocysteinemia but not to vascular disease: the result of a meta-analysis. *Circulation* 98:2520, 1998.

Cattaneo M: Hyperhomocysteinemia, atherosclerosis and thrombosis. *Thromb Haemost* 81:165, 1999.

den Heijer M et al: Hyperhomocysteinemia and venous thrombosis: A meta-analysis. *Thromb Haemost* 80:847, 1998.

Eichinger S et al: Hyperhomocysteinemia is a risk factor of recurrent venous thromboembolism. *Thromb Haemost* 80:566, 1998.

Eikelbloom JW et al: Homocyst(e)ine and cardiovascular disease: A critical review of the epidemiologic evidence. *Ann Intern Med* 131:363, 1999.

Evans RW et al: Homocyst(e)ine and risk of cardiovascular disease in the multiple risk factor intervention trial. *Arterioscler Thromb Vasc Biol* 17:1947, 1997.

Folsom AR et al: Prospective study of coronary heart disease incidence in relation to fasting total homocysteine, related genetic polymorphisms, and B vitamins. The Atherosclerosis Risk in Communities (ARIC) Study. *Circulation* 98:204, 1998.

Hankey GJ, Eikelboom JW: Homocysteine and vascular disease. *Lancet* 354:407, 1999.

Nappo F et al: Impairment of endothelial functions by acute hyperhomocysteinemia and reversal by antioxidant vitamins. *JAMA* 281:2113, 1999.

Nygard O et al: Plasma homocysteine levels and mortality in patients with coronary artery disease. *N Engl J Med* 337:230, 1997.

Perry IJ et al: Prospective study of serum total homocysteine concentration and risk of stroke in middle-aged British men. *Lancet* 346:1395, 1995.

Ridker PM et al: Homocysteine and risk of cardiovascular disease among postmenopausal women. *JAMA* 281:1817, 1999.

Ridker PM et al: Interrelation of hyperhomocyst(e)inemia, factor V Leiden, and risk of future venous thromboembolism. *Circulation* 95:1777, 1997.

Rimm EB et al: Folate and vitamin B6 from diet and supplements in relation to risk of coronary heart disease among women. *JAMA* 279:359, 1998.

Robinson K et al: Low circulating folate and vitamin B6 concentrations. Risk factors for stroke, peripheral vascular disease, and coronary artery disease. *Circulation* 97:437, 1998.

Selhub J et al: Association between plasma homocysteine concentrations and extracranial carotid-artery stenosis. *N Engl J Med* 332:286, 1995.

Stampfer MJ et al: A prospective study of plasma homocyst(e)ine and risk of myocardial infarction in US physicians. *JAMA* 268:877, 1992.

Stehouwer CDA et al: Serum homocysteine and risk of coronary heart disease and cerebrovascular disease in elderly men. A 10-year follow-up. *Arterioscler Thromb Vasc Biol* 18:1895, 1998.

Welch GN, Loscalzo J: Homocysteine and atherothrombosis. *N Engl J Med,* 338:1042, 1998.

CHAPTER 43

Antiphospholipid Antibodies

Antiphospholipid antibodies (APA) are IgG, IgM, or IgA antibodies that occur as a result of autoimmune disease or as a reaction to infections or drugs. The name APA is a misnomer because in most instances the true antigen is a protein (e.g., β_2-glycoprotein 1 or prothrombin), rather than phospholipid (PL). APA can be divided into two broad categories, anti-cardiolipin antibodies (ACA) and the lupus anticoagulant (LA)—distinct and separable groups of antibodies that are known by the tests used to identify them, rather than reflecting their function in vivo. ACA are detected by solid-phase assay systems (ELISA), whereas LA are fluid-phase antibodies that inhibit PL-dependent coagulation tests (Fig. 43-1). Both ACA and LA are associated with thrombosis, including deep venous thrombosis (DVT) and pulmonary emboli (PE), arterial occlusion (myocardial infarction, stroke), pregnancy loss (placental infarction), and microvascular thrombi (livido reticularis).

PATHOGENESIS

Clinically important APA are a result of autoimmune disease, either as a primary phenomenon (e.g., primary antiphospholipid antibody syndrome, PAPS) or secondary to a disorder such as systemic lupus erythematosis (SLE). Autoimmune APA are associated with thrombosis and vascular disease, whereas APA arising as a consequence of infection or drug reactions are typically asymptomatic, although notable exceptions occur (LA and protein S deficiency with major thromboses complicating varicella in children). The cause of autoimmune APA is unknown, but

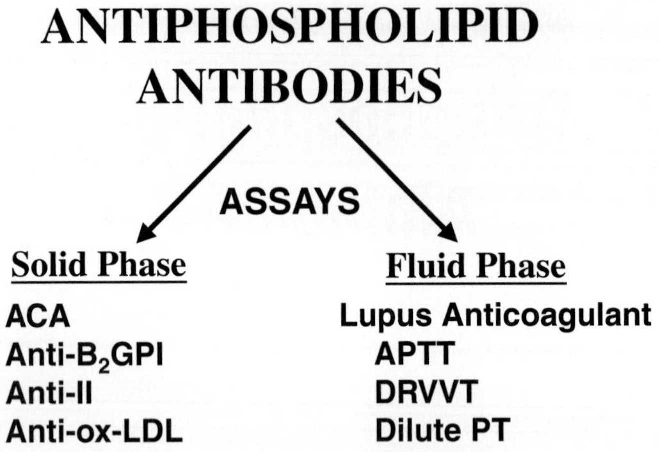

ANTIPHOSPHOLIPID ANTIBODIES

ASSAYS

Solid Phase

ACA
Anti-B$_2$GPI
Anti-II
Anti-ox-LDL

Fluid Phase

Lupus Anticoagulant
APTT
DRVVT
Dilute PT

FIGURE 43-1 Assays used to identify antiphospholipid antibodies.

could be a result of antibodies formed in response to vascular cell activation or injury.

As mentioned above, the major target antigen of ACA and some LA is β$_2$-glycoprotein I(β$_2$-GPI). β$_2$-GPI is a 50 kD lipophilic plasma protein (formerly called apolipoprotein H) that is composed of five fingerlike ("sushi") domains. The lipid-binding site resides in domain 5; APA appear to bind to amino acid sequences in domains 1, 4, or 5. β$_2$-GPI mildly inhibits prothrombinase formation (coagulation) and platelet function, activities that are probably not important clinically. In vivo, β$_2$-GPI rapidly binds to negatively charged PLs (e.g., phosphatidylserine). PL targets of β$_2$-GPI in vivo include activated or disrupted endothelial cells or platelets, interactions that could either stimulate autoantibody formation or serve as an antigen for circulating preexisting APA. In addition to β$_2$-GPI, LA also react with the clotting factor prothrombin (but not thrombin), which promotes the accumulation of prothrombin on cellular or other negatively charged PL surfaces.

APA may promote thrombosis by inhibiting the action of activated protein C (APC), which represents an acquired form of APC resistance (see Chap. 40), or by stimulating increased binding of prothrombin to PL surfaces. In both instances, excessive thrombin generation could occur at sites of cellular injury and promote thrombus formation. Other potential mechanisms include a fall in free protein S (see Chap. 39) or displacement of annexin V (a thromboprotective substance) from the surface of placental trophoblasts or endothelial cells. Table 43-1 lists additional possible mechanisms of thrombosis or vascular injury. Recently several studies

TABLE 43-1	

Possible Mechanisms of Thrombosis in Patients with Antiphospholipid Antibodies

Inhibition of Protein C System

    Decreased activation of protein C to activated protein C (APC)
    Inhibition of APC (persistence of factors Va, VIIIa)
    Decreased free protein S
    Inhibition of thrombin-thrombomodulin complex

Altered Platelet-Endothelial Balance

    Reduced endothelial prostacyclin synthesis
    Antibody-induced platelet activation
    Antibody-induced endothelial cell activation
    Endothelial cell microparticle formation
    Expression of P-selectin on platelets
    Decreased endothelial heparan sulfate
    Increased endothelial cell tissue factor

have suggested that APA (ACA, antibodies to oxidized LDL) may be associated with accelerated atherogenesis as well as thrombosis. For example, APA have been shown to accelerate β_2-GPI dependent uptake of oxidized LDL by macrophages.

LABORATORY DETECTION

APA are detected in the laboratory using either solid- or fluid-phase assays. Solid-phase assays (e.g., ELISA) are used to identify ACA and antibodies to β_2-GPI. In both instances the target antigen is β_2-GPI. The presence of the negatively charged PL cardiolipin, or irradiation of plastic microtiter plates, causes "clustering" of the β_2-GPI molecule, which facilitates bivalent antibody binding. This can then be quantified in the ELISA assay. Potential advantages of the anti-β_2-GPI assay over the classic ACA assay is an increased specificity for thrombosis (the anti-β_2-GPI test is negative in the presence of most infection-induced APA). Other solid-phase assays have been developed for measuring antibodies to prothrombin and oxidized LDL.

LA are detected by their ability to prolong PL-dependent coagulation tests such as the APTT, Russell Viper Venom Time (RVVT), or the PT (Table 43-2). These antibodies are heterogeneous, so that multiple tests must be performed to maximize their detection. The identification of a LA requires three steps: the prolongation of a PL-dependent coagulation test, mixing studies (with normal plasma) to show an inhibitory effect, and neutralization of the inhibitor with high concentrations of PL. Currently available assays may combine several of these steps. For example:

TABLE 43-2

Laboratory Identification and Characterization of the Lupus Anticoagulant

The following four steps should be satisfied for definitive identification of a LA:

Step 1: Multiple phospholipid-dependent screening tests are used to screen for the presence of the LA. Examples include the APTT, RVVT and dilute PT

Step 2: A mixing study (using normal plasma) will show that the abnormal screening test is due to an inhibitor rather than a clotting factor deficiency (see Chap. 4)

Step 3: The inhibitory activity will be neutralized by an excess of phospholipid

Step 4: Other coagulopathies should be excluded (e.g., acquired factor VIII inhibitor)

- APTT (+ hexagonal PL neutralization)
- RVVT with PL confirmation
- Dilute PT (using a LA-sensitive thromboplastin)

In each of these assays a LA will prolong the screening test; clotting times will then shorten after the addition of the PL in the first two tests. Results are expressed as the PL-induced shortening of the clotting time in seconds or as a ratio of the clotting times with and without added PL.

Distinguishing a LA from an acquired factor VIII inhibitor is important in patients presenting with a prolonged APTT and lack of correction with mixing studies (Table 43-3). Factor VIII levels are usually quite low in the presence of a factor VIII inhibitor (<10%). The LA inhibits intrinsic system factor assays (VIII, IX, XI, XII) because these tests are based on a APTT test system (see Chap. 2). However, coagulation factor assays for factor VIII activity are rarely <10% in the presence of a LA. Furthermore, the LA rapidly loses its inhibitory activity with dilution of the patient's plasma, so that the apparent clotting factor activity appears to increase ("titers up") as the test plasma is sequentially diluted in the clotting factor assay. This phenomenon is uncommon with factor VIII inhibitors. Finally, factor VIII inhibitors do not prolong the PT or RVVT, whereas LA frequently (but not always) does so.

APA do not cause bleeding, although several hemostatic defects occur in patients with the LA or ACA. Immune thrombocytopenia, platelet dysfunction (prolonged bleeding time), and isolated prothrombin deficiency (due to antiprothrombin antibodies with rapid clearance of the prothrombin–antiprothrombin complexes) have all been reported in patients with APA. Prothrombin deficiency should be suspected when the INR is >1.4 in a non-anticoagulated patient.

Monitoring anticoagulants in the presence of a LA is often difficult because the tests used for monitoring heparin (APTT) and warfarin (PT)

TABLE 43-3		
Differentiation of a Lupus Anticoagulant from an Acquired Factor VIII Inhibitor.		
	VIII Inhibitor	**Lupus Anticoagulant**
Symptoms	Bleeding	Thrombosis
VIII assay results	<10%	>10%
VIII assay with dilution	Stable	"Titers up"
PT & DRVVT	Normal	May be ↑

may both be prolonged, which could lead to under-anticoagulation and an increased risk of recurrent thromboembolism. In this situation, heparin levels can be monitored with an anti-Xa chromogenic heparin assay (note that -PL is not used in the test) or, alternatively, treatment can be instituted with low molecular weight heparin (LMWH) without laboratory monitoring. Although uncommon, a few patients will have LA that prolong the PT. Options for monitoring oral anticoagulant therapy in this situation include switching to a PT that uses a thromboplastin reagent that is not sensitive to the LA, or alternatively monitoring factor X levels (a vitamin K-dependent factor) using a chromogenic coagulation factor assay. INRs of 2 to 3 are approximately equivalent to factor X levels of 15 to 40%.

CLINICAL MANIFESTATIONS

APA are found in two broad categories of patients. Thrombosis, thrombocytopenia, and pregnancy loss are common in one group of patients (sometimes called the APA syndrome), whereas APA are usually of little clinical consequence in other individuals (e.g., normal blood donors, children with histories of infections, AIDS patients, and as a reaction to drugs, particularly phenothiazines). Nonpathologic APA are frequently low in titer, transient, and are more often IgM. In contrast, antibodies found in patients with thromboembolic disease tend to be high titer, persistent, and consist of IgG or IgA isotypes, although some studies have also linked IgM APA to thrombosis.

The medical literature is replete with case reports and series of patients that suggest an association of APA with thrombosis. These reports can be grouped into several more or less distinct clinical scenarios.

Primary Antiphospholipid Antibody Syndrome (PAPS)

These patients do not have evidence of SLE or other well-defined autoimmune disorder. The syndrome often occurs in young males with high titers of APA, thrombocytopenia, and recurrent arterial and venous thromboses. Livedo reticularis of the skin is common, and many patients have CNS infarction.

Recurrent Venous Thromboembolism

DVT is often associated with APA. Recent studies suggest that the thrombosis rate is ~2.4%/year in unselected patients with APA. As many as 15 to 20% of sequential patients presenting with thrombosis will be found to have APA, depending in part on case selection. The odds ratio for venous thrombosis in patients with APA is increased 6 to 10-fold. Recurrence rates are also very high and can approach 10 to 15%/year in the absence of anticoagulants. LA are stronger predictors of thrombosis than ACA.

Arterial Thromboembolism

APA are frequently discovered in young patients who have stroke or transient ischemic attacks (TIA) (Fig. 43-2). In one study, 47 percent of patients <45 years of age who were treated for acute stroke or TIA had

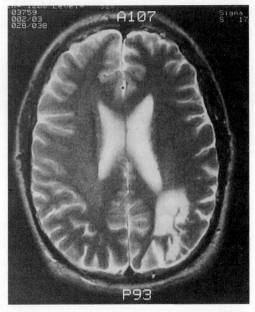

FIGURE 43-2 MRI scan showing a large infarct in a young man with APA.

either LA or ACA, compared to only 8 percent of patients who were seen for other neurologic disease. CNS infarcts are frequently small and show no evidence of vasculitis on biopsy (Fig. 43-3). The cardiac valves are a likely source of cerebral emboli causing ischemic symptoms (see later). In some patients, recurrent CNS thrombosis leads to multiinfarct dementia.

Cardiac Valvular Disease

Vegetations composed of fibrin and platelets occur frequently on the mitral and aortic cardiac valves in patients with APA. For example, studies using transthoracic echocardiography have documented vegetations in approximately 25 percent of patients with SLE who had APA on laboratory testing. In a group of patients with APA and recurrent cerebral ischemic events, over 75% had valvular vegetations or thickening when studied with transesophageal echocardiography.

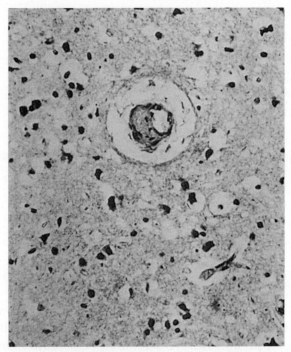

FIGURE 43-3 Section of brain frontal cortex obtained at autopsy that shows a platelet-fibrin thrombus within a small cerebral artery. There is no evidence of vasculitis. (H & E; × 40 before 2 percent enlargement.) (Used with permission from Briley DP et al: *Ann Neurol* 25:221, 1989.)

Recurrent Pregnancy Loss

First-trimester spontaneous abortion and second-trimester fetal loss have been associated with increased levels of APA in large clinical studies. The mechanisms that promote pregnancy loss are not entirely clear, but fetal wastage is most likely due to placental vascular insufficiency as a result of thrombosis or other vascular dysfunction. Studies have suggested that APA can displace annexin V (a thromboprotective agent) from the surface of trophoblasts, thereby promoting thrombosis. Pregnancy loss is more common when APA are persistent (over 3 to 4 months) and high in titer.

Other Associations

APA have been associated with a wide spectrum of other clinical disorders caused by vascular disease, including Addison's disease (adrenal cortical infarction), abdominal vein thrombosis, thrombotic pulmonary hypertension, livedo reticularis of the skin, retinal artery occlusion, migraine headache, acute ischemic encephalopathy, and myocardial infarction.

MANAGEMENT

Optimal management of patients with APA-associated thrombosis or pregnancy loss is controversial because of the lack of controlled prospective trials of antithrombotic or other therapies. However, until more data are available, recommendations for treatment include:

1. Patients with APA who do not have a history of thrombosis should not be treated. The risks of bleeding from anticoagulants are likely to outweigh any beneficial effects.
2. Immunosuppressive therapy (e.g., prednisone, cyclophosphamide) given in an effort to lower APA titers has not been shown to protect against thrombosis.
3. Because of high thrombotic recurrence rates, prolonged antithrombotic therapy should be considered for patients who have a history of thrombosis (arterial or venous) and who have persistently elevated levels of APA.
4. The best antithrombotic regimen for long-term therapy remains to be defined. Most data now suggest that warfarin therapy at INR 2 to 3 is sufficient for patients with venous thromboembolism. Somewhat higher-intensity therapy has been recommended for arterial thrombosis (e.g., INR 2.5 to 3.5), but a definitive recommendation awaits the results of prospective clinical trials.

5. The optimal therapy for the prevention of recurrent pregnancy loss is also a subject of ongoing study. At present, low-dose aspirin and prednisone appear ineffective, whereas the use of prophylactic levels of heparin or LMW heparin throughout pregnancy is likely to be beneficial. Heparin therapy should not be recommended to asymptomatic patients who have APA without a history of fetal loss. Low-dose aspirin (75 mg/day) was included with the low-dose heparin in most of the reported studies.
6. Immune thrombocytopenia is relatively common in patients with APA and thrombosis, and usually responds to standard approaches such as corticosteroids, intravenous gamma globulin, or splenectomy. In some cases, severe thrombocytopenia must be treated before antithrombotic therapy with heparin or warfarin can be safely administered.
7. Patients with APA and a history of thrombosis who require surgery should receive prophylactic anticoagulants (see Chap. 59).

BIBLIOGRAPHY

Arnout J et al: Optimization of the dilute prothrombin time for the detection of the lupus anticoagulant by use of a recombinant tissue thromboplastin. *Br J Haematol* 87:94, 1994.

Backos M et al: Pregnancy complications in women with recurrent miscarriage associated with antiphospholipid antibodies treated with low dose aspirin and heparin. *Br J Obstet Gynacol* 106:102, 1999.

Brandt JT at al: Laboratory identification of lupus anticoagulants: results of the Second International Workshop for identification of Lupus Anticoagulants. On behalf of the Subcommittee on Lupus Anticoagulants/Antiphospholipid Antibodies of the ISTH. *Thromb Haemost* 74:1597, 1995.

Field SL et al: Lupus anticoagulants form immune complexes with prothrombin and phospholipid that can augment thrombin production in flow. *Blood* 94:3421, 1999.

Finazzi G et al: Natural history and risk factors for thrombosis in 360 patients with antiphospholipid antibodies: A four-year prospective study from the Italian Registry. *Am J Med* 100:530, 1996.

Galli M et al: Antiprothrombin antibodies: Detection and clinical significance in the antiphospholipid syndrome. *Blood* 93:2149, 1999.

Gharavi AE et al: GDKV-induced antiphospholipid antibodies enhance thrombosis and activate endothelial cells in vivo and in vitro. *J Immunol* 163:2922, 1999.

Greaves M: Antiphospholipid antibodies and thrombosis. *Lancet* 353:1348, 1999.

Horbach DA et al: Lupus anticoagulant is the strongest risk factor for both venous and arterial thrombosis in patients with systemic lupus erythematosus. Comparison between different assays for the detection of antiphospholipid antibodies. *Thromb Haemost* 76:916, 1996.

Kutteh WH: Antiphospholipid antibody-associated recurrent pregnancy loss: Treatment with heparin and low-dose aspirin is superior to low-dose aspirin alone. *Am J Obstet Gynecol* 174:1584, 1996.

McNally T et al: The use of an anti-beta 2-glycoprotein-I assay for discrimination between anticardiolipin antibodies associated with infection and increased risk of thrombosis. *Br J Haematol* 91:471, 1995.

Pratico D et al: Ongoing prothrombotic state in patients with antiphospholipid antibodies: a role for increased lipid peroxidation. *Blood* 93:3401, 1999.

Rand JH et al: Pregnancy loss in the antiphospholipid-antibody syndrome—a possible thrombogenic mechanism. *N Engl J Med* 337:154, 1997.

Rao LVM et al: Mechanism and effects of the binding of lupus anticoagulant IgG and prothrombin to surface phospholipid. *Blood* 88:4173, 1996.

Rosove MH: Antiphospholipid thrombosis: clinical course after the first thrombotic event in 70 patients. *Ann Intern Med* 117:303, 1992.

Schulman S et al: Anticardiolipin antibodies predict early recurrence of thromboembolism and death among patients with venous thromboembolism following anticoagulant therapy. Duration of Anticoagulation Study Group. *Am J Med* 104:332, 1998.

Simioni P et al: Deep venous thrombosis and lupus anticoagulant. A case-control study. *Thromb Haemost* 76:187, 1996.

Triplett DA: Annotation. Laboratory identification of the lupus anticoagulant. *Br J Haematol* 72:139, 1989.

Tuhrim S et al: Elevated anticardiolipin antibody titer is a stroke risk factor in a multiethnic population independent of isotype or degree of positivity. *Stroke* 30:1561, 1999.

Verro P et al: Cerebrovascular ischemic events with high positive anticardiolipin antibodies. *Stroke* 29:2245, 1998.

CHAPTER 44

Myeloproliferative Disorders and Paroxysmal Nocturnal Hemoglobinuria

The clinical course of patients with myeloproliferative disorders (MPD) is often complicated by thrombosis, which is a major cause of death and disability. The thrombotic manifestations of MPD are covered in this chapter, whereas hemorrhagic problems are discussed in Chapter 33. Thrombosis is more common than bleeding, although both can occur in the same patient. The MPD commonly associated with thromboembolism include essential thrombocythemia (ET) and polycythemia rubra vera (PRV). Thrombosis typically involves a spectrum of vascular beds, including small and large vessels, arteries, and veins. Thrombosis is also frequent in paroxysmal nocturnal hemoglobinuria (PNH), a myeloid stem cell disorder, and is a cause of death in up to 40% of patients with the disease.

PATHOGENESIS

Myeloproliferative Disorders

For the most part, thrombotic events in patients with MPD are platelet-mediated, rather than a result of pathologic activation of coagulation or insufficient fibrinolysis. Although all of the MPD are commonly accompanied by thrombocytosis, abnormal function (rather than increased numbers) of platelets is more likely to be the cause of vascular occlusion.

Patients with reactive thrombocytosis and normally functioning platelets (e.g., as a result of splenectomy) rarely develop thromboembolism. A wide spectrum of platelet function defects, some seemingly predictive of bleeding and others of thrombosis, have been described in patients with MPD, but which, if any, of these disorders are responsible for arterial or venous thrombosis is not clear. The elevated concentration of red blood cells and increased blood viscosity in patients with PRV greatly magnifies the risk of thrombosis. Erythrocytosis may also contribute to enhanced platelet reactivity and platelet–vascular interactions. Increasing patient age, a history of prior thromboembolism, and the presence of underlying vascular disease are all highly predictive of future events.

Notably, excessive amounts of platelet-derived growth factor (PDGF) in both plasma and urine have been found in patients with MPD, although it is uncertain whether the growth factor is released from platelets or megakaryocytes. PDGF could be involved in the genesis of marrow fibrosis seen so commonly in MPD, and may also be responsible for the vascular proliferation that occurs in the digits of patients with severe erythromelalgia (see later).

Recently, studies of X-chromosome inactivation patterns in women with ET have shown that monoclonal myelopoiesis could be demonstrated in only about half the subjects. The remainder were found to have polyclonal myelopoiesis. There were no differences in clinical presentation or course between the two groups, with the exception that the polyclonal patients were significantly less likely to have thrombosis (Table 44-1).

TABLE 44-1

Comparison of Clinical Features of ET Patients with Monoclonal or Polyclonal Hematopoiesis

	Monoclonal Hematopoiesis (n = 10)	Polyclonal Hematopoiesis (n = 13)	Difference
Median age at diagnosis (yr)	48 (10–61)	40 (14–81)	NS
Median follow-up (mo)	83 (18–260)	32 (6–116)	NS
Median platelet count at diagnosis ($\times 10^9$/L)	722 (600–1457)	778 (600–1917)	NS
Hepatosplenomegaly	5 (50%)	2 (15%)	$0.05 < P < 0.1$
Thrombosis	6 (60%)	2 (15%)	$P < 0.05$
Hemorrhage	1 (10%)	0 (0%)	NS

Abbreviation: NS, not significant
(From Harrison CN et al: *Blood* 93:417, 1999)

Paroxysmal Nocturnal Hemoglobinuria

The thrombotic complications of PNH are also likely to be mediated by increased platelet reactivity. PNH platelets are extremely sensitive to certain aggregating agents; for example, only 1/1000 as much thrombin is required for maximal platelet aggregation in PNH as compared to normal controls. More recently, a group of 11 patients with PNH were found to have varying degrees of platelet activation using flow cytometry. Surface expression of activation dependent proteins, such as P-selectin, thrombospondin, and fibrinogen were increased (Gralnick ref). Defects in coagulation or fibrinolysis were not found. Finally, a recent study has suggested that procoagulant activity induced by complement may be enhanced in the red cells of patients with PNH, potentially contributing to thrombogenesis.

CLINICAL MANIFESTATIONS

Myeloproliferative Disorders

Thromboses complicating ET or PRV involve almost all levels of the vascular tree, including peripheral or abdominal veins, large arteries, and distal arterioles. Vascular occlusion occurs at some point during the course of the illness in 20 to 40 percent of patients. Although the disease is most common in older subjects, MPD occurs in younger patients as well. In one series of young adults (age <40 years) followed for 4.5 years, half had a thrombotic episode during the course of their illness, but the event was life threatening in <5 percent. Rarely ET or PRV is seen in children. Patients with untreated PRV and high hematocrits are especially likely to develop major thromboses following surgery. Several thrombotic syndromes merit special mention.

1. Central abdominal vein thrombosis: Some of the vasculature in the abdomen represents a special target for thrombosis and includes the hepatic veins (Budd-Chiari syndrome) and the portal, mesenteric, and splenic veins. On occasion, thromboses of these vessels predate a diagnosis of MPD by several years. In one study of patients who presented with portal vein thrombosis, MPD was identified in 50 percent of them using erythroid colony assays as a marker (see later).
2. Arterial occlusion: Patients with MPD have suffered thrombotic occlusions of almost every major artery, including myocardial infarction, peripheral artery thrombosis, and stroke. Other CNS symptoms of a vascular origin include transient ischemic attacks, amaurosis fugax, central retinal artery thrombosis, and headache (which have been ascribed to platelet thrombi within the cerebral microcircula-

tion). Cardiac valvular lesions resembling non-bacterial thrombotic endocarditis also occur, and may be the source of cerebral emboli.

3. Erythromelalgia: This syndrome often occurs in a subgroup of patients with MPD and consists of recurrent episodes of painful red feet (75 percent), hands (9 percent), or both (16 percent). Vascular occlusion is due to platelet clumping within the arterioles of the distal extremities. When the disorder is prolonged or severe, arteriolar inflammation, fibromuscular hyperplasia, and irreversible thrombosis can occur, culminating in necrosis of the digits (Fig. 44-1). As will be discussed later, low doses of aspirin or indomethacin often quickly and dramatically relieve symptoms of pain and erythema.

4. Pregnancy loss: Increased rates of first-trimester pregnancy loss and other complications (such as preeclampsia) have been reported in women with ET and PRV. Thrombosis of placental vessels is a likely cause. This disorder may well be analogous to the pregnancy loss associated with other hereditary and acquired thrombophilic states.

Paroxysmal Nocturnal Hemoglobinuria

The thromboses of PNH involve peripheral veins, but also frequently affect the veins of the portal and hepatic circulation as well. In one series, about 30 percent of young patients with PNH developed venous thrombosis, which included occlusion of the inferior vena cava, renal and pelvic veins, and the cerebral venous sinuses. In another report, 12 percent of 40 patients with PNH had Budd-Chiari syndrome. Thrombosis, along with infection, is a major clinical problem in patients with PNH and accounts for up to half the deaths in this disorder (Fig. 44-2).

LABORATORY TESTING

The diagnosis of MPD is usually not difficult when a patient has elevation of peripheral blood counts, splenomegaly, and hypercellularity of the myeloid elements of the bone marrow. However, in some instances, thrombosis is the presenting symptom and a diagnosis of MPD is much more difficult. An examination of the peripheral blood may be normal or show only a mild elevation in platelet count, slightly abnormal platelet morphology, or a minimal left shift in the granulocyte series. In difficult cases, a peripheral blood or bone marrow erythroid or megakaryocyte colony assay can be used to establish the correct diagnosis. Abnormal colony formation is a sensitive and specific marker for MPD and is often present before changes in peripheral blood counts or enlargement of the spleen. However these assays are not helpful in distinguishing the various subclasses of MPD.

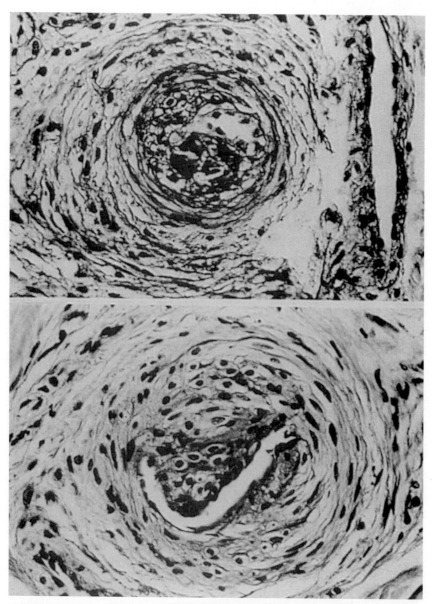

FIGURE 44-1 Biopsy of the skin from a patient with essential thrombocythemia and erythromelalgia. *Top:* Arteriole with pronounced cell proliferation of the inner layer of the media and degenerative cytoplasmatic swelling. *Bottom:* Thrombotic occlusions of an arteriole with proliferative vessel wall changes. (Hematoxylin and azophyloxine; original magnification × 380.) (Reproduced with permission from Michiels JJ et al: *Ann Intern Med* 102:466, 1985.)

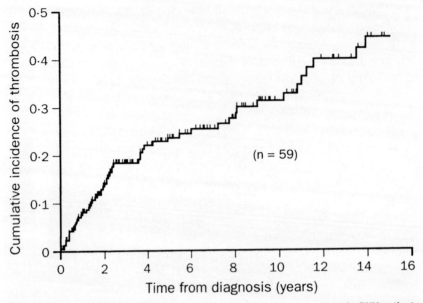

FIGURE 44-2 Kaplan-Meier estimates of rate of thrombosis development in PNH patients. (Used with permission from Socie et al. *Lancet* 348:573, 1996.)

Other laboratory procedures such as the platelet count, platelet aggregation tests, bleeding time, spontaneous platelet aggregation, circulating platelet aggregates, or plasma levels of platelet-specific proteins are rarely predictive of thrombosis. In several large series of patients, age >60 years, a prior history of thromboembolism and underlying vascular disease were the single best indicators of future vascular occlusion. Differentiating ET (primary thrombocytosis) from reactive thrombocytosis can usually be accomplished by a search for malignancy, infection, or inflammation; and measurement of C-reactive protein or IL-6 in the plasma. Elevated levels of these inflammatory markers are observed in reactive thrombocytosis. Tests are not yet available to determine mono- or polyclonality of patients with ET as a marker of thrombotic potential (discussed earlier).

MANAGEMENT

Myeloproliferative Disorders

Therapeutic options for the prevention and treatment of thrombosis in the MPD are increasing in number and complexity. Classical antithrombotic agents are used (anticoagulants, fibrinolytics, antiplatelet drugs), as well as measures to reduce elevated blood counts, which include: plateletpheresis or phlebotomy, myelosuppressive agents, interferon-α, and anagrelide. Finally, the best course of action for some patients may be to withhold treatment and observe, particularly young asymptomatic patients with ET. Several of these therapeutic options are discussed below:

1. Antithrombotic agents

   Acute major vessel thromboses in patients with MPD should be treated in standard fashion with anticoagulants (heparin, LMW heparin, warfarin). However fibrinolytic therapy should be strongly considered in patients who develop acute hepatic vein thrombosis (Budd-Chiari syndrome) because of its high mortality rate when treated with anticoagulants alone. Thrombolytic therapy may also be useful for other major life-threatening vascular occlusions.

   Antiplatelet therapy with low dose aspirin is particularly useful for patients suffering from erythromelalgia. Often dramatic relief occurs several days after a single dose. Aspirin (80–100 mg/day) may also be effective in treating neurological events such as transient ischemic events, amaurosis fugax or even headache due to intravascular platelet clumping. Early studies in patients with PRV reported a very high rate of gastrointestinal bleeding due to aspirin, but the doses used were high (900 mg/day). More recent studies have suggested that lower doses are safer.

2. Plateletpheresis and phlebotomy

   The treatment of choice for acute thrombosis (or major hemorrhage) in patients with very high platelet counts (e.g., >1 million) is repeated plateletpheresis to acutely lower the count to <600,000/μL. Apheresis should be combined with other agents (e.g., hydroxyurea, anagrelide) to inhibit platelet production and a rebound thrombocytosis.

   Repeated phlebotomy to reduce elevated hematocrits in patients with PRV are used to decrease symptoms of hyperviscosity. An increased risk of vascular thrombosis has been documented after phlebotomy by the PRV Study group. However, phlebotomy (plus a low dose of aspirin) should be considered for young asymptomatic PRV patients to avoid the side effects of myelosuppressive medications (see later).

3. Myelosuppressive agents

   The antimetabolite hydroxyurea (HU) has largely supplanted the use of radioactive phosphorus or alkylating agents to suppress thrombo- or erythropoiesis in patients with ET or PRV. Several studies have now shown that HU treatment also reduces the risk of thrombosis in patients with MPD (Fig. 44-3). However it is still unclear if platelet counts should best be maintained at <600,000/μL or reduced further to <350,000/μL. A concern with the use of HU is a low but now documented, increased risk of acute leukemia with long-term use. The benefits of therapy should outweigh this risk. Other problems include ulcerating skin lesions, gastrointestinal upset, and neutropenia. However, HU may be suitable for older (>60 yrs) patients with a history of prior thrombosis or major risk factors for vascular disease.

4. Interferon-α

   Interferon-α has been shown to reduce elevated platelet and red cell counts in patients with MPD, and to date has not been associated with an increased risk of leukemia. It is not yet clear if the reduced counts as a result of treatment with this agent are associated with a decreased risk of thrombosis. Side effects are frequent and include a flulike syndrome, fevers, and neurological symptoms, which may curtail treatment in up to 15% of patients. Interferon-α should be considered for patients who are <60 yrs of age and who are symptomatic or who have risk factors for vascular disease. Since interferon-α does not cross the placenta, it may be an option for treatment of severe, symptomatic ET or PRV during pregnancy.

5. Anagrelide

   Anagrelide is a selective inhibitor of platelet production that effectively lowers platelet counts in patients with ET and PRV. The drug

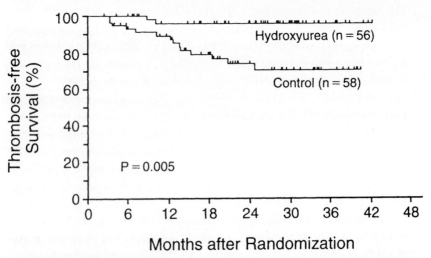

FIGURE 44-3 Probability of thrombosis-free survival in 114 patients with essential thromb-cythemia treated with hydroxyurea or left untreated. (Used with permission from Cortelazzo S et al. *N Engl J Med* 332:1132, 1995.)

does not reduce elevated red or white cell levels. There is no evidence to date that it is leukemogenic. Some data suggests that the risk of thrombosis is also reduced along with the platelet count. Side effects include fluid retention, cardiac arrhythmias, and headache, which may preclude its use, particularly in older patients with cardiac disease. Anagrelide should be considered in patients who are <60 years old but who have symptoms of vascular insufficiency.

6. No specific therapy

Patients with ET who are younger and asymptomatic have been shown to have a low risk of developing major thromboembolic events. In such patients, the side effects and complications of platelet suppressive therapies may be greater than their benefits. Consideration should be given to low-dose aspirin to try to prevent platelet-mediated thrombosis. If vascular occlusive symptoms should subsequently develop, then platelet-lowering therapy with anagrelide or interferon-α should be considered. Patients with reactive thrombocytosis (>1 million/μL) do not appear to have an increased risk of thrombosis and therefore do not warrant treatment.

BIBLIOGRAPHY

Anagrelide Study Group: Anagrelide, a therapy for thrombocythemic states: experience in 577 patients. *Am J Med* 92:69, 1992.

Besses C et al: Major vascular complications in essential thrombocythemia: a study of the predictive factors in a series of 148 patients. *Leukemia* 13:150, 1999.

Cortelazzo S et al: Hydroxyurea for patients with essential thrombocythemia and a high risk of thrombosis. *N Engl J Med* 332:1132, 1995.

Gralnick HR et al: Activated platelets in paroxysmal nocturnal haemoglobinuria. *Brit J Haematol* 91:697, 1995.

Griesshammer M et al: Etiology and clinical significance of thrombocytosis: analysis of 732 patients with an elevated platelet count. *J Intern Med* 245:295, 1999.

Gruppo Italiano Studio Policitemia: Polycythemia vera: the natural history of 1213 patients followed for 20 years. *Ann Intern Med* 123:656, 1995.

Harrison CN et al: A large proportion of patients with a diagnosis of essential thrombocythemia do not have a clonal disorder and may be at lower risk of thrombotic complications. *Blood* 93:417, 1999.

Hillmen P et al: Natural history of paroxysmal nocturnal hemoglobinuria. *N Engl J Med* 333:1253, 1995.

Hoffman R: Primary thrombocythemia, in *Hematology: Basic Principles and Practice*, 3rd ed, New York, Churchill Livingstone, 1999, p 1188.

Juvonen E et al: Megakaryocyte and erythroid colony formation in essential thrombocythaemia and reactive thrombocytosis: Diagnostic value and correlation to complications. *Brit J Haematol* 83:192, 1993.

Manoharan A et al: Thrombosis and bleeding in myeloproliferative disorders: identification of at-risk patients with whole blood platelet aggregation studies. *Brit J Haematol* 105:618, 1999.

Michiels JJ et al: Erythromelalgia caused by platelet-mediated arteriolar inflammation and thrombosis in thrombocythemia. *Ann Intern Med* 102:466, 1985.

Ninomiya H et al: Complement-induced procoagulant alteration of red blood cell membranes with microvesicle formation in paroxysmal nocturnal haemoglobinuria (PNH): implication for thrombogenesis in PNH. *Brit J Haematol* 106:224, 1999.

Rinder HM et al: Correlation of thrombosis with increased platelet turnover in thrombocytosis. *Blood* 91:1288, 1998.

Ruggeri M et al: No treatment for low-risk thrombocythaemia: results from a prospective study. *Brit J Haematol* 103:772, 1998.

Socie G et al: Paroxysmal nocturnal haemoglobinuria: long-term follow-up and prognostic factors. French Society of Haematology. *Lancet* 348:573, 1996.

Wadenvik H et al: The effect of alpha-interferon on bone marrow megakaryocytes and platelet production rate in essential thrombocythemia. *Blood* 77:2103, 1991.

Wang JC et al: Blood thrombopoietin levels in clonal thrombocytosis and reactive thrombocytosis. *Amer J Med* 104:451, 1998.

CHAPTER 45

Heparin-induced Thrombocytopenia

Heparin-induced thrombocytopenia (HIT) is an uncommon, but some-times devastating, clinical syndrome that consists of an immune-mediated fall in the platelet count in patients treated with heparin. The incidence of HIT is unknown, but it probably occurs in 1 to 3 percent of adult patients receiving heparin for a week or more. Approximately 10 to 15 percent of patients with the disorder develop arterial or venous throm-boses, and of these up to 30 percent will die or require amputation as a result of vascular occlusion. Early recognition is important because appropriate treatment may reduce morbidity and mortality.

PATHOGENESIS

Slight drops in the platelet count occur frequently in patients given heparin; this is a benign process that is probably due to a direct interac-tion of some component of the heparin with platelets. However, in other patients, heparin administration incites the formation of IgG antibodies, which react with heparin and low molecular weight proteins (e.g., platelet factor 4 [PF4]) to form immune complexes that bind to platelet Fc recep-tors. The complexes trigger platelet aggregation, the release reaction, and a subsequent fall in the circulating platelet count. The heparin dose, type of heparin, and patient platelet Fc receptor function influence the risk for the development of thrombocytopenia. Why some patients only become thrombocytopenic, whereas others develop life-threatening thromboses, is not yet clear.

Thrombin formation on the activated platelet surface or the generation of platelet microparticles is believed to play a major role in the genesis of vascular thrombosis. Injury to the endothelium via antibody binding to endogenous heparan-platelet factor 4 (PF4) complexes on the cell surface may result in the following changes: release of cytokines (IL-8), increased expression of endothelial and intercellular adhesion molecules (ECAM, ICAM), synthesis and expression of tissue factor (TF), and endothelial cell hyperplasia. Platelet aggregates (microthrombi) can occlude the microvasculature.

CLINICAL MANIFESTATIONS

The fall in the platelet count associated with HIT usually develops about 8 days (4 to 14 days of treatment) after a patient is given heparin for the first time. However, the syndrome may occur in only 1 to 3 days in patients who have had exposure to heparin in the recent past. Heparin-induced antibodies typically are undetectable 100 days after removal of heparin. Reductions in platelets are variable; the median platelet count is 60,000/μL, although counts sometimes drop to rather low levels (<20,000/μL). A minority of patients (10 to 15 percent) have nadirs that are >150,000/μL. Although somewhat arbitrary, abrupt decreases in the platelet count to <100,000/μL or the sudden fall in an elevated platelet count by half should raise the possibility of HIT. Once the heparin is stopped, the platelet count usually recovers in 2 to 5 days.

Another clue to the presence of HIT is an unexpected shortening of the APTT in patients receiving therapeutic concentrations of heparin for the treatment of thrombosis. An explanation for this finding is the release of the α-granule protein, PF4, into the plasma as a consequence of platelet activation in vivo. PF4 avidly binds heparin and neutralizes its anticoagulant activity.

The HIT syndrome occurs not only after full therapeutic doses of heparin, but also after minidose heparin prophylaxis (e.g., 5000 IU bid), or even as a consequence of the very small amounts of heparin used for flushing intravenous lines. Whether the frequency of HIT is less with patients who receive lower doses of heparin is unclear, but even small quantities may provoke the early onset of HIT after subsequent heparin exposure. HIT is less common (but still can occur) as a consequence of treatment with low molecular weight heparin (LMWH).

The spectrum of clinical manifestations of HIT is outlined in Table 45-1. Bleeding is rather unusual, probably because the thrombocytopenia is seldom profound and platelets are activated. In contrast, the effects of thrombosis can be sudden and devastating. Arterial, venous, and microvascular thrombosis have all been described, although venous thrombosis

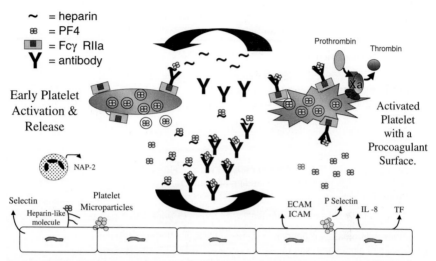

~ = heparin
⊞ = PF4
▣ = Fcγ RIIa
Y = antibody

Early Platelet Activation & Release

NAP-2

Selectin

Heparin-like molecule

Platelet Microparticles

Prothrombin

Thrombin

Xa

Activated Platelet with a Procoagulant Surface.

ECAM
ICAM

P Selectin

IL -8

TF

Endothelial Cell Activation, Release of Cytokines, Increased Endothelial Adhesion Proteins

FIGURE 45-1 Heparin-induced antibodies recognize a cryptic epitope on platelet factor 4 (PF4) that is exposed upon binding to heparin. The antigen–antibody complex then binds to the Fc receptor on the platelet, resulting in platelet activation and additional release of PF4 from the platelet alpha granules. The process is further amplified with the generation of additional antibody complexes. Other effects include the generation of platelet microparticles, exposure of endothelial and intercellular adhesion molecules (ECAM, ICAM) and platelet selectins, cytokine production (e.g., IL-8), and endothelial synthesis of tissue factor (TF).

is the most frequent. A particularly common clinical scenario is one of microvascular occlusion of the distil extremities leading to gradually progressive gangrene that begins in the digits, progresses proximally, and ultimately requires amputation. Peripheral arterial pulses are often intact despite extensive tissue injury.

The risk for thrombosis seems to vary in different patient populations. For example, postoperative orthopedic patients have a lower incidence of HIT with or without thrombosis than postoperative cardiac surgical patients. Infants and children rarely develop HIT, even though the use of heparin, especially in sick infants and after cardiopulmonary bypass, has been substantial.

DIAGNOSIS

A clinical suspicion of HIT and/or a documented drop in the platelet count should prompt the immediate discontinuation of heparin (including line flushes). Laboratory tests should be performed for confirmation of the clinical impression. However, current assays may fail to detect up

---

TABLE 45-1

Estimated Frequency of Clinical Syndromes Associated with HIT

Venous Thromboembolism

  Deep venous thrombosis (50%)
  Pulmonary embolism (25%)
  Venous limb gangrene* (5–10%)
  Cerebral sinus thrombosis (rare)
  Adrenal hemorrhagic infarction (rare)

Arterial Thrombosis

  Lower limb (distal aortic or iliofemoral) (5–10%) > "stroke" (3–5%) > myocardial infarction (3–5%) > miscellaneous (including intracardiac, upper limb, renal, mesenteric) (rare)

Acute Platelet-Activation Syndromes**

  Acute inflammatory reactions (e.g., fever/chills, flushing) (~25%)
  Transient global amnesia (rare)

Skin Lesions (erythematous plaques; necrosis) at Heparin Injection Sites (10–20%)

"Rare" indicates an estimated frequency of <3% of HIT patients
* Usually caused by high dose warfarin treatment of deep venous thrombosis complicating HIT.
** Usually occur following intravenous heparin bolus, and are associated with abrupt decreases in the platelet count.
Adapted from Warkentin TE: *Annu Rev Med* 50:129, 1999.

to 5 to 10 percent of HIT cases. None of the currently available assays lend themselves to rapid laboratory turn-around times. However, new tests that can be performed more quickly (e.g., <30 min) are being developed. The differential diagnosis of the hospitalized patient with thrombocytopenia includes drug reactions, consumption (postsurgical, DIC, massive thrombosis), destruction (splenic, dialysis, cardiopulmonary bypass), or dilution (blood products, IV fluids).

The currently available assays differ with regards to sensitivity, positive predictive value for thrombosis, and technical limitations. They can be divided into antigenic (enzyme-linked immunosorbent assay, ELISA) or functional (platelet aggregation, serotonin release, or flow cytometry) tests. The most commonly employed HIT tests are the ELISA and platelet aggregation. The ELISA typically has PF4 bound to a negative charged substance at the bottom of the well. It is an excellent screening test, but its limitations include a potential to be overly sensitive and its inability to detect non-PF4 antigens. The sensitivity of the platelet aggregation studies is dependent on the use of several well-characterized donor platelets (known to react with heparin-dependent antibodies), along with positive and negative controls. The serotonin-release assay is limited by the need for radiolabeled serotonin, a radioisotope that requires special handling and disposal. Flow cytometry assays detect heparin-stimulated platelet activation markers (P-selectin, CD 62, annexin v) and platelet microparticles. It has been demonstrated recently that this technology may be able to identify HIT complicated by thombosis (Jy ref). A strategy to identify populations at risk for thrombosis may be to screen with an antigenic assay and, if positive, perform a functional test.

THERAPY

Following the discontinuation of heparin, alternative anticoagulation therapy is usually substituted when the patient has recent thrombi or when extracorporal devices are required. Therapy is principally targeted at blocking thrombin generation. Hirudin and danaparoid have emerged as the most commonly used antithrombotic agents at this time.

Recombinant hirudin, lepirudin (Refludan®), is a thrombin inhibitor that has been FDA approved for the treatment of HIT with thrombosis. Dosing is a function of body weight (see Table 45-2) and renal function (Tables 45-3 and 45-4). Monitoring should be performed 4 hours after dosing using an APTT system; the therapeutic range is 1.5 to 2.5 times the mean normal APTT. For very low or very high doses, monitoring with an Ecarin clotting time may be necessary (Potzsch ref). Reduced dosing is recommended for patients with renal insufficiency (see Tables 45-3 and 45-4 for bolus and infusion rates). Anti-hirudin antibodies have been described. Concomitant use of thrombolytic therapy or warfarin places the patient at increased risk for serious bleeding. If warfarin therapy is

TABLE 45-2

Standard Refludan® Bolus (5 mg/mL Concentration) and Infusion Rate According to Body Weight (Manufacturers Recommendations)

		Infusion Rate at 0.15 mg/kg/h	
Body Weight (kg)	Bolus (Dosage 0.4 mg/kg)	(500-mL Infusion Bag 0.2 mg/mL)	(250-mL Infusion Bag 0.4 mg/mL)
50	4.0 mL	38 mL/h	19 mL/h
60	4.8 mL	45 mL/h	23 mL/h
70	5.6 mL	53 mL/h	26 mL/h
80	6.4 mL	60 mL/h	30 mL/h
90	7.2 mL	68 mL/h	34 mL/h
100	8.0 mL	75 mL/h	38 mL/h
≥110	8.8 mL	83 mL/h	41 mL/h

Start with IV bolus of 0.4 mg/kg body weight (up to 110 kg) over 15 to 20 sec. Follow with continuous infusion of 0.15 mg/kg body weight (up to 110 kg) per hour for 2 to 10 days or longer if clinically needed.

TABLE 45-3

Refludan® Bolus Volumes for Patients with Renal Insufficiency (5 mg/mL Concentration)

Body Weight (kg)	Injection Volume (Dosage 0.2 mg/kg)
50	2.0 mL
60	2.4 mL
70	2.8 mL
80	3.2 mL
90	3.6 mL
100	4.0 mL
≥110	4.4 mL

required, lepirudin infusions should be reduced to attain an APTT ratio of 1.5, and discontinued when an INR of at least 2.0 (due to the warfarin) has been reached. The most common adverse events include bleeding from puncture site or wounds (10.6%), anemia (12.4%), hematoma formation (10.6%), hematuria (4.4%), fever (4.4%), abnormal liver function (5.3%), and GI and rectal bleeding (5.3%) (data provided by manufacturer).

Danaparoid (Orgaran®), a heparanoid, shows a low (~10%) cross-reactivity with the antibodies in patients with HIT. Dosing of danaparoid for rapid full anticoagulation is as follows: 2,250 U intravenous bolus (1500 U if <60 kg, 3000 U if 75 to 90 kg, 3750 U if >90kg) followed by 400 U/h for 4 hours, then 300 U/h for 4 hours, then 150 to 200 U/h maintenance dose (see Hirsh ref). The therapeutic range is between 0.5 and 0.8 U/ml by a factor Xa inhibition assay obtained 4 hours after dosing. The drug is primarily metabolized by the kidneys and has a prolonged half-life of approximately 25 hours.

TABLE 45-4

Refludan® Reduced Infusion Rate in Patients with Renal Impairment

Creatinine Clearance (mL/min)	Serum Creatinine (mg/dL)	Adjusted Infusion Rate (% of Standard Initial Infusion Rate)	(mg/kg/h)
45–60	1.6–2.0	50%	0.075
30–44	2.1–3.0	30%	0.045
15–29	3.1–6.0	15%	0.0225
Below 15	Above 6.0	Avoid or STOP infusion!	

Additional intravenous bolus doses of 0.1 mg/kg body weight should be considered every other day only if the APTT ratio falls below the lower therapeutic limit of 1.5.

Occasionally a situation arises in which a patient has a history of HIT requires cardiac bypass surgery. Heparin-induced platelet antibody (HIPA) assays should be performed and, if negative, unfractionated heparin could be used during cardiopulmonary bypass. Heparin must be stopped immediately thereafter. If HIPA are present, then alternative anticoagulants must be used (discussed earlier).

Other Therapies

Argatroban (Novastan) is another anti-thrombin drug that has been used successfully in the treatment of HIT. Platelet IIb/IIIa inhibitors have been shown to be beneficial and could possibly be used an an adjunct to antithrombin therapy. Low molecular weight heparins cross-react with up to 80% of HIPAs and are therefore not recommended. Low-dose warfarin has been used successfully in the treatment of DVT; however, high-dose warfarin is contraindicated because a rapid drop in protein C in a susceptible patient could result in venous limb gangrene. Plasmapharesis may be beneficial if performed early following a thrombotic event.

BIBLIOGRAPHY

Bauer TL et al: Prevalence of heparin-associated antibodies without thrombosis in patients undergoing cardiopulmonary bypass surgery. *Circulation* 95:1242, 1997.

Carlsson LE et al: Heparin-induced thrombocytopenia: new insights into the impact of the FcgammaRIIa-R-H131 polymorphism. *Blood* 92:1526, 1998.

Cines DB et al: Immune endothelial-cell injury in heparin-associated thrombocytopenia. *N Engl J Med* 316:581, 1987.

Eichler P et al: First workshop for detection of heparin-induced antibodies: validation of the heparin-induced platelet-activation test (HIPA) in comparison with a PF4/heparin ELISA. *Thromb Haemost* 81:625, 1999.

Fischer KG et al: Recombinant hirudin (lepirudin) as anticoagulant in intensive care patients treated with continuous hemodialysis. *Kidney Int* 56:S46, 1999.

Greinacher A: Treatment of heparin-induced thrombocytopenia. *Thromb Haemost* 82:457, 1999.

Greinacher A et al: Recombinant hirudin (lepirudin) provides safe and effective anticoagulation in patients with heparin-induced thrombocytopenia: a prospective study. *Circulation* 99:73, 1999.

Griffiths E, Dzik WH: Assays for heparin-induced thrombocytopenia. *Transfusion Med* 7:1, 1997.

Hirsh J et al: Heparin and low-molecular-weight heparin: mechanisms of action, pharmacokinetics, dosing considerations, monitoring, efficacy, and safety. *Chest* 114:489S, 1998.

Jy W et al: A flow cytometric assay of platelet activation marker P-selectin (CD62P) distinguishes heparin-induced thrombocytopenia (HIT) from HIT with thrombosis (HITT). *Thromb Haemost* 82:1255, 1999.

Kelton JG: The clinical management of heparin-induced thrombocytopenia. *Semin Hematol* 36:17, 1999.

Kwaan HC, Sakurai S: Endothelial cell hyperplasia contributes to thrombosis in heparin-induced thrombocytopenia. *Semin Thromb Hemost* 25:23, 1999.

Laposata M et al: The clinical use and laboratory monitoring of low-molecular-weight heparin, danaparoid, hirudin and related compounds, and argatroban. *Arch Pathol Lab Med* 122:799. 1998.

Meyer O et al: Rapid detection of heparin-induced platelet antibodies with particle gel immunoassay (ID-HPF4). *Lancet* 354:1525, 1999.

Newman PM, Chong BH: Further characterization of antibody and antigen in heparin-induced thrombocytopenia. *Br J Haematol* 107:303, 1999.

Potzsch B et al: Monitoring of recombinant hirudin: assessment of a plasma-based ecarin clotting time assay. *Thromb Res* 86:373, 1997.

Vanholder R et al: Pharmacokinetics of recombinant hirudin in hemodialyzed end-stage renal failure patients. *Thromb Haemost* 77:650, 1997.

Warkentin TE: Heparin-induced thrombocytopenia: a ten-year retrospective. *Annu Rev Med* 50:129, 1999.

Warkentin TE: Heparin-induced thrombocytopenia: a clinicopathologic syndrome. *Thromb Haemost* 82:439, 1999.

Warkentin TE: Clinical presentation of heparin-induced thrombocytopenia. *Semin Hematol* 35(4 Suppl 5):9, 1998.

Warkentin TE: Heparin-induced thrombocytopenia: IgG-mediated platelet activation, platelet microparticle generation, and altered procoagulant/anticoagulant balance in the pathogenesis of thrombosis and venous limb gangrene complicating heparin-induced thrombocytopenia. *Transfusion Med Rev* 10:249, 1996.

Warkentin TE et al: Determinants of donor platelet variability when testing for heparin-induced thrombocytopenia. *J Lab Clin Med* 120:371, 1992.

Wilde MI, Markham A: Danaparoid. A review of its pharmacology and clinical use in the management of heparin-induced thrombocytopenia. *Drugs* 54:903, 1997.

CHAPTER 46

Thrombosis and Cancer

In a widely cited paper published in 1865, Trousseau highlighted the association of malignancy and vascular thrombosis. Since then, cancer has been recognized as one of the most common acquired causes of venous and arterial thrombosis. Although thromboembolism most often accompanies advanced malignancy, superficial or deep venous thrombosis (DVT) can be an early sign of the disease in asymptomatic patients (Fig. 46-1).

PATHOGENESIS

The cause of the thrombosis in cancer patients is most likely related to procoagulant activity of the malignant cells. For example, neoplastic cells can activate factor VII by a mechanism involving tissue factor, and tumor-associated mucin or cysteine proteases can directly activate factor X. Tumor cells have also been reported to shed plasma membrane vesicles that promote clot formation. Lastly, malignant cells may secrete cytokines that activate macrophages or endothelial cells that have prothrombotic activity. Direct effects of anti-cancer drugs on hemostasis may also be involved. For example, chemotherapeutic regimens or hormonal therapies used in the treatment of breast cancer are associated with increased rates of thromboembolism during early cycles of drug administration. Plasma levels of protein C and protein S are reduced in some of these patients.

Hypercoagulability in cancer patients varies widely. The majority of patients have minimal activation of hemostasis, which is usually asymptomatic. Moderate activation of hemostasis may present clinically as episodic venous or arterial thromboembolism, and marked stimulation

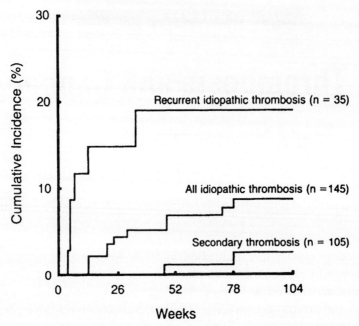

FIGURE 46-1 Cumulative incidence of cancer in patients with secondary thrombosis (predisposing factor), idiopathic thrombosis (no predisposing factor), and recurrent idiopathic thrombosis. (Reprinted by permission of *N Engl J Med* 327:1131, 1992.)

could produce overt disseminated intravascular coagulation, with bleeding, thrombosis, or both as the sequelae. Finally, antiphospholipid syndrome has been reported to accompany cancer.

CLINICAL MANIFESTATIONS

Several thrombotic syndromes occur in patients with malignancy. The risk tends to be higher during chemotherapy, hormonal therapy, and in the postoperative setting.

Migratory superficial phlebitis: While rare, the onset of apparently unprovoked thrombosis that involves the superficial veins of the extremities, chest, or abdomen was prominent in Trousseau's patients, and is strongly suggestive of malignancy.

DVT/PE: Venous thrombosis can occur at any time during the course of patients with cancer. Venous thrombosis is often recurrent and refractory to anticoagulation therapy. Several studies have shown an increased rate of cancer diagnosis during follow-up after a DVT, but the utility of extensive cancer screening in this situation is debatable.

Arterial thromboembolism: Arterial thrombosis often presents as stroke or acute peripheral artery occlusion. Vascular obstruction results either from in situ thrombosis at sites of preexisting atherosclerotic plaques or from emboli originating in the heart (see later).

Microvascular thrombosis: Small-vessel occlusion of the distal extremities can result in peripheral gangrene of the fingers and toes. Although digital ischemia can be due to large-vessel occlusion by thrombosis or embolism, disseminated intravascular coagulation (DIC) can also produce in situ microvascular thrombosis. Microangiopathic hemolytic anemia may also occur, particularly in the presence of widespread intravascular tumor cell emboli.

Nonbacterial thrombotic endocarditis: Vegetations composed of platelets and fibrin can form on mitral and aortic cardiac valves and embolize to the brain or other organs ("marantic endocarditis"). The kidney, spleen, liver, or extremities are other targets of the emboli.

Some cancers are more thrombogenic than others. In general, lymphoproliferative disease (e.g., lymphomas, Hodgkin's disease) rarely provoke thrombosis. Acute promyelocytic leukemia is often associated with DIC, brisk fibrinolysis, and bleeding, but clinically evident venous or arterial thromboembolism is unusual, and warrants further investigation. Chronic myeloproliferative disorders, such as polycythemia vera, are characteristically associated with thrombosis, but may also produce bleeding. Adenocarcinomas of abdominal organs such as the pancreas, stomach, or biliary tract appear to be the most potent in relation to thrombosis risk. Small cell carcinoma of the lung is also frequently complicated by thrombosis. Advanced prostate cancer has commonly been linked to hemostatic abnormalities such as chronic DIC or systemic fibrinolysis, but arterial or venous thrombosis is rare in the early stages of the disease.

Malignancy is often metastatic when it is associated with thrombosis. Less commonly, superficial venous thrombosis or DVT can be an early sign of cancer, particularly in malignancies that involve the tail of the pancreas or the biliary tract. In children, unexplained (acquired rather than hereditary) large-vessel thrombosis suggests malignancies such as neuroblastoma, histocytosis, or Hodgkin's disease.

Opinions vary as to whether previously healthy patients who present to their physicians with an acute thrombosis should be examined for malignancy. At least one randomized trial of screening compared to standard care is ongoing. Some generally accepted guidelines are as follows:

1. If thrombosis is associated with constitutional symptoms such as weight loss or new complaints that involve the chest or abdomen, additional diagnostic tests are indicated.
2. Patients with new-onset migratory superficial venous thrombosis or recurrent idiopathic DVT deserve further investigation.
3. At this time an extensive evaluation for occult cancer is not warranted in other patients presenting with an uncomplicated first episode of DVT. However, cancer diagnosis is more common in those with idiopathic, compared to secondary, DVT. Thrombosis in children is unusual, and secondary causes should always be considered (see Chap. 34).

If investigation for malignancy is warranted, a chest radiograph, a computed tomography scan of the chest (if a smoker) and abdomen, stool for occult blood (or colonoscopy depending on the patient's age), and laboratory tests to include a carcinoembryonic antigen, prostate specific antigen, and alpha-fetoprotein should be considered. In addition, a complete blood count should be obtained and the peripheral blood smear scrutinized for signs of marrow invasion by malignant cells. Hopefully, the relative benefit of diagnostic testing in terms of improved longevity and decreased morbidity in thrombosis patients will be better clarified.

LABORATORY TESTING

Screening tests of hemostasis in cancer patients often show elevated fibrinogen concentrations (Fig. 46-2), thrombocytosis, and a short APTT, which is a result of circulating activating clotting factors and elevated levels of factor VIII. These abnormalities often become more pronounced as the tumor progresses. If the APTT is prolonged, mixing studies to rule out clotting factor inhibitors or the lupus anticoagulant should be performed. Mild to moderate elevations of D-dimer are common, although markedly high levels are usually found only in patients with overt DIC. The role of inherited thrombophilic disorders in thrombosis in cancer patients is unknown, and extensive testing for these defects is usually not performed.

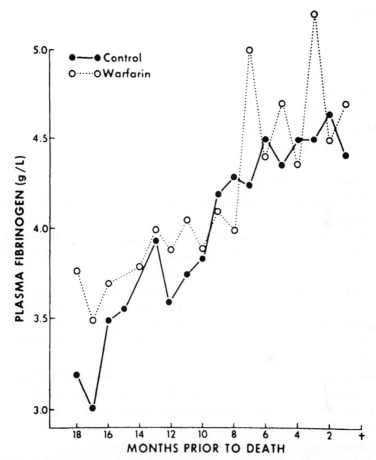

FIGURE 46-2 Sequential plasma fibrinogen levels in patients with cancer. The solid line represents the mean fibrinogen level for all patients in the control group who had fibrinogen determinations at the indicated time before death. The dashed line represents the mean fibrinogen level for anticoagulated patients (PT > 18 s) at the same time points. Plasma fibrinogen levels increased in both groups of patients as disease progressed. (Used with permission from Edwards RL et al: *Am J Clin Pathol* 88:596, 1987.)

A leukoerythroblastic picture with circulating nucleated red blood cells or immature white cells on the peripheral blood smear suggests marrow invasion by tumor. Fragmented red blood cells are commonly seen in patients with chronic DIC or disseminated tumor cell emboli in the microvasculature. Echocardiography, either transthoracic or transesophageal, can be used to identify vegetations on the mitral or aortic valves.

MANAGEMENT

Prophylactic Anticoagulation

Prophylactic anticoagulants; e.g., subcutaneous (SC) low-dose heparin, LMW heparin, or warfarin on a long-term basis are probably not indicated for cancer patients without a history of thrombosis. However, prophylaxis is warranted during periods of high risk such as surgery, prolonged immobilization, infections, and perhaps during chemotherapy (e.g., stage IV breast cancer; see Levine ref).

Therapeutic Anticoagulation

The initial treatment for thrombosis in patients with cancer is intravenous unfractionated or SC LWM heparin in full doses for a minimum of 5 days. Oral anticoagulation should be initiated concurrent with heparin, with a target INR of 2.0 to 3.0. Oral anticoagulants are given for 6 months, but may be continued for longer periods if the malignancy fails to respond to treatment. Some cancer patients will have recurrent thromboembolism on oral anticoagulants; alternative options include the use of SC LMW heparin or SC unfractionated heparin (in therapeutic doses). Unfractionated heparin is given q 12 h, with APTT or heparin level (anti-Xa) monitoring 6 hours after a dose. LMW heparin, if administered on a long-term basis, should also be monitored periodically using an anti-Xa LMW heparin assay. Serial platelet counts should be obtained along with heparin monitoring as surveillance for heparin-induced thrombocytopenia. The placement of an IVC filter should be considered if patients develop recurrent thromboembolism on full-dose heparin or LMW heparin, or if severe bleeding (or its potential) precludes effective anticoagulant therapy.

Superficial venous thromboses are often resistant to anticoagulants, antiplatelet agents, or anti-inflammatory drugs and must be treated symptomatically. Optimal therapy for nonbacterial thrombotic endocarditis is not established. Intravenous or LMW heparin is probably a preferable choice, despite the possibility of CNS bleeding due to metastatic or cerebral infarction. Intensive chemotherapy may provoke recurrent thromboembolic events in some cancer patients, possibly as a result of tumor cell stimulation or the release of procoagulant substances into the circulation. The use of heparin or LMW heparin prior to each cycle of treatment may be useful.

Because the hemostatic system is commonly activated in malignancy, and since fibrin formation has been shown to support the implantation of metastases, several clinical trials have been conducted in humans to determine if anticoagulant therapy can slow tumor progression. Some benefit has been observed following warfarin treatment in patients with small cell carcinoma of the lung. Recently, a review of clinical trials in which low molecular weight heparin was used for treatment of thrombosis suggested that the number of cancer deaths was lower among patients treated with low molecular weight heparin compared to those who received standard (unfractionated) heparin. However, clinical studies specifically designed to study this question will be needed for a definitive answer to this important question.

BIBLIOGRAPHY

Baron JA et al: Venous thromboembolism and cancer. *Lancet* 351:1077, 1998.

Barosi G: Testing for occult cancer in patients with idiopathic deep vein thrombosis—a decision analysis. *Thromb Haemost* 78:1319, 1997.

Bona RD et al: Efficacy and safety of oral anticoagulation in patients with cancer. *Thromb Haemost* 78:137; 1997.

Drewinko B et al: Untreated prostatic carcinoma is not associated with frequent thrombohemorrhagic disorders. *Urology* 30:11, 1987.

Edwards RL et al: Abnormalities of blood coagulation tests in patients with cancer. *Am J Clin Pathol* 88:596, 1987.

Goldberg RJ et al: Occult malignant neoplasm in patients with deep venous thrombosis. *Arch Intern Med* 147:251, 1987.

Green D et al: Lower mortality in cancer patients treated with low-molecular-weight versus standard heparin. *Lancet* 339:1476, 1992.

Griffin MR et al: Deep venous thrombosis and pulmonary embolism. Risk of subsequent malignant neoplasms. *Arch Intern Med* 147:1907, 1987.

Gugliotta L et al: Hypercoagulability during L-asparaginase treatment: The effect of antithrombin III supplementation in vivo. *Br J Haematol* 74:465, 1990.

Kakkar AK at al: Prevention of venous thromboembolism in cancer using low-molecular-weight heparins. *Haemostasis* 27:32, 1997.

Levine MN et al: Double-blind randomized trial of a very-low dose warfarin for prevention of thromboembolism in stage IV breast cancer. *Lancet* 343:886, 1994.

Monreal M: Occult cancer in patients with venous thromboembolism: which patients, which cancers. *Thromb Haemost* 78:1316, 1997.

Monreal M et al: Venous thromboembolism as a first manifestation of cancer. *Sem Thromb Hemost.* 25:131, 1999

Nand S et al: Hemostatic abnormalities in untreated cancer: Incidence and correlation with thrombotic and hemorrhagic complications. *J Clin Oncol* 5:1998, 1987.

Piccioli A et al: Cancer and venous thromboembolism. *Am Heart J* 132:850, 1996.

Prandoni P et al: Cancer and venous thromboembolism: an overview. *Haematologica* 84:437, 1999.

Rogers JS et al: Chemotherapy for breast cancer decreases plasma protein C and protein S. *J Clin Oncol* 6:276, 1988.

Rogers LR: Cerebrovascular complications in cancer patients. *Neuro Clin* 9:889, 1991.

CHAPTER 47

Atherosclerosis and Thrombosis

Myocardial infarction, stroke, and other chronic cardiac conditions due to atherosclerosis are major causes of disability and death in Western societies; e.g., in the United States just under one-half of all deaths are cardiovascular in nature, and most have an atherosclerotic and/or thrombotic basis. Acute arterial occlusion is most often due to the formation of a fresh thrombus overlying a ruptured or eroded atherosclerotic plaque. Evidence for coronary artery thrombosis is based on pathologic examination at autopsy, the effectiveness of thrombolytic therapy, and direct visualization of thrombi by established techniques such as angioscopy, and emerging techniques such as coronary MRI. A major research effort is underway to learn more about the pathogenesis of atherosclerosis and thrombosis, along with controlled clinical trials to determine the most effect methods for prevention and treatment of these disorders.

PATHOGENESIS

Atherosclerosis is the culmination of a complex process involving vascular injury, lipid deposition, and the activation and/or proliferation of monocytes/macrophages, smooth muscle cells, and platelets. As the initial atherosclerotic plaque enlarges due to lipid accumulation, it becomes "vulnerable" to rupture. When this occurs, lipids and other sub-endothelial components are exposed, which results in localized thrombus formation. If the thrombus is sufficiently large, acute vascular occlusion and tissue infarction will ensue. However, if the clot is smaller and non-occlusive, fibrinolytic resolution occurs, followed by the incorporation of any remaining thrombus into the now somewhat enlarged and complex atherosclerotic lesion. This may culminate in further luminal narrowing (Fig. 47-1). More complex lesions may also become "destabilized" and either rupture (thrombus observed extending into the plaque structure) or erode (thrombus observed on the surface of the plaque only), causing repeated thrombosis at the same site and progressive luminal narrowing. Even if this process does not result in an acute ischemic syndrome, it may lead to a chronic condition such as congestive heart failure and/or, ultimately, sudden cardiac death due to a fatal arrhythmia.

The atherosclerotic vessel is not only morphologically abnormal but also has functional defects that predispose to thrombosis and/or excessive vasoconstriction. The endothelium overlying an atherosclerotic lesion synthesizes reduced amounts of prostacyclin (which inhibits platelet function and produces vasodilatation), tissue-type plasminogen activator (t-PA, initiates fibrinolysis), and nitric oxide (endothelium-derived relaxing factor). Moreover, blood flowing through vascular stenoses causes increased shear forces that promote platelet activation. In addition to vascular dysfunction, abnormalities in the blood have been reported to predispose patients to arterial thrombosis; these will be discussed.

Coagulation Factors

Elevated levels of plasma fibrinogen have been repeatedly and strongly linked to an increased risk of myocardial infarction, stroke, peripheral vascular disease, and death. The predictive power of a high fibrinogen concentration is approximately the same as that of elevated serum cholesterol. It is unclear whether high fibrinogen causes an increased procoagulant potential, whether it reflects an underlying inflammatory condition (fibrinogen is a acute-phase reactant), or both. Other acute-phase proteins, such as C-reactive protein, also predict future atherothrombotic events.

Initial epidemiologic studies suggested that increased levels of factor VII were associated with future cardiovascular disease events, but more recent studies have been inconclusive. In general, genetic factors related to venous thrombosis risk (e.g., Factor V Leiden) have not proven to be important in predicting arterial events, with the possible exception of certain high-risk subgroups, such as young women smokers who are obese, hypertensive, or have diabetes (see Chap. 40). More work is needed to definitively determine if markers of procoagulant factor activation, such as the thrombin marker F1.2 or the activation peptides of factor X, factor IX, and/or protein C, are related to future events.

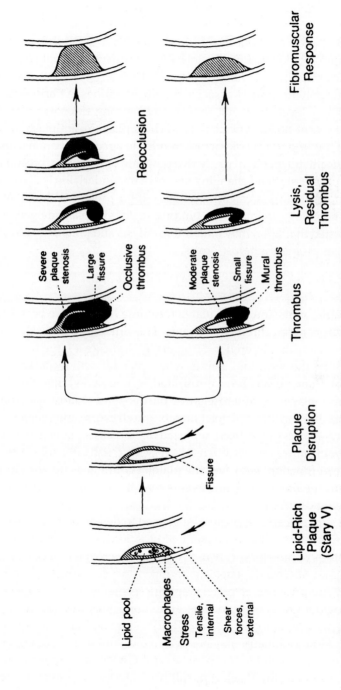

FIGURE 47-1 Typical dynamic evolution of the complicated disrupted plaque. (Reprinted by permission of the *N Engl J Med* 326:242, 1992.)

Fibrinolytic Factors

Some clinical studies have described a link between elevated levels of plasminogen activator inhibitor-1 (PAI-1, the major fibrinolytic inhibitor in blood) and atherothrombotic events, but others have failed to confirm this finding. Interpretation is difficult since PAI-1 levels are strongly related to triglyceride levels and insulin levels, and PAI-1 is also an acute-phase protein. Genetic polymorphisms associated with alterations in fibrinolytic factor or inhibitor levels have not proven to be strong risk factors to date. Markers of recent fibrinolytic activity, such as plasmin–antiplasmin complexes, are not important risk factors in middle-aged populations, but do have significant independent predictive power in older adults, presumably due to the progressive and changing nature of the underlying lesions. Since lipoprotein (a) [Lp(a)] is essentially LDL with a protein adduct that has structural homology to important binding regions in plasminogen, it has been suggested that Lp(a) may inhibit fibrinolysis and potentiate thrombosis, as well as promote atherosclerosis.

Platelets

High platelet counts and mean platelet volume (MPV) have been linked to risk of future atherothrombotic events. This link may be causal, since a) studies of myocardial infarction "triggering" indicate a large increase in event rates in the morning, a time when platelet activity is known to increase; b) smoking has been implicated in both activating circulating platelets and increasing atherosclerotic burden; and c) fatty acid composition of the diet can affect platelet membrane structure and platelet function: saturated fats have been reported to increase platelet reactivity, while monounsaturated fats and n-3 fatty acids ("fish oil") appear to suppress platelet function. However the platelet count goes up with inflammation, and the link to ischemic events may be due to platelet reactions to underlying disease.

Several sophisticated tests have been used to detect increased platelet–vascular interactions that result from atherosclerosis, including radioisotope measures of platelet survival, the urinary excretion of metabolites of thromboxane A2 (from platelets) and prostacyclin (from endothelial cells), and the presence of platelet-specific proteins in plasma, such as β-thromboglobulin. When platelets and monocytes interact with each other and with endothelial cells, cell adhesion molecules (CAMs) are expressed. Flow cytometry may be used to measure these proteins on circulating cells, and soluble forms of several CAMs may be measured in plasma (e.g., E-selectin, P-selectin, soluble ICAM-1), representing recent interactions between cells. To date, however, none of these tests are sufficiently sensitive and/or specific to be of value in individual patients.

Other Plasma Factors

The homozygous inborn error of metabolism homocysteinuria has long been associated with premature atherothrombotic disease, as well as recurrent venous thrombosis. Recently, homocysteinemia (as a result of a genetic condition or of dietary deficiencies of folic acid or other B vitamins) has been linked clearly to increased risk of venous thrombosis and implicated as a risk factor in arterial disease. Homocysteine may promote atherosclerosis and/or thrombosis by chronically altering the vessel wall in a prothrombotic direction (see Chap. 42). Also, C-reactive protein has been shown to be an important, independent risk marker, reflecting circulating levels of the proinflammatory cytokine interleukin-6. Recent work has shown that the major effect of aspirin in preventing first myocardial infarction is in those with higher CRP levels, suggesting aspirin may work via an anti-inflammatory mechanism instead of, or in addition to, an anti-platelet mechanism.

CLINICAL MANIFESTATIONS

The clinical expressions of atherothrombotic disease are diverse, but fall into four general areas:

1. The most dramatic and serious complication of atherosclerosis is plaque rupture/erosion with acute thrombotic vascular occlusion and tissue infarction. For example, this sequence might result in coronary artery occlusion, producing a massive (Q wave) myocardial infarction, or carotid artery occlusion followed by a large hemispheric stroke.
2. If the plaque rupture/erosion is less severe, subocclusive platelet-mediated thrombosis may be of sufficient size to temporarily stop or slow blood flow to produce reversible ischemia, which then regresses, possibly to reoccur at another time. Intermittent vasoconstriction could augment the ischemic symptoms. A classic example is unstable angina or perhaps stroke-in-evolution when it involves the cerebral vasculature.
3. Even smaller vascular lesions may result in the accumulation of small platelet thrombi that do not disrupt blood flow, but embolize to the distal circulation with intermittent occlusion of the microvasculature. A clinical example is transient ischemic attack or amaurosis fugax in patients with carotid artery atherosclerosis. In addition, cholesterol

crystals from the lesion itself may embolize and cause similar symptoms. Origins for emboli to the cerebral vasculature include the carotid arteries, the ascending aorta, and, in the case of non-atherosclerotic thrombi, a dysfunction atrium in atrial fibrillation. For the peripheral vasculature, the descending or distal aorta may provide the emboli seen in "purple toe syndrome," occurring in some patients given warfarin.

4. Progressive narrowing of an atherosclerotic artery may not result in infarction, but can reduce blood flow to a point where deficits produce reversible organ ischemia when stressed. Examples include angina on exertion and exercise-induced ischemia in the legs of patients with extensive iliofemoral atherosclerosis.

5. Finally, the extent of atherosclerotic disease is a leading risk factor for more chronic disease such as congestive heart failure, as well as for sudden cardiac death, including non-thrombotic cardiac death. It is likely that chronic insufficient blood flow, possibly when coupled with genetic predisposition towards electrical dysfunction caused by alterations in sodium and potassium channel proteins ("channelopathies"), ultimately leads to non-fatal and fatal arrhythmias associated with these conditions.

LABORATORY TESTING

Unfortunately, blood tests are not available to detect or localize atherosclerosis, measure its extent, or identify plaques that are likely to rupture. However, some laboratory tests involving coagulation, fibrinolysis, platelet function, or inflammation might ultimately prove helpful as predictors of future atherothrombotic complications. These tests were developed in epidemiological studies, and it remains to be seen whether they can be applied to individual patients, as some have suggested. The following assays appear to hold the most promise: fibrinogen, C-reactive protein, PAI-1, platelet count and MPV, platelet reactivity either by flow cytometry of through soluble CAMs, homocysteine, and Lp(a) (see Chap. 35). However, all of are being intensively investigated, with fibrinogen, CRP, and homocysteine the closest to clinical application.

MANAGEMENT

Therapy of Atherosclerosis

The National Cholesterol Education Panel Report—II outlines a therapeutic approach to atherosclerotic risk. Regression of established atherosclerosis has been documented by quantitative coronary angiography in groups of patients treated extensively over several years with pharmaceutical agents (e.g., lovastatin, simvastatin) to lower blood cholesterol levels. Nonpharmacological approaches, mostly based on the recommendations of the American Heart Association step I and II diets, have also been successful in certain cases. Other lifestyle modifications that have been shown to have benefit in certain subjects include smoking cessation, exercise, and weight loss.

Thrombolytic Therapy for Acute Myocardial Infarction

Since many myocardial infarctions are caused by blood clots occluding a coronary artery, thrombolytic therapy (e.g., streptokinase, t-PA) was developed to assure prompt reperfusion and the resumption of blood flow, salvage of myocardium, and improved survival. This approach has been most successful when patients have been treated with a plasminogen activator within 6 hours of onset of chest pain. Vascular surgeons and interventional radiologists and cardiologists have also been successful in reestablishing blood flow through the use of angioplasty or catheter-directed low-dose thrombolytic therapy for lesions not amenable to other approaches. Thrombolytic therapy has also proven efficacious in certain patients with thrombotic stroke. Thrombolytic therapy is used in conjunction with an anticoagulant such as heparin and/or an antiplatelet drug such as aspirin.

Anticoagulation and Antiplatelet Therapy

Anticoagulants for prevention of thrombosis in arterial disease are gaining acceptance. Heparin or low molecular weight heparin is commonly used in the initial treatment of unstable angina with or without low-dose aspirin (Chap. 59). Since there may be a "rebound" effect when heparin is stopped, antiplatelet agents such as aspirin may also be used. Much research is currently underway exploring a wide variety of established antiplatelet drugs (aspirin) and new antiplatelet agents (glycoprotein IIb-IIIa inhibitors, ADP receptor inhibitors, etc) (Chap. 62). Oral agents such as warfarin may be given in higher doses to prevent recurrent myocardial infarction, and lower doses to prevent stroke. A recent clinical trial has shown that low-dose warfarin may be used in men at high risk to prevent first myocardial infarction. In a recent population-based study, aspirin was shown to effectively prevent first myocardial infarction, especially in men with higher CRP concentrations, suggesting that aspirin's effect may be anti-inflammatory. There are a wide variety of clinical conditions in which aspirin may be an effective therapeutic agent, as shown in Table 48-1. Newer agents (e.g., clopidogrel) may be useful for some indications or in patients who are aspirin failures (see Chap. 62).

BIBLIOGRAPHY

Adjusted-dose warfarin versus low-intensity, fixed-dose warfarin plus aspirin for high-risk patients with atrial fibrillation: Stroke Prevention in Atrial Fibrillation III randomized clinical trial. *Lancet* 348:633, 1996.

Brown BG, Maher V: Reversal of coronary heart disease by lipid-lowering therapy. Observations and pathological mechanisms. *Circulation* 89:2928, 1994.

Burke AP et al: Coronary risk factors and plaque morphology in men with coronary disease who died suddenly. *N Engl J Med* 336:1276, 1997.

Danesh J et al: Association of fibrinogen, C-reactive protein, albumin, or leukocyte count with coronary heart disease: meta-analyses of prospective studies. *JAMA* 279:1477, 1998.

Fuster V: Lewis A. Conner memorial lecture: Mechanisms leading to myocardial infarctions: insights from studies of vascular biology. *Circulation* 90:2126, 1994.

Goodnight SH et al: Antiplatelet therapy—Part I. *West J Med* 158:385, 1993; Part II. *West J Med* 158:506, 1993

TABLE 47-1

Clinical Conditions in which Antiplatelet Therapy Is, or May Be, of Benefit for Treatment of Atherosclerosis

Coronary Heart Disease

- Primary prevention of myocardial infarction in middle-aged men
- Primary prevention of macrovascular disease in diabetes*
- Secondary prevention of myocardial infarction
- Unstable angina
- Chronic stable angina
- Following coronary thrombolysis
- Coronary artery bypass grafts
- Percutaneous transluminal coronary angioplasty

Cerebrovascular Disease**

- Primary prevention of stroke in patients with coronary artery disease
- Secondary prevention of stroke following transient ischemic attack

Chronic Lower Extremity Ischemia

- Infrainguinal artery bypass graft

* Recommendation of the American Diabetes Association
** May not be appropriate in older patients

Gotto AM Jr: Lipid lowering, regression, and coronary events. A review of the Interdisciplinary Council on Lipids and Cardiovascular Risk Intervention, Seventh Council meeting. *Circulation* 92:646, 1995.

Grundy SM et al: Rationale of the diet-heart statement of the American Heart Association. Report of Nutrition Committee. *Circulation* 65:839A, 1982.

Iacoviello L et al: The 4G/5G polymorphism of PAI-1 promoter gene and the risk of myocardial infarction: a meta-analysis. *Thromb Haemostas* 80:1029, 1998.

Muller JE et al: Triggers, acute risk factors and vulnerable plaques: the lexicon of a new frontier. *J Am Coll Cardiol* 23:809, 1994.

National Cholesterol Education Program. Second Report of the Expert Panel on Detection, Evaluation, and Treatment of High Blood Cholesterol in Adults (Adult Treatment Panel II). *Circulation* 89:1333, 1994.

Ornish D et al: Can lifestyle changes reverse coronary heart disease? The Lifestyle Heart Trial. *Lancet* 336:129, 1990.

Ridker PM et al: Inflammation, aspirin, and the risk of cardiovascular disease in apparently healthy men. N *Engl J Med* 336:973, 1997.

Ross R: Atherosclerosis—an inflammatory disease. N *Engl J Med* 340:115, 1999.

Ross R: The pathogenesis of atherosclerosis: a perspective for the 1990s. *Nature* 362:801, 1993.

Scheffer MG et al: Thrombocythemia and coronary artery disease. *Am Heart J* 122:573, 1991.

Thrombosis Prevention Trial: Randomized trial of low-intensity oral anticoagulation with warfarin and low-dose aspirin in the primary prevention of ischemic heart disease in men at increased risk. The Medical Research Council's General Practice Research Framework. *Lancet* 351:233, 1998.

Tracy RP: Inflammation in cardiovascular disease: cart, horse, or both. *Circulation* 97:2000, 1998.

Tracy RP et al: The relationship of fibrinogen and factors VII and VIII to incident cardiovascular disease and death in the elderly: results from the cardiovascular health study. *Arterioscler Thromb Vasc Biol* 19:1776, 1999.

Trip MD et al: Platelet hyperreactivity and prognosis in survivors of myocardial infarction. N *Engl J Med* 322:1549, 1990.

Willard JE et al: The use of aspirin in ischemic heart disease. N *Engl J Med* 327:175, 1992.

CHAPTER 48

Vascular Disorders Associated with Thrombosis

Vasculitis (angiitis) can be produced by inflammation, infection, metabolic disease, immunologic disorders, and degenerative processes in the vascular wall that often result in vascular insufficiency and thrombosis. This chapter discusses vascular disorders that may be associated with changes in hemostasis or that should be considered in the differential diagnosis of arterial (and occasionally venous) thrombosis.

Most of the disorders affect large and medium-sized vessels, whereas the small-vessel or cutaneous vasculitis syndromes more commonly produce palpable purpura or petechiae (considered in Chap. 21). In general, most of the vasculitic syndromes are either directly caused by, or closely associated with, an immunopathogenetic mechanism. Circulating immune complexes (CIC) are deposited in the vascular wall, producing increased permeability (via platelet-derived vasoactive amines) with trapping of CIC along basement membranes of the vessel wall and activation of the complement system. The complement-derived chemotactic factors cause release of lysosomal enzymes (collagenases, elastase) from polymorphonuclear cells, which in turn produce necrosis, thrombotic occlusion, and hemorrhage in the vessel wall. Table 48-1 lists the vasculitic syndromes associated with thrombotic disease; each is discussed below. The thrombotic complications noted include thrombosis in arterial aneurysms, coronary artery disease, ischemic and hemorrhagic strokes, and peripheral gangrene.

TABLE 48-1

Vasculitides Associated with Thrombotic Disease

Disorder	Major Thrombotic Manifestations
Takayasu's arteritis	Stroke, pulmonary hypertension, peripheral arterial insufficiency, coronary artery disease
Giant cell arteritis	Ocular involvement
Polyarteritis nodosa	Necrotizing glomerulonephritis, necrotic skin lesions, spontaneous visceral hemorrhage, myocardial infarction
Kawasaki syndrome	Coronary artery thrombosis, peripheral gangrene
Moyamoya disease	Ischemic stroke, subarachnoid and intracranial hemorrhage
Behcet's syndrome	Venous and arterial thromboses
Connective tissue disorders (RA, SLE, scleroderma)	Venous and arterial thromboses
Buerger's disease	Claudication, skin ulcers, gangrene

RA, rheumatoid arthritis; SLE, systemic lupus erythematosis.

TAKAYASU'S DISEASE

Aortoarteritis (Takayasu's disease) is a rare, idiopathic, chronic inflammatory disease affecting all races and involving the aorta, arteries arising from the aorta, and pulmonary and coronary arteries. Clinical findings may vary in different ethnic groups. Granulomatous inflammation progresses to fibrosis of the intima and adventitia, resulting in focal or segmental stenosis and occasional aneurysm formation. Four major complications are hypertension, retinopathy, aortic regurgitation, and arterial aneurysm. Upper extremity claudication and gradual obliteration of peripheral pulses are seen in most cases ("pulseless disease"). Other complicating events include dissecting aneurysm, cerebral thrombosis-embolism, subarachnoid hemorrhage, massive hemoptysis (pulmonary hypertension), blindness, and coronary artery disease. While hemostatic activation has been reported, this doesn't seem to correlate with disease activity. Treatment has included corticosteroids and anticoagulation therapy. In one series of 88 patients, the overall survival and event-free survival rates at 20 years after onset were 80 and 60 percent, respectively.

GIANT CELL ARTERITIS (TEMPORAL ARTERITIS)

Although temporal arteritis characteristically involves one or more branches of the carotid artery, particularly the temporal artery, the disease may be widespread and any medium or large artery can be involved. The syndrome of temporal arteritis is common and easily recognized by the classic picture of fever, anemia, elevated sedimentation rate, and polymyalgia rheumatica syndrome (stiffness; aching; pain in muscles of neck, shoulders, back, hips, and thighs), headache, and jaw claudication. A serious complication is ocular involvement (central retinal artery occlusion) leading to sudden blindness in some patients. The disease must be differentiated from Takayasu's disease, another giant cell arteritis. Diagnosis is confirmed by temporal artery biopsy. Corticosteroids are highly effective and treatment should be started early to preserve vision.

POLYARTERITIS NODOSA

The pathologic lesion characteristic of polyarteritis nodosa (PAN) is a focal segmental vasculitis and fibrinoid necrosis of medium and small arteries associated with microaneurysms. Sometimes arterioles and even venules are involved, whereas large vessels are not. The key clinical features suggestive of PAN include skin lesions (palpable purpura, livedo reticularis, necrotic lesions, infarcts of tips of the digits), peripheral neuropathy, and renal involvement (proteinuria, sediment abnormalities). These features and evidence of other organ involvement in a patient with vague constitutional symptoms of fever, fatigue, anorexia, weight loss, joint and muscle pain, and laboratory evidence of anemia of chronic disease with acute-phase reaction (elevated fibrinogen, thrombocytosis) are suggestive of PAN. Diagnosis is confirmed by biopsy of involved tissue (usually skin, sural nerve, skeletal muscle).

KAWASAKI SYNDROME

Kawasaki syndrome or mucocutaneous lymph node syndrome is a distinctive multisystem vasculitis that occurs in children (80 percent <4 years of age). Epidemic and endemic groups of cases have been reported in Japan, Korea, Europe, and the United States, although a racial predisposition in Asians is striking. The etiology is unknown, but the epidemiology, age susceptibility, evidence for immune complex formation, and elevated DNA polymerase activity in patients strongly suggest an infectious agent. About 30 percent of patients develop evidence for cardiac disease (frequently coronary artery aneurysm), and death from myocardial infarction has been reported in about 2 percent of cases.

The principal diagnostic criteria include: (1) fever for 5 or more days, (2) rash (scarlatiniform, morbilliform, or erythema multiforme), (3) conjunctival injection, (4) changes in mouth (erythema, fissures of lips, strawberry tongue, diffuse oropharyngeal redness), (5) acute cervical lymphadenopathy, and (6) changes in peripheral extremities (erythema of palms and soles, induration of hands and feet, desquamation of fingertips and toetips 2 weeks after onset). At least five of the six criteria should be present for the diagnosis of Kawasaki syndrome; however, infants have developed complicating coronary aneurysms with only four of the signs present. The acute phase of the illness lasts about 11 days (untreated). Complications include urethritis, abdominal pain and diarrhea, myocarditis, myocardial infarction, obstructive jaundice, hydrops of the gallbladder, and formation of aneurysms in medium-sized arteries (usually in coronary arteries).

Laboratory abnormalities include leukocytosis and a striking thrombocytosis (may last for 3 to 4 weeks); a rare patient may have thrombocytopenia. In addition, acute-phase reactants (factor VIII, fibrinogen, von Willebrand factor) are elevated acutely; initially low antithrombin (AT) levels and decreased fibrinolytic activity are seen in about half the patients. Thus, a hypercoagulable state is present in many patients during the acute phase of the disease, and can be correlated with the formation of coronary aneurysm and thrombosis in a few patients.

Current recommendations for treatment include intravenous gamma globulin, 2 g/kg given in a 10 to 12-hour infusion or 400 mg/kg/day for 5 consecutive days. Aspirin, in an anti-inflammatory dose of 100 mg/kg/day is given until fever has abated (or to day 14) followed by ASA 5 to 10 mg/kg/day for about 2 months, until all laboratory signs are normal. Patients with transient or small aneurysms are treated with low doses of ASA until resolution of lesions or indefinitely; patients with large aneurysms, myocardial infarction, or peripheral gangrene may be anticoagulated with heparin followed by warfarin therapy until stabilization of lesions. Maintenance therapy (after heparin-warfarin) is individualized, but has frequently involved antiplatelet agents. Prognosis and follow-up are discussed in the reference by Melish and Hicks.

MOYAMOYA DISEASE

Moyamoya disease is an idiopathic, progressive cerebral arterial occlusive disorder involving stenosis or occlusion of the terminal internal carotid arteries. This is associated with the formation of an abnormal collateral vascular network, resulting in an angiographic appearance to which the Japanese expression for "something hazy such as a puff of cigarette smoke drifting in the air" or "moyamoya" has been applied. The disorder is most often seen in children. Childhood moyamoya presents with ischemic cerebrovascular episodes, whereas in adults, subarachnoid and intracranial hemorrhage from the small arteries is the prevailing presentation. Some have suggested that ischemic stroke may be a more common presentation in adults in the Western hemisphere.

The etiology of moyamoya disease is unknown, although approximately 10 percent occur as familial cases and a genetic locus has been proposed. A role for excess TGF beta-1 has also been proposed. The characteristic angiographic signs (but unilateral) may appear in other conditions, such as neurofibromatosis, tuberous sclerosis, PAN, congenital heart disease, and after radiation therapy.

Treatment is either surgical (revascularization) or medical, with little data available comparing these. Anticoagulation has not been consistently applied, except as an adjunct to surgery or in the acute management of acute hemiplegia or childhood stroke.

BEHCET'S SYNDROME

Behcet's disease is due to a systemic vasculitis manifest clinically by oral and genital ulcers, iritis, and thrombosis (in 30 to 45 percent of patients). The disorder is most common in the Mediterranean, Middle East, and Asia. The thrombotic manifestations include venous thrombosis (~65 percent), arterial thrombosis (25 percent), or both (10 percent). Venous thromboses include deep veins, superficial veins, central veins of the abdomen including the vena cava, and the cerebral sinus veins (10 percent of patients in one series). The pathogenesis of thrombosis is not clear, but may relate to vascular injury from inflammation. Antiphospholipid antibodies and impaired fibrinolysis have been implicated, but these findings may be secondary to the chronic inflammatory process. Protein C and protein S deficiencies or factor V leiden do not seem to be increased in frequency in Behcet's patients with thrombosis.

CONNECTIVE TISSUE DISORDERS

Connective tissue or collagen-vascular disorders such as systemic lupus erythematosus (SLE), rheumatoid arthritis (RA), and scleroderma have long been associated with thrombotic complications. Antiphospholipid antibodies are found in many of these patients with thrombosis. Other mechanisms for thrombosis may play a role in these patients, including vasculitis and endothelial cell damage, platelet activation by immune complexes, and acquired deficiencies of coagulation proteins (AT, protein C, protein S). Antiphospholipid syndrome is discussed in Chapter 43.

BUERGER'S DISEASE

Thromboangiitis obliterans (Buerger's disease) is a vasculitis of medium and small arteries leading to gangrene, which involves mainly the extremities (rarely cerebral and visceral vessels). It usually affects men under 50 years of age and is considered an autoimmune reaction triggered and made worse by tobacco use. The presentation includes claudication, rest pain, digital gangrene, and ischemic ulcers. Patients with hematologic disorders, connective tissue disease, ergot overuse, thoracic outlet syndromes, embolic disease, and cold injury may have vascular disease features resembling Buerger's disease.

Over the course of the illness, most affected patients develop lesions in sites that are separate from their initial presentation. Amputation is common, especially of the forefoot. Smoking cessation appears to be the most effective therapy; amputation rates are much higher in those who continue smoking. The prostacyclin analogue iloprost was reported to reduce rest pain, but not to improve ulcer healing in Buerger's patients. Any association of this disease with hypercoagulable states has not been systematically assessed.

BIBLIOGRAPHY

Akazawa H et al: Hypercoagulable state in patients with Takayasu's arteritis. *Thromb Haemost.* 75:712, 1996.

Borner C, Heidrich H: Long-term follow up of thromboangiitis obliterans. *Vasa* 27:80, 1998.

Burns JC et al: Coagulopathy and platelet activation in Kawasaki syndrome: identification of patients at high risk for development of coronary artery aneurysms. *J Pediatr* 105:206, 1984.

Chiu D et al: Clinical features of moyamoya disease in the United States. *Stroke* 29:1347, 1998.

The European TAO Study Group: Oral iloprost in the treatment of thromboangiitis obliterans (Buerger's disease): a double-blind, randomised, placebo-controlled trial. *Eur J Vasc Endovasc Surg* 15:456, 1998.

Hall S, Buchbinder R: Takayasu's arteritis. *Rheum Dis Clin North Am* 16:411, 1990.

Hojo M et al: Role of transforming growth factor-beta 1 in pathogenesis of moyamoya disease. *J Neurosurg* 89:623, 1998.

Ikeda H et al: Mapping of a familial moyamoya disease gene to chromosome 3p24.2-p26. *Am J Hum Genet* 64:533, 1999.

Joyce JW: Buerger's disease (thromboangiitis obliterans). *Rheum Dis Clin North Am* 16:463, 1990.

Koc Y et al: Vascular involvement in Behcet's disease. *J Rheumatol* 19:402, 1992.

Krowchuk DP: Kawasaki disease presenting with thrombocytopenia. *Am J Dis Child* 144:19, 1990.

Melish ME, Hicks RV: Kawasaki syndrome: clinical features, pathophysiology, etiology and therapy. *J Rheumatol* 17(suppl 24):2, 1990.

Rizzi R et al: Takayasu's arteritis: a cell-mediated large-vessel vasculitis. *Int J Clin Lab Res* 29:8, 1999.

Sagdic K et al: Venous lesions in Behcet's disease. *Eur J Vasc Endovasc Surg* 11:437, 1996.

Scott JP et al: Evidence for intravascular coagulation in systemic onset, but not polyarticular, juvenile rheumatoid arthritis. *Arthr Rheum* 28:256, 1985.

Subramanyan R et al: Natural history of aortoarteritis (Takayasu's disease). *Circulation* 80:429, 1989.

CHAPTER 49

Cardiac Disease and Thrombosis

The most frequent cause of thrombosis that involves the heart in adults is coronary artery disease, whereas congenital heart defects and Kawasaki syndrome are more common in infants and children (see Chaps. 47 and 48). Advanced cardiac disease also predisposes to other forms of thrombosis (Fig. 49-1). Left ventricular thrombi occur in patients with cardiomyopathy, ventricular aneurysm, and transmural myocardial infarction. Thrombosis can complicate mechanical or tissue cardiac valves, and systemic emboli are common in patients with chronic atrial fibrillation. Thromboembolism related to cardiac disease is an important clinical problem that can be treated successfully with oral anticoagulants or other antithrombotic agents.

PATHOGENESIS

The pathogenesis of cardiac thromboembolism is complex, but is likely to involve one or more of the following: endocardial injury, stasis of blood, the generation of activated clotting factors, or defects in fibrinolysis (Table 49-1).

Damage to the endothelium that covers the interior surface of the left ventricle is an important factor in the pathogenesis of mural thromboses following a full-thickness myocardial infarction. Endothelial cell injury creates a thrombogenic surface due to the synthesis and expression of tissue factor and the loss of protective mechanisms from the cardiac surface, such as the platelet inhibitor prostacyclin, the effects of anticoagulants such as protein C and antithrombin, and fibrinolytic enzymes such as tissue plasminogen activator. In children, damage to the heart can also

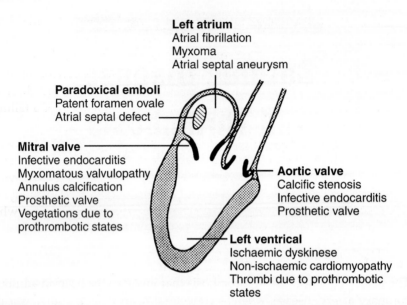

Left atrium
Atrial fibrillation
Myxoma
Atrial septal aneurysm

Paradoxical emboli
Patent foramen ovale
Atrial septal defect

Mitral valve
Infective endocarditis
Myxomatous valvulopathy
Annulus calcification
Prosthetic valve
Vegetations due to
prothrombotic states

Aortic valve
Calcific stenosis
Infective endocarditis
Prosthetic valve

Left ventrical
Ischaemic dyskinese
Non-ischaemic cardiomyopathy
Thrombi due to prothrombotic
states

FIGURE 49-1 Sources of cardiogenic emboli. (Used with permission from Hart RG: _Lancet_ 339:589, 1992.)

occur as a consequence of endocardial tissue injury from long-term indwelling parenteral nutrition catheters.

Stasis of blood due to cardiac chamber enlargement or abnormal cardiac rhythms allows the accumulation of circulating prothrombotic substances, which can overwhelm local concentrations of antithrombotic proteins and promote thrombosis. In many instances, recently formed thrombi are not firmly attached to cardiac surfaces, thus facilitating systemic embolization to the brain or other organs. Prime examples of disturbed cardiac blood flow include atrial fibrillation, advanced cardiomyopathy with stasis of blood in the dilated ventricles, and congenital heart disease in infants and children.

TABLE 49-1

Mechanisms of Thrombosis in Cardiac Disease

Mechanism	Example
Endocardial injury	Transmural myocardial infarction with mural thrombus
Sluggish or disturbed blood flow	Atrial fibrillation with embolic stroke
Activated clotting factors or platelets	Pancreatic cancer with nonbacterial thrombotic endocarditis
Fibrinolytic defects	Coronary artery disease and myocardial infarction

Activated coagulation factors (e.g., thrombin, factor Xa) or platelets can be generated in the heart, particularly at sites of tissue damage (following myocardial infarction or on the surface of a damaged heart valve in subacute bacterial endocarditis). Alternatively, activated clotting factors could be generated at sites of inflammation or malignant disease elsewhere in the body, and then accumulate in the chambers of a failing heart because of stasis or disturbed blood flow.

Some evidence suggests that patients with premature coronary artery disease could have impaired fibrinolysis due to elevated circulating levels of plasminogen activator inhibitor, which in some cases is associated with increased concentrations of plasma triglyceride. Local fibrinolysis may also be impaired in individuals with coronary artery disease who have high levels of lipoprotein(a) (see Chap. 47).

CLINICAL MANIFESTATIONS

Acute Coronary Syndromes

The etiology of patients presenting with acute coronary syndromes is a two-step process. The first step takes place over many years, if not decades, during growth of the coronary artery plaque. The second step is a sudden increase in thrombogenicity of the plaque due to rupture of the fibrous cap, leading to thrombosis via the activation of platelets and coagulation. Patients with transmural myocardial infarctions, as well as those with unstable angina and non-Q wave infarction, have evidence of fresh thrombosis on pathologic exam or angioscopy.

In the past, as many as 50 percent of patients suffering a large anterior transmural myocardial infarction developed left ventricular thrombi. The recent use of more aggressive antithrombotic treatment of myocardial infarction has appeared to decrease this risk. The clinical course in about 10 percent of these patients treated without anticoagulation is complicated by cerebral embolization. Half of these take place during the first week following infarction, with the remainder occurring over the next 2 to 12 weeks.

Cardiomyopathy and Congestive Heart Failure

Advanced cardiac muscle dysfunction of any cause is frequently associated with intracardiac thrombi. In one series, 75 percent of patients had thrombi discovered in the heart at autopsy. Systemic emboli occur at a rate of approximately 2 to 3 percent per year in cardiomyopathy patients. After a recent systemic embolus, rates of subsequent emboli may be as high as 10 to 20 percent per year. Deep venous thrombosis and pulmonary emboli are common (up to 35 percent) in both children and adults with advanced cardiac failure.

Atrial Enlargement and Atrial Fibrillation

Patients with dilated left atria (greater than 5 cm in diameter) or chronic atrial fibrillation due to rheumatic heart disease, coronary artery disease, or other cardiac disorders have a high incidence of systemic embolization. For example, untreated patients with chronic nonrheumatic atrial fibrillation have been found to have embolic complications (usually associated with stroke) at a rate of 6 to 8 percent per year; this risk is increased up to 20 percent per year in patients with rheumatic heart disease.

Valve Replacement

Patients who require artificial (mechanical) heart valves are almost always treated with anticoagulants to prevent valvular thrombosis and subsequent systemic embolization. Despite these precautions, mechanical valves in the mitral position continue to generate emboli at a rate of approximately 2 to 3 percent per year, whereas aortic valves have a lower risk (approximately 1 percent per year). Heterotopic tissue valves (e.g., of porcine origin) have lower rates of embolic complications, particularly when implanted in the aortic position.

LABORATORY TESTING

As of yet, laboratory tests are not available that predict thrombosis in patients with advanced cardiac disease, so that management decisions are still based largely on clinical parameters. Studies are needed to determine if tests reflecting activation of coagulation such as F1.2, thrombin–antithrombin complexes, fibrinopeptide A, or plasmin–antiplasmin complexes will prove to be of clinical value. Careful laboratory or point-of-care monitoring of oral anticoagulant therapy is essential to avoid recurrent thrombosis or excessive bleeding.

MANAGEMENT

Ischemic Heart Disease

Primary Prevention and Stable Angina

Three of four clinical trials have established that aspirin is effective in primary prevention of coronary thrombosis (Chap. 62). Aspirin prophylaxis is indicated in men and women >50 years of age with known risk factors for coronary disease (e.g., family history, hyperlipidemia). Patients < age

50 with atherosclerotic vascular disease or multiple strong risk factors should also be treated. Treatment of very low risk subjects is probably not indicated because aspirin is associated with a small, but statistically significant, increased risk of gastrointestinal hemorrhage, and a borderline elevated risk of intracranial bleeding. Patients with stable angina or clinical evidence of coronary artery disease should receive aspirin 75 to 325 mg/day indefinitely.

Unstable Angina

All patients with unstable angina should receive aspirin 160 to 325 mg as soon as possible, and a dose of 75 to 325 mg continued indefinitely thereafter. The rapid initiation of aspirin therapy has proven to be the single most effective step in the management of patients with acute coronary syndromes. In addition, those with persistent pain, EKG changes, elevated levels of troponin I or T, or non-Q wave myocardial infarction should receive additional antithrombotic therapy. Clinical trials have indicated improved outcomes with either the use of low molecular weight heparin (LMWH) or the glycoprotein (GP) IIb/IIIa inhibitors. Further studies are underway to determine if the combination of LMWH and the GP IIb/IIIa inhibitors will provide additional benefit.

The ESSENCE and TIMI 11B trials demonstrated that the use of enoxaparin had both short- and long-term beneficial effects in patients with severe unstable angina when compared to standard heparin. Studies have also been performed with dalteparin (FRIC) and nadroparin (FRAXIS) in which these LMWH were found to be equivalent to standard heparin.

The GP IIb/IIIa inhibitors (Chap. 62) have also been shown useful in unstable angina syndromes. Tirofiban, a synthetic non-peptide antagonist, reduced myocardial infarction and death by 22 percent at 30 days when used with heparin and aspirin. Another IIb/IIIa inhibitor, eptifibatide, showed an improvement in 30-day outcome in patients with unstable angina.

Although management guidelines continue to evolve, most cardiologists recommend aspirin for all patients with unstable angina. Patients requiring hospitalization can be treated with LMWH, and those undergoing percutaneous coronary interventions or who have refractory pain may be candidates for the GP IIb/IIIa inhibitors.

Acute Myocardial Infarction

Patients with acute myocardial infarction (AMI) are at risk for thrombotic complications, including re-infarction, stroke, and venous thromboembolism. Some form of antithrombotic therapy is indicated in most patients: the type and intensity of therapy depends on the clinical circumstances. Aspirin should be continued at 80 to 160 mg indefinitely, even if heparin is used acutely. However, if long-term warfarin is necessary (see below), aspirin should not be given until after the course of warfarin has been completed. Patients with contraindications to post-AMI aspirin should be treated with warfarin to an INR of 2.5 to 3.5. The use of warfarin following myocardial infarction has been shown to reduce re-infarction and mortality rates.

The following groups of patients are candidates for therapeutic heparin or LMWH, followed by warfarin (INR 2 to 3):

- Severe LV dysfunction
- Advanced congestive heart failure
- History of systemic or pulmonary embolism
- Mural thrombus on echocardiography
- Atrial fibrillation (indefinite warfarin therapy)
- Large anterior Q-wave infarction

Other patients with AMI should be given heparin 7,500 U every 12 h or LMWH in prophylactic doses for either 7 days or until fully ambulatory.

Percutaneous Coronary Intervention

Therapeutic doses of heparin are recommended for 2 to 4 h after simple procedures and up to 24 h in complicated patients. Aspirin at 325 mg should be given before the procedure and continued indefinitely at a dose of 75 to 325 mg/day. GP IIb/IIIa inhibitor (abciximab) therapy has been shown to be of benefit for all groups of patients undergoing coronary angioplasty, and its use should be strongly considered in high-risk patients. The likelihood of bleeding due to abciximab is reduced using lower doses of heparin without loss of antithrombotic efficacy. Currently the recommended heparin dose for coronary intervention procedures is 70 U/kg (maximum 7000 U) bolus with additional doses to achieve an ACT of 200 sec. Excess bleeding was also lessened by early sheath removal at a time when the ACT < 175 sec.

Cardiomyopathy

Patients with severe dilated cardiomyopathy are usually treated with low-intensity warfarin (INR 2 to 3) when these are risk factors such as ejection fractions under 25 percent, a history of a prior systemic embolic event, the presence of atrial fibrillation, or a history of venous thromboembolism. The use of anticoagulation in other patients with heart failure is less clear and must be based on individual risk-benefit ratios. The management of anticoagulant therapy is often difficult in patients with chronic congestive heart failure because of poor diets, congestive hepatomegaly with liver dysfunction, and interactions of warfarin with the multitude of other drugs that are required for the treatment of advanced heart disease.

Rheumatic Heart Disease

Patients with rheumatic heart disease complicated by a large left atrium, chronic atrial fibrillation, a history of embolization, or advanced congestive heart failure should be treated with warfarin at low intensity (INR 2 to 3). If a recent systemic embolus has occurred, then the INR should probably be higher (i.e., 2.5 to 3.5) for the next year, with subsequent reduction to an INR ratio of 2 to 3. Alternatively, aspirin (160 mg/day) could be added to low-intensity warfarin in these high-risk patients.

Non-Rheumatic Atrial Fibrillation

Recently seven well-designed studies have clarified the role of anticoagulant therapy in the prevention of stroke in patients with nonvalvular atrial fibrillation. The use of warfarin clearly reduces the risk of stroke from cerebral embolism by 60 to 70 percent. The risk of serious bleeding is approximately 2 percent per year and that of fatal bleeding is 0.6 percent per year. The role of aspirin is more controversial. It is not effective in high-risk patients, particularly those over age 75 or who have had a prior stroke. The SPAF III trial data indicates that low-risk patients can safely be managed with aspirin alone.

Risk factors for stroke in atrial fibrillation patients include a history of congestive heart failure, previous stroke, age over 75, hypertension, and diabetes. Patients with none of these risk factors have a stroke risk of less than 1 percent per year and are therefore candidates for aspirin treatment. However, the presence of even one risk factor greatly increases the stroke risk to 6 to 7 percent, which makes warfarin a prudent choice if the likelihood of bleeding is low. Patients over age 75 years, who have a history of stroke, or who have two or more risk factors are at very high risk of emboli (up to 20 percent/year), and should receive long term warfarin therapy (Table 49-2).

Mechanical or Tissue Valves

Adults and children with mechanical cardiac valves should be treated indefinitely with oral anticoagulants. The optimal INR range that produces the lowest risks of embolization and bleeding is currently being

---

TABLE 49-2

Treatment Guidelines for Atrial Fibrillation

No Risk Factors
Aspirin

One Risk Factor
Warfarin INR 2–3 unless bleeding risk present

Two or More Risk Factors
Warfarin INR 2–3

Risk Factors include:
History of congestive heart failure
Previous stroke*
Age over 75*
Diabetes
Hypertension

* Strongly consider warfarin therapy

reevaluated. In the past, all patients were given high-intensity warfarin (INR 3 to 4.5), but now lower levels are recommended (e.g., an INR of 2.5 to 3.5) for patients with mechanical valves without a history of systemic emboli. Similar ranges are probably appropriate for children, although applicable clinical trials are not available. Patients can also be stratified by the type and the position of the valve (see Table 49-3).

TABLE 49-3

Anticoagulation for Cardiac Prosthetic Valves.

Mechanical Valves

Bileaflet mechanical valve in aortic position: INR 2–3 (normal left atrial size, ejection fraction, sinus rhythm)

Bileaflet or tilting disk mechanical valves in the mitral position: INR 2.5–3.5

Caged ball valve: INR 2.5–3.5 (consider adding 80–100 mg/day aspirin in high-risk patients)

Mechanical prosthetic valves in patients with systemic embolism despite adequate anticoagulation: INR 2.5–3.5 plus 80 mg/day aspirin

Bioprosthetic Valves

Mitral or aortic position: INR 2–3 for first 3 months after insertion, followed by aspirin 160 mg daily

Bioprosthetic valves with atrial fibrillation: INR 2–3 (long term)

Bioprosthetic valves with history of systemic embolism: INR 2–3

From Stein PD et al: *Chest* 114:602S, 1998.

When tissue valves are inserted in the mitral position, low-intensity warfarin is usually given for a period of 3 months and then stopped. Anticoagulation is optional for aortic bioprostheses. Some patients with tissue valve prostheses require long-term warfarin therapy, especially if the left atrium is dilated or if atrial fibrillation is present.

BIBLIOGRAPHY

Antman EM et al: Enoxaparin prevents death and cardiac ischemic events in unstable angina/non-Q-wave myocardial infarction. Results of the thrombolysis in myocardial infarction (TIMI) 11B trial. *Circulation* 100:1593, 1999.

Braunwald E et al: Redefining medical treatment in the management of unstable angina. *Am J Med* 108:41, 2000.

Cairns JA et al: Antithrombotic agents in coronary artery disease. *Chest* 114:611S, 1998.

Comparison of two treatment durations (6 days and 14 days) of a low molecular weight heparin with a 6-day treatment of unfractionated heparin in the initial management of unstable angina or non-Q wave myocardial infarction: FRAXIS. (FRAxiparine in Ischaemic Syndromes). *Eur Heart J* 20:1553, 1999.

DeLoughery TG: Antithrombotic Therapy for Cardiac Disease, in Hemostasis and Thrombosis. Landes Bioscience, Austin TX, 1999, p150.

Hart RG: Cardiogenic embolism of the brain. *Lancet* 339:589, 1992.

Hsu DT et al: Acute pulmonary embolism in pediatric patients awaiting heart transplantation. *J Am Coll Cardiol* 17:1621, 1991.

Jagasia DH et al: Clinical implication of antiembolic trials in atrial fibrillation and role of transesophageal echocardiography in atrial fibrillation. *Curr Opin Cardiol* 15:58, 2000.

Klein W et al: Comparison of low-molecular-weight heparin with unfractionated heparin acutely and with placebo for 6 weeks in the management of unstable coronary artery disease. Fragmin in unstable coronary artery disease study (FRIC). *Circulation* 96:61, 1997.

Kong DF, Califf RM: Glycoprotein IIb/IIIa receptor antagonists in non-ST elevation acute coronary syndromes and percutaneous revascularisation: a review of trial reports. *Drugs* 58:609, 1999.

Koniaris LS, Goldhaber SZ: Anticoagulation in dilated cardiomyopathy. *J Amer Coll Cardiol* 31:745, 1998.

Kujovich J, Goodnight SH: Pathogenesis and therapy of thrombosis in patients with congestive heart failure. In: *Congestive Heart Failure: Pathophysiology, Differential Diagnosis and Comprehensive Approach to Therapy*, 2nd Ed., Hosenpud JD, Greenberg BH (eds), New York, Springer Verlag, 2000.

Platelet Receptor Inhibition in Ischemic Syndrome Management in Patients Limited by Unstable Signs and Symptoms (PRISM-PLUS) Study Investigators. Inhibition of the platelet glycoprotein IIb/IIIa receptor with tirofiban in unstable angina and non-Q-wave myocardial infarction. *N Engl J Med* 338:1488, 1998.

Roberts WC et al: Idiopathic dilated cardiomyopathy: Analysis of 152 necropsy patients. *Am J Cardiol* 60:1340, 1987.

Salem DN et al: Antithrombotic therapy in valvular heart disease. *Chest* 114 (Suppl):590S, 1998.

Saour JN et al: Trial of different intensities of anticoagulation in patients with prosthetic heart valves. *N Engl J Med* 322:428, 1990.

The SPAF III Writing Committee for the Stroke Prevention in Atrial Fibrillation Investigators. Patients with nonvalvular atrial fibrillation at low risk of stroke during treatment with aspirin: Stroke Prevention in Atrial Fibrillation III Study. *JAMA* 279:1273, 1998.

Stein PD et al: Antithrombotic therapy in patients with mechanical and biological prosthetic heart valves. *Chest* 114:602S, 1998.

Yeghiazarians Y et al: Unstable angina pectoris. *N Engl J Med* 342:101, 2000.

Zed PJ et al: Low-molecular-weight heparins in the management of acute coronary syndromes. *Arch Intern Med* 159:1849, 1999.

CHAPTER 50

Cerebrovascular Disease and Thrombosis

Ischemic stroke has many causes, as indicated in Fig. 50-1, which includes atherosclerotic vascular disease, emboli from cardiac sources, and hereditary or acquired thrombophilic states. Hematologic disorders complicated by stroke are covered elsewhere and include cancer (non-bacterial thrombotic endocarditis), Chapter 46; myeloproliferative disorders (polycythemia rubra vera and essential thrombocythemia), Chapter 44; heparin-induced thrombocytopenia, Chapter 45; and thrombotic thrombocytopenic purpura, Chapter 28. This chapter will focus on those hereditary and acquired hypercoagulable states associated with stroke such as antiphospholipid antibodies (APA), homocysteinemia, and the hereditary thrombophilic states.

THROMBOPHILIC DISORDERS ASSOCIATED WITH STROKE

Antiphospholipid Antibodies

Although APA are frequently associated with venous thrombosis, ischemic stroke is the most common form of arterial thromboembolism in this disorder. Anticardiolipin antibodies (both IgG and IgM) were identified in 34 percent of a multiethnic urban population presenting with stroke (compared to 11 percent in controls) (adjusted odds ratio [OR] = 4.0) (Tuhrim ref). Other studies have also shown that about one-third of new strokes in young patients (<50 yr) are associated with the lupus anticoagulant or anticardiolipin antibodies. Recurrences of transient ischemic attacks (TIA) and stroke are high in this group of patients; e.g., TIA: 25 percent/yr, stroke: 5 percent/yr (Verro ref). The great majority (>75 percent) will be found to have valvular or other abnormalities on

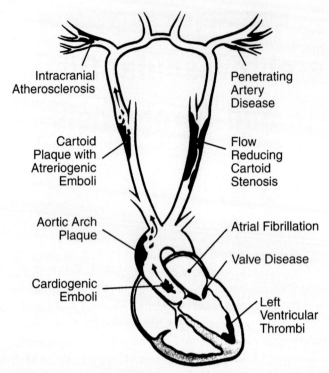

FIGURE 50-1 The most frequent sites of arterial and cardiac abnormalities causing ischemic stroke. (Used with permission from Albers GW et al: *Chest* 114: 683, 1998.)

transesophageal echocardiography (TEE), suggesting that most cerebral ischemic events are the result of cardiac emboli.

A subgroup of patients with APA have Sneddon's syndrome (stroke, livido reticularis, and Raynaud's phenomenon). Patients are also seen who have high-intensity punctate subcortical cerebral lesions on magnetic resonance imaging. These lesions are also seen in the elderly, patients with hypertension or multiple sclerosis, but are particularly prominent in some patients with APA (Fig. 50-2). The pathogenesis of these lesions is uncertain but could be due to microinfarcts or vascular injury.

Homocysteinemia

Early studies indicated that approximately 30 percent of young patients (<50 yr) with stroke had elevated levels of plasma homocysteine (HC). More recent reports have confirmed this observation in the general population and in older individuals, with ORs for stroke of 1.82 (HC levels > 14.2 µmol/L) to 2.53 (HC levels > 18.6 µmol/L). Elevated plasma HC (but

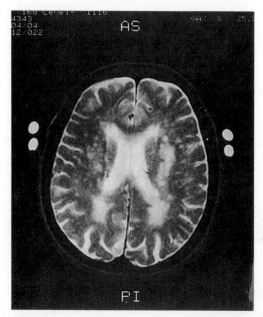

FIGURE 50-2 MRI scan showing puntate lesions in a patient with high-titer APA.

not methylene tetrahydrofolate reductase genotype) is also associated with the extent of carotid artery stenosis in both young and older individuals. Of interest, low levels of plasma vitamin B_6 (pyridoxine) were also found to be an independent risk factor for carotid atherosclerosis. These studies indicate that homocysteinemia is associated with both atherosclerosis and thrombosis. Possible mechanisms include direct vascular injury as well as the conversion of vascular endothelium from an antithrombotic to a prothrombotic phenotype (Chap. 42). As of yet, results of trials attempting to slow the progression of atherosclerosis or reduce the incidence of arterial thrombosis with vitamin therapy are not yet available.

Hereditary Thrombophilia

The great majority of studies in patients with stroke have not documented an increased incidence of hereditary thrombophilic states, such as factor V Leiden or the prothrombin gene mutation. It is not yet clear whether hereditary thrombophilia might contribute to an increased risk of stroke when present in concert with other major risk factors for vascular disease, such as hypertension, smoking, or diabetes. However, there are three settings in which hereditary thrombophilia has been associated with cerebral ischemia: right to left cardiac shunts with paradoxical emboli, cerebral vein thrombosis, and stroke in children.

Paradoxical emboli to the brain can occur in patients with a patent foramen ovale or other communication between the right and left sides of the heart, particularly in patients with multiple small pulmonary emboli (PE) with intermittent pulmonary hypertension or sudden changes in intrathoracic pressure. In one study, 30 percent of patients had APC-resistance or APA, a rate that may be even higher if additional thrombophilia tests were to be performed. The identification of this subgroup of patients has potential therapeutic ramifications; e.g., the use of anticoagulant rather than antiplatelet therapy (see later).

Hereditary thrombophilic states are commonly associated with cerebral vein thrombosis (CVT), particularly in conjunction with other risk factors such as oral contraceptive (OC) use or pregnancy. Virtually all of the thrombophilic disorders have been implicated in cerebral sinus vein thrombosis, particularly factor V Leiden and the prothrombin gene mutation. ORs for thrombosis increase dramatically with the use of oral contraceptives. For example, in a group of 40 patients with CVT, the prothrombin gene mutation was found in 20 percent and factor V Leiden in 15 percent. The OR for thrombosis was 10.2 in the prothrombin gene mutation subjects, which increased to 150 for women with the mutation who are also on OCs (Martinelli ref).

Finally, although childhood stroke is rare, most reports suggest that factor V Leiden, protein C deficiency, homocysteinemia, elevated lipoprotein (a), and other thrombophilic states are increased in frequency in these children (up to 50 percent of patients). It is not clear whether these events reflect in situ thrombosis, or perhaps paradoxical emboli via a patent foramen ovale or from other cardiac lesions.

LABORATORY DIAGNOSIS

An appropriate laboratory evaluation for stroke patients is predicated in part on the presence or absence of vascular disease. Patients with atherosclerosis of the aorta, carotid arteries, or cerebral vessels may benefit from assessment of plasma lipids [± lipoprotein(a)] and homocysteine. Both of these disorders are treatable, which could decrease the risk of future ischemic vascular events.

Patients with a thrombotic or embolic stroke not due to atherosclerosis are more likely to have a hereditary or acquired thrombophilic state that can be identified on laboratory testing. Assays to be considered include APA (Chap. 43), HC (Chap. 42), and tests to rule out a myeloproliferative disorder—CBC, erythroid, or megakaryocyte colony assays (Chap. 44). A panel of tests usually reserved for venous thrombophilia

(Chaps. 34 and 35) is appropriate for patients with a documented right-to-left cardiac shunt, cerebral vein thrombosis, or children with stroke. In our opinion, tests such as APC-resistance, factor V Leiden, or the prothrombin gene mutation are not appropriate in most adults with strokes due to documented arterial disease. As mentioned previously (Chap. 35), acute thrombosis and its attendant inflammatory state may produce alterations in thrombophilia assay results, so that if initial tests are abnormal, repeat testing should be performed several weeks after the acute event.

ANTITHROMBOTIC MANAGEMENT

Acute and long-term management of ischemic stroke is covered in the chapters on thrombolytic (Chap. 61) and antiplatelet agents (Chap. 62). The reference by Albers et al is an important resource. Therapeutic recommendations for patients with stroke-related to thrombophilic disorders are discussed below.

Antiphospholipid Antibodies

At this point in time, it is not entirely clear what constitutes optimal treatment for patients with APA and stroke, because of the lack of controlled prospective clinical trials. The uncontrolled but large retrospective studies of Rosove and Khamashta (see refs) suggested that higher intensity warfarin (INR 2.5 to 3.5) prevented recurrent thrombotic events in these patients, whereas lower intensity warfarin (INR <2.5) or aspirin did not. Until more data is available, higher intensity warfarin is a reasonable alternative for stroke patients with primary antiphospholipid antibody syndrome (PAPS), high-titer ACA/anti-β_2-glycoprotein I antibodies and/or lupus anticoagulant, documented intracardiac lesions, and recurrent events while on other therapies. Even more difficult is the situation in which an older individual suffers a stroke associated with atherosclerotic vascular disease and is found to have low titers of ACA or other APA. It is not known whether such patients would benefit from oral anticoagulant therapy. Standard antiplatelet therapy might be more appropriate in these patients until the results of prospective studies are available to provide guidance.

Homocysteinemia

As previously mentioned, prospective controlled studies are not yet available to show whether vitamin therapy (folic acid, vitamin B_6, vitamin B_{12}) will reduce the risk of recurrent stroke or slow the progression of carotid or cerebral atherosclerosis in patients with homocysteinemia. Until such studies are available, treatment with low doses of folic acid (e.g., 1 to 2 mg/day), and vitamin B_6 (e.g., 50 mg/day) seems to be a reasonable course of action, based on the low cost of therapy and negligible side effects. It is important to exclude vitamin B_{12} deficiency in these patients as the cause of the increased levels of homocysteine (with a plasma methylmalonic acid or vitamin B_{12} assay) (see Chap. 42). Standard treatment with antiplatelet agents should be used if indicated.

Other Thrombophilic Defects

Patients with ischemic stroke and thrombophilia may be candidates for oral anticoagulant therapy. In particular, those with stroke due to paradoxical emboli should receive long-term treatment with warfarin (INR 2 to 3). It is not yet clear whether repair of a patent foramen ovale will improve upon the risk–benefit ratio associated with anticoagulant therapy. In the future, catheter-guided repair of the intracardiac lesion may reduce the cost and the risk of such procedures. Long-term oral anticoagulants are usually indicated for patients with cerebral vein thrombosis associated with APA or hereditary thrombophilic states. If a major associated risk factor can be eliminated (e.g., oral contraceptives), then a shorter course of therapy (e.g., 6 to 12 months), would be an option. The optimal treatment of children with stroke and thrombophilia has not been established; acute heparin therapy followed by long-term oral anticoagulants is often used, along with a search for treatable sources of the thrombi (e.g., cardiac lesions).

BIBLIOGRAPHY

Albers GW et al: Antithrombotic and thrombolytic therapy for ischemic stroke. *Chest* 114:683S, 1998.

Becker S et al: Thrombophilic disorders in children with cerebral infarction. *Lancet* 352:1756, 1998.

Bostom AG et al: Nonfasting plasma total homocysteine levels and stroke incidence in elderly persons: the Framingham Study. *Ann Intern Med* 131:352, 1999.

Bots ML et al: Homocysteine and short-term risk of myocardial infarction and stroke in the elderly. *Arch Intern Med* 159:38, 1999.

Chaturvedi S: Coagulation abnormalities in adults with cryptogenic stroke and patent foramen ovale. *J Neuro Sci* 160:158, 1998.

Deschiens MA et al: Coagulation studies, factor V Leiden, and anticardiolipin antibodies in 40 cases of cerebral venous thrombosis. *Stroke* 27:1724, 1996.

Espinola-Zavaleta N et al: Echocardiographic evaluation of patients with primary antiphospholipid syndrome. *Am Heart J* 137:974, 1999.

Frances C et al: Sneddon syndrome with or without antiphospholipid antibodies. A comparative study in 46 patients. *Medicine* 78:209, 1999.

Khamashta MA et al: The management of thrombosis in the antiphospholipid-antibody syndrome. *N Engl J Med* 332:993, 1995.

Levine SR et al: IgG anticardiolipin antibody titer >40 GPL and the risk of subsequent thrombo-occlusive events and death. A prospective cohort study. *Stroke* 28:1660, 1997.

Ludemann P et al: Factor V Leiden mutation is a risk factor for cerebral venous thrombosis. A case-control study of 55 patients. *Stroke* 29:2507, 1998.

Martinelli I et al: High risk of cerebral-vein thrombosis in carriers of a prothrombin-gene mutation and in users of oral contraceptives. *N Engl J Med* 338:1793, 1998.

McColl MD et al: Factor V Leiden, prothrombin 20210 G$\rightarrow$A and the MTHFR C677T mutations in childhood stroke. *Thromb Haemost* 81:690, 1999.

McQuillan BM et al: Hyperhomocysteinemia but not the C677T mutation of methylenetetrahydrofolate reductase is an independent risk determinant of carotid wall thickening. The Perth Carotid Ultrasound Disease Assessment Study (CUDAS). *Circulation* 99:2383, 1999.

Nojima J et al: Risk of arterial thrombosis in patients with anticardiolipin antibodies and lupus anticoagulant. *Br J Haematol* 96:447, 1997.

Nowak-Gottl et al: Lipoprotein (a) and genetic polymorphisms of clotting factor V, prothrombin, and methylenetrahydrofolate reductase are risk factors of spontaneous ischemic stroke in childhood. *Blood* 94:3678, 1999.

Perry IJ et al: Prospective study of serum total homocysteine concentration and risk of stroke in middle-aged British men. *Lancet* 346:1395, 1995.

Robinson K et al: Low circulating folate and vitamin B_6 concentrations. Risk factors for stroke, peripheral vascular disease, and coronary artery disease. *Circulation* 97:437, 1998.

Rosove MH et al: Antiphospholipid thrombosis: clinical course after the first thrombotic event in 70 patients. *Ann Intern Med* 117:303, 1992.

Selhub J et al: Association between plasma homocysteine concentrations and extracranial carotid-artery stenosis. *N Engl J Med* 332:286, 1995.

Spence JD et al: Plasma homocyst(e)ine concentration, but not MTHFR genotype, is associated with variation in carotid plaque area. *Stroke* 30:969, 1999.

Tanne D et al: Anticardiolipin antibodies and their associations with cerebrovascular risk factors. *Neurology* 52:1368, 1999.

Tuhrim S et al: Elevated anticardiolipin antibody titer is a stroke risk factor in a multiethnic population independent of isotype or degree of positivity. *Stroke* 30:1561, 1999.

van Beynum IM et al: Hyperhomocysteinemia. A risk factor for ischemic stroke in children. *Circulation* 99:2070, 1999.

Verro P et al: Cerebrovascular ischemic events with high positive anticardiolipin antibodies. *Stroke* 29:2245, 1998.

Zenz W et al: Factor V Leiden and prothrombin gene G 20210A variant in children with ischemic stroke. *Thromb Haemost* 80:763, 1998.

CHAPTER 51

Thrombosis and Pregnancy

Thrombosis is a leading cause of maternal morbidity and mortality throughout the world. Pregnancy-related thromboses include venous thromboembolism (VTE), cerebral sinus vein thrombosis, and pregnancy loss or other complications due to placental infarction. Pregnancy can be considered a "pre-thrombotic" state, which is often complicated by hereditary or acquired thrombophilia. This chapter will discuss the diagnosis and management of thrombosis in pregnancy as well as the increased thrombotic risk associated with oral contraceptives and hormone replacement therapy.

PATHOPHYSIOLOGY OF PREGNANCY-RELATED THROMBOSIS

Venous Thromboembolism

The risk off VTE is increased approximately fivefold during pregnancy; thrombosis occurs at a rate of 1 in 1000 to 2000 pregnancies. This elevated risk is related in part to an increased prothrombotic potential found in normal pregnancy. Von Willebrand factor (vWF), factors VIII and V, and fibrinogen are all increased; protein S is decreased by 40 percent; acquired activated protein C-resistance (APC-R) is present and fibrinolysis is inhibited with decreased plasminogen activator inhibitor-1 (PAI-1) and PAI-2 (a placental-derived fibrinolytic inhibitor). Other thrombotic risk factors operative in normal pregnancy include venous stasis (maximum at 34 wks gestation) and potential pelvic vascular endothelial injury at time of delivery. Other entities that increase the risk of thrombosis include uterine sepsis, caesarean section (especially emergency), parity >gravida 4, and possibly increased maternal age (>35 yr) (Fig. 51-1). Pre-eclampsia also increases the risk of postpartum VTE by a factor of three.

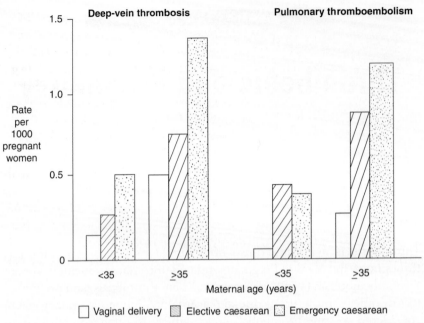

FIGURE 51-1 Incidence of postpartum deep vein thrombosis by maternal age and method of delivery. (Used with permission from Greer IA: *Lancet* 353:1258, 1999.)

Most thromboses occur prepartum (65 percent) with thrombotic events distributed throughout pregnancy (first trimester, 21.9 percent; second trimester, 33.7 percent; third trimester, 65.5 percent). Although only 35 percent of VTE occur postpartum, the risk per day is 20 to 30-fold increased compared to the prepartum incidence. Pulmonary embolism (PE) is also more likely to occur postpartum. The left leg is involved 90 percent of the time (compared to 55 percent in non-pregnant women), possibly due to compression of the left iliac vein by other vascular structures in the pelvis. The great majority of DVT involve the iliofemoral veins (72 percent), which increases the risk of PE. Other thromboses associated with pregnancy include cerebral venous stroke (8 to 9 events/100,000 deliveries, especially after C-section). Ovarian vein thrombosis (1/2,000 to 5,000 pregnancies) is also common, occurring postpartum (average ~ 7 days) and presenting with pelvic pain and fever, but negative blood cultures.

The risks of VTE are further increased by hereditary and acquired thrombophilia. Hereditary defects include factor V Leiden, the prothrombin gene mutation, deficiency of protein C, protein S, and antithrombin, dysfibrinogenemia, and homocysteinemia. Acquired prothrombotic disorders include antiphospholipid antibodies (APA) and myeloprolifera-tive disorders such as essential thrombocythemia (ET). Retrospective stud-ies have suggested that pregnancy-related thrombosis in women with hereditary thrombophilia from symptomatic families are rather high (e.g., 44 percent in AT deficiency, 24 percent in PC deficiency, 28 percent in PS defi-ciency and 2 to 8 percent in subjects with factor V Leiden). However, these rates probably overestimate the frequency of thrombosis during pregnancy; prospective studies are likely to show lower event rates. In a recent study, factor V Leiden was found in 43.5 percent of women with a pregnancy-related thrombosis (compared to 7.7 percent in normal women). The overall risk of thrombosis for carriers of the V Leiden mutation is 0.2 percent (i.e., 1/500 pregnancies). The prothrombin gene mutation was identified in 16.9 percent of pregnancies with thrombosis (1.3 percent in controls) with a like-lihood of thrombosis in pregnancy of 0.5 percent (1/200 pregnancies). Both defects were found in 9.3 percent of thrombotic pregnancies and the risk rose to 1/20 pregnancies (Gerhardt ref).

Fetal Loss and Other Complications of Pregnancy

APA have long been linked to pregnancy loss, but recently most other thrombophilic defects have been implicated as well. The mechanism of fetal loss most likely relates to placental vascular insufficiency due to thrombosis. The risks are substantially higher for stillbirth (odds ratio [OR] = 3.6) with OR recorded of 5.2 for AT deficiency, 2.3 for PC defi-ciency, 3.3 for PS deficiency, and 2.0 for factor V Leiden. If combined defects were present, the relative risk increased to 14.3. In contrast, OR for first-trimester miscarriage are substantially lower (averaging 1.27) with values of 1.7, 1.4, 1.2, and 0.9 in the respective subgroups cited above (Preston ref).

An increased likelihood of thrombophilic defects has also been reported in women with other complications of pregnancy, such as pre-eclampsia, placental abruption, and intrauterine fetal growth retardation. In one recent study, APC-R, homocysteinemia, and anticardiolipin anti-bodies were four times as common in women with a history of severe preeclampsia (van Pampus ref). Other studies did not find this associa-tion however (deGroot ref).

DIAGNOSIS OF VENOUS THROMBOEMBOLISM

The diagnosis of DVT and PE during or after pregnancy is similar in approach to non-pregnant subjects (see Chap. 36), although there are some significant differences. An evaluation is indicated if unilateral pain or swelling occurs in the leg or inguinal region (especially left-sided) during any trimester or postpartum. Doppler ultrasound (US) is the first-line diagnostic test for DVT; if positive, therapy can be started immediately. If it is negative, and diagnostic suspicion remains high, then repeat US can be performed, followed, if needed, by limited venography with pelvic shielding. Perfusion ventilation (V/Q) scans are used for diagnosis of PE, with the perfusion phase often performed first. Rarely, pulmonary angiography will be required. A diagnostic evaluation that includes chest x-ray, V/Q lung scanning, and limited venography (with shielding) provides minimal irradiation exposure to the fetus. D-dimer testing and measurement of other coagulation activation markers have not been studied in pregnancy, but are not likely to provide useful diagnostic information.

LABORATORY EVALUATION

A laboratory evaluation for thrombophilia can be performed during pregnancy, although there are several limitations. As in non-pregnant patients, some studies may be misleading if obtained immediately following a major thromboembolism or during full-dose heparin therapy (e.g., fall in AT, PC, PS). However, DNA testing for factor V Leiden and the prothrombin gene mutation will be informative at any time. Protein S levels (free and total) decline during normal pregnancy (by 40 percent or more) making it very difficult to identify hereditary PS deficiency during pregnancy. AT and PC levels remain generally normal, but AT may decrease in patients with severe preeclampsia. First-generation APC-R assays (without dilution of patient plasma in factor V-deficient plasma) are frequently abnormal in pregnancy, most likely as a result of elevated levels of factors VIII and V (see Chap. 40). Homocysteine levels decline during pregnancy, in part due to dilution and in part a result of folic acid supplementation. As mentioned above, factor VIII levels are high, making a diagnosis of thrombophilia due to elevated levels of factor VIII problematic (see Chap. 40). Lupus anticoagulant and solid-phase assays for APA are valid in pregnant patients (see Chap. 43).

Screening normal asymptomatic women for thrombophilia prior to pregnancy is usually not warranted. However, high-risk individuals (past history of VTE, strong family history of thrombosis) should be tested, particularly if management will be modified (e.g., prophylactic anticoagulants during pregnancy and peripartum). The likelihood of finding a hereditary or acquired thrombophilic state in high-risk subjects probably exceeds 50 percent. The question of whether to screen women with a history of pregnancy loss is even more difficult, in part because there is as yet no clinical data that demonstrates that prophylactic antithrombotic therapy prevents fetal loss. However, testing should be considered for women with a history of stillbirth (particularly multiple), intrauterine fetal growth retardation, or severe preeclampsia, especially if a trial of heparin or low molecular weight heparin (LMWH) is being considered (see below). The association of thrombophilia with first-trimester miscarriage is weak, which makes testing in this setting less productive.

MANAGEMENT

Antithrombotic Agents

Unfractionated heparin (IV and SC) has been used during pregnancy to treat or prevent VTE for many years. Heparin does not cross the placenta and has been shown to be as effective and safe. However, problems include poor bioavailability, heparin-induced thrombocytopenia (HIT), osteoporosis, and variability of APTT reagents used for monitoring therapy. Increasing doses of unfractionated heparin (UH) are needed as pregnancy progresses to maintain APTT or anti-factor Xa heparin levels in the therapeutic range.

Some of these problems are reduced with the use of LMWH. LMWH does not cross the placenta and studies have suggested a lower rate of HIT and osteoporosis than UH. Importantly, it has a more stable and longer half-life (4 h), and a substantially more predictable dose-response curve. Monitoring is still required using an anti-Xa LMWH assay (but at less frequent intervals than UH) because increasing doses of the anticoagulant are required as pregnancy proceeds (see Fig. 51-2). Prophylaxis or treatment of VTE in pregnancy with LMWH has not been approved by the Food and Drug Administration (FDA) in the United States. However, multiple studies have shown it to be at least as safe and effective as UH in pregnancy (see ACOG, Sanson refs).

Warfarin crosses the placenta and can cause an embryopathy that affects 4 to 5 percent of fetuses if it is administered between 6 and 12 weeks gestation. Later in pregnancy, central nervous system lesions can occur as a result of fetal intracerebral hemorrhage. Therapeutic levels of anticoagulation in the mother produces supratherapeutic warfarin effects on the fetus, in part because of liver immaturity, which can lead to fetal hemorrhage during the birthing process. Breastfeeding is not a contraindication to maternal warfarin treatment.

Other anticoagulants include hirudin and heparinoids that are used to treat some patients with HIT. Hirudin crosses the placenta and should

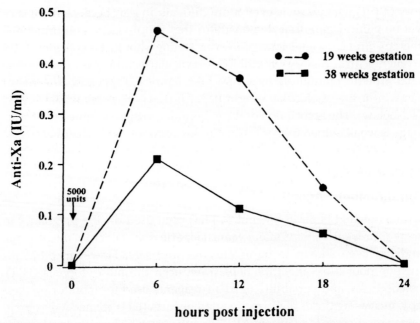

FIGURE 51-2 Pregnant women showing anti-Xa heparin levels at 19 weeks and 38 weeks gestation following LMWH (5000 U tinzaparin) by subcutaneous injection. Levels at 38 weeks are substantially lower, indicating reduced bioavailability in late pregnancy. (Used with permission from Bonnar J et al: *Semin Thromb Hemost* 25:481, 1999.)

not be used in pregnancy. Heparinoids (e.g., danaperoid) have been administered to a few pregnant patients who have developed HIT without complication.

Acute DVT and PE

VTE that occurs during pregnancy is managed in standard fashion using IV UH or SC LMWH in therapeutic doses with monitoring, preferably with an anti-Xa heparin assay (see Chaps. 36 and 59). Anticoagulation is continued throughout the remainder of the pregnancy. Some studies have suggested that the half-lives of both heparin and LMWH lengthen just prior to parturition, so that doses may need to be reduced (guided by frequent laboratory tests). Prophylactic doses of UH or LMWH can be used during labor and delivery. Postpartum, heparin concentrations can be increased to therapeutic levels (depending on the risks of bleeding) and oral anticoagulants started on postpartum day one or two. Heparin should be continued until the INR is from 2 to 3 r for 24 to 48 h. Warfarin should be continued for at least 3 months postpartum.

Epidural anesthesia is a concern during anticoagulation therapy because of the risk of spinal hematoma and neurologic damage. In patients receiving prophylactic doses of LMWH, peak values occur 2 to 4 h after injection; insertion or removal of the canula should be delayed for at least 12 h after a dose, and longer if heparin levels are higher (e.g., >0.2 U/mL). LMWH should not be restarted until at least 2 h have elapsed after catheter removal.

Peripartum AT concentrates should be strongly considered in women with hereditary AT deficiency. The first dose can be administered prior to delivery, and continued postpartum until warfarin is effective. Plasma AT levels should be monitored to assure concentrations between 80 to 120 percent.

Antithrombotic Prophylaxis During Pregnancy

Prophylactic UH or LMWH during pregnancy is indicated for women at a high risk of thrombosis (e.g., a past history of VTE or perhaps a more severe thrombophilic state, such as AT deficiency). Prophylaxis is usually not warranted in asymptomatic women (i.e., no history of thrombosis) who have other forms of thrombophilia. Other possible indications include a diagnosis of thrombophilia in conjunction with a history of stillbirth, intrauterine growth retardation, or preeclampsia. Prophylaxis can be accomplished with SC heparin, 5000 U or more given q 12 h with monitoring (at 4–6 h) to keep the APTT at the upper end of the normal range (or preferably an anti-Xa heparin assay at 0.1–0.2 U/mL). LMWH can also be used once or twice daily to obtain LMWH heparin levels (anti-Xa assay) at 0.2 to 0.4 U/mL 4 hours postinjection.

Women with APA having two or more fetal losses (regardless of duration of pregnancy) are candidates for prophylactic antithrombotic therapy. Current recommendations include heparin 5,000 U q 12h (or LMWH) plus low doses of aspirin (80 mg) started after confirmation of pregnancy and continued until delivery. In some instances heparin or warfarin can be continued for 6 to 12 weeks thereafter to prevent possible VTE (Lockshin ref).

Women who are taking warfarin prior to conception can either switch to UH or LMWH, or continue warfarin with frequent pregnancy testing. The warfarin is stopped immediately after pregnancy is confirmed followed by UH or LMWH.

Heart Valves

Optimal antithrombotic therapy during pregnancy is a major dilemma for women who have mechanical or bioprosthetic heart valves. Several studies have suggested that twice-daily SC full-dose UH has not been fully protective against systemic embolization, although concern has been raised that heparin levels were not optimal. One course of action is to treat with heparin throughout pregnancy, with care taken to ensure therapeutic heparin levels. Alternatively, heparin can be administered from the time of conception until 13 weeks (past the point of highest risk of warfarin embryopathy), then warfarin administered (INR 2.5 to 3.5) until the middle of the third trimester, followed again by full-dose heparin. The use of therapeutic doses of LMWH could also be considered (with monitoring), but clinical trials of efficacy are lacking at present.

ORAL CONTRACEPTIVES AND THROMBOSIS

Oral contraceptives (OCs) have been associated with an increased risk of VTE. The OR for thrombosis is increased 4.2 to 6-fold with the absolute increase in risk rising from 0.8 to 3.0/10,000 women/year. Third-generation OCs (e.g., containing a progestogen component such as desogestrel or gestodene) are twice as likely to provoke thrombosis than second-generation agents. The presence of thrombophilia substantially increases the risk; e.g., rates for women with factor V Leiden alone have been shown to be 5.7/10,000 women/year, which is increased to 28.5/10,000 woman/year when OCs are added. The highest risk is in the first year of use.

Similar data has been reported for the combination of the prothrombin gene mutation and OCs in respect to the rate of cerebral sinus vein thrombosis (OR increases to 150). The mechanisms underlying the increased risk of thrombosis with estrogen-containing OCs are undoubtedly multifactorial, but recent studies have shown acquired APC resistance using a modified assay based on the endogenous thrombin potential. Greater APC resistance was associated with third- versus second-generation OCs (Fig. 51-3). Widespread screening of women for thrombophilia prior to starting OCs is unlikely to be cost-effective and is not warranted. However, women with a personal or family history of VTE should undergo diagnostic testing, particularly if alternative measures of birth control are being considered.

At least four studies have now shown that hormone replacement therapy (HRT) in postmenopausal women is associated with a 2 to 4-fold increased risk of VTE. However the absolute increased risk is only 2 to 3/10,000 woman/year. It is likely that women with thrombophilia or a past history of thrombosis are at higher risk, but studies are not yet available to quantitate the magnitude of the increase, or to compare the benefits of estrogen replacement therapy with the risk of thromboembolism.

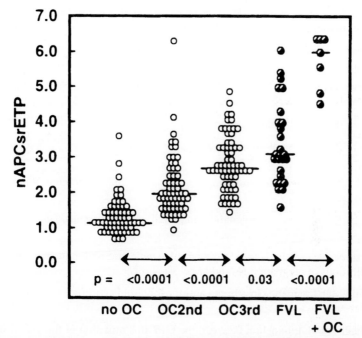

FIGURE 51-3 Effect of oral contraceptive (OC) use on normalized APC sensitivity ratios (nAPCsr) as determined using an endogenous thrombin potential (ETP) based APC-resistance test. Subjects tested include: no OC (n = 62), second-generation OC (n = 62), third generation OC (n = 64), heterozygous factor V leiden (FVL) not on OC (n = 26), and FVL heterozygotes on OC (n = 7). (Used with permission from Curvers J et al: *Br J Haematol* 105:88, 1999.)

The added likelihood of thrombosis from HRT in women who are taking warfarin is likely to be low.

BIBLIOGRAPHY

ACOG: Anticoagulation with low-molecular-weight heparin during pregnancy. *Intl J Gynecol/Obstet* 65:89, 1999.

Ballem P: Acquired thrombophilia in pregnancy. *Semin Thromb Hemost* 24 (Suppl 1):41, 1998.

Bonnar J et al: Perinatal aspects of inherited thrombophilia. *Semin Thromb Hemost* 25:481, 1999.

Brenner B: Inherited thrombophilia and pregnancy loss. *Thromb Haemost* 82:634, 1999.

Brenner B et al: Thrombophilic polymorphisms are common in women with fetal loss without apparent cause. *Thromb Haemost* 82:6, 1999.

Curvers J et al: Acquired APC resistance and oral contraceptives: differences between two functional tests. *Br J Haematol* 105:88, 1999.

De Groot CJM et al: Preeclampsia and genetic risk factors for thrombosis: a case-control study. *Am J Obstet Gynecol* 181:975, 1999.

Gerhardt A et al: Prothrombin and factor V mutations in women with a history of thrombosis during pregnancy and the puerperium. *N Engl J Med* 342:374, 2000.

Ginsberg JS: Thromboembolism and pregnancy. *Thromb Haemost* 82:620, 1999.

Ginsberg JS et al: Use of antithrombotic agents during pregnancy. *Chest* 114:524S, 1998.

Greer IA: The challenge of thrombophilia in maternal-fetal medicine. *N Engl J Med* 342:424, 2000.

Greer IA: Thrombosis in pregnancy: maternal and fetal issues. *Lancet* 353:1258, 1999.

Kupferminc MJ et al: Increased frequency of genetic thrombophilia in women with complications of pregnancy. *N Engl J Med* 340:9, 1999.

Lockshin MD: Pregnancy loss in the antiphospholipid syndrome. *Thromb Haemost* 82:641, 1999.

Martinelli I et al: Interaction between the G20210A mutation of the prothrombin gene and oral contraceptive use in deep vein thrombosis. *Arterioscler Thromb Vasc Biol* 19:700, 1999.

Martinelli I et al: High risk of cerebral-vein thrombosis in carriers of a prothrombin-gene mutation and in users of oral contraceptives. *N Engl J Med* 338:1793, 1998.

Preston FE et al: Increased fetal loss in women with heritable thrombophilia. *Lancet* 348:913, 1996.

Ray JG, Chan SW: Deep vein thrombosis during pregnancy and the puerperium: a meta-analysis of the period of risk and the leg of presentation. *Obstet Gynecol Surv* 54:265, 1999.

Ridker PM et al: Factor V Leiden mutation as a risk factor for recurrent pregnancy loss. *Ann Intern Med* 128:1000, 1998.

Rosendaal FR: Thrombosis in the young: epidemiology and risk factors. A focus on venous thrombosis. *Thromb Haemost* 78:1, 1997.

Rosing J, Tans G: Effects of oral contraceptives on hemostasis and thrombosis. *Am J Obstet Gynecol* 180:S375, 1999.

Ruiz-Irastorza G et al: Treatment of the antiphospholipid syndrome in pregnancy. *Scand J Rheumatol* 107:44, 1998.

Sanson BJ et al: Safety of low-molecular-weight heparin in pregnancy: a systematic review. *Thromb Haemost* 81:668, 1999.

Van Pampus MG et al: High prevalence of hemostatic abnormalities in women with a history of severe preeclampsia. *Am J Obstet Gynecol* 180:1146, 1999.

Walker MC et al: Changes in homocysteine levels during normal pregnancy. *Am J Obstet Gynecol* 180:660, 1999.

Waselenko JK et al: Women with thrombophilia: assessing the risks for thrombosis with oral contraceptives or hormone replacement therapy. *Semin Thromb Hemost* 24:33, 1998.

Treatment Modalities

CHAPTER 52

Platelet Transfusions

Platelet transfusion is used to treat or prevent bleeding due to significant thrombocytopenia or platelet dysfunction. Clinical characteristics of platelet-type bleeding include diffuse oozing from trauma sites (wounds, punctures), mucosal hemorrhage (gingival or oral bleeding, epistaxis, hematuria, melena, menorrhagia), formation of petechiae and ecchymoses, and spontaneous intracranial hemorrhage.

THERAPEUTIC TARGETS AND CLINICAL CONSIDERATIONS

Most patients will not have bleeding at platelet counts of 40,000 to 50,000/µL unless there is concomitant platelet dysfunction or other hemostatic defect. This level is the usual therapeutic target for treatment of active bleeding, as well as for prophylaxis perioperatively and prior to invasive procedures. In bleeding patients with platelet dysfunction (e.g., drug-induced, post-cardiopulmonary bypass) infusion of platelets to raise the platelet count by 40,000 to 50,000/µL is indicated. For central nervous system or life-threatening bleeding, higher targets (75,000 to 100,000/µL) are often used. Studies in adults and children with thrombocytopenia due to marrow failure suggest the risk of serious bleeding is minimal at platelet counts of 10,000 to 20,000/µL, and rises markedly only when the platelet count is <5000/µL. Therefore, for prophylaxis of hemorrhage in clinically stable patients, a "transfusion trigger" of <10,000/µL is normally indicated, although a threshold of <20,000/µL is reasonable in selected high-risk settings (e.g., infants, disseminated intravascular coagulation, coincident coagulation factor deficiencies, sepsis).

Relative contraindications to platelet transfusion include idiopathic thrombocytopenic purpura (ITP), unless clinically dangerous bleeding is present, as well as thrombotic thrombocytopenic purpura/hemolytic uremic syndrome (TTP/HUS) and heparin-induced thrombocytopenia. Platelet transfusion in the latter two conditions may precipitate or worsen thrombosis. Intravenous or intranasal DDAVP should be considered as a possible alternative or adjunct to platelet transfusion in some patients with congenital or acquired platelet dysfunction (drug-induced, uremia, hepatic dysfunction). Keeping the hematocrit at about 30 percent (in platelet dysfunction, uremia), and use of conjugated estrogens (in uremia) or antifibrinolytic agents (for oral bleeding) may also be helpful. Other investigational alternatives to platelet transfusion include the use of thrombopoietin and infusions of platelet membrane (both in early clinical trials), as well as fibrinogen-coated albumin microspheres (preclinical trials).

STORAGE AND CHOICE OF PLATELET PRODUCTS

In North America two basic platelet products are manufactured: whole-blood-derived ("random donor") platelets (minimum 5.5×10^{10} platelets/U in about 50 mL plasma) and apheresis ("single donor") platelets (minimum 3×10^{11} platelets/U in about 300 mL plasma). Both use acid-citrate dextrose (ACD) anticoagulant, have a pH $\approx$ 7.0, a 5-day outdate, and require 22°C (room temperature) storage with gentle agitation (refrigeration results in platelet dysfunction). One apheresis unit is generally equivalent to 5 to 6 random donor units. Apheresis platelets generally have lower white-cell and red-cell contamination, and many apheresis products are now prestorage leukoreduced (see later). Use of apheresis platelets decreases donor exposures, although it provides less flexibility in dosing.

In patients requiring ongoing platelet transfusion, risk of alloimmunization can be minimized by use of prestorage or poststorage high-efficiency leukoreduction (LR). LR random-donor pools appear equivalent to single-donor apheresis products for prevention of alloimmunization. However prestorage LR (performed in the blood center at the time of collection by either filtration or apheresis technology) is superior to poststorage LR (performed in the hospital transfusion service or by bedside leukofiltration) for minimizing febrile reactions.

Testing using nucleic acid amplification (polymerase chain reaction, PCR) technology indicates that 1 to 4% of cytomegalovirus (CMV)-seronegative donors are in fact PCR positive for CMV, and clinical studies suggest these platelet products are capable of transmitting the virus.

Because CMV is leukocyte-associated, prestorage LR (and probably also poststorage LR) results in a CMV-safe product equivalent or superior to CMV-seronegative products for prevention of transfusion-transmitted CMV. CMV-safe or CMV-seronegative products are indicated for CMV-seronegative recipients of CMV-seronegative bone marrow transplants (BMT) as well as for intrauterine transfusion and in premature infants <1250 g. They are also frequently provided to other CMV-seronegative immunocompromised recipients (e.g., pregnant women, AIDS patients).

Irradiation (usual dose: 2500 centagrays) prevents transfusion-transmitted graft vs host disease. This procedure is indicated for platelet transfusions in BMT and Hodgkin's patients, many lymphoma and other intensive tumor regimens, high-grade congenital immunodeficiencies, for HLA-matched or platelet cross-matched products, and for directed donations from any blood relative (including maternal platelets transfused to the thrombocytopenic neonate in neonatal alloimmune thrombocytopenia).

GENERAL DOSAGE GUIDELINES

Table 52-1 shows standard dosage guidelines for platelet transfusions. These guidelines assume sequestration of about one-third of transfused platelets in the spleen, and will generally be adequate to raise the 1 h posttransfusion platelet count by at least 50,000/μL. In the absence of accelerated platelet consumption, about 80 percent of the transfused platelets should be circulating 24 hours later. Although the dosage in Table 52-1 are those in standard use, there is preliminary data suggesting 1 to 2 random donor U/day in the adult may be sufficient to maintain vascular integrity and prevent spontaneous bleeding. Other studies suggest that if a higher dose of platelets is given to patients at a set prophylactic transfusion trigger, the interval between platelet transfusions may

---

TABLE 52-1
Dosage Guidelines for Platelet Transfusions
Newborn Infant
10 ml/kg should raise the platelet count by 75,000–100,000/μL
Older Child and Adult
1 apheresis unit (or 1 U random donor platelets/10 kg body weight) should raise the 1 h post-platelet count by 50,000/μL

be longer and the patients may need fewer overall platelet transfusions. Both these issues require further confirmation. Because individual response will vary according to the recipient's size, the number of platelets transfused (which can vary from unit to unit), and the presence of accelerated consumption or alloimmunization, platelet recovery can be quantified using the corrected count increment (CCI). The CCI is based on pre- and 1 h postplatelet counts (10 to 15 min counts are comparable to 1 h post counts), the recipient's body surface area (m^2), and the number of platelets transfused (marked on some apheresis units; otherwise a value of 5.5×10^{10}/random donor unit and 3×10^{11}/apheresis unit can be used). A CCI of $20,000/\mu L$ is considered adequate:

$$\text{Corrected count increment (CCI)} = \frac{(\text{Post-Precount})(\text{Body surface area})}{\text{Number platelets transfused } (\times 10^{10})}$$

REFRACTORINESS AND ALLOIMMUNIZATION

Refractoriness may be defined as failure to achieve a 1 h posttransfusion increase in the platelet count of at least $5000/\mu L$. In identifying and treating refractoriness to platelets, 1 h post counts (not just daily counts) should be monitored. Insufficient platelet dosing should be excluded—recipient size, number of platelets given (there is wide unit-to-unit variability especially with "split" apheresis bags), and the CCI should be considered. The differential diagnosis of refractoriness includes clinical factors (hypersplenism, accelerated consumption, sepsis, DIC, bleeding), infusion of a suboptimal platelet product (ABO mismatch, especially A into O; product > 48 h old), and alloimmunization.

Alloimmunization may be due to development of alloantibodies to HLA antigens or to platelet-specific antigens. HLA sensitization is more common than platelet-specific sensitization, and can result from recipient exposure to leukocytes in previously transfused products or through prior pregnancy. In the TRAP (Trial to Reduce Alloimmunization to Platelets) study, lymphocytotoxic antibodies developed in 45% of patients with acute myelogenous leukemia receiving unmodified random donor platelets and in ~19 percent of patients receiving leukoreduced (LR) or apheresis products. Platelet-specific alloantibodies developed in 6 to 11% of recipients with the rate unaffected by LR. The primary alloimmunization rate for previously unexposed patients was 13% and was decreased to 3 to 4% by either the use of LR or apheresis products. Ultraviolet (UV-B) irradiation was equally effective, but is not generally available.

A suggested scheme for prevention and management of platelet refractoriness that alloimmunization should be minimized by giving LR products to chronically transfused patients. If refractoriness appears, verify that an adequate dose of product is being given and give ABO matched platelets that are < 48 h old. If the patient is still refractory, as evidenced by low 1h post counts, screen for the presence of anti-HLA and anti-platelet antibodies. The solid-phase assay (SPA), which will detect both types of antibodies, can be used as an initial screening test. If the SPA is negative, the refractoriness is presumed *not* to be antibody-mediated, and continued support with fresh ABO-matched platelets can be used, increasing the dose as clinically appropriate. If the SPA is positive, a lymphocytotoxicity assay (LCT) against a lymphocyte panel to define the presence or absence of anti-HLA antibodies can be performed. If the SPA is positive and the LCT negative, or if only mild-moderate HLA sensitization is present (<70% LCT panel reactivity), platelet support can be provided with platelet-crossmatched products. Platelet crossmatching is faster and cheaper than HLA-matching and has given equivalent results in this setting. If high levels of HLA sensitization are present (>70% LCT), HLA-matched (+/− platelet-crossmatched) products are used.

TRANSFUSION REACTIONS AND COMPLICATIONS

Febrile reactions occur in 20 to 30% of patients receiving unmodified random donor platelet pools. The major cause of these reactions is leukocyte-derived cytokines (especially IL-6), although alloimmunization to contaminating leukocytes also causes a significant percentage. Prestorage leukoreduction (LR) is the most effective strategy for prevention of febrile reactions, followed by plasma reduction and poststorage LR, in that order. About 1 in 2000 to 12,000 platelet products have positive bacterial cultures on outdate, and sepsis should be considered in all severe febrile reactions, especially if hypotension is present or if the transfused product is 4 to 5 days old or has been pooled (sterility outdate is 4 h for pooled platelet products). If sepsis is suspected, both the patient and the platelet unit should be cultured, and broad-spectrum gram-positive and gram-negative antibiotic coverage provided. Less frequent complications include allergic reactions (most to plasma proteins), transfusion-related acute lung injury (due to neutrophil-activating factor generated during product storage or to passive transfer of anti-leukocyte antibodies in the donor plasma), circulatory overload, transfusion-transmitted infection, and graft vs host disease.

BIBLIOGRAPHY

AABB Bulletin #97-2. Leukocyte reduction for the prevention of transfusion-transmitted cytomegalovirus (TT-CMV), AABB Press, Bethesda, 1997 (web site: *http://www.aabb.org*).

AABB Bulletin #99-7. Leukocyte reduction, AABB Press, Bethesda, 1999 (web site: *http://www.aabb.org*).

Friedberg RC: Transfusion therapy in hematopoietic stem cell transplantation. In *Transfusion Therapy: Clinical Principles and Practice*, Mintz PD, ed, Bethesda, AABB Press, 1999, pp 233–249.

Heddle NM et al: A randomized controlled trial comparing plasma removal with white cell reduction to prevent reactions to platelets. *Transfusion* 39:231, 1999.

Herman JH: Platelet transfusion therapy. In *Transfusion Therapy: Clinical Principles and Practice*, Mintz, PD ed, Bethesda, AABB Press, 1999, pp 65–79.

Murphy S et al: Selecting platelets for transfusion of the alloimmunized patient. *Immunohematology* 14:117, 1998.

Slichter SJ: Optimizing platelet transfusions in chronically thrombocytopenic patients. *Semin Hematol* 269, 1998.

The Trial to Reduce Alloimmunization to Platelets (TRAP) Study Group: Leukoreduction and ultraviolet B irradiation of platelets to prevent alloimmunization and refractoriness to platelet transfusions. *N Engl J Med 337:* 1861, 1997.

Vamvakis EC: Meta-analysis of randomized controlled trials of the efficacy of white cell reduction in preventing HLA-alloimmunization and refractoriness to random-donor platelet transfusions. *Trans Med Rev* 12:258, 1998.

CHAPTER 53

Plasma

TYPES OF FROZEN PLASMA PRODUCTS AND STORAGE CONDITIONS

Several types of plasma products are currently available in North America. These products differ in their local availability and include:

Fresh frozen plasma (FFP): FFP is prepared either by separating the liquid portion of 1 U of whole blood (WB-FFP) or by collecting the liquid portion of the blood by apheresis technology (A-FFP) and freezing it within 8 h of collection. Each WB-FFP unit averages about 250 mL and contains 200–450 mg/dL of fibrinogen and about 1 U/mL of all normal coagulation factors and naturally occurring inhibitors of coagulation. WB-FFP units may be sterilely separated into 4×60 mL mini-bags for pediatric use prior to freezing. Each A-FFP unit averages about 500 mL and is equal to 2 U of WB-FFP.

Other plasma products prepared from whole blood: Frozen plasma, liquid plasma, and source plasma are other plasma preparations that are processed and frozen at varying times (up to 24 h) after collection. With storage times of greater than 8 h prior to freezing, there is some loss of labile factors V and VIII. However recent data suggest that storage of up to 24 h prior to freezing is associated with significant decreases (28 to 33%) in factor VIII only. Cryosupernant plasma (CSP) is plasma refrozen after removal of cryoprecipitate and is relatively poor in von Willebrand factor, factor VIII, and fibrinogen. CSP is used mainly for therapy of thrombotic thrombocytopenic purpura (TTP), especially refractory TTP.

Donor-retested or delayed-release plasma (DRP): This is WB-FFP or A-FFP that is held in quarantine for a minimum of 112 days, at which time the original donor returns for further donation and repeat testing for transfusion-transmitted disease is again negative. The 112-day hold period exceeds the average "window period" (time from acquisition of viral infection to seropositivity) for HIV, HBV, HCV, and HTLV and is thought to decrease the residual risk of viral transmission by > 95%. DRP is not available in all areas and is more expensive than FFP. The recent implementation of experimental nucleic acid amplification testing (NAT) (pending FDA licensure) for HCV and HIV by most blood centers has reduced the margin of safety provided by DRP over FFP.

Solvent-detergent treated plasma (SDP): This is an ABO-group–specific product produced from plasma pools of up to 2500 donors that have been treated with solvent and detergent (later removed) to eliminate lipid-enveloped viruses (HIV, HBV, HCV). The product is provided in uniform volumes of 200 mL. Mini-bags are unavailable. Non-lipid enveloped viruses (HAV and B19 parvovirus) are unaffected by SD treatment, but neutralizing antibody to these is present in the product. Asymptomatic B19 parvovirus viremia has been reported and SDP is now also tested serologically for both HAV and B19 parvovirus. Theoretical concern exists regarding a possible emerging pathogen not inactivated by the SD process.

SDP is recommended for the same indications as FFP. However there is less clinical experience with it and existing controlled studies are too small at present to permit conclusion that it is equivalent to FFP for all indications. To date, there have been no specific controlled studies of the product in the pediatric and neonatal setting. SDP lacks high molecular weight von Willebrand multimers and has lower in vitro activity levels of protein C, protein S, and α-2 antiplasmin than does FFP. It is more expensive than FFP. As with DRP, the recent implementation of experimental NAT for HCV and HIV by most blood centers has reduced the previous margin of safety provided by SDP over FFP.

General coagulation factor characteristics in plasma products are shown in Table 53-1. All frozen plasmas can be stored for 12 months at –18°C or colder. Plasma must be thawed under controlled conditions (thaw time is about 30 min for a 200 to 250 mL unit and 45 min for a 500 mL unit) and once thawed must be used within 24 h for sterility reasons. All plasmas except SDP should be refrigerated post-thaw; SDP should be stored at room temperature. All plasma must be ABO compatible with the recipient's red cells.

TABLE 53-1

Coagulation Factor Characteristics in Plasma

Coagulation Factor	T½ in Vitro*	T½ Postinfusion (h)*
Fibrinogen	Stable	96
II	Stable	60
V	3–5 days	24
VII	Stable	4–6
VIII	1–2 weeks	11–12
IX	Stable	22
X	Stable	35
XI	Stable	60
XIII	Stable	144
vWF	Stable	8–12

* T½—half-disappearance time of the clotting factor in vitro or in vivo

INDICATIONS FOR USE

The major indications for use of plasma are given in Table 53-2.

Plasma is also sometimes used to prepare "reconstituted whole blood" for exchange transfusion in infants and small children. Plasma should *not* be used as a volume expander in shock (use crystalloid or albumin), as a nutritional supplement, or for non-urgent correction of vitamin K deficiency or warfarin reversal (pharmaceutical preparations of vitamin K will usually reverse this in 6 to 12 h). Hypofibrinoginemia (DIC, massive transfusion) is best corrected with cryoprecipitate (see Chap. 54). Although plasma is frequently given to correct mild to moderate prolongations of the PT and APTT to <1.5× normal prior to invasive procedures (line placements, paracentesis, biopsies), there is little data to support this practice,

TABLE 53-2

Major Indications for Use of Plasma

Urgent clinical correction of multifactorial coagulopathy (Vit K deficiency, warfarin reversal, severe liver disease, DIC)

Factor replacement for known factor deficiencies for which specific plasma-derived or recombinant factor concentrates are unavailable (Factor II, V, VII*, X, XI* and XIII* deficiencies; Protein C* and protein S deficiencies)

Correction of microvascular bleeding (when the PT or APTT are >1.5× normal or when the patient has been transfused >1 blood volume and the PT and PTT are not available in a timely fashion—see Chap. 26)

Plasmapheresis or plasma infusion in TTP

*Concentrates available in some areas

and the skill of the operator doing the procedure is more predictive of bleeding. It should also be noted that increasing coagulation factor levels by 10 percent will have a significant effect on the PT and APTT when they are prolonged >2× mid-normal range, but will have only a minimal effect on more modest prolongations. Plasma is also usually ineffective in correction of the coagulopathy in severe liver disease because the T½ of factor VII (4 to 6 h) makes it very difficult to infuse the product fast enough; DDAVP (for the bleeding time defect) or plasma exchange (for low coagulation factors) may be helpful in this setting.

DOSE

The administration of ~20 mL/kg of plasma will usually achieve a coagulation factor concentration of ~30 percent of normal in children and adults. Correction of a clinically significant coagulopathy in an adult usually requires infusion of multiple bags of plasma; doses should be infused rapidly (within an hour if possible, depending on cardiovascular status) for maximal effect, which can be monitored with screening or specific coagulation factor assays. Repeat doses are indicated as a function of the T½ of the factor deficiency being treated (Table 53-1).

COMPLICATIONS

For standard plasma products that test seronegative by present FDA-mandated tests, the risk of transfusion-transmitted infection per million donor exposures is 0.4 to 0.5 for HIV, 4 to 36 for HCV, and 7 to 32 for HBV. HTLV has not been transmitted by any frozen plasma products. Use of DRP or SDP will provide an additional margin of safety compared to other plasma products (discussed earlier), although the recent implementation of NAT for HCV and HIV by most blood centers has further reduced risks for these viruses and narrowed this margin. Allergic reactions occur in up to 5 percent of plasma infusions. Most are mild (urticaria, rash) and can be treated with antihistamines, with the infusion continued at a slower rate. Generalized urticaria, bronchospasm, and anaphylaxis are uncommon; if they occur the infusion must be stopped and appropriate therapy instituted. Severe allergic reactions are common in patients with IgA deficiency (about 1:800 to 900) and anti-IgA antibodies (about 10 to 15 percent of those with IgA-deficiency). Plasma from IgA-deficient donors can be used for such patients. Plasma-associated transfusion-related acute lung injury (TRALI) reactions (about 1:5000 transfusions) are mediated by anti-leukocyte antibodies in donor plasma that react with recipient leukocytes to cause non-cardiogenic pulmonary edema.

BIBLIOGRAPHY

American Society of Anesthesiologists: Practice guidelines for blood component therapy: A report by the American Society of Anesthesiologists task force on blood component therapy. *Anesthesiology* 84:732, 1996.

Beck H et al: In vitro characterization of solvent/detergent-treated human plasma and of quarantine fresh frozen plasma. *Vox Sang* 74:219, 1998.

College of American Pathologists: Practice parameter for the use of fresh-frozen plasma, cryoprecipitate and platelets. *JAMA* 271:777, 1994.

Dzik S: The use of blood components prior to invasive bedside procedures: A critical appraisal. In *Transfusion Therapy: Clinical Principles and Practice*, Mintz PD, ed, Bethesda, AABB Press, 1999, pp 151–169.

Freeman JW et al: A randomized trial of solvent/detergent and standard fresh frozen plasma in the treatment of the coagulopathy seen during orthotopic liver transplantation. *Vox Sang* 74:225, 1998.

Goodnough LT et al: Transfusion medicine: blood transfusion. (First of two parts). *N Engl J Med* 340:438, 1999.

Horowitz MS et al: SD plasma in TTP and coagulation factor deficiencies for which no concentrates are available. *Vox Sang* 74:231, 1998.

Humphries JE: Treatment of acquired disorders of hemostasis. In *Transfusion Therapy: Clinical Principles and Practice,* Mintz PD, ed, Bethesda, AABB Press, 1999, pp 129–149.

Klein HG et al: Current status of solvent/detergent-treated frozen plasma. *Transfusion* 38:02, 1998.

Lusher JM: Treatment of congenital coagulopathies. In *Transfusion Therapy: Clinical Principles and Practice,* Mintz PD, ed, Bethesda, AABB Press, 1999, pp 97–128.

Makris M et al: Emergency oral anticoagulant reversal: the relative efficacy of infusions of fresh frozen plasma and clotting factor concentrate on the correction of the coagulopathy. *Thromb Haemost* 77:477, 1997.

Mast AE et al: Solvent/detergent-treated plasma has decreased antitrypsin activity and absent antiplasmin activity. *Blood* 94:3922, 1999.

O'Neill EM et al: Effect of 24-hour whole-blood storage on plasma clotting factors. *Transfusion* 39:488, 1999.

Office of Medical Applications of Research, National Institutes of Health Consensus Conference: Fresh frozen plasma: indications and risks. *Trans Med Rev* 1:201, 1987.

Pereira A: Cost-effectiveness of transfusing virus-inactivated plasma instead of standard plasma, *Transfusion* 39:479, 1999.

Schreiber GB et al, for the Retrovirus Epidemiology Donor Study: The risk of transfusion-transmitted viral infections *N Engl J Med* 334:1685, 1996.

Spence RK et al: Transfusion in surgery and trauma. In *Transfusion Therapy: Clinical Principles and Practice*, Mintz PD, ed, Bethesda, AABB Press, 1999, pp 171–197.

CHAPTER 54

Cryoprecipitate

PRODUCT PREPARATION AND CHARACTERISTICS

A one U bag (10–15 mL) of cryoprecipitate (cryo) is produced by thawing one U of fresh frozen plasma at 1 to 6°C and refreezing the precipitate, which may be stored at −18°C or lower for up to one year. Some blood suppliers also supply cryo in 5 U pools. Cryo is rich in fibrinogen, factor VIII, von Willebrand factor (vWF), and factor XIII (see Table 54-1). To use, an appropriate number of bags are thawed at 37°C, filtered, and usually pooled in a syringe or another bag. After thawing, cryo should be stored at room temperature and transfused within 6 h (4 h if pooled) for sterility reasons. Cryo should be ABO and Rh type-specific whenever possible and should be infused through a standard blood filter to prevent infusion of fibrin or particulate matter.

INDICATIONS FOR USE

Cryo is used in patients with congenital and acquired hypofibrinogen-emia (fibrinogen <100 mg/dL: DIC, obstetrical catastrophe) or dysfibrino-genemia with microvascular bleeding. Factor concentrates (which are treated to inactivate viruses or made by recombinant technology) and DDAVP (which does not carry a risk of transfusion-transmitted disease) are the currently preferred first-line therapy for hemophilia A and von Willebrand disease (VWD). However cryo is suitable for VWD unrespon-sive to DDAVP if von Willebrand factor concentrates are unavailable, and for treatment of moderate-to-severe factor VIII deficiency where DDAVP is ineffective and recombinant or purified factor concentrates are unavail-able. Factor XIII deficiency is usually treated with frozen plasma, although

TABLE 54-1

Major Plasma Proteins Contained in a Single 10–15 mL Bag of Cryoprecipitate

Constituent	Amount per Bag	Half-Life (h)
Fibrinogen	150–250 mg	100–150 h
von Willebrand factor (normal multimeric pattern)	100–150 U (40–70% of original plasma)	12
Factor VIII	80–150 U	12
Factor XIII	50–75 U	150–300

cryoprecipitate could also be used. Although its efficacy is not confined by randomized clinical trials, cryo has been used to treat platelet dysfunction (uremia, drug-induced) unresponsive to DDAVP. It is ineffective and contraindicated for the treatment of multiorgan failure.

Fibrin Glue

Allogeneic or autologous cryo may also be used to prepare fibrin glue. To make this hemostatic product, cryo is mixed with a commercial topical source of thrombin (usually bovine) at the time of use. Fibrin glue is useful surgically for slow venous-type bleeding, diffuse oozing, and lymphatic leaks; it is used most commonly in cardiothoracic and vascular surgery, neurosurgery, and maxillofacial surgery. It has been used extensively in Europe for over 20 years and is becoming increasingly popular in the United States. Commercially-manufactured fibrin sealant preparations were FDA approved in the United States in May 1998, and may have some advantages over locally produced fibrin glue; however, they are substantially more costly.

DOSING

See Table 54-2

COMPLICATIONS

Transfusion reactions and disease risks for cryoprecipitate are the same as those for fresh frozen plasma. The risk of bacterial contamination increases if post-thaw, post-pooling storage time for the product is exceeded. "Paradoxical" bleeding has been described despite adequate levels of factor VIII and VWF in patients receiving large amounts of cryo

TABLE 54-2

Dosing Guidelines for Cryoprecipitate

Clinical Condition	Usual Dose	Minimal Hemostatic Level
Fibrinogen replacement	Adult (70 kg): 10 bags Child: 1 bag/10 kg will increase fibrinogen by 60–100 mg/dL Neonate: 1 bag will increase fibrinogen by >100 mg/dL	Minimal fibrinogen of 75 –100 mg/dL (measure post infusion—dosing frequency can vary from every 8–12 h in active DIC to days
von Willebrand disease Note: 2nd line therapy (see text)	Adult: 10–12 bags q 12 h Child: 1 bag/6 kg q 12 h	Stated dose will usually assure hemostasis (bleeding time may not always correct)
Hemophilia A (Factor VIII deficiency) Note: 2nd line therapy (see text)	Use dosage guidelines for concentrates (Chap. 55) assuming 1 bag cryo contains 100 U factor VIII (1 bag/6 kg will usually give a factor VIII level of about 35%	Factor VIII of 35–100% depending on clinical setting (see Chap. 55)
Factor XIII deficiency	1 bag/10 kg every 7–14 days	Low levels (2–3%) of factor XIII are hemostatic

Note: Fresh frozen plasma is often used for prophylaxis.

over an extended period of time for treatment of hemophilia A. This appears to be related to prolongation of the bleeding time associated with high fibrinogen concentrations and increased fibrin degradation products. Due to small quantities of erythrocyte isohemagglutinins in cryo, a positive direct antiglobulin test, or more rarely hemolysis (usually mild) can result if large volumes of ABO-incompatible cryo are used.

BIBLIOGRAPHY

Alving BA et al: Fibrin sealant: Summary of a conference on characteristics and clinical uses. *Transfusion* 35:783, 1995.

College of American Pathologists: Practice parameter for the use of fresh-frozen plasma, cryoprecipitate and platelets. *JAMA* 271:777, 1994.

Gribble JW, Ness PM: Fibrin glue: the perfect operative sealant? *Transfusion* 30:741, 1990.

Hathaway WE et al: Paradoxical bleeding in intensively transfused hemophiliacs: alteration of platelet function. *Transfusion* 13:6, 1973.

Humphries JE: Treatment of acquired disorders of hemostasis. In *Transfusion Therapy: Clinical Principles and Practice,* Mintz PD, ed, Bethesda, AABB Press, 1999, pp. 129–149.

Lusher JM: Treatment of congenital coagulopathies. In *Transfusion Therapy: Clinical Principles and Practice,* Mintz PD, ed, Bethesda, AABB Press, 1999, pp. 97–128.

Poon MC: Cryoprecipitate: Uses and alternatives. *Transfus Med Rev* 7:180, 1993.

Reiner AP: Fibrin glue increasingly popular for topical surgical hemostasis. *Labora Med* 30:189, 1999.

Spence RK et al: Transfusion in surgery and trauma. In *Transfusion Therapy: Clinical Principles and Practice,* Mintz PD, ed, Bethesda, AABB Press, 1999, pp. 171–198.

Spotnitz WD, Welker RL: Clinical uses of fibrin sealant. In *Transfusion Therapy: Clinical Principles and Practice,* Mintz PD, ed, Bethesda, AABB Press, 1999, pp. 199–222.

CHAPTER 55

Coagulation Factor Concentrates

During the past 30 years steady advances have been made in the development and manufacture of coagulation factor concentrates for clinical use. Viral complications of plasma-derived concentrate therapy (HIV, hepatitis viruses) have been catastrophic, but in the last decade advances in methodology have all but eliminated this threat. At the present time adequate studies do not exist to document removal of more resistant viruses (non-lipid enveloped) such as parvovirus. The advent of recombinant protein technology (established for factors VII, VIII, and IX) should provide the means for the ultimate pure and safe products. Both recombinant factor VIIa and IX do not include added albumin for stabilization in the final preparation. Second-generation recombinant factor VIII concentrates, including a mutated B-domainless protein, are without added albumin and are in clinical trials. A great deal of the progress is due to systematic safety testing of new products as they become available. Since 1984, guidelines prepared by the International Committee on Thrombosis and Hemostasis (ICTH) have been available for the use of investigators and manufacturers in testing new products. Physicians using replacement products should be aware of the results of clinical studies performed to determine the occurrence of adverse events such as viral transmissions or inhibitor development.

CONCENTRATE DESCRIPTION AND PRINCIPLES OF THERAPY

Although it is beyond the scope of this discussion to review methodology for preparation of concentrates, a few general remarks are in order. Current production of plasma-derived clotting factor concentrates requires a large starting pool of carefully screened donor plasma that is processed to produce as pure a clotting factor(s) as practical. Affinity chromatography using monoclonal antibodies currently provides the purest plasma-derived products (Table 55-1). Viral inactivation procedures (pasteurization, solvent-detergent treatment, chemical disruption with sodium thiocyanate, or ultrafiltration) are effective against HIV and hepatitis viruses. The final product is assayed against international coagulation factor standards and labeled accordingly. A unit is the coagulant activity in 1 mL fresh normal plasma (the standard); for instance, 100 U factor VIII is the amount of clotting activity in 100 mL fresh plasma.

FACTOR VIII

Table 55-1 lists several factor VIII-containing concentrates available for clinical use. The dose of factor concentrate to achieve a desired level of correction is estimated by the following formula:

$$\text{\# units required} = \text{weight (kg)} \times \text{volume of distribution} \times \text{level desired}$$

For factor VIII the volume of distribution is ≈ 0.5. The level desired should be placed in the formula as a whole number (e.g., "100" representing a level of 100%).

For example, to raise the plasma level to 0.40 u/mL or 40% in a severe hemophilia A child weighing 10 kg, 200 U ($10 \times 0.5 \times 40 = 200$) of factor VIII product should be given.

The type of bleeding episode dictates the level required. To arrest bleeding in a patient with an early joint or muscle bleed, a hemostatic level of approximately 30 to 40 percent is adequate to achieve hemostasis and prevent recurrent hemorrhage. With more severe musculoskeletal bleeding, and if a longer period of correction is desired, levels of 60 to 80 percent are needed. To achieve hemostasis for major surgical procedures, an initial level of 60 to 100 percent is obtained, followed by a prophylactic level of 30 to 50 percent until the wound is healed (10 to 14 days). Most orthopedic surgery can be managed postoperatively with levels of at least 30 percent except at times of wound or joint manipulation (removal of drains, early physical therapy) when a 50 percent level is necessary.

Severe oral pharyngeal bleeding and CNS hemorrhage require higher levels (50 to 100 percent correction) for longer periods of time (usually until the lesion is deemed "healed" or resolved). Realizing that infused factor VIII concentrate has a half-disappearance time of about 12 h, post-surgical prophylaxis is accomplished by bolus infusions every 12 h or by continuous therapy (a continuous infusion of factor VIII concentrate of

TABLE 55-1

Products Licensed for Use in United States

Product	Manufacturer	Preparation	Viral Attenuation/Inactivation	SP ACT IU/mg	PD/R, +/−Alb
Factor VIII					
Humate-P*	Centeon	Multiple precipitation	Pasteurization 60°C, 10 h	40	PD, +Alb
Koate HP*	Bayer	Multiple precipitation, chromatography	TNBP / polysorbate 80	75–125	PD, +Alb
Alphanate*	Alpha	Heparin chromatography	TNBP / polysorbate 80, dry heat 80° C 72 h	140	PD, +Alb
Monoclate-P	Centeon	Monoclonal Ab affinity chromatography	Pasteurization 60°, 10 h	3000	PD, +Alb
Hemofil M	Baxter-Immuno	Monoclonal Ab affinity chromatography	TNBP / Triton X 100	>2000	PD, +Alb
Monarc-M	American Red Cross	Monoclonal Ab affinity chromatography	TNBP / Triton X 100	>2000	PD, +Alb
Recombinate (=Bioclate)	Baxter-Immuno	Recombinant, ion exchange, monoclonal Ab chromatography	Viral attenuation through purification	1650–19000	R, +Alb
Kogenate (=Helixate)	Bayer	Recombinant, ion exchange, monoclonal Ab affinity chromatography	Viral attenuation through purification	3000	R, +Alb
Factor IX					
Bebulin	Baxter-Immuno	DEAE-Sephadex	Vapor heat 60°C 10 h, 80°C 1 h	1.9	PD
Proplex T	Baxter-Immuno	Tricalcium phosphate absorption, PEG fractionation	Dry heat 60°C 144 h	↑FVII, ~3 FVII:FIX	PD

TABLE 55-1 CONTINUED

Products Licensed for Use in United States

Product	Manufacturer	Preparation	Viral Attenuation/Inactivation	SP ACT IU/mg	PD/R, +/–Alb
Konyne 80	Bayer	DEAE absorption	Dry heat 80°C 72 h	1–3	PD, –Alb
Profilnine SD	Alpha	DEAE cellulose adsorption	TNBP / polysorbate 80	4	PD, –Alb
Alphanine SD	Alpha	Ion exchange, carbohydrate ligand chromatography	TNBP / polysorbate 80, nanofiltration	210	PD, –Alb
Mononine	Centeon	Immunoaffinity chromatography	Sodium thiocyanate, ultrafiltration	190	PD, –Alb
BeneFIX	Genetics Institute	Recombinant, Q Sepharose FF, Cellufine sulfate, Ceramic hydroxyapatite, chelate-EMD-Cu(II)	Nanofiltration	200 or >	R, –Alb
Inhibitor Products					
NovoSeven	Novo-Nordisk	Recombinant, ion exchange and monoclonal antibody chromatography	Viral attenuation through purification	50,000	R, –Alb
FEIBA	Baxter-Immuno	Ehtanol, DEAE-Sephadex, surface-activated PCC	Vapor heat 60°C 10 h, 80°C 1 h	Not applicable	PD
Autoplex T	NABI	TriCa PO₄, PEG fractionation, surface-activated PCC interaction chromatography from porcine plasma	20% ethanol, dry heat 60°C 144 h	Not applicable	PD
Hyate C	Speywood	Polyelectrolyte resin ion-exchange/hydrophobic interaction chromatography from porcine plasma	Viral attenuation through purification	100	Animal PD

(Modified from Kasper and Costa e Silva) PD = plasma derived; R = recombinant; SP ACT = specific activity; Alb = albumin; * can be used to treat vWD

approximately 2 U/kg/h maintains a mean level of about 50 percent). Continuous infusion offers the advantage of consistent levels, less frequent monitoring due to concern of troughs with bolus infusion, and decreased factor utilization.

RECOMBINANT FACTOR VIII

The first hemophilia A patients to be successfully treated with recombinant factor VIII were reported in early 1989. Collaborative clinical trials have demonstrated excellent efficacy with the recombinant factor VIII concentrates produced by two companies, Baxter-Immuno (Recombinate®) and Bayer (Kogenate®). Safety trials to date reveal no evidence for viral transmission and excellent recovery and half-life studies. Inhibitor development in previously untransfused patients has averaged about 25 to 30 percent for both products. Many of the inhibitors in these patients may be transient or responsive to immune tolerance. The higher incidence of inhibitors documented with the recombinant products is most likely associated with the increased intensity of monitoring performed in these prospective studies. Despite this, there does appear to be an increased number of observations of inhibitors in moderate and mildly deficient patients (see Chap. 20).

FACTOR IX

The plasma levels of factor IX needed for hemostasis in hemophilia B are similar to those for hemophilia A. Unlike factor VIII, factor IX readily diffuses into the extravascular spaces, therefore approximately twice the amount per dose is needed.

$$\text{\# units required} = \text{weight (kg)} \times \text{volume distribution} \times \text{level desired}$$

The volume of distribution for plasma derived factor IX $\simeq 1.0$, and for recombinant factor IX $\simeq 1.2$ The level desired should be placed in the formula as a whole number (e.g. "100" representing a level of 100%).

Factor IX has a half-disappearance time of 18 to 20 h. In surgical interventions, daily bolus infusion may be utilized, as well as continuous infusion except for the day of surgery when two doses (every 12 h) are often administered.

BeneFIX®, a genetically engineered factor IX concentrate, was licensed in 1997. BeneFIX® has been shown to have a volume of distribution of at least 1.2 due to a difference in sulfation and phosphorylation of the recombinant product compared to plasma-derived factor IX. Although the average volume of distribution is 1.2 for this product, there exists con-

TABLE 55-2

Products in Clinical Trials in United States

Product	Manufacturer	Clinical Trials / Indications	PD/R, +/–Alb
Factor VII concentrate	Baxter-Immuno	Factor VII deficiency	PD
Refacto	Genetics Institute	Factor VIII deficiency	R, –Alb
Kogenate SF	Bayer	Factor VIII deficiency	R, –Alb
Protein C concentrate	Baxter-Immuno	Protein C deficiency (homozygous)	PD
Activated protein C	Lilly	Sepsis, compassionate use	R

PD = plasma derived, R = recombinant; Alb = albumin

siderable variability in recovery in individual patients. Therefore, in the young child, for hemorrhagic episodes not responding to infusion therapy, or in the preoperative patient, it is recommended that individual recovery be determined.

The products listed in Table 55-1 are currently available; those in Table 55-2 are clinical trials. BeneFIX® (Genetics Institute) is a recombinant product that has been genetically engineered by insertion of the human factor IX gene into a Chinese Hamster Ovary cell line. BeneFIX® has been proven to be safe and effective in the treatment of patients with hemophilia B. The two plasma-derived coagulation factor IX concentrates (Mononine®, Alphanine SD®) are of high purity, free of thrombogenic risk, and utilize proven virucidal safety measures. These three or similarly pure products should always be used for previously untreated patients (infants and children) and for patients undergoing surgery. The products providing the highest degree of viral safety and least associated risk should be considered for all patients.

The licensed prothrombin-complex concentrate (PCC) products, although relatively safe in regards to viral transmission, have varying amounts of copurified factors II, VII, and X, in activated and inactivated forms, with a resultant clinical thrombogenic risk. PCCs have been noted to provide bypassing activity and currently may be utilized more commonly for the treatment of factor VIII inhibitor patients. Presently licensed PCCs include Bebulin®, Proplex-T®, Profiline SD®, and Konyne 80® (listed in Table 55-1). PCCs may also be used to treat hereditary deficiencies of factors II, VII, and IX when no better product is available.

VON WILLEBRAND FACTOR

Several concentrates have been advocated for use in patients with von Willebrand disease who cannot be treated with DDAVP. Although these concentrates raise the factor VIII level efficiently, they do not uniformly correct the bleeding time. In fact, studies indicate decreased amounts of high molecular weight multimers in all the products, with some variability in the same products from lot to lot. Currently the product that most efficiently corrects the bleeding time and multimeric pattern is Humate P® (Centeon). The dosage of Humate P® is based on the ristocetin cofactor assay: to achieve the best correction of the bleeding time, 50 to 60 U/kg is given over 5 to 10 min. For surgery, the dose is repeated every 12 h. Alphanate SD® is also available, but has a lower concentration of high molecular weight multimers compared to Humate-P®, therefore, twice the dose is recommended. Koate HP® (Bayer) has been evaluated in the treatment of patients with vWD. Despite absence of high molecular weight multimers and lack of correction of the bleeding time, clinical hemostasis was obtained.

A purification procedure based on conventional chromatographic methods has been developed in France (Biotransfusion) allowing simultaneous preparation from cryoprecipitate of a factor VIII concentrate and a von Willebrand factor concentrate. The pure vWf concentrate was effective in raising the factor VIII levels, correcting the bleeding time, and restoring a normal multimeric pattern in patients with von Willebrand disease. The American Red Cross conducted clinical trials in the United States with this product, with results similar to those obtained in Europe. However, the IND for this product currently is not being pursued.

CONCENTRATES FOR FACTOR II, VII, X, XI, AND XIII DEFICIENCY

Several concentrates are available for the treatment of other coagulation factor deficiencies; in almost all instances they are available mainly in Europe, not in the United States. Factor VII concentrate has been developed as a spin-off of the purification of factor IX. A factor VII concentrate (Baxter-Immuno) will be made available for use in the United States. Clinical experience has accrued with the use of a factor XI concentrate (prepared by Bio-Products Laboratory, Oxford, UK) for patients with factor XI deficiency who bleed excessively after surgery or trauma. The concentrate is dry heated at 80°C for 72 h, an established viral inactivation step. The mean recovery of factor XI was about 2 percent/U/kg, with an estimated overall half-disappearance time of 52 h. The concentrate was used for 45 invasive procedures with normal hemostasis achieved in all but one. This product has been associated with increased thrombogenic potential compared to FFP, in spite of the copurification of AT and addition of heparin. Hemoleven® (LFB, France), a factor XI concentrate containing C-1 inhibitor, has similar (~2%) recovery per unit per kilogram administered and a half-disappearance time of 45.5 ± 7.9 h. There was no excessive bleeding in 32 reported procedures. Thrombosis has been reported with this concentrate prior to addition of C-1 inhibitor as an antithrombotic agent.

Experience in Europe with a plasma-derived factor XIII concentrate (Fibrogammin®, HS, Centeon, Marburg, Germany) indicates that the concentrate is as effective as the previous placenta-derived product in treatment and prophylaxis of severe factor XIII deficiency. The T½ is 9.3 days. The plasma factor XIII concentrate contains both the active α-subunit and the carrier β-subunit, and has replaced the previous placenta-derived product. No evidence of increased incidence of antibody formation or viral transmission was noted after use for over 10 years in several patients. The pharmacokinetics and tolerability of plasma- versus placenta-derived product were compared in a non-randomized crossover study, which revealed the plasma-derived product to be as efficient as treatment with the placenta-derived preparation.

CONCENTRATES USED IN MANAGEMENT OF INHIBITOR PATIENTS

Table 55-1 summarizes the concentrates available for use in bleeding factor VIII and factor IX inhibitor patients. Because inhibitor antibodies are partially species specific, porcine factor VIII has been used to treat patients with auto- and alloantibodies to factor VIII. A number of studies with porcine factor VIII, Hyate-C®, (Speywood) indicate that hemostatic levels of factor VIII activity can be achieved in factor VIII inhibitor patients, even when the human antibody titer is high. Treatment of the bleeding episode is more apt to be successful when the porcine Bethesda assay is low in titer (<10 BU) (the porcine Bethesda titer is performed like the human assay except that porcine VIII is used as the target antigen). Adverse reactions of fever, chills, and hives may occur, and may require antihistamines and steroids, but are less frequent now than in the past due to improvements in the purification process; mild to severe thrombocytopenia has also been documented, especially in association with large doses. An anamestic rise in the inhibitor titer can occur to porcine VIII (18 percent). The usual dose is 50 to 150 U/kg per dose depending on the clinical and laboratory response. The dose may also be calculated based upon the porcine Bethesda titer.

FEIBA® (Baxter-Immuno) and Autoplex® (Nabi) are activated PCCs (aPCCs) that have similar hemostatic effects in bleeding factor VIII or factor IX inhibitor patients. The aPCCs are prepared by controlled activation to contain "bypassing" activity, and are indicated for use only in inhibitor patients. The product is usually given as a bolus of 50 to 100 U/kg for a specific bleeding episode. The dose may be increased or repeated in 12 h if necessary, but "prophylactic" use is not recommended. If hemostasis is achieved, no further product is given unless bleeding recurs. The repeated use and increased dosage of the bypassing products have been associated with fatal myocardial infarction, venous thromboembolism, and disseminated intravascular coagulation (DIC). Other PCC products (Konyne-80®, Proplex T®, Bebulin®, Profilnine SD®) have variable bypassing activity and have also been used to halt bleeding in inhibitor patients.

Both plasma-derived and recombinant-activated factor VII (rFVIIa, NovoSeven®, Novo Nordisk) have been used to treat hemorrhage in inhibitor patients. NovoSeven® was licensed in March 1999. Doses of 70 to 90 µg/kg every 2 to 3 h have been effective in halting bleeding. Under therapy, the PT and APTT shorten, and factor VII activity greatly increases. A prospective surgical study has been performed that showed a significant difference in favor of the high-dose group (90 µg/kg/dose) as compared to the low-dose (30 µg/kg/dose) group, especially in the major surgery category. A home-treatment study was also performed with NovoSeven® using 90 µg/kg every 3 h for up to four total injections for mild to moderate bleeding episodes. Hemostasis was rated as effective in 92 percent of bleeding episodes. Thrombotic complications appear to be much decreased with the use of NovoSeven® compared to PCCs and aPCCs. The use of NovoSeven® should be considered in patients with intractable bleeding, even when the underlying diagnosis may be unclear or not yet established.

COMPLICATIONS

The major complications of clotting factor therapy have been related to the transmission of viral disease, mainly HIV or hepatitis viruses. The current use of donor screening, virucidal techniques (solvent-detergent, pasteurization, vapor heating, sodium thiocyanate), the insistence on safety testing when the product is first used, and the advent of recombinant products has led to a generation of products that have been proven to be at extremely low risk of viral transmission. A nonlipid envelope virus (B19 parvovirus) is currently the exception to elimination by dry, wet, and steam-heated methods. Parvovirus has been transmitted to hemophilics in factor VIII concentrates and has even caused mild hypoplastic anemia in a solvent-detergent–treated concentrate recipient. Hepatitis A has also been transmitted via plasma-derived products.

Concern exists regarding infectious agents for which no screening tests or known method to remove or inactivate the transmissible agent are available. Such agents include Creutzfeldt-Jakob Disease (CJD) and new variant (nv) CJD. CJD and nvCJD are forms of transmissible spongiform encephalopathies. The incubation period for CJD in general is long, but may vary depending on the route of transmission (direct CNS, oral, intramuscular, or intravenous exposure) and the exposure material (dura mater, red or white blood cells, plasma, or plasma fractions). To date, case-control studies have not linked transmission of CJD to blood or blood-product–derivative transfusion. Ongoing research and surveillance continues in this area.

Ultrapure products (monoclonally derived, recombinant) have been shown to preserve or stabilize the immunologic status in HIV-positive hemophilics. Plasma-derived coagulation products contain substances known to inhibit a variety of immune reactions when assessed in vitro. It is now clear that in choosing a replacement product, purer is better. Additional evidence for this concept comes from the observations that high-purity factor IX products have distinctly fewer thrombogenic properties than previous intermediate-purity materials. The major obstacles to the widespread use of high-purity and recombinant products are related to availability and cost.

CONCENTRATES OF ANTICOAGULANT AND OTHER FACTORS

Two anticoagulant proteins are available in concentrate form, antithrombin (AT) and protein C. Viral inactivation usually has been by pasteurization or wet heat, and has not been associated with transmission of hepatitis or HIV agents. The composition of the final product (ATnativ®, Baxter-Immuno; Thrombate®, Bayer) is >95 percent AT. Vials of the lyophilized product are labeled in international units (IU). A dose of 1 U/kg will produce a rise of approximately 2 percent, with a half-disappearance time of approximately 60 h. In patients with heterozygous AT deficiency requiring surgery (in whom heparinization increases hemorrhagic risk), a dose of 25 U/kg should increase base levels by 50 percent (AT activity assay).

However, in ill patients, in pregnancy, and in preeclampsia, only a 1 percent rise/U/kg may be seen (use 50 U/kg); the half-disappearance time may also be less (29 h) so that a daily dose may be required.

Other clinical situations where AT concentrates have shown efficacy include fulminant hepatic failure (patients with liver failure requiring hemodialysis need less heparin and platelets when supplemented with AT concentrate), posttrauma shock and DIC, acute fatty liver of pregnancy, HELLP (hemolysis, elevated liver enzymes, low platelet count) syndrome in preeclampsia, neonatal ECMO procedures, and veno-occlusive disease in transplant patients.

Protein C concentrate has been produced by Baxter-Immuno and has been used with success in cases of severe protein C deficiency, and both hereditary and acquired infectious purpura fulminans (see Chap. 38). Future uses may include prophylaxis for thrombotic episodes in heterozygous protein C deficiency at time of surgery. Recombinant activated protein C concentrate (Lilly) is now in clinical trials in patients with purpura fulminans associated with sepsis. Plasminogen concentrate (Lys-Plasminogen, Baxter-Immuno, Vienna) has been used effectively in the treatment of a homozygous plasminogen-deficient child with ligneous conjunctivitis.

BIBLIOGRAPHY

Bjorkman S et al: Pharmacokinetics of factor VIII in humans; obtaining clinically relevant data from comparative studies. *Clin Pharmacokinet* 22:385, 1992.

Bolton-Maggs PHB: The management of factor XI deficiency. *Haemophilia* 4:683, 1998.

Brackmann HH et al: Pharmacokinetics and tolerability of factor XIII concentrates prepared from human placenta or plasma: A crossover randomised study. *Thromb Haemost* 74:622, 1995.

Bray G et al: A multicenter study of recombinant fVIII (Recombinate): Safety, efficacy and inhibitor risk in previously untreated patients with haemophilia A. *Blood* 83:2428, 1994.

Bucur SZ at al: Uses of antithrombin III concentrate in congenital and acquired deficiency states. *Transfusion* 38:481, 1998.

Goldsmith JC et al: Coagulation factor IX. Successful surgical experience with a purified factor IX concentrate. *Am J Hematol* 40:210, 1992.

Gootenberg JC: Factor concentrates for the treatment of factor XIII deficiency. *Curr Opin Hematol* 5:372, 1998.

Hay CM et al: Factor VIII inhibitors in mild and moderate-severity haemophilia A. *Thromb Haemost* 79:762, 1998.

Hay CM et al: Porcine factor VIII in patients with congenital hemophilia and inhibitors: Efficicay, patient selection and side effects. *Semin Hematol* 31:20, 1994.

Kasper CK, Costa e Silva M: Registry of clotting factor concentrates. World Federation of Hemophilia. No. 6, 1998.

Key NS et al: Home treatment of mild to moderate bleeding episodes using recombinant factor VIIa (NovoSeven) in haemophiliacs with inhibitors. *Thromb Haemost* 80:912, 1998.

Liebman HA et al: Activated recombinant human coagulation factor VII (rFVIIa) therapy for abdominal bleeding in patients with inhibitory antibodies to factor VIII. *Am J Hematol* 63:109, 2000.

Martinovitz U et al: Adjusted dose continuous infusion of factor VIII in patients with haemophilia. *Br J Haemat* 82:729, 1992.

Menache D, Aronson DL: New treatments of von Willebrand disease: Plasma derived von Willebrand factor concentrates. *Thromb Haemost* 78:566, 1997.

Morfini M et al: Hypoplastic anemia in a hemophiliac first infused with a solvent/detergent treated factor VIII concentrate: The role of human B19 parvovirus. *Am J Hematol* 39:149, 1992.

Peerlinck K, Vermylen J: Acute myocardial infarction following administration of recombinant activated factor VII (Novo Seven) in a patient with haemophilia A and inhibitor. *Thromb Haemost* 82:1775, 1999.

Pearson HJL et al: TGF-beta is not the principal immunosuppressive component in coagulation factor concentrates. *Brit J Haematol* 106:971, 1999.

Roberts H: Clinical experience with recombinant factor VIIa (NovoSeven): Summary of efficacy and safety. *Haemophilia* 2:63, 1996.

Schott D et al: Therapy with a purified plasminogen concentrate in an infant with ligneous conjunctivitis and homozygous plasminogen deficiency. *N Engl J Med* 339:1679, 1998.

Serementis SV et al: Three-year randomized study of a high-purity or intermediate-purity factor VIII concentrates in symptom-free HIV-seropositive haemophiliacs: Effects on immune status. *Lancet* 342:700, 1993.

Shapiro AD et al: Prospective, randomized trial of two doses of rFVIIa (NovoSeven) in haemophilia patients with inhibitors undergoing surgery. *Thromb Haemost* 80:773, 1998.

Shapiro AD et al: Safety and Efficacy of monoclonal antibody purified factor IX concentrate in previously untreated patients with hemophilia B. *Thromb Haemost* 75:30, 1996.

Smith JK: Factor XI deficiency and its management. *Haemophilia* 2:128, 1996.

Smith OP, White B: Infectious purpura fulminans: diagnosis and treatment. Annotation. *Brit J Haematol* 104:202, 1999.

Turner M: The impact of new-variant Creutzfeldt-Jacob disease on blood transfusion practice. Review. *Brit J Haematol* 106:842, 1999.

White G et al: Clinical evaluation of recombinant factor IX. *Semin Hematol* 35:33, 1998.

CHAPTER 56

Therapeutic Apheresis and Exchange Transfusion

TYPES OF THERAPEUTIC APHERESIS

Therapeutic apheresis is a procedure for removal of whole blood from the patient, with separation and removal of a pathological blood component and return of the remaining portion of the blood to the patient. Therapeutic apheresis is normally performed using sophisticated programmed apheresis machines that separate the blood components centrifugally. High flow rates (30 to 80 mL/min) are usual, and adequate vascular access is necessary (usually achieved by placement of a wide-bore double-lumen central venous catheter). During the procedure the patient is anticoagulated with citrate and/or heparin and is connected to a sterile set of collection and infusion bags that fit into the apheresis machine. Therapeutic apheresis normally takes 1 to 2 h or more to complete. Procedures include the following.

Plasmapheresis (plasma exchange): The patient's plasma is removed and replaced with normal donor plasma or with a solution to maintain colloid osmotic pressure (usually a 1:1 mix of 5 percent albumin and isotonic saline). Depending on the condition being treated, therapeutic efficacy may be due to removal of pathogenic antibodies, circulating immune complexes, paraproteins, or other substances, and/or replacement of a normal plasma component that is absent or reduced in the patient's plasma. A 1.0 to 1.5× plasma volume exchange is usual.

Cytapheresis: The patient's pathological red cells, white cells, or platelets are removed. Apart from red cell exchange transfusion, most cytapheresis procedures require no volume replacement beyond the anticoagulant and saline priming solution.

Extracorporeal immunoadsorption: The patient's plasma is passed over a specific adsorption column such as staphylococcal protein A (SpA), which will bind IgG and circulating immune complexes. The treated plasma is returned to the patient.

Exchange transfusion: Although therapeutic apheresis can be performed in children, the small size of neonates and young infants precludes use of this procedure. However, similar physiological effects can be achieved by exchange transfusion with the use of reconstituted or whole blood.

INDICATIONS FOR THERAPEUTIC APHERESIS AND EXCHANGE TRANSFUSION

Table 56-1 lists hemostatic and thrombotic disorders in which therapeutic apheresis and exchange transfusion may be used. For plasmapheresis the usual replacement fluid and frequency of apheresis are indicated. Generally a 1 volume plasma exchange will decrease immunoglobulins by about 60 to 65% (with a 45% recovery 48 h afterwards), paraproteins by 30 to 60% (with variable recovery 48 h later), and immune complexes and C_3 complement by 75 to 80% (with C_3 recovery in 3 to 4 days). IgM is more readily removed than IgG due to its lesser extravascular distribution. Exchanges larger than 1.5 plasma volumes should generally be avoided due to diminishing efficiency. Indication Categories (IC) for therapeutic apheresis (based largely on American Association of Blood Banks Guidelines) are also shown in the table. These categories are as follows:

Category I: Standard/acceptable under certain circumstances, including primary therapy

Category II: Sufficient evidence to suggest efficacy: acceptable on an adjunctive basis

Category III: Inconclusive efficacy or uncertain risk–benefit ratio

Category IV: Lack of efficacy in controlled trials

COMPLICATIONS OF THERAPEUTIC APHERESIS AND NEONATAL EXCHANGE TRANSFUSION

A one plasma volume exchange is usually associated with loss of about 30 mL of red cells and a fall in the platelet count of 25 to 30% (with recovery in 2 to 4 days). When non-plasma replacement fluid is used, a one vol-

TABLE 56-1		

Disorders of Hemostasis and Thrombosis in Which Therapeutic Apheresis and Exchange Transfusion May be Used

Plasmapheresis

Disorder	IC*	Comments
Thrombotic thrombocytopenic purpura (TTP) (including HIV-related TTP)	I	TTP/HUS: 1–1.5 PV daily replaced with FFP or CSP (see Chap. 28) (SDP also appears effective, but less clinical experience)
Hemolytic uremic syndrome (HUS)	II	
Cryoglobulinemia	I	1 PV daily replaced with 5% albumin +/–NS (warm room, patient and replacement fluid)
Goodpasture's syndrome	I	1 PV daily replaced with 5% albumin +/–NS
Posttransfusion purpura (PTP)	I	1 PV q 1–2 d replaced with 5% albumin +/–NS
Coagulation factor inhibitors	II	2–3 PV replaced with FFP daily
Plasma hyperviscosity syndromes (macroglobulinemia, myeloma, HIV)	I	PV replaced with 5% albumin +/–NS—individualize frequency; may need 3–7×/ week for 1–4 weeks
Refractory ITP	II	1–1.5 PV 3–5 × week × 1–2 weeks; 5% albumin +/–NS
Catastrophic antiphospholipid syndrome	II	
Meningococcemia	II	
Quinine-quinidine thrombocytopenia	II	
Fulminant liver failure	IV	Replace with FFP. Advocated by some clinicians as "bridging" therapy prior to transplantation
Chronic ITP	IV	Replace with 5% albumin/NS

Cytapheresis

Disorder	IC*	Comments
Sickling disorders including: - Acute chest syndrome - Acute splenic sequestration - Cerebrovascular accident (CVA) (children) - Acute, severe priapism Note: For routine perioperative cases simple transfusion to Hct ~30 as effective as exchange with fewer complications	I	Automated red cell exchange transfusion—final target Hct usually ~30% - Sequestration: 2-vol exchange—final Hct 22–25% - CVA: reduce HbS to <30% for 3–5 yrs, then to <50% if no recurrence - Priapism: early exchange best

(Continued on next page)

Cytapheresis		
Disorder	**IC***	**Comments**
Leukemia with hyperleukocytosis (WBC> 100,000/µL and leukostasis or retinal hemorrhage)	I	Leukapheresis to decrease WBC to <100,000/µL. Note: recent data show poor correlation of cytoreduction with early mortality
Severe symptomatic thrombocytosis (platelets >1,000,000/µL with bleeding or thrombosis)	I	Plateletpheresis to decrease platelets to <1,000,000/µL (e.g., 400,000–500,000/µL)
Hyperparasitemia (cerebral malaria, babesiosis)	II	2 volume red cell exchange transfusion
Neonatal alloimmune thrombocytopenia	I	Plateletpheresis: Neonate receives washed irradiated maternal platelets
Immunoadsorption (SpA Column)		
Disorder	**IC***	**Comments**
Refractory ITP	II	1–3×/week for total of six treatments
TTP associated with cancer chemotherapy	I	SpA column preferred by some clinicians to plasmapheresis
Exchange Transfusion		
Disorder		**Comments**
Severe hemolytic disease of the newborn, fetal hydrops		Double-volume exchange with washed or red cells reconstituted in FFP. (Red cells should be <5 d old, "CMV safe," and sickle cell negative; also irradiated if a directed donation from a blood relative or if recipient is a premature or is immunocompromised). If available CPD-A anticoagulated whole blood <48 h old is also suitable. Platelet concentrates are given at the end of the procedure to correct significant thrombocytopenia
Severe liver disease; disseminated intravascular coagulation		Component replacement may be preferable to exchange

IC* = Indication Category (see text). Abbreviations: PV, plasma volume; FFP, fresh frozen plasma; CSP, cryosupernatant plasma; SDP, solvent/detergent treated plasma; NS, normal saline; 5% albumin +/–NS—usual ratio used for replacement is 1:1

ume exchange will reduce fibrinogen by 60 to 65%, and coagulation proteins and inhibitors (including V, VII, IX, X and contact factors, antithrombin, and plasminogen) by variable amounts. The PT, APTT, and TCT may be transiently prolonged, although most factors, with the exception of fibrinogen, recover within hours and bleeding complications are very rare.

Other complications of therapeutic apheresis include rare deaths (older estimates: 3/10,000 procedures), hypotension (most common in children and the elderly), and hypocalcemic symptoms (perioral dyesthesias, tremors, cramps, tetany) from the rapid return of large volumes of citrated blood. In addition, allergic reactions (especially with plasma exchange), respiratory distress, rare mechanical hemolysis or equipment failure, lowering of therapeutic drug doses, infection, sclerosis of veins, Thrombosis, embolism, and hemorrhage (the latter four are usually access-site related) occasionally can occur. Many centers routinely administer calcium to patients during therapeutic apheresis to avoid hypocalcemia, especially if impaired liver function is present. Anaphylactoid reactions may be more frequent in patients on acetylcholine esterase (ACE) inhibitors, so discontinuing ACE inhibitors 24 to 48 h prior to apheresis should be considered.

In a recent study by McLeod et al involving 3429 procedures in 18 centers, the overall incidence of side effects was 4.75%, with most being reversible. Procedure-specific complication rates were 8/78 (10.26%) for red cell exchange, 89/1140 (7.81%) for plasma exchange with plasma replacement, 42/1255 (3.35%) for plasma exchange without plasma, 4/70 (5.71%) for leukapheresis, and 0/18 for plateletpheresis. Recent data from the Canadian Apheresis Study Group (CASG) suggest that the frequency of complications is declining, probably because of improvements in technology and better patient selection. Current CASG data based on 78,161 procedures show that severe reactions (patient was clinically unstable and physician intervention was required) occurred in only 0.4% of procedures (2.5% of patients) treated.

Complications of exchange transfusion are largely related to the use of umbilical vessels and operator inexperience (improper catheter placement, liver necrosis, hemoperitoneum, necrotizing enterocolitis, air embolism), hypocalcemia (from citrated blood), local catheter problems (thrombosis, infection), and complications related to use of improper blood, including hyperkalemia (old blood), hyperviscosity (use of packed cells with very high hematocrits), or graft vs. host disease (due to failure to irradiate blood products appropriately).

BIBLIOGRAPHY

Asherson RA et al: Catastrophic antiphospholipid syndrome: Clinical and laboratory features of 50 patients. *Medicine* 77:195, 1998.

Barnard DR et al: Blood for use in exchange transfusion in the newborn. *Transfusion* 20:401, 1980.

Berkman EM et al: Use of plasmapheresis and partial plasma exchange in the management of patients with cryoglobulinemia. *Transfusion* 20:171, 1980.

Canadian Apheresis Group: Guidelines for therapeutic apheresis. (Suite 206, 435 St. Laurent Blvd, Ottawa, Ontario, KIK 2Z8), 1997.

Clark WF et al: Therapeutic plasma exchange: an update from the Canadian Apheresis Group. *Ann Intern Med* 131:453, 1999,

Klein HG: Therapeutic hemapheresis. In: *Clinical Practice of Transfusion Medicine* 3rd ed., Petz LD et al, eds., New York, Churchill Livingstone, 1996, pp 1011–22.

Luban NL et al: Commentary on the safety of red cells preserved in extended-storage media for neonatal transfusions. *Transfusion* 31:229, 1991.

Maurer HS et al: The effect of initial management of hyperleukocytosis on early complications and outcome of children with acute lymphoblastic leukemia. *J Clin Oncol* 6:425, 1988.

McLeod BC et al, eds: *Apheresis: Principles and Practice,* Bethesda, AABB Press, 1997.

McLeod BC et al: Frequency of immediate adverse effects associated with therapeutic apheresis. *Transfusion* 39:282, 1999.

Porcu P et al: Therapeutic leukapheresis in hyperleukocytic leukemias: Lack of correlation between degree of cytoreduction and early mortality rate. *Br J Haematol* 98:433, 1997.

Rao AK et al: The hemostatic system in children undergoing intensive plasma exchange. *J Pediatr* 100:69, 1982.

Rock G, Sutton DMC: Apheresis: man versus machine. *Transfusion* 37:993, 1997.

Rock GA et al: Comparison of plasma exchange with plasma infusion in the treatment of thrombotic thrombocytopenic purpura. Canadian Apheresis Study Group. *N Engl J Med* 325:393, 1991.

Snyder HW et al: Experience with protein A-immunoadsorption in treatment-resistant adult immune thrombocytopenic purpura. *Blood* 79:2237, 1992.

Steinberg MH: Management of sickle cell disease. *N Engl J Med* 340:1021, 1999.

Sutton DM et al: Complications of plasma exchange. *Transfusion* 29:124, 1989.

CHAPTER 57

Intravenous Immunoglobulin

Initially introduced for the treatment of immunodeficiency diseases, intravenous immunoglobulin (IVIG) has become an important tool in the treatment of autoimmune and inflammatory syndromes. Clinical trials have demonstrated benefit for patients with such diverse diseases as inflammatory demyelinating neuropathies, Guillain–Barre syndrome, myasthenia gravis, and Kawasaki disease. Several hemostatic disorders also respond to IVIG (Table 57-1); the best established of these are discussed in the following.

Several mechanisms of action have been proposed to explain the efficacy of IVIG in the autoimmune diseases. These include 1) reversible blockade of Fc receptors on cells of the reticuloendothelial system and on cellular effectors of antibody-dependent cytotoxicity by Fc fragments of injected IVIG; 2) inhibition of autoantibody synthesis through Fc-dependent or anticlass II-dependent modulation of T-cell and B-cell function; 3) saturation of a transport receptor for IgG (FcRn), leading to increased catabolism of IgG nonspecifically (in proportion to its presence in plasma); 4) anti-idiotype activity against disease-associated autoantibodies, and 5) interference of IVIG with complement (C3)-mediated damage or cytokine secretion.

INDICATIONS FOR USE IN HEMOSTATIC DISORDERS

Immune Thrombocytopenia

Intravenous immunoglobulin plays an important role in the treatment of severe thrombocytopenia in patients with immune thrombocytopenia (ITP), especially in children, where the majority of cases are self-limited

---

TABLE 57-1

Uses of Intravenous Immunoglobulin in Disorders of Hemostasis

Established benefit
  Immune thrombocytopenia purpura (childhood and adult)
  Neonatal alloimmune thrombocytopenia
  Wiscott-Aldrich syndrome
Potential benefit
  Factor VIII acquired autoantibodies
  Anticardiolipin antibodies and recurrent abortions
  Acquired von Willebrand disease
  HIV-induced thrombocytopenia
  Immune tolerance treatment—hemophilia
  Thrombotic thrombocytopenia purpura

---

and only a single course of therapy is needed. The major use in adult ITP is for rapid control of acute bleeding episodes, preparation of patients for surgery, and when steroids or splenectomy are contraindicated (elderly, pregnancy, diabetes mellitus). Its use has proven efficacious in both acute and chronic ITP (to delay or to be used instead of splenectomy), and in passively transferred autoantibody-induced thrombocytopenia in offspring of mothers with ITP. IVIG is effective in the treatment of thrombocytopenia in HIV-infected individuals. The advantages of using IVIG include its rapid onset of action (1 to 2 days) and the fact that it does not exacerbate previously existing immunodeficiencies. IVIG has few side effects, but requires slow intravenous infusion and is expensive.

Intravenous immunoglobulin has been demonstrated to be effective in neonatal alloimmune thrombocytopenia, both as a treatment for the severely thrombocytopenic newborn and as prevention for intracranial bleeding by raising the platelet count in the fetus when the IVIG is administered to the mother in the weeks before delivery. IVIG is generally ineffective for improving the response to platelet transfusions in patients who have become alloimmunized to HLA or platelet antigens, and who are platelet refractory after repeated transfusions.

Acquired Factor VIII Inhibitors and von Willebrand Disease

Administration of IVIG has reduced the level of factor VIII autoantibody, leading to recovery of factor VIII levels in some patients with acquired or spontaneous factor VIII autoantibodies. This effect is likely due, at least in part, to suppression of the autoantibodies by the anti-idiotypic antibodies contained in the IVIG. In contrast, IVIG has had little effect in lowering factor VIII antibody titers in hemophilia patients with inhibitors. IVIG can also ameliorate acquired von Willebrand disease associated with monoclonal gammopathies of unknown significance; infusions have been shown to improve bleeding time and FVIII/vWF levels in some of these patients.

DOSAGE GUIDELINES

Intravenous immunoglobulin is a therapeutic preparation of polyspecific IgG obtained from plasma pools of 8000 to over 20,000 healthy blood donors. Current preparations are made of intact IgG with low amounts of IgA (2 to 610 g/mL) and a normal distribution of IgG subclasses. Immunoglobulin fragments and aggregates are present. The lyophylized product is reconstituted and slowly given intravenously. IVIG has a half-life of 3 weeks.

A dose of 1 g/kg daily for 2 days is now a standard dose of IVIG, although 2 g/kg given in divided doses over 2 to 5 days is still commonly used. In ITP or neonatal alloimmune thrombocytopenia, a prompt rise in platelet count is expected in the first few days. A single maintenance dose of 400 mg/kg may be given for ITP in children, or in adults with severe ITP for whom other therapies are inappropriate or ineffective.

COMPLICATIONS

While reactions to IVIG preparations are common, they generally cause only mild discomfort, and are often related to the speed of administration. Symptoms include pallor, sweating, nausea, chills, low-grade fever, back discomfort, muscle aches, chest tightening, and blood pressure changes. Temporary slowing or stopping of the infusion leads to disappearance of symptoms. Rarely, a true anaphylactic reaction will occur due to anti-IgA antibodies. Serum sickness can also occur. The direct antiglobulin test may become positive. Rapid hemolysis due to anti-A and anti-B antibody, with fever and disseminated intravascular coagulation, has been reported after IVIG in a patient with Kawasaki disease. Acute renal failure has infrequently been attributed to IVIG, with a higher incidence with re-peated administration of sucrose-containing products in some regimens for ITP.

INTRAVENOUS ANTI-D TREATMENT

An intravenous preparation of anti-D immunoglobulin(e.g., WinRho®) has been used successfully in Rh-positive ITP patients to produce reticu-loendothelial cell blockade and to increase the platelet count (see Chap.

9). Mild alloimmune hemolysis is the major toxicity. Although not as predictably effective as IVIG or corticosteroids, anti-D immunoglogulin can be given rapidly and has a therapeutic role for some patients with chronic ITP. HIV-infected patients respond as well as ITP patients; platelet counts can be maintained at adequate levels with a mean interval of 24 days between infusions.

BIBLIOGRAPHY

Ahsan N: Intravenous immunoglobulin induced-nephropathy: A complication of IVIG therapy. *J Nephro* 11:157, 1998.

Blanchette VS et al: Role of intravenous immunoglobulin G in autoimmune hematologic disorders. *Sem Hematol* 29:72, 1992.

Bussel JB et al: Intravenous anti-D treatment of immune thrombocytopenic purpura; analysis of efficacy, toxicity, and mechanism of effect. *Blood* 77:1884, 1991.

Bussel JB et al: Antenatal treatment of neonatal alloimmune thrombocytopenia. *N Engl J Med* 319:1374, 1988.

Clark AL et al: Pregnancy complicated by the antiphospholipid syndrome: Outcomes with intravenous immunoglobulin therapy. *Obstet Gynecol* 93:437, 1999.

Dietrich G et al: Modulation of autoimmunity by intravenous immune globulin through interaction with the function of the immune/idiotypic network. *Clin Immunol Immunopathol* 62:S73, 1992.

Epstein JS, Zoon KC: Important Drug Warning, Department of Health and Human Services, Food & Drug Administration. Sept 29, 1999.

Federici AB et al: Treatment of acquired von Willebrand syndrome in patients with monoclonal gammopathy of uncertain significance: Comparison of three different therapeutic approaches. *Blood* 92, 2707, 1998.

George JN et al: Idiopathic thrombocytopenic purpura: A practice guideline developed by explicit methods for the American Society of Hematology. *Blood* 88: 3, 1996.

Green D, Kwaan HC: An acquired factor VIII inhibitor responsive to high-dose gamma globulin. *Thromb Haemost* 58:1005, 1987.

Kaveri SV et al: Intravenous immunoglobulins (IVIg) in the treatment of autoimmune diseases. *Clin Exp Immunol* 86:192, 1991.

Law C et al: High-dose intravenous immune globulin and the response to splenectomy in patients with idiopathic thrombocytopenic purpura. *N Eng J Med* 336: 1494, 1997.

Majluf-Cruz A et al: Usefulness of a low-dose intravenous immunoglobulin regimen for the treatment of thrombocytopenia associated with AIDS. *Am J Hematol* 59:127, 1998.

Nydegger UE et al: Adverse effects of intravenous immunoglobulin therapy. *Drug Safety* 21:171, 1999.

Pietz J et al: High-dose intravenous gamma globulin for neonatal alloimmune thrombocytopenia in twins. *Acta Paediatr Scand* 80:129, 1991.

Simpson KN et al: Idiopathic thrombocytopenia purpura: Treatment patterns and an analysis of cost associated with intravenous immunoglobulin and anti-D therapy. *Sem Hematol* 35:58, 1998.

Suarez CR, Anderson C: High-dose intravenous gamma globulin (IVG) in neonatal immune thrombocytopenia. *Am J Hematol* 26:247, 1987.

Sultan Y et al: Anti-idiotypic suppression of autoantibodies to factor VIII (antihaemophilic factor) by high-dose intravenous gamma globulin. *Lancet* i:765, 1984.

Tarantino MD et al: Treatment of childhood acute immune thrombocytopenic purpura with anti-D immune globulin or pooled immune globulin. *J Peds* 134:21, 1999.

Tarantino MD et al: Treatment of acute immune thrombocytopenic purpura. *Sem Hematol* 35:28, 1998.

Yu Z, Lennon V: Mechanism of intravenous immune globulin therapy in antibody-mediated autoimmune diseases. *N Engl J Med* 340: 227, 1999.

CHAPTER 58

Use of Desmopressin, Antifibrinolytics, and Conjugated Estrogens in Hemostasis

As noted in previous chapters, several pharmacologic agents have a role in achieving hemostasis in many clinical bleeding syndromes. The efficacy of these agents (desmopressin, antifibrinolytics, and conjugated estrogens) has now been well established by controlled trials and should be a major part of the armamentarium of the physician dealing with the bleeding patient.

DESMOPRESSIN

Mechanism of Action

Desmopressin (1-desamino-8-D-arginine vasopressin, DDAVP) is a synthetic analogue of the antidiuretic hormone L-arginine vasopressin, AVP. As shown in Fig. 58-1, DDAVP differs from AVP by two structural changes. These changes increase the antidiuretic effect that is mediated through the V2 receptor and a calcium-independent cyclic adenosine monophosphate (AMP)-dependent second messenger; factor VIII and von Willebrand factor release is also apparently mediated by the V2-receptor mechanism. DDAVP has little effect on the V1 receptor, which mediates vascular smooth muscle contraction and is responsible for the pressor effects of AVP. Thus, DDAVP exhibits superior antidiuretic effects

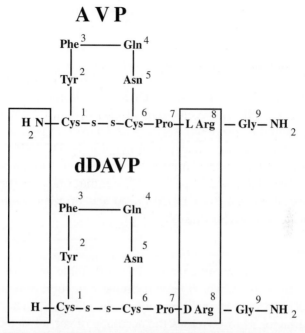

FIGURE 58-1 Comparison of the structure of arginine vasopressin (AVP) with the synthetic analogue (DDAVP). The boxes enclose the differences between the two peptide molecules: deamination of hemicysteine at position 1 and substitution of the D-isomer of arginine for L Arg at position 8. (Used with permission from Richardson DW, Robinson AG: *Ann Intern Med* 103:228, 1985.)

without the undesirable pressor and uterotonic side effects, and is responsible for the almost immediate release through the V2-receptor mechanism of factor VIII, von Willebrand factor, and t-PA from endothelial cells without increasing plasma levels of other endothelial cell constituents (fibronectin, antithrombin III, platelet factor 4). DDAVP does not increase factor VIII and von Willebrand factor release when incubated with cultured or perfused endothelial cells; this observation and others suggest that a "second messenger" is involved in the raised plasma levels of clotting factors after DDAVP. The concept that desmopressin exerts its effects directly through its strong V2 agonist effect is supported by the finding that patients with nephrogenic diabetes insipidus (who lack V2 receptors) had no increase factor VIII and von Willebrand factor levels after DDAVP.

Several studies in normal adults have indicated that pharmacologic doses of DDAVP produce shortening of the bleeding time, a three- to fivefold increase in factor VIII and von Willebrand factor (antigen and activity), and a three- to fourfold increase in t-PA without significant changes in fibrinogen, plasminogen, and α_2-antiplasmin (α_2-AP). However, plasmin-α_2-AP inhibitor complex increases and fibrin degradation products are normal or slightly increased. Plasminogen activator inhibitor (PAI) decreases. Although clinically significant fibrinolysis with bleeding is not produced, the relevance of these findings to thrombosis has been questioned (see Complications section). Of interest is the observation that patients with type III von Willebrand disease do not release t-PA (even though it is stored in endothelial cells) after DDAVP or venous occlusion. The marked increase of platelet adhesiveness to DDAVP is not fully understood, but has been shown to be dependent of the presence of platelet-vWF and platelet receptor IIb/IIIa, rather than just the quantitative increase of plasma vWF. DDAVP also acts on platelets to generate microparticles and enhance procoagulant activity.

Clinical Use

In addition to the therapeutic uses of DDAVP (Table 58-1), several diagnostic uses are known, which have included detection of hemophilia A carriers (using a post-DDAVP instead of the standard factor VIII/von Willebrand factor ratio increases the accuracy of carrier detection to 95 percent) and of acquired and hereditary defects in t-PA release. (DDAVP in a standard dose can be used instead of venous occlusion.) Test doses of DDAVP are frequently used to confirm responses in von Willebrand disease.

Desmopressin is the major hemostatic therapy for bleeding episodes and for surgical procedures in mild hemophilia A, hemophilia A carriers with low levels, and type 1 von Willebrand disease. Test doses are used in hemophilia A when the baseline level is <10 percent. Responses can vary substantially within families. The expected factor VIII rise (from two- to sixfold, mean of threefold) will produce a hemostatic level of at least 20 percent in almost all mild hemophilia A patients (base level of 6 percent or above) and an occasional moderately severe (4 to 5 percent) patient. In general, if the base level is at least 10 percent, adequate hemostasis is ensured; patients with levels of 4 to 9 percent may also respond but should be monitored for effect. The factor VIII level may also be increased to hemostatic levels without an anamnestic rise in antibody titer.

As noted in Chapter 12, DDAVP is usually effective in the common type of von Willebrand disease (type 1), is sometimes effective in type 2A, is ineffective in type 3 and Normandy variant, and is contraindicated in type 2B and platelet-type disease. Factor VIII and ristocetin cofactor levels increase with variable bleeding time correction (up to 6 h) in patients responding with good clinical hemostasis; however, hemostasis may be

TABLE 58-1

Hemostatic Use of Desmopressin (DDAVP)

Hemophilia (factor VIII deficiency)
   Hereditary, mild
   Carriers
   Acquired (inhibitors)

von Willebrand disease (see Chap. 12)
   (not types IIB and III)

Acquired von Willebrand disease

Hereditary platelet function defects
   Storage pool deficiencies (occasionally)
   Secretion defects
   Bernard-Soulier syndrome

Acquired bleeding disorders
   Uremia
   Liver disease
   Cardiovascular surgery
   ASA-induced defects
   Vascular defects
   Glycogen storage diseases

Other disorders
   Heparin-induced bleeding
   Thrombocytopenic bleeding
   Myeloproliferative disorders
   Unexplained prolonged bleeding time
   Ehlers-Danlos syndrome

adequate, even though only partial or little correction of the bleeding time occurs.

Bleeding episodes in many hereditary platelet function defects also respond to DDAVP; the notable exceptions are thrombasthenia, delta storage pool deficiency, and congenital afibrinogenemia. The responses are not related to correction of the platelet aggregation defects (usually they do not correct), but rather to improvement in the bleeding time. Bleeding times and clinical hemostasis are improved in many acquired bleeding disorders, in particular in uremia and liver disease (cirrhosis, biliary atresia, Alagille's syndrome), despite the presence of elevated baseline levels of factor VIII and von Willebrand factor. Other acquired platelet function defects where DDAVP has been effective in shortening the bleeding time or decreasing bleeding include myeloproliferative syndromes (see Chap. 33); some forms of acquired von Willebrand disease; after drugs like aspirin, dextran, and heparin; and glycogen storage disease type 1. Several controlled studies have shown that routinely used DDAVP may slightly or not decrease blood loss in cardiovascular surgical procedures, spinal fusion for scoliosis, and total joint arthroplasty; however, the occasional patient with severe postoperative hemorrhage may respond to DDAVP administration.

Although tranexamic acid or ε-aminocaproic acid has been used with DDAVP (to prevent excess fibrinolysis), our experience is that the hemostatic effect is good, not requiring antifibrinolytic agents in most instances. The exceptions are oral bleeding or dental surgery in which antifibrinolytic agents are used in von Willebrand disease or mild hemophilia A; in addition, adenotonsillectomy has been managed (DDAVP, EACA) without the use of blood products in children with vWD (see Derkay ref).

Dosage Guidelines

Desmopressin causes a transient increase in the factor VIII–von Willebrand factor complex; an optimal response (all ages) occurs with the dose of 0.3 µg/kg in 15 to 30 mL isotonic saline given by slow intravenous push or drip over 15 to 30 min. The peak effect is in 30 to 60 min and the duration of raised clotting factors is similar to that seen in administered cryoprecipitate. DDAVP or desmopressin is available for intravenous, subcutaneous, or nasal administration (see Table 58-2). The intranasal form of DDAVP is currently widely used in the treatment of bleeding in mild factor VIII deficiency and von Willebrand disease.

The response to repeated doses of DDAVP is of four patterns: equally good responses to doses every 12 h, gradually less response with each dose, essentially no response after the first dose, and, most commonly, reduced but steady responses after the first dose. About half the responses to repeated doses will show resistance or tachyphylaxis; thus, when higher factor levels are needed for longer periods of time (i.e., major surgery), von Willebrand factor concentrate therapy may be needed. Often only one or two doses are needed for surgical procedures in patients with mild hemophilia or von Willebrand disease. The initial dose should be timed so that the procedure is started within 30 to 60 min after administration of the DDAVP. DDAVP has been used effectively at all ages and immediately following delivery; the response in small infants is sometimes less than optimal.

Side Effects and Complications

For a drug with such wide use in difficult clinical situations, only a few adverse effects have been observed with desmopressin. Probably the

TABLE 58-2

Dosage Guidelines for DDAVP and Antifibrinolytics

Drug	Dose
DDAVP	
Desmopressin acetate (DDAVP, intravenous)	0.3 µg/kg in 50 mL normal saline over 20 min IV
Desmopressin acetate (Stimate Nasal Spray)	One spray (150 µg) - child Two sprays (300 µg) - adult
Desmopressin acetate (EMOSINT, SCAVO, Siena) for subcutaneous use	0.3 µg/kg SC
ANTIFIBRINOLYTICS	
EACA (Amicar, Lederle)	Load: 100 mg/kg IV or PO (often 5 g in adults) Maint: 500–1000 mg/h*
Tranexamic acid (TA) (Cyklokapron, Kabi)	Load: 10 mg/kg IV Maint: 10 mg/kg IV q 6–8 h 25 mg/kg po q 6–8 h
Aprotinin (Trasylol, Bayer)	Load: 2.0 million KIU IV Maint: 500,000 KIU/h IV
Cardiopulmonary Bypass	
EACA	Load: 150 mg/kg IV Maint: 15 mg/kg over 6 h
TA**	Load: 10 mg/kg IV Maint: 1 mg/kg over 6 h
Aprotinin KIU	Load: 2.0 million KIU IV plus 2.0 million KIU pump prime Maint: 500,000 KIU IV/h during procedure

* In children, a loading dose of 200 mg/kg of EACA is followed by 100 mg/kg q 6 h po up to a total of 6 g per 6 h.
** For children, a loading dose of TA, 100 mg/kg followed by 10 mg/kg/h during the procedure has been used.

most frequent side effect is facial flushing due to mild skin vasodilation. A few patients complain of headache; some patients show slight increases in heart rate and minor alterations in blood pressure; the concomitant use of pressor agents should be avoided. The most serious complication is hyponatremia, which occurs in a few patients, usually after repeated doses of intravenous DDAVP in conjunction with excessive intakes of hypotonic fluids (intravenous fluids with surgical procedures). The hyponatremia (serum sodium 114 to 123 meq/L) was usually associated with tonic-clonic convulsions and altered mental status; the lowest sodium level occurred 6 to 21 h after multiple doses of DDAVP. Young children, especially those under the age of 2 years, are especially prone to develop symptomatic hyponatremia and should be monitored carefully. Serum sodium concentration should be checked every 12 h, or more frequently if the level is falling; total fluid intake should be restricted by one-third. Avoid repeated doses of DDAVP if the serum sodium level is decreasing. Based on multiple clinical trials in patients undergoing major cardiovascular surgery, no significant increase in risk of thrombotic complications has been documented with the use of desmopressin.

ANTIFIBRINOLYTIC AGENTS

Antifibrinolytic agents are used for treatment or prevention of bleeding in two clinical settings: to block systemic fibrinolysis or to inhibit local fibrinolysis at sites of vascular injury. Three drugs are available for use in the United States. ε-aminocaproic acid (EACA) and tranexamic acid (TA) inhibit the fibrinolytic enzymes tissue plasminogen activator (t-PA) and plasmin. Aprotinin inhibits plasmin, as well as other serine proteases such as trypsin or kallikrein.

Mechanism of Action

Both EACA and TA are similar in structure to the amino acid lysine (Fig. 58-2). Since lysine-binding sites are required for binding of plasminogen and t-PA to fibrin, these agents competitively inhibit these interactions and thereby effectively block fibrinolysis. In contrast, aprotinin blocks the serine site within the active center of the plasmin molecule.

EACA and TA are small molecules (Mr 131 and 157 D) and are readily absorbed with peak blood concentrations at 2 (EACA) and 4 (TA) h after oral ingestion. Both agents have short plasma half-lives and are rapidly cleared from the plasma and concentrated in the urine; EACA urinary levels are 100 times higher than those in plasma. Moreover, because of their small size, they cross the blood–brain barrier and enter most tissues and body cavities. Both can be given intravenously, used topically, or administered orally. TA differs from EACA in at least two respects, both of which have therapeutic implications. TA provides equivalent antifibrinolytic therapy at only one-tenth the concentration, and has a slower renal clearance (6 to 8 h compared to <3 h for EACA). Therefore, TA is used in lower doses and given at less frequent intervals than EACA (Table 58-2).

Aprotinin (Mr 6512 D), extracted from bovine lung, inhibits the action of several serine proteases, such as trypsin, plasmin, and kallikrein without

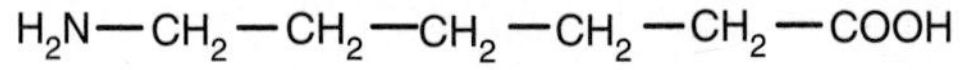

$$H_2N-CH_2-CH_2-CH_2-CH_2-CH_2-COOH$$

ε-Aminocaproic acid

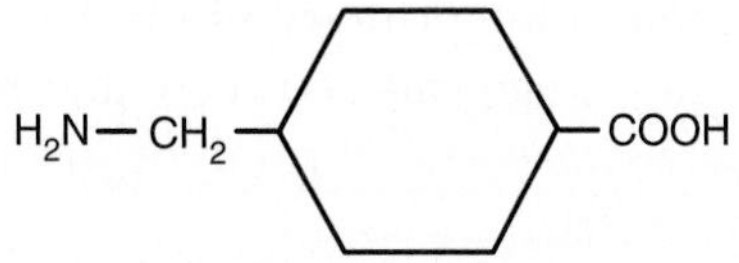

$$H_2N-CH_2-\bigcirc-COOH$$

Tranexamic Acid
(*trans*-4-aminomethylcyclohexane carboxylic acid)

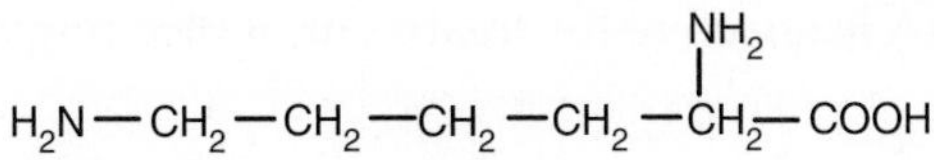

$$H_2N-CH_2-CH_2-CH_2-CH_2-\overset{\overset{\displaystyle NH_2}{|}}{CH_2}-COOH$$

Lysine

FIGURE 58-2 Lysine and the lysine analogue antifibrinolytic drugs. (Reprinted with permission from Horrow JC: *Int Anesthesiol Clin* **28:230, 1990.)**

affecting platelet function. It is not adsorbed from the gastrointestinal tract, is cleared from the plasma in two phases (half-lives of 2 and 7 h), and undergoes degradation to small polypeptides or amino acids before excretion into the urine. It is administered only by intravenous injection or used topically (Table 58-2). Aprotinin is 10 times more costly than EACA or TA.

Laboratory Monitoring

Laboratory tests are not used to monitor the clinical effects of the anti-fibrinolytic agents. Instead, control of bleeding is the best therapeutic end point. During cardiopulmonary bypass, whole-blood heparin measurements are unaffected by aprotinin, and correlate well with anti-Xa heparin assays. Evidence of circulating fibrinolytic activity (e.g., shortened euglobulin lysis time and/or low α_2-antiplasmin levels) should be sought, and disseminated intravascular coagulation (DIC) excluded before EACA or TA are used to treat bleeding in patients with systemic fibrinolysis.

Clinical Uses

Treatment of Systemic Fibrinolysis

Antifibrinolytic agents are used to treat or prevent bleeding due to systemic fibrinolysis. Although the primary fibrinolytic syndromes are distinctly uncommon, hemorrhage can be severe and refractory to clotting factor replacement therapy. Several fibrinolytic disorders in which treatment may be useful are listed.

Hereditary a2-Antiplasmin or Plasminogen Activator Inhibitor Deficiencies. Deficiencies of the natural fibrinolytic inhibitors result in bleeding due to excessive fibrinolysis (see Chap. 25). Chronic or intermittent therapy with EACA or TA is effective for treatment of bleeding episodes in these patients.

Bleeding Following Thrombolytic Therapy. Antifibrinolytic agents are seldom needed because of the very short half-life of most of the thrombolytic agents (e.g., 5 to 30 min). Consequently, continued bleeding is more likely to be due to clotting factor depletion, platelet function defects, or structural lesions, rather than persistent systemic fibrinolysis.

Acute Promyelocytic Leukemia (APL). A subset of patients with APL have systemic fibrinolysis with or without DIC. Antifibrinolytic agents are used for treatment of isolated primary fibrinolysis, or can be administered in conjunction with heparin when patients have concurrent DIC and systemic fibrinolysis. Patients with excessive fibrinolysis often show levels of α_2 antiplasmin less than 40 percent of normal.

Anhepatic Phase of Liver Transplantation. A rapid rise in plasma levels of t-PA frequently occurs during liver transplantation surgery after the removal of the diseased liver (anhepatic phase). In some instances, severe systemic fibrinolysis produces massive hemorrhage. Intravenous TA or aprotinin has reduced bleeding and has been associated with decreased requirements of plasma and platelets; however, the routine use of these agents cannot be recommended on basis of recent investigations.

Systemic Amyloidosis with Primary Fibrinolysis. Some patients with widespread amyloidosis have severe and recurrent fibrinolytic bleeding that responds to chronic oral antifibrinolytic therapy.

Severe Hemorrhagic Events Associated with Systemic Fibrinolysis. Examples include heat stroke, amniotic fluid embolism, persistent bleeding in cancer patients, and intractable gastrointestinal hemorrhage. Often these syndromes involve DIC with rapid changes in the character of the hemostatic defects from hour to hour. Laboratory tests should be performed to implicate systemic fibrinolysis and exclude DIC before treatment with antifibrinolytic agents is instituted (see Chap. 25).

Cardiopulmonary Bypass. All three antifibrinolytic agents (EACA, TA, and aprotinin) have been effective in the reduction of bleeding and transfusion requirements in patients undergoing cardiac surgery with cardiopulmonary bypass. In over 1000 patients treated with TA or EACA, results have indicated that either drug reduces blood loss by 30 to 40 percent as compared to placebo. Double-blind studies involving more than 500 patients given aprotinin have demonstrated similar effectiveness in cardiac valve replacement and coronary artery bypass grafting.

Prevention of Local Fibrinolysis

The presence of a hemostatic defect (e.g., hemophilia) and excessive local fibrinolysis (e.g., release of plasminogen activators in the genitourinary tract or saliva) can accentuate bleeding from sites of injury. Local fibrinolysis can be blocked by the systemic administration of the antifibrinolytic agents and occasionally by direct topical application to an injury site (particularly for dental surgery). Examples are listed below.

Bleeding from the Mouth and Upper Respiratory Tract. The antifibrinolytic agents effectively control bleeding from the mouth in patients with hereditary or acquired hemostatic defects. Controlled clinical trials have shown that the oral administration of EACA or TA can substitute for continued infusions of clotting factor concentrates in children or adults undergoing dental extractions. Patients with severe hemophilia who require dental surgery are usually given a single dose of clotting factor concentrate along with EACA or TA, which is continued for 4 to 7 days. Patients with mild or moderate hemophilia A and many patients with von Willebrand disease can be managed with antifibrinolytic agents with or without the addition of DDAVP. Mouthwashes (swish and swallow) containing TA has been used effectively for prevention of oral bleeding in mild hemophiliacs and those on oral anticoagulants who require dental extractions (see Sindet-Pedersen ref). Mucosal hemorrhage in thrombocytopenic patients may be controlled by oral TA or EACA.

Subarachnoid Hemorrhage and Hyphema. Patients who survive a subarachnoid hemorrhage due to rupture of a cerebral artery aneurysm often have recurrent bleeding before surgical repair can be safely attempted. Recent studies indicate the usefulness of antifibrinolytic therapy in reducing rebleeding when given before early surgery. Ophthalmologists have used antifibrinolytic agents for the prevention of persistent bleeding in patients with traumatic hyphema, but randomized clinical trials are needed to prove benefit.

Bleeding from the Gastrointestinal Tract. Antifibrinolytic therapy has occasionally been used for treatment of patients with persistent bleeding from the upper gastrointestinal tract (e.g., diffuse gastritis, peptic ulcer disease, and esophageal varices). TA has been shown to reduce recurrent bleeding by 20 to 30 percent, the need for surgery by 30 to 40 percent, and mortality by 40 percent. Intractable lower gastrointestinal bleeding due to ulcerative colitis (often with associated hemostatic defects) has also been treated with possible benefit, although the development of thrombosis in patients with inflammatory bowel disease is a major concern.

Bleeding from the Urinary Tract. Antifibrinolytic agents have been advocated for treatment of patients who have persistent bleeding from the kidney. Subjects at risk include patients with hemophilia or sickle cell disease, or patients following renal biopsy. A major problem is the formation and retention of large blood clots in the renal collecting system, which require surgical removal to preserve renal function. Because of this, antifibrinolytic drugs are rarely indicated in upper urinary tract bleeding, even if only microscopic hematuria is present. However, if the bleeding is intractable and no other alternatives are available, then these risks may be acceptable in selected patients.

Prolonged severe bleeding from the prostatic bed can occur following prostate resection. Because the operative site is bathed in plasminogen activator (e.g., urokinase in the urine and prostatic tissues), antifibrinolytic therapy has been used to control hemorrhage. Randomized clinical trials have shown that prophylactic administration of EACA or TA reduces blood loss in patients after prostatectomy, although postoperative venous thrombosis remains a concern.

Uterine Bleeding. Excessive bleeding from the uterine cervix following cone biopsy, refractory hemorrhage in women with intrauterine contraceptive devices, and postpartum hemorrhage have responded to antifibrinolytic drugs. TA reduced blood loss in women with primary menorrhagia by 40 to 50 percent in one recent study. Standard approaches, including hormone therapy, should be tried before antifibrinolytic agents are considered.

Complications and Side Effects

Thrombosis

Pharmacologic blockade of the fibrinolytic system can accelerate thrombus growth or allow clots to persist in an unwelcome location. The possibility of thrombosis should be weighed each time the use of antifibrinolytic agents is considered. If, for example, a patient with carcinoma has DIC, then antifibrinolytic therapy can precipitate glomerular thrombosis and acute renal failure. Deep venous thrombosis is always a concern in patients who are bedridden or those who have had recent abdominal or pelvic surgery. No significant increase in thromboembolic complications has been reported in the many clinical trials of TA, EACA, or aprotinin, although an occasional case report of thrombi in association with the drugs is known.

Other Side Effects

Patients given large oral doses or rapid intravenous infusions of EACA have developed symptomatic orthostatic hypotension. This complication is more frequent in older individuals and can persist for several hours. Symptoms are relieved by recumbency and a reduction in dose. Since aprotinin is extracted from bovine lungs, hypersensitivity reactions may occur after repeated use. Also, the possibility that Creutzfeldt-Jakob disease may be transmitted to patients has been raised in Italy, where the drug was subsequently withdrawn. No other country has taken this step.

Nausea, vomiting, diarrhea, headache, conjunctival suffusion, skin rash, and stuffy nose have all been reported. Rarely, visual symptoms can occur; these agents are not recommended for persons with impaired color vision. Other patients have developed significant liver damage. Importantly, because EACA and TA are largely excreted by the kidney, high plasma levels can occur in patients with renal insufficiency. Doses must be reduced in this setting.

CONJUGATED ESTROGENS

Conjugated estrogens (CEs) (sodium estrone sulfate, equilin sulfate, and others as found in equine urine) are naturally occurring compounds that have been used as hemostatic agents. Although the mechanism of CEs effect on shortening of the BT and cessation of hemorrhage is unknown, the drug has shown efficacy in several clinical situations. Uremia-associated bleeding was controlled and sustained shortening of the BT achieved by either intravenous infusion of CE (0.6 mg/kg, repeated every 4 to 5 days if needed) or a daily oral dose of 50 mg for 7 days. If an immediate effect on bleeding tendency is required, the use of DDAVP is recommended. Patients undergoing orthotopic liver transplantation used significantly less FFP, platelets, and red blood cells than untreated controls when given 100 mg CE iv at the beginning of the procedure and repeated after reperfusion of the new graft. CEs are well tolerated; for the short-term use for the control of hemostasis, essentially no adverse effects are known.

BIBLIOGRAPHY

Avvisati G et al: Tranexamic acid for control of haemorrhage in acute promyelocytic leukaemia. *Lancet* 2:122, 1989.

Bartholomew JR et al: Control of bleeding in patients with immune and nonimmune thrombocytopenia with aminocaproic acid. *Arch Intern Med* 149:1959, 1989.

Bonnar J, Sheppard BL: Treatment of menorrhagia during menstruation: randomised controlled trial of ethamsylate, mefenamic acid, and tranexamic acid. *BMJ* 313:579, 1996.

Byrnes JJ et al: Thrombosis following desmopressin for uremic bleeding. *Am J Hematol* 28:63, 1988.

Cattaneo M et al: The effect of desmopressin on reducing blood loss in cardiac surgery—a meta-analysis of double-blind, placebo-controlled trials. *Thromb Haemost* 74:1064, 1995.

Cox FL et al: Conjugated estrogen reduces transfusion and coagulation factor requirements in orthotopic liver transplantation. *Anesth Analg* 86: 1183, 1998.

Dean A et al: Fibrinolytic inhibitors for cancer-associated bleeding problems. *J Pain Symptom Manage* 13:20, 1997.

de la Fuente B et al: Response of patients with mild and moderate hemophilia A and von Willebrand's disease to treatment with desmopression. *Ann Intern Med* 103:6, 1985.

Derkay CS et al: Management of children with von Willebrand disease undergoing adenotonsillectomy. *Am J Otolaryn* 17:172, 1996.

Despotis GJ et al: Effect of aprotinin on activated clotting time, whole blood and plasma heparin measurements. *Ann Thorac Surg* 59: 106, 1995.

Havel M et al: Aprotinin does not decrease early graft patency after coronary artery bypass grafting despite reducing postoperative bleeding and use of donated blood. *J Thorac Cardiovasc Surg* 107:807, 1994.

Horstman LL et al: Desmopressin (DDAVP) acts on platelets to generate platelet microparticles and enhanced procoagulant activity. *Thromb Res* 79: 163, 1995.

Kane MJ et al: Myonecrosis as a complication of the use of epsilon amino-caproic acid: A case report and review of the literature. *Am J Med* 85:861, 1988.

Karnezis TA et al: The hemostatic effects of desmopressin on patients who had total joint arthroplasty. *J Bone Joint Surg* 76A: 1545, 1994.

Kim HC et al: Patients with prolonged bleeding time of undefined etiology, and their response to desmopressin. *Thromb Haemost* 59:221, 1988.

Kobrinsky NL et al: Absent factor VIII response to synthetic vasopressin analogue (DDAVP) in nephrogenic diabetes insipidus. *Lancet* i:1293, 1985

Kufner RP: Antifibrinolytics and orthotopic liver transplantation. *Transplant Proc* 30:692, 1998.

Lethagen S: Desmopressin—a hemostatic drug: a state-of-the-art review. *Europ J Anaesthesiol* 14:1, 1997.

Letts M et al: The influence of desmopressin on blood loss during spinal fusion surgery in neuromuscular patients. *Spine* 23:475, 1998.

Mannucci PM: Hemostatic drugs. *N Eng J Med* 339: 245, 1998.

Mannucci PM et al: Patterns of development of tachyphylaxis in patients with haemophilia and von Willebrand disease after repeated doses of desmopressin (DDAVP). *Br J Haematol* 82:87, 1992.

Rao AK et al: Mechanisms of platelet dysfunction and response to DDAVP in patients with congenital platelet function defects. A double-blind placebo-controlled trial. *Thromb Haemost* 74:1071, 1995.

Ravensbaek Jensen A et al: Variability of the factor VIII response to DDAVP in a large kindred with mild haemophilia A. *Haemophilia* 3:259, 1997.

Reid RW et al: The efficacy of tranexamic acid versus placebo in decreasing blood loss in pediatric patients undergoing repeat cardiac surgery. *Anesth Analg* 84:990, 1997.

Rodeghiero F et al: Prospective multicenter study on subcutaneous concentrated desmopressin for home treatment of patients with von Willebrand disease and mild or moderate hemophilia A. *Thromb Haemost* 76:692, 1996.

Rose EH, Aledort LM: Nasal spray desmopressin (DDAVP) for mild hemophilia A and von Willebrand disease. *Ann Intern Med* 114:563, 1991.

Schultz M, van der Lelie H: Microscopic haematuria as a relative contraindication for tranexamic acid. *Br J Haematol* 89: 663, 1995.

Sindet-Pedersen S et al: Hemostatic effect of tranexamic acid mouthwash in anti-coagulant-treated patients undergoing oral surgery. *N Engl J Med* 320:840, 1989.

Slaughter TF, Greenberg CS: Antifibrinolytic drugs and perioperative hemostasis. *Am J Hematol* 56:32, 1997.

Smith TJ et al: Hyponatremia and seizures in young children given DDAVP. *Am J Hematol* 31:199, 1989.

Stefanini M et al: Safe and effective, prolonged administration of epsilon aminocaproic acid in bleeding from the urinary tract. *J Urol* 143:559, 1990.

Stine KC, Becton DL: DDAVP therapy controls bleeding in Ehlers-Danlos syndrome. *J Pediat Hem/Onc* 19:156, 1997.

Sutor AH: DDAVP is not a panacea for children with bleeding disorders. Review. *Br J Haematol* 108:217, 2000.

Theroux MC et al: A study of desmopressin and blood loss during spinal fusion for neuromuscular scoliosis. *Anesthesiology* 87:260, 1997.

Waldenstrom E et al: Bernard-Soulier syndrome in two Swedish families: Effect of DDAVP on bleeding time. *Eur J Haematol* 46:182, 1991.

CHAPTER 59

Heparins

For over 40 years heparin has been standard therapy for the initial treatment of vascular thrombosis. When used appropriately, heparin prevents recurrent thromboembolism with an acceptable risk of major bleeding. Recently, however, the dominance of unfractionated heparin (UH) in our antithrombotic armamentarium has been overtaken by the low molecular weight heparins (LMWH). The data from current clinical trials suggest that LMWH are at least as safe and effective as standard heparin, and are easier to administer.

PHARMACOLOGY

Standard heparin is a complex glycosaminoglycan isolated and purified from animal tissues (porcine intestinal mucosa or bovine lung). It functions as an anticoagulant by inducing a conformational change in the structure of antithrombin (AT) that dramatically augments the ability of AT to neutralize thrombin and, to a lesser extent, factor Xa and other serine proteases that participate in the formation of fibrin. Standard heparin binds to endothelial cells and macrophages, as well as to several plasma proteins (such as platelet factor 4 and von Willebrand factor), which explains the substantial variability in plasma heparin activity observed after parenteral injection. Platelet function is also impaired by heparin due to inhibition of platelet aggregation mediated by collagen and von Willebrand factor.

The LMWH are prepared from UH by enzymatic or chemical hydrolysis, procedures that substantially alter the biologic properties and clinical attributes of the anticoagulant (Table 59-1). For example, LMWH inhibits factor Xa more potently than thrombin, whereas UH predominantly

TABLE 59-1

Standard Heparin versus Low Molecular Weight Heparin

Standard Heparin	Low Molecular Weight Heparin
Binds nonspecifically to plasma proteins	Lacks nonspecific binding
Increased plasma half-life with increased dose of drug	Stable plasma half-life
Binds platelet factor 4	Does not bind platelet factor 4
APTT used to monitor therapy	Most patients can be treated without monitoring
APTT or anti-Xa heparin assay used to monitor therapy	Anti-Xa heparin assay
Neutralized by protamine	Only ~50% neutralized by protamine
Half-life 30 min to 4 h (dose-related)	Half-life ~4 h

inhibits thrombin. A major stimulus for the development of these new heparins has been the hope that the low molecular weight preparations will provide equal or greater antithrombotic effects with less bleeding than UH. At least in part, these expectations have been realized; LMWH have more predictable biologic availability and are administered in a subcutaneous dose once or twice daily without the need for laboratory monitoring. Because of these attributes, LMWH are now being used in multiple settings, including home therapy in patients with uncomplicated venous thrombosis and in hospitalized patients with unstable angina.

CLINICAL USE

UH and LMWH have been rigorously tested in clinical trials and both are effective anticoagulants. At least five preparations of LMWH are available throughout the world and four are now or soon to be released for use in the United States. Recommended doses vary depending on methods of manufacture and the results of human clinical trials (Table 59-2).

Deep Venous Thrombosis and Pulmonary Embolism

Clinicians now have the option of UH or LMWH for treatment of venous thrombosis. Given UH's variability in terms of absorption, bioavailability, and dosing, LMWH are now being more widely used to treat patients with venous thromboembolism. If UH is used one should strive to achieve a therapeutic APTT as rapidly as possible. Since APTT reagents have differing sensitivities to heparin, laboratories must insure that their therapeutic APTT ranges have been calibrated to reflect anti-Xa heparin

---

TABLE 59-2

Agents and Dosing for Adults*

HEPARIN (given SC or IV)

Prophylactic: 5,000 U q 12 h SC. Higher doses used in some settings (see text)
Therapeutic: 1–2,000 U/h IV to achieve APTT's equivalent to 0.3–0.7 U/mL
  anti-Xa heparin levels

LOW MOLECULAR WEIGHT HEPARIN (given SC)

Ardeparin

Orthopedic lower extremity surgery: 50 anti-Xa U/kg q 12 h starting 12–24 h after
  surgery

Dalteparin

Prophylactic: 2500 U daily (low risk); 5000 U daily (high-risk abdominal surgery)
Therapeutic: 100 U/kg q 12 h

Enoxaparin

Prophylactic: 40 mg daily or 30 mg q 12 h (orthopedic indications)
Therapeutic: 1 mg/kg q 12 h or 1.5 mg/kg daily (low risk patients)

Nadroparin

Prophylactic: 3100 U 2 h before surgery and once daily thereafter
        Orthopedic surgery: 40 U/kg 2 h before surgery and once daily for 3
        days post operatively; 60 U/kg daily thereafter
Therapeutic: <55 kg: 12,500 U q 12 h; 55–80 kg: 15,000 U q 12 h; >80 kg: 17,500 U q
        12 h

Tinzaparin

Prophylactic: General surgery: 3500 U 2 h before surgery and daily thereafter
        Orthopedic: 50 U/kg 2 h before surgery and daily thereafter
Therapeutic: 175 U/kg daily

---

* For pediatric dosing, see Chapter 34.
Data from Clagett GP et al: Prevention of venous thromboembolism. *Chest* 114:531S, 1998; and Hyers TM
et al: Antithrombotic therapy for venous thromboembolic disease. *Chest* 114:561S, 1998.
Product literature should be consulted for dosage changes.

levels of 0.3 to 0.7 anti-Xa U/mL. LMWH can be dosed by weight in most patients. Patients with > than 150 percent or <75 percent ideal body weight, renal failure, or pregnancy, and infants, children, and the very old should have LMWH heparin levels monitored using an anti-Xa heparin assay (discussed later). Even in the very obese, the dose of LMWH should be calculated using true, not ideal, body weight.

In patients with DVT, oral anticoagulants should be started on the first day of heparin therapy, so that the total duration of heparin or LMWH is approximately 5 days. The PT should be prolonged into the therapeutic range by the warfarin (INR 2 to 3) for at least 24 h before discontinuing the heparin or LMWH. If the heparin is stopped prematurely, risks of recurrent thrombosis may be increased because of lower levels of AT (due to the heparin), reduced protein C (due to the warfarin), and the persistence of a highly thrombogenic clot. Warfarin causes a rapid fall in factor VII (T½ ~ 5 h), which prolongs the PT, but reductions in clotting factors II, and X (T½ = 24 to 48 h) are necessary for optimal anticoagulation.

Other Venous Thromboses

Although controlled clinical trials are not available, heparin is effective for treatment of venous thromboses in sites other than the extremities, which include the hepatic, mesenteric, and portal veins. Heparin has been shown to be safe and effective in the treatment of most patients with acute cerebral vein thrombosis.

Cardiac Disorders

Clinical trials have convincingly shown that the combination of LMWH and aspirin is superior to UH and aspirin for reduction of chest pain, subsequent myocardial infarction, and mortality in patients with unstable angina. UH is used routinely following thrombolytic therapy with t-PA for acute coronary artery thrombosis in an attempt to maintain arterial patency following resolution of the clot. Lastly, UH in doses of at least 7500 U twice daily or LMWH in prophylactic doses are recommended for patients with transmural anterior myocardial infarction to prevent the formation of mural thrombi in the left ventricle.

Cardioembolic Stroke

Following an embolic stroke, the rate of recurrent cerebral embolization has been estimated to be as high as 1 percent per day for the next 2 weeks. Because a feared complication of heparin therapy is CNS bleeding, anticoagulants should be withheld for 24 to 48 h and a CT scan obtained. If the cerebral infarct is not large (i.e., not greater than 4 to 5 cm), and there is no evidence of hemorrhagic transformation, intravenous heparin can be begun at a rate of 1000 U/h without a loading dose. Unlike other indications, clinical trials have not yet shown an advantage for LMWH in the treatment of stroke.

Prophylaxis for Venous Thromboembolism in Surgical and Medical Patients

Unfractionated heparin has been shown to prevent DVT following surgery and other high-risk situations. However, a dose of 5000 U bid may not be sufficient for all patients, with larger amounts needed for effective prophylaxis in some. LMWH has the advantage of rapid complete absorption and excellent bioavailability; it has been shown to be effective in medical, surgical, orthopedic, and trauma patients.

Heparin in Infants and Children

Venous thrombosis is uncommon in infants, but arterial occlusion is relatively frequent (1 to 5 percent or more) in newborns who require umbilical catheters. Optimal heparin therapy is difficult due to its large volume of distribution in neonates (compared to adults) and its accelerated clearance from the blood. Other problems include low levels of AT (as low as 25 percent in premature infants), difficulties in obtaining accurate blood samples for laboratory monitoring, and the risk of intraventricular hemorrhage. See Chapter 34 for details of heparin therapy in children.

Pregnancy

See Chapter 51 for additional discussion.

Therapy for Acute Venous Thrombosis

Heparin is used for two reasons during pregnancy: therapeutic anticoagulation for women with an acute venous thromboembolism or for prophylactic anticoagulation in patients with a history of thrombosis in the past. It is becoming increasingly clear that LMWH are safe and effective in pregnancy, are easier to administer and monitor, and cause less osteoporosis than UH. LMWH is started in therapeutic doses for treatment of acute thrombosis and then continued for the remainder of the pregnancy. If possible, the last dose of LMWH should be 12 h or more before delivery to allow adequate time for clearance from the blood and tissues. If desired, prophylactic doses of heparin can be given during labor, delivery, and immediately postpartum, although caution must be exercised if epidural anesthesia is employed. Oral anticoagulants (warfarin) are usually begun following delivery (with heparin overlap) and continued for at least 6 to 12 weeks.

If UH is chosen for long-term treatment following initial intravenous heparin for acute thrombosis, doses of heparin are usually given every 12 h as subcutaneous injections, with monitoring 4 h later to keep the anti-Xa heparin assay in the therapeutic range. Available data suggest that either LMWH or UF is effective, and both have low rates of bleeding and are not harmful to the fetus.

Prophylaxis

Prophylactic heparin protocols for women with a past history of venous thromboembolism include the use of UH or LMWH during pregnancy.

Several studies have suggested that 5000 U of UH given subcutaneously twice daily may not be fully protective. An alternative approach is to administer the heparin subcutaneously at 12-hour intervals at doses adjusted to keep the 4 h post-injection APTT at the upper limit of normal, or the heparin assay (using an anti-Xa method) between 0.10 and 0.15 U/mL. Alternatively, once or twice daily LMWH is effective and reduces the need for laboratory monitoring. Some preliminary studies have suggested that LMWH may be beneficial in prevention of thrombosis and recurrent pregnancy loss in women with hereditary or acquired thrombophilia (see Chap. 51).

LABORATORY MONITORING

Activated Partial Thromboplastin Time

The APTT is routinely used to monitor the therapeutic effects of UH, although recently heparin assays are being used more frequently, particularly in complicated patients (see below). It is important to recall that heparin also prolongs the TCT and PT. With low doses of heparin, the dilute thrombin time (normal, 20 to 25 sec) is rapidly prolonged to >150 sec; with larger doses of heparin the APTT increases, followed thereafter by prolongation of the PT. Several of the PT thromboplastin reagents that use recombinant tissue factor now include polybrene as an agent to neutralize heparin. An arbitrary APTT therapeutic range (such as 1½–2× control) should not be used to monitor heparin. Instead, each laboratory's APTT must be calibrated to a heparin concentration of 0.3 to 0.7 U/mL by a factor-Xa inhibition heparin assay using plasma obtained from patients receiving heparin. Studies have shown that "therapeutic" APTT ranges can vary substantially depending on the APTT reagents and coagulometers.

Heparin Assays

Heparin assays such as the factor Xa inhibition test are increasingly used to monitor heparin therapy in patients with complex hemostatic disorders that can independently alter the APTT. In this assay, a known quantity of purified factor Xa (and an excess of AT) is added to patient plasma containing heparin or to normal plasmas that contain heparin standards. The ability of heparin-AT to inhibit cleavage of a chromogenic substrate by factor Xa is then measured in a spectrophotometer. Heparin standards are used to assay UH or the LMWH. The therapeutic range for UH is 0.3 to 0.7 U/mL of anti-Xa activity for treatment of venous thrombosis. The provisional therapeutic range for LMWH is approximately 0.6 to 1.0 anti-Xa U/mL.

Heparin assays are extremely useful for monitoring heparin therapy in difficult clinical situations in which the APTT may be unreliable, such as in patients with a lupus anticoagulant or during pregnancy. Other conditions include concomitant warfarin therapy, associated intrinsic coagulation system defects and in infants who often have prolonged APTTs for various reasons. Since LMWH anticoagulant effect cannot be measured by the APTT, heparin levels must be used if monitoring is desired. Indications for LMWH assays include extremes of body weight, renal failure, pregnancy, long-term therapy (e.g., cancer-induced thrombosis), infants and children, and patients at very high risk of bleeding or thrombosis.

Platelet Counts

Platelet counts are recommended in patients receiving therapeutic doses of heparin for early recognition and treatment of heparin-induced thrombocytopenia (HIT). Hematocrits should be obtained at the same time to detect occult bleeding.

SIDE EFFECTS AND COMPLICATIONS

Bleeding

Rates of serious hemorrhage with heparin therapy are low and average 3 to 5 percent in most clinical trials. Bleeding has been shown to be higher in patients with one or more risk factors, such as low performance status, recent trauma or surgery, or a history of a bleeding diathesis (Table 59-3). If bleeding is severe, protamine sulfate can be used for immediate neutralization of the anticoagulant. When the heparin has been given very recently, then 1 mg protamine sulfate neutralizes approximately 100 U heparin. However, lesser doses of protamine (e.g., 10 to 20 mg) are often effective, particularly when several hours have elapsed since heparin was administered. The relative prolongations of the PT and APTT and heparin assays are useful for estimating the quantity of circulating heparin and the need for protamine. If extremely large doses of heparin have been given in error, repeated infusions of protamine sulfate may be required because the survival of heparin in the plasma is dose related; that is, the T½ is longer with larger doses of heparin. The efficacy of protamine neutralization of heparin is assessed by repeated measurement of the APTT.

Protamine sulfate is less effective in neutralizing LMWH heparin. One approach is to give 1 mg of protamine for every 1 mg or 10 anti-Xa units

TABLE 59-3
Clinical Conditions that Increase the Risk of Bleeding with Heparin Therapy
Advanced age (women >60, men >70) Surgery within 10 days Elevated serum creatinine Recent intracranial hemorrhage or stroke Active peptic ulcer disease Hypertension (diastolic pressure >120 mm Hg) Recent CPR History of bleeding diathesis Multiple comorbid conditions APTT >2 times control

of LMWH. For example, if a patient has been given 90 mg of enoxaparin they should receive 90 mg of protamine. Given the longer half-life of LMWH, one-half of this dose can be repeated in 4 hours if necessary.

Heparin-Induced Thrombocytopenia (HIT)

This important clinical problem is discussed in detail in Chap. 45.

Osteopenia

Long-term full-dose and prophylactic levels of heparin have been reported to cause osteopenia. In series of pregnant women treated with UH heparin, 20 to 30 percent had measurable bone loss and 1 to 2 percent developed overt fractures. Fortunately, the osteopenia was reversible in 6 to 12 months. Several clinical trials in pregnant women have demonstrated that LMWH is associated with a lesser degree of bone loss.

Reduction in Antithrombin Levels

The concentration of circulating AT often falls acutely after a large thrombosis, but then drops further as a result of heparin therapy (by as much as 20 to 30 percent). Although usually of little consequence, lowered levels of AT could predispose to recurrent thrombosis if heparin is stopped prematurely before oral anticoagulants are fully effective.

Heparin Resistance

Some patients are resistant to the effects of heparin and require large doses of the anticoagulant to prolong the APTT into the therapeutic range. Possible explanations include shortened heparin survival associated with large thrombi, short preheparin APTTs due to elevated levels of factor VIII or circulating activated clotting factors, hereditary or acquired AT deficiency, and HIT (due to heparin neutralization by platelet factor 4 released from aggregating platelets). Frequent APTTs during the first 24 h of therapy may be necessary, and in complex situations, heparin assays, HIT tests, and AT measurements are useful.

BIBLIOGRAPHY

Dahlman T et al: Osteopenia in pregnancy during long-term heparin treatment: A radiological study post partum. *Br J Obstet Gynaecol* 97:221, 1990.

Dahlman TC et al: Thrombosis prophylaxis in pregnancy with use of subcutaneous heparin adjusted by monitoring heparin concentration in plasma. *Am J Obstet Gynecol* 161:420, 1989.

Einhaupl KM et al: Heparin treatment in sinus venous thrombosis. *Lancet* 338:597, 1991.

Gould MK et al: Low-molecular-weight heparins compared with unfractionated heparin for treatment of acute deep venous thrombosis. A meta-analysis of randomized controlled trials. *Ann Intern Med* 130:800, 1999.

Harrison L et al: Assessment of outpatient treatment of deep-vein thrombosis with low-molecular-weight heparin. *Arch Intern Med* 158:2001, 1998.

Hirsh J et al: Heparin and low-molecular-weight heparin: mechanisms of action, pharmokinetics, dosing considerations, monitoring, efficacy, and safety. *Chest* 114:489S, 1998.

Landefeld CS et al: A bleeding risk index for estimating the probability of major bleeding in hospitalized patients starting anticoagulant therapy. *Am J Med* 89:569, 1990.

Litin SC et al: Use of low-molecular-weight heparin in the treatment of venous thromboembolic disease: answers to frequently asked questions. The Thrombophilia Center Investigators. *Mayo Clin Proc* 73: 545, 1998.

Nieuwenhuis HK et al: Identification of risk factors for bleeding during treatment of acute venous thromboembolism with heparin or low molecular weight heparin. *Blood* 78:2337, 1991

Noble S et al: Enoxaparin. A review of its clinical potential in the management of coronary artery disease. *Drugs* 56:259, 1998.

Noble S et al: Enoxaparin. A reappraisal of its pharmacology and clinical applications in the prevention and treatment of thromboembolic disease. *Drugs* 49:388, 1995.

Nurmohamed MT et al: Low-molecular-weight heparin versus standard heparin in general and orthopaedic surgery: A meta-analysis. *Lancet* 340:152, 1992.

O'Brien B et al: Economic evaluation of outpatient treatment with low-molecular-weight heparin for proximal vein thrombosis. *Arch Intern Med* 159:2298, 1999.

Sanson BJ et al: Safety of low-molecular-weight heparin in pregnancy: a systematic review. *Thromb Haemost* 81: 668, 1999.

Turpie AG: Anticoagulants in acute coronary syndromes. *Am J Cardiol* 84: 2M, 1999.

Warkentin TE: Heparin-induced thrombocytopenia. Pathogenesis, frequency, avoidance and management. *Drug Safety* 17:325, 1997.

Weitz JI: Low-molecular-weight heparins. *N Engl J Med* 337(10):688, 1997.

Wilde MI, Markham A: Danaparoid. A review of its pharmacology and clinical use in the management of heparin-induced thrombocytopenia. *Drugs* 54(6):903, 1997.

CHAPTER 60

Oral Anticoagulants

Oral anticoagulants such as warfarin are highly effective antithrombotic agents with relatively low risks of serious bleeding. Although available for decades, clinical uses and applications have evolved over the years. Recent changes include:

- The development of clinical guidelines for management of oral anticoagulants based on evidence derived from controlled trials (see Fifth ACCP Consensus Conference on Antithrombotic Therapy. *Chest* 114 (Suppl), 1998).
- Standardization of laboratory monitoring so intensities of anticoagulation are more equivalent around the world.
- New indications and protocols for treatment have emerged from prospective controlled clinical trials; for example, prophylaxis of embolic stroke in patients with chronic nonrheumatic atrial fibrillation.
- The development of point-of-care prothrombin time (PT) monitoring instruments for use in the clinic and home.

PHARMACOLOGY

Warfarin is a 4-hydroxycoumarin derivative that exerts an antithrombotic effect by blocking the regeneration of vitamin K from its epoxide (Fig. 60-1). Vitamin K is necessary for the addition of γ-carboxyglutamic acid (Gla) residues to clotting factors II, VII, IX, and X (and also proteins C, S, and Z).

Gla residues bind metal ions such as calcium and undergo a conformational change that is necessary for the protein to attach to their cofac-

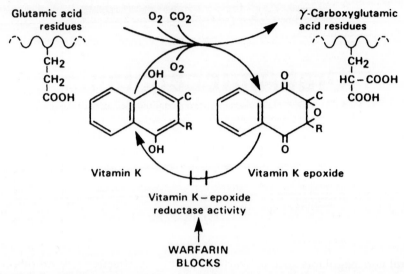

FIGURE 60-1 Interactions of warfarin and vitamin K. (Reprinted with permission from *Sem Thromb Hemost* 12:1, 1986.)

tors on phospholipid surfaces and participate in coagulation. Warfarin treatment reduces the number of Gla residues (normal 10 to 13) per clotting factor molecule with a concomitant fall in coagulant activity. When the number of residues decreases to 9, only 70 percent of the activity of the clotting factor remains; when there are 6, only 2 percent activity is present.

Warfarin is rapidly absorbed from the gastrointestinal tract in 1.5 to 2 h, is 99 percent bound to albumin, and has a prolonged half-life of ~40 h in the circulation. The effects of warfarin on coagulation are dependent on the half-life of the vitamin K clotting factors in plasma. Thus, factor VII activity (half-life, 5 h) falls quickly following initiation of therapy and prolongs the PT. The remaining three vitamin K-dependent coagulation factors (II, IX, X) have half-lives ranging from 24 to 48 h and therefore fall more slowly, only gradually contributing to the lengthening of the PT and APTT. Reductions in these longer-lived clotting factors, especially factors II and X, are most likely responsible for the antithrombotic effects of warfarin. The relationships between oral doses of warfarin and the prolongation of the PT are complex and sometimes unpredictable. Variables include patient compliance, vitamin K content of the diet, genetics, concurrent illness, liver function, and certain genetic mutations in vitamin K dependent clotting factors (Chu et al ref). The effects of warfarin are also significantly modified by the use of many pharmaceutical agents (Table 60-1).

TABLE 60-1

Medication Effects of Warfarin

Increased Effect

Acetaminophen
Allopurinol
Aminodarone* (may last for months after drug is stopped)
Anabolic Steroids*
Aspirin*
Cephalosporins (Nmtt group)
Cimetidine*
Clofibrate*
Cyclophosphamide
Disulfiram
Erythromycin*
Fluconazole*
Furosemide
Gemfibrozil
Isoniazid
Itraconazole*
Ketoconazole*
Metronidazole*
Micronase*
Omeprazole
Propafenone
Propranolol
Quinidine*
Quinine*
Quinolones
Serotonin uptake inhibitors
Sulfinpyrazone*
Sulfonylureas*
Tamoxifen*
Tetracycline*
Thyroid Hormones*
Tricyclics
Vitamin E*

Decreased Effect

Alcohol
Barbiturates*
Carbamazepine
Corticosteroids
Cholestyramine
Estrogens
Griseofulvin
Phenytoin (may potentiate warfarin with initiation of drug)
Rifampin
Sucralfate
Vitamin K

* Major Effect; **Bold**, strongest evidence for effect

LABORATORY TESTING

Prothrombin Time

Both the PT and the APTT are prolonged in patients who are treated with long-term oral anticoagulants. Shortly after the initiation of therapy, the PT lengthens due to the rapid fall in factor VII activity, followed in several days by an increase in the APTT as factors II, IX, and X are reduced. The TCT and fibrinogen concentration is not altered by warfarin treatment.

Traditionally, the PT has been used to monitor the antithrombotic affects of oral anticoagulants. The test is performed by the addition of a thromboplastin (a combination of tissue factor and phospholipid) to recalcified plasma. The sensitivity of the thromboplastin to warfarin-induced reductions in clotting factor activity is a critical variable in the assay. Some thromboplastins are very sensitive (produce long PTs for a given intensity of anticoagulation), whereas others are insensitive. Consequently, a patient could receive substantially different doses of an oral anticoagulant depending on the thromboplastin used in the PT test if using a therapeutic range based on seconds of prolongation or a PT ratio.

To address this important clinical problem, the PT ratio (patient PT/control PT) is now modified by a factor (the International Sensitivity Index or ISI) that reflects the "sensitivity" of the thromboplastin used in the assay. Highly sensitive thromboplastins are assigned low ISIs (1.0 to 1.8), whereas insensitive reagents have high ISIs (e.g., 2.8). After correction of the PT ratio by the ISI assigned to the thromboplastin, the result is termed the International Normalized Ratio (INR). The calculation is performed as follows:

$$INR = (PT\ ratio)^{ISI}$$

Thus, a patient taking warfarin who has a PT of 18 sec (with a mean normal PT performed in the same laboratory of 12 sec) would have an PT ratio of 1.5. If the ISI of the thromboplastin being used for the assay is 2.0, then the INR is 2.25; that is, $(1.5)^2 = 2.25$. There is now a major worldwide trend toward the use of thromboplastins with ISI values close to 1.0, as exemplified by the development of reagents that utilize recombinant tissue factor.

Whole Blood Prothrombin Time Instruments

Small portable instruments that have been designed to measure a PT and INR on finger-stick blood samples are now available for use in point-of-care testing in the hospital or in patients' homes. Studies have confirmed the accuracy and reliability of these instruments as compared to centralized laboratories.

Recently, evidence is accumulating that self-management of oral anticoagulant therapy in selected patients is feasible and results in similar INR values and rates of bleeding or recurrent thrombosis, compared to office or clinic-based management.

COMPUTERIZED PREDICTION OF WARFARIN DOSAGE

Computer-assisted dosing of warfarin is gaining acceptance, with several programs now being tested in clinical trials. In general, the automated programs have proven equivalent or superior to empiric dose adjustment by office-based physicians or anticoagulation clinics (see Poller ref).

CLINICAL USE

Institution of Therapy

Warfarin is usually started with a dose of 5 to 10 mg daily for the first 2 days in adult patients who have been treated with heparin for an acute thrombosis. Two clinical trials suggest that a lower loading dose of 5 mg more rapidly achieves a stable INR. Daily PTs are obtained and subsequent warfarin orders are based on the results with a goal of attaining an INR of 2 to 3. The heparin infusion should not be stopped until the INR has remained in the therapeutic range for 24 h, which allows clotting factors II and X to decrease to antithrombotic levels. Dosing protocols for 5 and 10 mg warfarin levels are given in Tables 60-2 and 60-3.

Most clinicians give oral anticoagulants in the evening and obtain the PT the following morning; this practice allows time for absorption of the prior dose of warfarin and the return of laboratory test results. Each dose should be ordered daily and only after the results of the laboratory tests and the clinical status of the patient have been reviewed. When patients are electively anticoagulated as outpatients (e.g., for atrial fibrillation), loading doses of warfarin are omitted; 5 to 7.5 mg is given daily with adjustments as needed.

Warfarin treatment of children poses several problems. Children often have variable response to therapy, and younger children require increased warfarin doses, a longer time to achieve target INR ranges, and frequent dose adjustments (see Chap. 34). An initial loading dose of 0.2 mg/kg may be used followed by dose adjustments based on the INR.

TABLE 60-2		
Nomogram for Warfarin Loading in Adults—5 mg Dose		
Day	**INR**	**Dosage (mg)**
1		5.0
2	<1.5	5.0
	1.5–1.9	2.5
	2.0–2.5	1.0–2.5
	>2.5	0.0
3	<1.5	5.0–10.0
	1.5–1.9	2.5–5.0
	2.0–2.5	0.0–2.5
	2.5–3.0	0.0–2.5
	>3.0	0.0
4	<1.5	10.0
	1.5–1.9	5.0–7.5
	2.0–3.0	0.0–0.5
	>3.0	0.0
5	<1.5	10.0
	1.5–1.9	7.5–10.0
	2.0–3.0	0.0–5.0
	>3.0	0.0
6	<1.5	7.5–12.5
	1.5–1.9	5.0–10.0
	2.0–3.0	0.0–7.5
	>3.0	0.0

From Crowther MA et al. *Ann Intern Med* 127:333, 1997

Therapeutic Ranges

Most patients with thromboembolism require low-intensity anticoagulation which corresponds to an INR of 2 to 3. Examples are patients with deep venous thrombosis and pulmonary embolism, atrial fibrillation, and tissue valves. Higher-intensity therapy (INR of 2.5 to 3.5) is suggested for most patients with artificial valves. Higher-intensity therapy may also be appropriate for treatment of infants and children with homozygous protein C or protein S deficiency (see Chap. 34).

Maintenance Therapy

Because of the long half-life of warfarin, changes in therapy should be based on a percent of the total weekly dose in patients on chronic anticoagulants rather than an alteration of each daily dose. An effective strategy is to make an initial adjustment to bring the PT rapidly into the therapeutic range, and then alter the weekly dose as necessary. A proto-

TABLE 60-3

Nomogram for Warfarin Loading in Adults—10 mg Dose

Day	INR	Dosage (mg)
1		10.0
2	<1.5	7.5–10.0
	1.5–1.9	2.5
	2.0–2.5	1.0–2.5
	>2.5	0.0
3	<1.5	5.0–10.0
	1.5–1.9	2.5–5.0
	2.0–2.5	0.0–2.5
	2.5–3.0	0.0–2.5
	>3.0	0.0
4	<1.5	10.0
	1.5–1.9	5.0–7.5
	2.0–3.0	0.0–5.0
	>3.0	0.0
5	<1.5	10.0
	1.5–1.9	7.5–10.0
	2.0–3.0	0.0–5.0
	>3.0	0.0
6	<1.5	7.5–12.5
	1.5–1.9	5.0–10.0
	2.0–3.0	0.0–7.5
	>3.0	0.0

From Crowther MA et al: *Ann Intern Med* 127:333, 1997

col for management of long term outpatient anticoagulation therapy is shown in Table 60-4. Alternatively a computerized warfarin-dosing program can be used to guide therapy in stable outpatients.

Problems in Management

Unstable Prothrombin Times

The great majority of patients on long-term anticoagulants require only minor adjustments in dose. However, some patients have widely fluctuating PTs that pose major challenges in management. Changes in the vitamin K content of the diet can sometimes be responsible (e.g., salads in the summer, use of olestra; see Harrell and Kline and Booth et al refs, Table 60-5), or intercurrent illness can be a problem. Heart failure, liver disease, and diarrhea all lower anticoagulant requirements. Viral illnesses are a particular challenge in infants and children, who often have a dramatic increase in INR a day or two following an upper respiratory

TABLE 60-4

Protocol for Warfarin Dosage Adjustment in Outpatients with a Target INR of 2 to 3

INR	Adjustment
1.1–1.4	*Day 1:* Add 10–20% of TWD* *Weekly:* Increase TWD by 10–20% *Return:* 1 wk
1.5–1.9	*Day 1:* Add 5–10% of TWD *Weekly:* Increase TWD by 5–10% *Return:* 2 wks
2–3	No change *Return:* 4 wks
3.1–3.9	*Day 1:* Subtract 5–10% of TWD *Weekly:* Reduce TWD by 5–10% *Return:* 2 wks
4.0–5.0	*Day 1:* No warfarin *Weekly:* Reduce TWD by 10–20% *Return:* 1 wk
>5	Stop warfarin; monitor INR until 3.0, reinstitute at lower TWD—e.g., decrease by 20–50%. *Return:* daily

* TWD, Total weekly dose of warfarin. A patient taking 5 mg on Monday, Wednesday, and Friday, and 7.5 mg on the remaining days, would have a TWD of 45 mg.

TABLE 60-5

Vitamin K Content of Foods

Item	Vitamin K Content (µg/100 ug)
Green tea	712
Avocado	634
Turnip greens	408
Brussels sprouts	317
Chickpeas	220
Broccoli	200
Cauliflower	192
Lettuce	129
Cabbage	125
Kale	125
Beef liver	92
Spinach	89
Watercress	57
Asparagus	57
Lettuce (iceberg)	26
Green beans	14

infection or gastrointestinal upset. Drug interactions as a cause of instability are common (especially antibiotics), and excessive use of alcohol can alter dietary patterns as well as compliance. Older or mentally impaired patients can become confused about tablet size or therapeutic regimen. Warfarin sensitivity has occurred in subjects with a mutation in the factor IX propeptide (Chu et al ref). Finally, if no other cause for instability is identified, patient compliance could be less than optimal.

Intercurrent Surgical Procedures

Surgical or invasive diagnostic procedures such as dental extractions, biopsies, or gastrointestinal endoscopy are often necessary in patients on oral anticoagulants. Relatively minor procedures can often be safely performed by allowing the PT to drift toward normal, with subsequent replacement of missing warfarin doses (Table 60-6). Major surgical procedures in patients at high risk for thrombosis pose a bigger problem. Most surgeons are comfortable operating when the INR is below 1.5; however, during the period of time when the warfarin effect is diminishing, the risk of thromboembolic events increases. The likelihood of thrombosis in this setting is not well established, but is probably less than 1 percent per day. However, an acute thromboembolic event in the perisurgical setting may be catastrophic. High-risk patients, such as those with mechanical heart valves or atrial fibrillation with a previous embolic event can be covered with "bridging therapy." The use of low molecular weight heparin (LMWH) in the outpatient setting has simplified the treatment of patients on long-term oral anticoagulant therapy and has lessened the

---

TABLE 60-6

Management of Warfarin for Minor Surgical Procedures

Step 1: Obtain INR 5–7 days before procedure.

Step 2: Stop warfarin 1–4 days before the procedure depending on INR (e.g., INR 2–3 = 2 days; INR 3–4 = 3–4 days; INR > 4 = 5 days).

Step 3: On the evening following the surgical procedure, reinstitute warfarin if no bleeding.

Replace missing doses of warfarin on a day to day basis; e.g.,

Th	F	Sa	S	M	T	W	Th	F	Sa
5 mg	5 mg	5 mg	5 mg	0	0	10 mg	10 mg	5 mg	5 mg

(INR 2.5) ↑ (procedure)

Step 4: Check INR 5–7 days after procedure.

need for prolonged hospital stays and the use of intravenous heparin. One approach is outlined in Table 60-7.

Pregnancy and Lactation

Oral anticoagulants are usually not recommended during pregnancy because of the risks of warfarin-induced embryopathy, particularly during weeks 6 to 12. Fetal neural disorders can occur in mid-trimester, as well as bleeding in the neonate at time of delivery. Maternal warfarin therapy does not pose a problem for nursing infants as long as they are not vitamin K deficient (the infant should have had parenteral or repeated oral neonatal prophylaxis, see Chap. 22).

Refractory Patients

Most recurrent thrombosis occurs when the INR is allowed to fall to less than 2.0. However, some patients (particularly with cancer, myeloproliferative disease, or antiphospholipid antibodies) develop thrombo-embolism despite an adequate intensity of anticoagulation. In such instances, treatment with heparin or LMWH should be considered.

Lupus Anticoagulants

The lupus anticoagulant (LA) can occasionally prolong the PT (elevate the INR) in patients with thrombosis, which leads to undertreatment with warfarin and an increased risk of thrombosis (see Chap. 43). In general, this is an uncommon problem that occurs only sporadically with many different thromboplastins. Alternatives include switching to a prothrombin reagent that is insensitive to the patients LA, monitoring with chromogenic factor X assay levels (INR 2 = ~40% factor X activity; INR 3 = ~15% factor X activity), or using the prothrombin and proconvertin (P & P) test, if it is available.

TABLE 60-7	
Protocol for Very High Risk Patients Scheduled for Major Surgery	
Day −5	Stop warfarin, begin therapeutic doses of LMW heparin
Day −4 to −2	Continue LMW heparin
Day −1	Give last dose of LMW heparin in AM (daily dosing) or PM (q 12 hr dosing)
Surgery	No heparin (or prophylactic doses of LMWH), use pneumatic stockings
Day 2–3	Restart LMW heparin at therapeutic doses, if risk of bleeding is high use prophylactic doses. Restart warfarin when patient can take oral fluids
Day 7–8	Stop LMW heparin when INR > 2.0 for 24 h

SIDE EFFECTS AND COMPLICATIONS

Hemorrhage

Major hemorrhage is directly related to increases in the INR, so that low-intensity anticoagulation has a lower rate of bleeding than higher-intensity therapy. Most studies in unselected groups of patients suggest that the risk of major bleeding (as defined by need to discontinue warfarin, or necessitate hospitalization or blood transfusion) is approximately 2 percent per year (2 of 100 patients treated for 1 year). CNS hemorrhage occurs at a rate of 0.1 to 0.5 percent per year. Risk factors for bleeding on warfarin include being female, concurrent use of multiple drugs, associated serious illness such as renal failure or congestive heart failure, and intercurrent illnesses in small children. Advanced age does not appear to increase bleeding, but elderly patients require up to one-third less warfarin to maintain a target INR.

The management of excessively anticoagulated patients who are not bleeding depends in part on the prolongation of the INR. Mild elevations are simply treated with appropriate dose adjustments, whereas moderately increased INR (4 to 6) require discontinuation of the anticoagulant for 1 to 2 days. More marked INR prolongations can be corrected with small oral doses of vitamin K (0.5 to 2 mg). In each case, frequent INR determinations are essential, so that anticoagulants can be restarted at an appropriate time.

Minor bleeding in patients with INRs in the low-intensity range can usually be managed with local measures alone. However, more serious bleeding associated with an excessively prolonged INR requires larger doses of oral vitamin K (2 to 5 mg), IV vitamin K (rarely), or infusions of frozen plasma if bleeding is life-threatening. Prothrombin-complex concentrates are rarely necessary, except perhaps in the unusual patient with CNS hemorrhage and neurologic deterioration.

Poisoning or surreptitious ingestion of coumarins are treated as indicated above. However, long-acting agents such as those found in some rodenticides (e.g., brodificoum) usually require repeated large doses of vitamin K over long periods of time (weeks) to avoid a rebound in the PT at a later date.

Warfarin Skin Necrosis

Most, but not all, episodes of warfarin skin necrosis have occurred in patients with hereditary protein C (and occasionally protein S) deficiency. The pathogenesis of this often devastating complication involves a warfarin-induced rapid fall in protein C activity, from levels of about 50 percent (heterozygote levels) to less than 5 percent, which is a consequence of the short plasma half-life of protein C. Infants with homozygous or compound heterozygous protein C deficiency also have extremely low levels of protein C activity and develop a similar syndrome in the absence of warfarin, termed neonatal purpura fulminans (see Chaps. 34 and 38). Concurrent inflammation or other prothrombotic states, such as surgery or cancer, may predispose patients to this syndrome via cytokine-induced downregulation of thrombomodulin on the surface of vascular endothelium, with impaired activation of any remaining protein C. Because of the risks of warfarin skin necrosis, patients who have a history of venous thrombosis should be tested for deficiencies of protein C and protein S before oral anticoagulants are electively given (i.e., without heparin pre-treatment).

Anticoagulation of patients with protein C deficiency or a history of warfarin skin necrosis can be accomplished by the use of concomitant full-dose heparin, or LMWH in high-risk patients, or by the administration of very low doses of warfarin with gradual increases in an attempt to slow the fall in protein C relative to other vitamin K-dependent clotting factors. One strategy involves starting warfarin at 0.5 mg/day for 3 days and then sequentially increasing the dose at 3-day intervals (0.5 mg/day for 3 days, 1 mg/day for 3 days, 2 mg, 4 mg, etc.) until therapeutic anticoagulation has been achieved. Both approaches can be used together if necessary. In severe protein C deficiency, the use of protein C concentrates may be necessary during the initiation of therapy.

Other Complications

Other side effects of warfarin therapy include alopecia, skin rash, and diarrhea. One rare but striking complication is purple toe syndrome, which is thought to be due to warfarin-induced embolization of cholesterol particles from atherosclerotic plaques in the aorta or another major artery to the microvasculature of the toes.

BIBLIOGRAPHY

Aithal GP et al: Association of polymorphisms in the cytochrome P450 CYP2C9 with warfarin dose requirement and risk of bleeding complications. *Lancet* 353:717, 1999.

Baglin T: Management of warfarin (coumarin) overdose. *Blood Rev* 12:91, 1998.

Bentley DP et al: Investigation of patients with abnormal response to warfarin. *Brit J Clin Pharm* 22:37, 1986.

Beyth RJ et al: Prospective evaluation of an index for predicting the risk of major bleeding in outpatients treated with warfarin. *Am J Med* 105:91, 1998.

Booth SL et al: Dietary vitamin K_1 and stability of oral anticoagulation: proposal of a diet with constant vitamin K_1 content. *Thromb Haemost* 77:504, 1997.

Boulis NM et al: Use of factor IX complex in warfarin-related intracranial hemmorhage. *Neurosurgery* 45:1113, 1999.

Butler AC, Tait RC: Management of oral anticoagulant-induced intracranial haemorrhage. *Blood Rev* 12:35, 1998.

Chu K et al: A mutation in the propeptide of factor IX leads to warfarin sensitivity by a novel mechanism. *J Clin Invest* 98: 1619, 1996.

Cleland JG et al: Should all patients with atrial fibrillation receive warfarin? Evidence from randomized clinical trials. *Euro Heart J* 17:674, 1996.

Crowther MA et al: A randomized trial comparing 5-mg and 10-mg warfarin loading doses. *Arch Intern Med* 159:46, 1999.

DeLoughery TG: Anticoagulant therapy in special circumstances. *Curr Cardiol Rep* 2:74, 2000.

Glover JJ, Morrill GB: Conservative treatment of overanticoagulated patients. *Chest* 108:987, 1995.

Harrell CC, Kline SS: Vitamin K-supplemented snacks containing olestra: implication for patients taking warfarin. *JAMA* 282:1133, 1999.

Hirsh J et al: Oral anticoagulants: mechanism of action, clinical effectiveness, and optimal therapeutic range. *Chest* 114:445S, 1998.

Hulse ML: Warfarin resistance: diagnosis and therapeutic alternatives. *Pharmacotherapy* 16:1009, 1996.

Kearon C, Hirsh J: Management of anticoagulation before and after elective surgery. *N Engl J Med* 336:1506, 1997.

Levine MN et al: Hemorrhagic complications of anticoagulant treatment. *Chest* 114:511S, 1998.

Poller L et al: Multicentre randomised study of computerised anticoagulant dosage. European Concerted Action on Anticoagulation. *Lancet* 352:1505, 1998.

Raj G et al: Time course of reversal of anticoagulant effect of warfarin by intravenous and subcutaneous phytodione. *Arch Intern Med* 159: 2721, 1999.

Streif W, Andrew ME: Venous thromboembolic events in pediatric patients. Diagnosis and management. *Hem Oncol Clin North Amer* 12:1283, 1998.

Tiede DJ et al: Modern management of prosthetic valve anticoagulation. *Mayo Clinic Proc* 73:665, 1998.

Weibert RT et al: Correction of excessive anticoagulation with low-dose oral vitamin K1. *Ann Intern Med* 126:959, 1997.

Weitzel JN et al: Surreptitious ingestion of a long-acting vitamin K antagonist/ rodenticide, brodifacoum: clinical and metabolic studies of three cases. *Blood* 76: 2555, 1990.

Zivelin A et al: Mechanism of the anticoagulant effect of warfarin as evaluated in rabbits by selective depression of individual procoagulant vitamin K-dependent clotting factors. *J Clin Invest* 92:2131, 1993.

CHAPTER 61

Thrombolytic Agents

Acute coronary artery thrombosis, venous thromboembolism, ischemic stroke, and peripheral artery occlusion have all been successfully treated with systemic or local infusions of fibrinolytic agents. Although thrombolysis is an attractive therapeutic modality, potential problems include a risk of serious bleeding and recurrent thrombosis of newly reperfused vessels. Streptokinase (SK), urokinase (UK), acylated plasminogen streptokinase activator complex (APSAC), and tissue plasminogen activator (t-PA) are currently available for clinical use. New generations of thrombolytic agents are being developed to maximize clot lysis with lower rates of hemorrhage and reocclusion. Adjunctive antithrombotic and antiplatelet therapies are used with all thrombolytic agents to prevent rethrombosis.

PHARMACOLOGY

Thrombolytic agents are plasminogen activators that promote clot lysis by converting plasminogen to the fibrinolytic enzyme plasmin. Plasmin cleaves fibrin, breaks down the clot, and generates soluble fibrin degradation products (FDP), which are subsequently cleared by the kidney and reticuloendothelial system. The various fibrinolytic drugs differ as to mechanisms of plasminogen activation, their survival time in the circulation, and specificity for fibrin, as outlined in Fig. 61-1.

Unfortunately, all currently available thrombolytic agents can produce marked impairment of hemostasis and bleeding as a result of the induced "lytic" state. Fibrinolytic enzymes cannot distinguish pathologic thromboses (e.g., obstructing a coronary artery) from hemostatic plugs that prevent bleeding from a critical vascular defect (e.g., a small injury to a

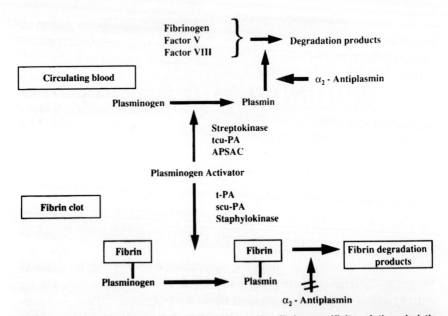

FIGURE 61-1 Molecular interactions determining the fibrin specificity of thrombolytic agents. Non-fibrin-specific agents (streptokinase, tcu-PA, APSAC) extensively activate plasminogen in the circulating blood, whereas fibrin-specific agents (t-PA, scu-PA, staphlokinase) preferentially activate fibrin-associated plasminogen. (Used with permission from *Cardiovascular Thrombosis: Thrombocardiology and Thromboneurology. Second Edition.* Verstraete M, Fuster V, and Topol EJ, eds. Philadelphia: Lippincott-Raven. p 302, 1998.)

cerebral vessel). Effective clot lysis leads to potentially lifesaving vascular reperfusion in the former instance, but to catastrophic bleeding in the latter. Plasminogen activators, in particular those that are not fibrin specific, not only act on plasminogen bound to fibrin but also on circulating plasminogen, which generates plasmin and produces subsequent systemic fibrinolysis. Circulating plasmin destroys fibrinogen, factor V, and factor VIII. Platelet function is compromised because of inhibition of platelet aggregation by FDP and to impaired platelet adhesion by plasmin-induced proteolysis of glycoprotein Ib and von Willebrand factor.

Thrombolytic agents must be administered by intravenous or intra-arterial routes. Protocols for clinical use include short-term intravenous infusion, often with an initial bolus (for acute coronary artery thrombosis); continuous long-term intravenous infusion (for deep venous thrombosis [DVT]); catheter-directed thrombolysis of peripheral arterial occlusions and DVT; and rapid early infusion for massive pulmonary embolism with hemodynamic compromise. Although fibrinolytic agents are usually administered in large amounts designed to produce rapid clot lysis, lower doses are sometimes administered directly into the clot in an attempt to destroy thrombi without producing a systemic fibrinolytic state and to achieve higher local concentrations throughout the clot. Dosage and schedules of administration differ depending on the fibrinolytic agent and its intended use and are evolving at the present time. Thus, current pharmaceutical product information must be consulted for details of therapy.

ADJUVANT THERAPIES

Heparins and aspirin (ASA) are the mainstays of adjunctive therapy to prevent rethrombosis; however, they have little effect on the rate of clot lysis. Ten percent of treated patients suffer acute coronary reocclusion in spite of adjuvant therapy. Consequently, major efforts are presently focused on developing new drugs to prevent rethrombosis. Specific antiplatelet agents such as monoclonal antibodies, as well as small peptides containing an Arg-Gly-Asp sequence that blocks the platelet glycoprotein IIb/IIIa receptor, are presently in clinical trials. Selective thrombin inhibitors such as the leach anticoagulant hirudin, and synthetic peptides such as argatroban have been shown to be more effective than heparin/ASA, but unfortunately these thrombin inhibitors have been associated with unacceptable rates of intracranial hemorrhage. Researchers are now focusing on novel protease inhibitors targeted higher in the coagulation cascade, for example at factors Xa and VIIa.

NEW THROMBOLYTIC AGENTS

Novel thrombolytic agents are now under development primarily as a consequence of the widespread use and success of thrombolytics in acute myocardial infarction (MI). In the setting of acute MI the goals of therapy are to increase the rate of clot lysis and to decrease rethrombosis. Variant forms of t-PA have been produced with altered fibrin binding/activation properties, reduced plasma clearance, and resistance to natural plasminogen activator (PA) inhibitors. These variants of t-PA include the deletion mutants reteplase (missing the finger, epidermal growth factor [EGF], and kringle 1 domains) and lanoteplase (missing the finger and EGF domains) and structurally altered versions like TNK-rt-PA with specifically altered amino acid structure. Clinical trials have shown these variants to alter pharmacodynamic and biochemical properties, but to provide generally little or no improvement over t-PA in respect to clinical outcomes. The latter finding is not surprising as they have not altered the catalytic machinery of the variant plasminogen activators and have been examined in trials designed to evaluate equivalence with t-PA.

Presumably new mechanistic approaches might be more effective. Three candidates are the PA derived from the vampire bat (*Desmodus rotundus*) (bat-PA), the bacterial-derived agent staphylokinase, and chimeric molecules combining the PA with an antibody-derived, highly specific antigen recognition site to concentrate the PA at the thrombus. Staphylokinase has the advantage of novel mechanistic characteristics, including fibrin specificity, together with a low cost, although it, like streptokinase, is a foreign protein that can incite inactivating antibodies and hypotension. These agents are all currently being evaluated in clinical trials.

LABORATORY MONITORING

Fibrinolytic therapy alters most laboratory measurements of hemostatic function, but few tests predict either efficacy of thrombolysis or the risks of bleeding (Table 61-1). Most of the assays reflect a systemic fibrinolytic state; for example, a short euglobulin lysis time (ELT), hypofibrinogen-

TABLE 61-1

Laboratory Tests in Thrombolytic Therapy

Test	Primary Use	Comments
Thrombin time	Identify persistent lytic state	Heparin also prolongs
Partial thromboplastin time	Identify persistent lytic state	Alternative to thrombin time; heparin also prolongs
Reptilase time	Identify persistent lytic state in heparinized patients	
Fibrinogen	Guide therapy with cryoprecipitate	Check to ensure adequate repletion; clotting rate assay (Clauss) method preferred
Bleeding time		Not generally useful
Factors V and VIII	Identify specific factor deficiencies	Not generally useful
Fibrin degradation Products (D-dimer)	Modest elevations only	Not useful in therapy
α_2-Antiplasmin	Depletion confirms lytic state	Not useful in therapy

Modified and used with permission from Sane DC et al: *Ann Intern Med* 111:1010, 1989.

emia, and a long thrombin clotting time (TCT), prothrombin time (PT), and activated partial thromboplastin time (APTT). Impaired platelet function is suggested by prolongation of the bleeding time. Older generations of FDP tests that measure both fibrinogen- and fibrin-degradation products are markedly elevated, although more current assays that detect only cross-linked fibrin degradation products (D-dimer) show somewhat less elevation. Some studies have suggested that lower platelet counts are also associated with bleeding.

Most short-term infusions of thrombolytic agents do not require laboratory monitoring. However, the dilute thrombin time (normal range of 20 to 30 sec) is sometimes used to ensure continued fibrinolysis in patients treated with long-term SK (e.g., 3 days) for DVT. Tests that can be used to document the presence of a systemic fibrinolytic state in children and adults include shortening of the ELT, prolongation of the TCT, and a fall in the concentration of fibrinogen. Unfortunately, levels of the fibrin degradation product, D-dimer, have not been helpful as a marker of reperfusion success because lysis of circulating soluble fibrin complexes and fibrin in atherosclerotic lesions from other arterial locations can also elevate D-dimer.

Finally, the use of adjunctive anticoagulant and antiplatelet therapies must be considered in the interpretation of laboratory tests during and after thrombolytic therapy. The new adjunctive therapies just entering clinical trials will likely need novel monitoring strategies to ensure efficacy and limit bleeding.

CLINICAL USE

Coronary Thrombolysis

Angiographic and pathologic studies have shown that the great majority of acute transmural myocardial infarctions are caused by a thrombus located on the surface of a ruptured atherosclerotic plaque in a diseased coronary artery. Intraarterial or intravenous fibrinolytic therapy produces vascular reperfusion in 55 to 90 percent of patients, particularly if treatment is administered within 6 h of the onset of symptoms, although only about 50 percent achieve brisk TIMI 3 grade flow. The intravenous route is now preferred because patients can be treated rapidly with less bleeding, although reperfusion rates are slightly lower. Clinical studies have convincingly shown that early thrombolytic therapy is of benefit for acute coronary artery occlusion; salvage of myocardium, improved left ventricular function, and most importantly, reduction in both short-term and 1-year mortality rates have all been documented. A major problem is acute rethrombosis, an event that occurs in 10 percent of patients. Because of this, most patients are treated with aspirin and heparin antcoagulants; some may also require coronary artery revascularization procedures following thrombolysis.

Controversy persists as to the optimal fibrinolytic agent for coronary thrombolysis, and debate centers on rates of reperfusion or rethrombosis, hemorrhage, and cost. However, the GUSTO trial (see reference) demonstrated that early, rapid (TIMI 3) flow and persistent recanalization are predictors of a good clinical outcome. Finally, GUSTO and other studies have clearly demonstrated the importance of initiating thrombolytic therapy as soon after the onset of symptoms as possible with mortality being 4.3 percent if treatment is started within 2 h versus 8.9 percent if it is begun between 4 and 6 h.

Peripheral Arterial Thrombosis

Acute occlusion of peripheral arteries (usually in the lower extremities) is most often related to emboli from the heart or more proximal vessels, or to thrombosis at sites of advanced atherosclerotic disease. Unlike acute MI and ischemic stroke, the therapeutic window is wider, with the time of acute onset of symptoms to treatment defined as less than 14 days. Intravenous systemic thrombolytic therapy has been disappointing in this condition, and more recent studies have focused on catheter-directed thrombolysis, which has been shown to achieve up to 85 percent successful recanalization rates. Successful passage of a guidewire through the thrombus suggests a soft recent clot. A specially designed catheter with multiple side ports is then fed through the thrombus to allow the lytic agent to permeate the clot. At the present time urokinase appears to be the drug of choice in peripheral artery occlusion, edging out t-PA, with marginally fewer complications and proving superior to SK in all measured parameters. Clinical studies such as the STILE trial, which compared surgery and thrombolysis, suggested that patients with acute occlusion treated with thrombolysis had lower amputation rates and shorter hospital stays. Therapeutic thrombolysis not only reperfuses occluded vessels, but also uncovers other lesions that can be treated by surgical or percutaneous approaches, thus simplifying future surgical procedures. Results of thrombolytic therapy, with respect to long-term patency in the lower extremity, are somewhat equivocal compared to a surgical approach. As with acute MI, these results will likely improve with the advent of more effective adjunctive therapies to prevent rethrombosis of the treated vessel.

Deep Venous Thrombosis

Initial fibrinolysis for DVT achieves clot lysis fourfold more frequently than heparin alone, but bleeding complications tend to negate the positive impact of thrombolytic therapy during the acute phase of DVT. However, recent evidence suggests that increased rates of clot lysis may reduce the incidence of post-phlebitic syndrome. At the present time the only unequivocal indication for thrombolytic therapy in DVT is massive venous thrombosis with obstruction and incipient gangrene in spite of conventional therapy. Many clinicians consider thrombolytic therapy in the setting of massive proximal venous thrombosis, even in the absence of gangrene. The risks of hemorrhagic complications must be carefully weighed against the benefits of treatment in these settings, with careful attention to exclusion criteria. Thrombolytic agents are most effective in the acute phase of DVT, which is variably defined as 7 to 14 days.

Recent anecdotal studies support the use of catheter-directed thrombolysis for DVT. The basic approach is similar to that described earlier for peripheral arterial thrombosis. There are fewer systemic complications and some indication that there are fewer chronic post-phlebitic complications. However, the definitive role of catheter-directed therapy awaits the results of well-designed clinical trials.

Pulmonary Embolism

Thrombolytic therapy can be life-saving in the setting of massive pulmonary embolism (PE) with cardiogenic shock, and should be administered as soon as possible. The indications for early thrombolytic therapy in massive PE may be extended to individuals with evidence of right-heart hemodynamic compromise, even without evident hypotension and before the onset of the metabolic sequelae of shock. In the setting of massive PE the choice to use thrombolytic agents must be carefully tempered with the risk of bleeding complications. In less serious PE the advantage of more rapid lysis of the clot compared with heparin is less evident, and by 5 days the degree of clot lysis is no different, with bleeding complications outweighing the benefits of early lysis. There is some evidence that long-term pulmonary function, as reflected by pulmonary capillary blood volume and diffusing capacity, is better following thrombolytic than heparin therapy. The clinical significance of these latter findings awaits further study.

Successful lysis of pulmonary emboli has been observed with SK, UK, and t-PA. Earlier trials with SK and UK used infusions (either intravenous or via pulmonary artery catheters) that lasted for 12 to 24 h or more. More recently, investigators have successfully used short-term high-dose infusion regimens to induce brisk fibrinolysis with lower risks of bleeding. UK and t-PA appear to be equivalent and both superior to SK.

Acute Stroke

Large clinical trials over the past decade have demonstrated that early (under 3 to 6 h) thrombolytic therapy with t-PA reduces death and disability from ischemic stroke by about 30 percent (OR 0.67, 95 percent CI 0.56 to 0.8). SK was ineffective in this setting. The benefits are most evident in patients treated within 3 h of symptom onset, and this is the presently accepted therapeutic window. Careful attention to inclusion and exclusion criteria is essential in this patient group. To treat ischemic stroke with t-PA, institutional protocols must be carefully designed and implemented to allow for rapid assessment for exclusion of hemorrhagic stroke and of individuals with an elevated risk of bleeding complications.

Other Indications

A myriad of individual case reports or small clinical series have appeared in the medical literature that describe thrombolytic therapy for a wide range of vascular occlusions, including thrombosis of cerebral, retinal, and abdominal veins. Prompt catheter-directed thrombolytic therapy has also been reported to preserve vision in patients with central retinal artery occlusion. Both arterial and venous thromboses have resolved in infants and children after fibrinolytic therapy. Recent reports encourage the greater use of thrombolytic agents in children (see Chap. 34).

SIDE EFFECTS AND COMPLICATIONS

Hemorrhage has occurred in virtually all the clinical trials in which large doses of fibrinolytic agents have been used. Most bleeding occurs at sites of vascular injury (e.g., in vessels punctured for diagnostic procedures) or in surgical wounds, and may be severe. Rates of major bleeding in large clinical trials vary from 5 to 20 percent or more, and depend on patient selection, duration of therapy, and dose of thrombolytic agents. In general, the risk of serious hemorrhage is at least two to three times greater than that of heparin for the same indication. Because of the risks of bleeding, careful patient selection is important.

One of the most feared complications of thrombolytic therapy is intracranial hemorrhage, which occurs in 0.5 to 1.0 percent of patients and is fatal at least two-thirds of the time. Bleeding risks must be care-

TABLE 61-2
Contraindications to Thrombolytic Therapy
Absolute Contraindications
Recent neurosurgery, head trauma, or CNS hemorrhage Intracranial/intraspinal neoplasm or aneurysm Stroke within 6 months Active or recent internal bleeding Uncontrolled hypertension (diastolic pressure > 110 mm Hg) Suspected aortic dissection
Relative Contraindications
Surgery or organ biopsy in prior 2 weeks Recent trauma (including cardiopulmonary resuscitation) Puncture of major non-compressible vessel within 10 days Infective endocarditis, pericarditis Pregnancy or recent delivery Hemostatic defects Active peptic ulcer disease

fully considered before decisions are made about the use of fibrinolytic agents in clinical practice. In some cases, the potential benefit may be substantial (e.g., the treatment of acute coronary artery occlusion), so that the risks of CNS bleeding are clearly acceptable. However, the risk/benefit ratio does not seem reasonable in a patient with a venous thrombosis limited to the popliteal vein in the leg. Additional controlled clinical trials will help provide the information needed for physicians and patients to make accurate and informed decisions about the risks and benefits of thrombolytic therapy.

Treatment of serious bleeding associated with fibrinolytic therapy requires immediate cessation of the infusion and rapid correction of residual hemostatic defects. The management of systemic fibrinolysis is discussed in Chapter 25, and a therapeutic strategy for major hemorrhage that complicates thrombolytic therapy of coronary artery occlusion is shown in Fig. 61-2.

BIBLIOGRAPHY

Bovill EG et al: Future directions in antiplatelet and anticoagulant therapy (part of College of American Pathologists International Consensus Conference on laboratory monitoring of anticoagulant therapy). *Arch Pathol Lab Med* 122:808, 1998.

Bovill EG et al: Monitoring thrombolytic therapy. *Prog Cardiovasc Dis* 34:279, 1992.

Bovill EG et al: Hemorrhagic events during therapy with recombinant tissue-type plasminogen activator, heparin and aspirin for acute myocardial infarction: results

Management for Patients with Bleeding from Thrombolytic Therapy

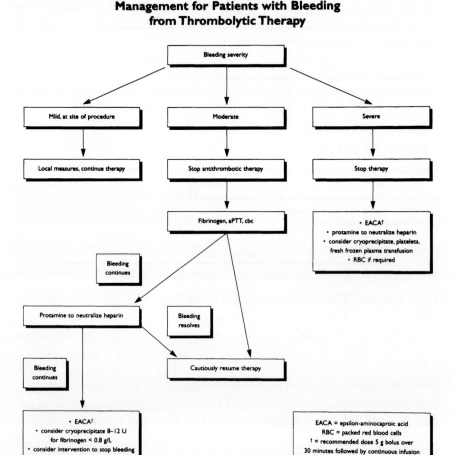

FIGURE 61-2 A protocol for management of bleeding patients receiving thrombolytic therapy. (Used with permission from Ginsberg J. et al, eds. Ontario, Canada: Decker p 172, 1998.)

of the Thrombolysis in Myocardial Infarction (TIMI), Phase II Trial. *Ann Int Med* 115:256, 1991.

Braunwald E: The open artery theory is alive and well—again. *N Engl J Med* 329:1615, 1993.

Chalmers EA et al: Thrombolytic therapy in the management of paediatric thromboembolic disease. *Br J Haematol* 104:14, 1999.

Collen D: Staphylokinase: a potent, uniquely fibrin-selective thrombolytic agent. *Nat Med* 4:279, 1998.

Collen D, Haber E: The fibrinolytic system and thrombolytic therapy. In: Chien KR (ed), *Molecular Basis of Cardiovascular Disease,* Philadelphia, Saunders, 1998, pp 537–565 (includes discussion of antibody/PA chimeras).

Del Zoppo DJ: Antithrombotic treatments in acute ischemic stroke. *Thromb Haemost* 82:938, 1999.

Ginsberg J et al: *Critical Decisions in Thrombosis and Hemostasis* (Chaps. 12, 28, 31), Ontario, Canada, Decker, 1998.

Goldhaber SZ: Contemporary pulmonary embolism thrombolysis. In: Goldhaber SZ (ed), *Cardiopulmonary Diseases and Cardiac Tumors, Vol III,* in Braunwald E (series ed): *Atlas of Heart Diseases.* Philadelphia, *Current Medicine* 6.1–6.12, 1995.

GUSTO angiographic investigators: The effects of tissue plasminogen activator, streptokinase, or both on coronary-artery patency, ventricular function, and survival after acute myocardial infarction. *N Engl J Med* 329:1615, 1993.

Hacke W et al: Thrombolysis in acute cerebrovascular disease; indications and limitations. *Thromb Haemost* 82:983, 1999.

Kandarpa K: Catheter-directed thrombolysis of peripheral arterial occlusions and deep vein thrombosis. *Thromb Haemost* 82:987, 1999.

Lincoff AM, Topol EJ (eds): *Platelet Glycoprotein IIb/IIIa Inhibitors in Cardiovascular Disease.* Totowa, NJ, Humana, 1999.

Sane DC et al: Bleeding during thrombolytic therapy for acute myocardial infarction: mechanisms and management. *Ann Intern Med* 111:1010, 1989.

Timmis GC (ed): *Thrombolytic Therapy.* Armonk, NY, Futura, 1999.

Verstraete M et al: Specific thrombin inhibitors. In: *Cardiovascular Thrombosis: Thrombocardiology and Thromboneurology,* 2nd ed, Verstraete M et al (eds), Philadelphia, Lippincott-Raven, 1998, pp 141–172.

Weitz JI et al: Mechanism of action of plasminogen activators. *Thromb Haemost* 82:974, 1999.

CHAPTER 62

Antiplatelet Agents

A major goal of antiplatelet therapy is to block platelet deposition on the surface of disrupted atherosclerotic plaques in order to prevent acute vascular occlusion or embolization of thrombotic debris. Clinical trials have shown that antiplatelet therapy significantly reduces arterial thrombosis rates in patients with coronary, cerebral, or peripheral vascular disease. Aspirin is the most commonly used antiplatelet agent because it is inexpensive, widely available, relatively safe, and demonstrably effective. An alternative to aspirin, clopidogrel, is also an effective platelet inhibitor that has recently been tested in clinical trials for vascular disease. The use of sulfinpyrazone and dipyridamole has diminished substantially because they are less effective and more costly than aspirin. Finally, a new class of antiplatelet drugs, the GP IIb/IIIa inhibitors, are now coming into widespread use as an adjunct for the treatment of acute coronary occlusion.

PHARMACOLOGY

Aspirin's antithrombotic effects are due to inhibition of platelet aggregation (but not platelet adhesion). A key platelet enzyme, cyclooxygenase-1 (COX-1), is permanently acetylated by aspirin, which impairs the synthesis of thromboxane A_2, a prostanoid with potent platelet-aggregating properties. Aspirin also inhibits the cyclooxygenase of endothelial cells, and therefore reduces the synthesis of prostacyclin (PGI_2), a prostaglandin that inhibits platelet function. In contrast to platelets, however, endothelial cell cyclooxygenase is renewable, so that PGI_2 synthesis recovers in 24 to 48 h. Platelet cyclooxygenase may also be more sensitive than the endothelial cell enzyme to the inhibitory affects of aspirin.

Recently, a new class of anti-inflammatory agents have been developed to specifically inhibit cyclooxygenase-2 (COX-2), an enzyme inducible by inflammation, without blocking COX-1. These COX-2 inhibitors (e.g., celecoxib) are effective anti-inflammatory agents that do not inhibit thromboxane-dependent platelet aggregation (McAdam ref), and produce less gastrointestinal toxity than the COX-1 inhibitors (i.e., non-steroidal anti-inflammatory agents). COX-2 inhibitors do not have antithrombotic properties.

Since aspirin permanently inhibits platelet cyclooxygenase, abnormalities in laboratory tests of platelet function (platelet aggregation) persist for a week or more after a single dose of the drug. The bleeding time, however, is less sensitive, returning to normal in most people within 2 to 3 days. Ideally aspirin should be stopped for at least a week prior to surgical procedures in which excessive bleeding could lead to complications.

In the past, substantial controversy surrounded the dose of aspirin that provides an optimal antithrombotic effect. Based the results of recent clinical trials, current recommendations are for the use of 60 to 325 mg aspirin daily or 160–325 mg every other day. Higher doses do not appear to improve clinical outcomes and are associated with higher rates of bleeding and gastrointestinal symptoms.

Clopidogrel is a thienopyridine derivative that blocks platelet aggregation possibly by inhibition of a putative ADP receptor on the platelet membrane (Table 62-1). Clopidogrel is rapidly absorbed and transformed by the liver into a short-lived platelet inhibitor of unknown structure. Maximal platelet inhibition is noted in 4–7 days, which returns to normal approximately 7 days after the last dose of the drug. Clopidogrel is associated with rash and diarrhea, but does not cause neutropenia. A related drug, ticlopidine, is falling from favor due to uncommon but serious hematological side effects (e.g., neutropenia and thrombotic thrombocytopenic purpura-TTP).

CLINICAL USE

Aspirin is used for prevention of thrombosis in patients with atherosclerosis (Table 62-2). The antithrombotic benefits of aspirin are greatest in those patients with the highest risks of vascular complications (Fig. 62-1). Antiplatelet therapy does not seem to be of benefit for treatment of deep venous thrombosis or pulmonary embolism. However, low-dose aspirin has been shown to provide some protection against embolic stroke in low risk patients with chronic non-rheumatic atrial fibrillation.

TABLE 62-1	
Newer Antiplatelet Agents	
Ticlopidine	
Dose:	250 mg bid
Indications:	Secondary prevention of ischemic disease in patients intolerant of aspirin or aspirin failures. Prevention of coronary stent thrombosis in combination with aspirin.
Toxicities:	Gastrointestinal upset (10%) Neutropenia (1%) Thrombotic thrombocytopenic purpura (0.1%)
Clopidogrel	
Dose:	75 mg daily
Indications:	Secondary prevention of ischemic disease in patients intolerant of aspirin or aspirin failures. Prevention of coronary stent thrombosis in combination with aspirin.
Toxicities:	Gastrointestinal upset (10%)
Abciximab	
Dose:	0.25 mg/kg plus 0.125 µg/kg/min (maximum 10 µg/min) for twelve hours after PTCA. Heparin dose: 70 units/kg (maximum 7000 units) bolus with additional bolus to achieve an ACT of 200 seconds.
Tirofiban	
Dose:	0.4µg/kg/min for 30 minutes plus an infusion of 0.1 µg/kg/min until resolution of the pain syndrome or for 12–24 hours after angiography. Given with aspirin and heparin.
Eptifibatide	
Dose:	For unstable angina, 180 µg/kg bolus followed by a continuous infusion of 2µg/kg/min for up to 72 hours. For PTCA, 135µg/kg bolus followed by 0.5µg/kg/min for 20–24 hours after the procedure.

Modified from Deloughery TG: Antiplatelet Agents. In Hemostasis and Thrombosis. *Landes Bioscience*, Austin TX, 1999. p. 183.

As discussed above, the most appropriate dose of aspirin for management of patients with atherosclerosis is a matter of controversy. Aspirin has proven successful in therapeutic trials in doses ranging from as low as 30 mg once daily to as high as 650 mg twice a day. A reasonable clinical practice is to treat most patients with a single standard low dose of aspirin (80–160 mg once daily).

TABLE 62-2
Indications for Aspirin Therapy
Primary prevention of myocardial infarction
Secondary prevention of myocardial infarction
Secondary prevention of stroke after TIA or stroke
Acute therapy of myocardial infarction
Acute therapy of unstable angina
Prevention of saphenous vein bypass thrombosis

Myocardial Infarction

Primary Prevention

Four large prospective clinical trials of low-dose aspirin in male physicians and in patients with risk factors for myocardial infarction showed that first attacks of fatal or nonfatal myocardial infarction were significantly reduced by at least one-third, although overall mortality was unchanged. A similar reduction in risk was found in a prospective but nonrandomized trial of aspirin in nurses. Based on these data, males (and

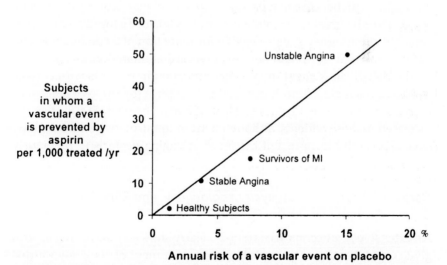

Annual risk of a vascular event on placebo

FIGURE 62-1 The absolute risk of vascular complications is the major determinant of the absolute benefit of antiplatelet prophylaxis. Data are plotted from placebo-controlled trials in different clinical settings. For each category of patients, the abcissa denotes the absolute risk of experiencing a major cardiovascular event as recorded in the placebo arm of the trial(s). The absolute benefit of antiplatelet treatment is reported on the ordinate as the number of subjects in whom an important vascular event (nonfatal MI, nonfatal stroke, or vascular death is actually prevented by treating 1000 subjects with aspirin for 1 year. Used with permission from Patrono C et al: Chest 114:470S, 1998.

most likely females) over 40 years of age with a predisposition to coronary atherosclerosis, such as a family history of coronary heart disease, hyperlipidemia or diabetes should be treated with aspirin. However, aspirin therapy should not substitute for effective management of coronary risk factors such as smoking, hyperlipidemia, lack of exercise, or hypertension.

Secondary Prevention of Myocardial Infarction

A meta-analysis that included 25 trials of antiplatelet therapy in patients with a history of coronary artery disease showed that aspirin significantly reduced all cause mortality, vascular mortality, and stroke or myocardial infarction. In each instance, event rates were reduced by 15 to 30 percent. Low doses of aspirin were as effective as higher doses. Accordingly, long-term low-dose aspirin therapy is now recommended for all patients who have had an acute myocardial infarction.

Unstable and Chronic Stable Angina

Aspirin is a mainstay in the treatment of cardiac ischemic syndromes. Aspirin prevents myocardial infarction and death in patients with unstable angina with benefits that persist for at least a year. The antithrombotic agent with the greatest absolute benefit is aspirin. Ticlopidine and, presumably clopidogrel, is also effective for reduction of a combination end point of vascular death and nonfatal myocardial infarction.

The risk of subsequent myocardial infarction in patients with chronic stable angina is significantly reduced with aspirin (by up to 70 percent or more) as noted in the Physicians' Health Study. The relative risk of stroke increased in these patients, although none of the strokes were fatal. However, aspirin did not prevent the onset of angina pectoris in previously asymptomatic men.

Coronary Artery Thrombolysis, Angioplasty, and Saphenous Vein Bypass Grafts

An extensive multicenter trial (ISIS-2) clearly showed that 160 mg aspirin given concurrently with streptokinase for treatment of acute myocardial infarction produced a 42 percent decline in vascular deaths by 5 weeks, a benefit that persisted for the next 10 years. Other studies have substantiated these findings. Daily low-dose aspirin has also been shown to reduce saphenous vein graft occlusion in patients undergoing coronary artery bypass surgery. In contrast, aspirin has not reduced late restenosis following coronary angioplasty. Long-term aspirin can be recommended in each of these clinical situations for the prevention of future coronary artery occlusion.

Stroke

Primary Prevention

Most cerebral vascular accidents are caused by thrombotic or embolic occlusion of cerebral vessels. The benefit of aspirin in the primary prevention of stroke is a matter of some controversy. At the present time, based on a meta-analysis of reported trials showing a subsequent reduction of nonfatal stroke of 40 percent, most would recommend low-dose aspirin for the prevention of stroke in patients who are known to have coronary artery disease. Nevertheless, patients with risk factors for atherosclerosis such as hypertension or diabetes should probably receive aspirin to prevent coronary artery thrombosis.

Secondary Prevention

A series of individual studies as well as a meta-analysis of a large number of clinical trials have suggested that low-dose aspirin therapy reduces subsequent stroke and death in patients with transient ischemic attacks (TIA). The data is also strong for the use of antiplatelet therapy following a completed stroke. Two trials have suggested that very low doses of aspirin (30 mg and 75 mg daily) are as effective as 325 mg in preventing future vascular events. Clopidogrel has also been shown to be effective in patients with either TIA or completed stroke.

Carotid Endarterectomy

A clinical trial suggested that antiplatelet therapy with aspirin does not prevent restenosis following carotid endarterectomy. However, because most patients with carotid atherosclerosis have coronary artery disease, aspirin therapy is recommended for prevention of myocardial infarction.

Atrial Fibrillation

Patients with chronic nonrheumatic atrial fibrillation have a risk of cerebral vascular accident that ranges from 2 to 8 percent per year. A series of trials have shown that warfarin reduces the risk of stroke from 5 to 1 percent/year. A recent trial (SPAF III) has shown that aspirin is effective stroke prevention in low risk patents with atrial fibrillation. Included in this group are those with lone atrial fibrillation, patients without heart failure or hypertension, patients without a history of stroke and women less than the age of 75 years.

Chronic Lower Extremity Ischemia

The efficacy of antiplatelet therapy for prevention of thrombotic vascular occlusion in patients with lower extremity atherosclerosis or to prevent occlusion of saphenous vein or prosthetic vascular grafts following surgery is not yet established. Limited data suggest that antiplatelet therapy with aspirin is of benefit if it is started preoperatively in patients undergoing infrainguinal bypass surgery and also in patients with chronic lower extremity ischemia who are treated non-operatively. An additional indication for antiplatelet therapy is for the prevention of coronary or cerebral vascular thrombosis, which is exceedingly common in patients with peripheral artery disease.

Other Indications for Antiplatelet Therapy of Vascular Disease

Aspirin has been used in a wide variety of other vascular disorders. Examples include Kawasaki disease, myeloproliferative disorders (particularly erythromelalgia), and pre-eclampsia.

COMPLICATIONS AND SIDE EFFECTS

Although often considered a harmless drug, aspirin can cause gastrointestinal symptoms and hemorrhagic events. Gastrointestinal symptoms (including bleeding) are related to the dose of aspirin; higher event rates are observed with doses of aspirin greater than 3 tablets daily.

Bruising, gastrointestinal bleeding, postoperative hemorrhage, and epistaxis are also more common in patients taking aspirin and have been reported with all doses. Rates of bleeding may be greater when aspirin is combined with alcohol. Template bleeding times were greatly prolonged (>30 min) in 40 percent of a group of normal subjects given both drugs. When aspirin was given at a dose of 325 mg every other day in the Physicians Health Study, bleeding occurred in 27 percent of patients, compared to 20 percent of patients who received placebo. A small but not statistically significant increase in CNS hemorrhage has been reported in two large trials of low-dose aspirin in asymptomatic men.

Ticlopidine has been associated with side effects that include severe neutropenia (which is usually reversible) in 1 percent, diarrhea in up to 20 percent, and elevations of plasma cholesterol in 10 percent of patients. As many as 1/1600 subjects treated with ticlopidine have developed a severe thrombotic thrombocytopenia purpura-like syndrome, which is often fatal. Clopidogrel has fewer side effects (rash, diarrhea).

Aspirin should be stopped 7 to 10 days before elective surgical procedures, particularly those where small amounts of bleeding could cause major complications. Patients with other defects of hemostasis (e.g., liver disease, thrombocytopenia, hemophilia, warfarin therapy) should avoid the use of aspirin because of an increased risk of major hemorrhage. If the antiplatelet effect of aspirin is thought to contribute to severe bleeding, DDAVP can be used followed by platelet transfusions, if necessary.

Glycoprotein IIb/IIIa Inhibitors

A powerful addition to the antithrombotic armamentarium has been the introduction of the glycoprotein IIb/IIIa (GP IIb/IIIa) inhibitors (table 62-1). These drugs prevent fibrinogen binding to GP IIb/IIIa and block platelet aggregation producing profound platelet inhibition. GP IIb/IIIa inhibitors are most widely used in conjunction with percutaneous coronary interventions (PCI), but clinical trials are ongoing in other types of vascular disease.

Abciximab is a novel antibody that blocks the crucial GP IIb/IIIa platelet receptor for fibrinogen and von Willebrand factor. The antibody is a chimeric human-mouse antibody with its Fc portion is deleted, so that it binds to platelets and inhibits their function. Abciximab must bind to more than 80 percent of the GP IIb/IIIa sites to significantly impair platelet aggregation. Soon after an infusion is ended, the antibody undergoes rapid redistribution. Recovery of platelet function recovers over time, with bleeding times returning to normal by 12 hr.

Abciximab has consistently been shown to be beneficial in patients undergoing PCI including intra-coronary stent placement and in patients with refractory unstable angina prior to PCI. Use of this agent reduces unfavorable outcomes by 30–50 percent. This initial benefit is sustained for at least three years.

During PCI abciximab is usually given in conjunction with the anticoagulant heparin. Early studies showed an increased risk of bleeding with this combination of agents. However, the recent EPILOG study indicated that the risk of bleeding with abciximab was lowered if the dose of heparin was reduced, but without loss of effectiveness. Excess bleeding was also lessened by early sheath removal (when the activated clotting time was under 175 sec).

Tirofiban is the first of a large number of non-antibody GP IIb/IIIa inhibitors to be approved by the FDA. Tirofiban is a synthetic non-peptide derivative of tyrosine which is administered intravenously. In trials in patients with unstable angina, tirofiban in combination with aspirin and heparin reduced myocardial infarction and death by 22 percent at 30 days. In conjunction with PCI, tirofiban was initially effective in patients presenting with unstable angina or myocardial infarction, but the beneficial effect appeared to dissipate after 30 days.

Eptifibatide is a second non-antibody anti-GP IIb/IIIa agent. In patients undergoing PCI there was a trend for better outcomes with eptifibatide. In patients with unstable angina, the 30 day outcome was improved.

GP IIb/IIIa Inhibitors: Side Effects

The major side effects of the GP IIb/IIIa inhibitors are bleeding and thrombocytopenia. Bleeding is treated by platelet transfusions, which will promote redistribution of antibody and hasten return of platelet function. Severe thrombocytopenia has been reported in 0.5 percent of patients receiving abciximab. The mechanism of the thrombocytopenia is unknown but is thought to be related to conformational changes in GP IIb/IIIa induced by the inhibitor leading to binding of naturally occurring antibodies that occur in 1 percent of the population. Experience with abciximab has shown that infusion of intravenous immunoglobulin is not helpful in treatment of abciximab induced thrombocytopenia. Platelet transfusions result in a prompt rise in platelet count. Thrombocytopenia has also been seen in 0.5–2 percent of patients receiving other non-antibody GP IIb/IIIa inhibitors, suggesting this is complication is common to this class of antiplatelet agents.

BIBLIOGRAPHY

Alexander JH, Harrington RA: Recent antiplatelet drug trials in the acute coronary syndromes. Clinical interpretation of PRISM, PRISM-PLUS, PARAGON A and PURSUIT. *Drugs* 56:965, 1998.

Baigent C et al: ISIS-2: 10 year survival among patients with suspected acute myocardial infarction in randomised comparison of intravenous streptokinase, oral aspirin, both, or neither. The ISIS-2 (Second International Study of Infarct Survival) Collaborative Group. *Brit Med J* 316:1337, 1998.

Coller BS: Platelet GPIIb/IIIa antagonists: the first anti-integrin receptor therapeutics. *J Clin Invest* 100 (11 Suppl):S57, 1997.

Coukell AJ, Markham A: Clopidogrel. *Drugs* 54:745, 1997.

Frishman WH et al: Novel antiplatelet therapies for treatment of patients with ischemic heart disease: inhibitors of the platelet glycoprotein IIb/IIIa integrin receptor. *Am Heart J* 130:877, 1995.

Goa KL, Noble S: Eptifibatide: a review of its use in patients with acute coronary syndromes and/or undergoing percutaneous coronary intervention. *Drugs* 57:439, 1999.

Goodnight SH: Aspirin therapy for cardiovascular disease. *Curr Opin Hematol* 3:355, 1996.

Kong DF et al: Clinical outcomes of therapeutic agents that block the platelet glycoprotein IIb/IIIa integrin in ischemic heart disease. *Circulation* 98:2829, 1998.

Lefkowith JB: Cyclooxygenase-2 specificity and its clinical implications. *Am J Med* 106: 43S, 1999.

Lincoff AM et al: Complementary clinical benefits of coronary-artery stenting and blockade of platelet glycoprotein IIb/IIIa receptors. Evaluation of Platelet IIb/IIIa Inhibition in Stenting Investigators. *N Engl J Med* 341:319, 1999.

Madan M et al: Bleeding complications with platelet glycoprotein IIb/IIIa receptor antagonists. *Curr Opin Hematol* 6:334, 1999.

McAdam BF et al: Systemic biosynthesis of prostacyclin by cyclooxygenase (COX)-2: the human pharmacology of a selective inhibitor of COX-2. *Proc Natl Acad Sci USA* 96:272, 1999.

Noble S et al: Enoxaparin. A reappraisal of its pharmacology and clinical applications in the prevention and treatment of thromboembolic disease. *Drugs* 49:388, 1995.

Patrono C et al: Platelet-active drugs: the relationships among dose, effectiveness, and side effects. *Chest* 114:(Suppl) 470S, 1998.

Schafer AI: Effects of nonsteroidal anti-inflammatory therapy on platelets. *Am J Med* 106: 25S, 1999.

Schror K: Antiplatelet drugs. A comparative review. *Drugs* 50:7, 1995.

Steinhubl SR et al: Incidence and clinical course of thrombotic thrombocytopenic purpura due to ticlopidine following coronary stenting. EPISTENT Investigators. Evaluation of Platelet IIb/IIIa Inhibitor for Stenting. *JAMA* 281:806, 1999.

The International Stroke Trial (IST): a randomised trial of aspirin, subcutaneous heparin, both, or neither among 19435 patients with acute ischaemic stroke. International Stroke Trial Collaborative Group. *Lancet* 349:1569, 1997.

Verstraete M, Zoldhelyi P: Novel antithrombotic drugs in development. *Drugs* 49:856, 1995.

Vorchheimer DA et al: Platelet glycoprotein IIb/IIIa receptor antagonists in cardiovascular disease. *JAMA* 281:1407, 1999.

Subject Index

ISBN 0-07-134834-4

90000

9 780071 348348

GOODNIGHT / DISORDERS OF HEMOSTASIS
AND THROMBOSIS: A CLINICAL GUIDE